ATLAS OF GYNECOLOGIC SURGICAL PATHOLOGY

ATLASES IN
DIAGNOSTIC SURGICAL PATHOLOGY

Consulting Editor
Gerald M. Bordin, M.D.
Department of Pathology
Scripps Clinic and Research Foundation

Published:

Wold, McLeod, Sim, and Unni:
Atlas of Orthopedic Pathology

Colby, Lombard, Yousem, and Kitaichi:
Atlas of Pulmonary Surgical Pathology

Wenig:
Atlas of Head and Neck Pathology

Kanel and Korula:
Atlas of Liver Pathology

Owen and Kelly:
Atlas of Gastrointestinal Pathology

Virmani, Burke, and Farb:
Atlas of Cardiovascular Pathology

Ro, Grignon, Amin, and Ayala:
Atlas of Surgical Pathology of the Male Reproductive Tract

Wenig, Heffess, and Adair:
Atlas of Endocrine Pathology

Ferry and Harris:
Atlas of Lymphoid Hyperplasia and Lymphoma

Kern, Silva, Laszik, Bane, Nadasdy, and Pitha:
Atlas of Renal Pathology

Forthcoming Titles:

Naiem:
Atlas of Blood and Bone Marrow Pathology

Brooks:
Atlas of Soft Tissue Pathology

ATLAS OF GYNECOLOGIC SURGICAL PATHOLOGY

Philip B. Clement, M.D.
Professor of Pathology
University of British Columbia and
Department of Pathology
Vancouver General Hospital and
Health Sciences Center
Vancouver, British Columbia

Robert H. Young, M.D., F.R.C.Path.
Professor of Pathology
Harvard Medical School and
Department of Pathology
Massachusetts General Hospital
Boston, Massachusetts

W.B. SAUNDERS COMPANY
A Harcourt Health Sciences Company
Philadelphia ■ London ■ New York ■ St. Louis ■ Toronto ■ Sydney

W.B. SAUNDERS COMPANY
A Harcourt Health Sciences Company

The Curtis Center
Independence Square West
Philadelphia, Pennsylvania 19106

Editor: Marc Strauss
Designer: Maria Gardocky Clifton
Production Manager: Frank Polizzano
Illustration Coordinator: Francis J. Moriarty

ATLAS OF GYNECOLOGIC SURGICAL PATHOLOGY   ISBN 0-7216-2458-8

Printed in the United States of America.

Last digit is the print number: 9   8   7   6   5   4   3   2   1

To Robert E. Scully, M.D.
A great pathologist,
a wonderful mentor,
and a good friend

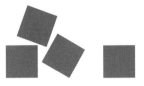

PREFACE

This book is intended as an easy-to-use practical guide to the diagnosis of lesions involving the female reproductive system and female peritoneum. As with other works in this series, the text material is extensive. It is the intent of both the publisher and ourselves that the reader will find in this volume more information than is generally available in other atlases of gynecologic pathology. The manner of presentation of the written material will, we hope, help the reader quickly assimilate the essential information about the numerous processes discussed and illustrated.

The emphasis is on the diagnosis of neoplastic and pseudoneoplastic lesions, with a broad interpretation of "pseudoneoplastic" to include all lesions that could be misinterpreted as tumors on clinical, gross, or microscopic examination. Although the focus is on common lesions, less common and even rare lesions are discussed when appropriate. Diagnosis of the lesions covered can in most cases be accomplished by careful evaluation of routinely stained slides, and, accordingly, the vast majority of illustrations are of such preparations. Gross examination plays an important role in evaluating specimens from the female genital tract, and we have included many gross illustrations, although space constraints precluded illustrating every lesion conceivably of merit. Immunohistochemical findings are also included, but only when useful in establishing a diagnosis, the use of this technique in this area of pathology often being out of proportion to the benefits obtained except in a number of particular situations. The clinical background may also be important when evaluating gynecologic tumors: basic features such as the age of the patient and clinical history may be crucial in formulating a reasonable differential diagnosis, especially when dealing with an ovarian tumor. A detailed knowledge of the normal histology of the female reproductive system is important as a background to evaluating the pathology of this area. Some such aspects are discussed briefly where appropriate but are not considered in great detail because a standard text in this area is readily available.[1]

The twenty chapters are organized by site within the female genital tract and peritoneum. As in previous volumes in this series, the text is organized in concise, point form that highlights the cardinal clinical, gross, and microscopic features and the differential diagnosis of the various lesions. Also included are the most commonly used staging systems for tumors in each major site. The classifications used are those of the recently revised World Health Organization classifications of tumors of the female genital tract[2] and ovary.[3] The text is illustrated with gross and microscopic figures (two thirds of which are in color), largely derived from the extensive consultation material available to us, much of it courtesy of Dr. Robert E. Scully. Selected references, with emphasis on those from the recent literature, are provided. A final section of the book is devoted to appendices, most of which pertain to a pattern-based approach to ovarian tumors, a feature that we hope will facilitate the approach to the differential diagnosis of this complex group of tumors. A separate appendix is also devoted to the intriguing group of ovarian tumors referred to as "tumors with functioning stroma." The dedication of the book speaks for itself with regard to the person to whom we are most indebted for enabling us to have the material and background to prepare this contribution.

We hope that the practitioner in general community practice will find this work helpful in evaluating the numerous, often perplexing patterns that may be seen in female genital tract specimens, such material accounting for a considerable proportion of the volume seen in daily practice. Additionally, we hope that the academic surgical pathologist with a particular interest in this area will find this work a good source of helpful information and reference material.

PHILIP B. CLEMENT, M.D.
ROBERT H. YOUNG, M.D.

References

1. Sternberg SS (ed). Histology for Pathologists, 2nd ed. New York: Lippincott-Raven, 1997.
2. Scully RE, Bonfiglio TA, Kurman RJ, et al. Histological Typing of Female Genital Tract Tumours. World Health Organization International Histological Classification of Tumours. Berlin: Springer-Verlag, 1994.
3. Scully RE. Histological Typing of Ovarian Tumours. World Health Organization International Histological Classification of Tumours. Berlin: Springer-Verlag, 1999.

CONTENTS

CHAPTER 1

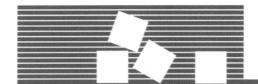

Nonneoplastic Lesions and Benign Tumors of the Vulva

NONNEOPLASTIC LESIONS

Viral Lesions

Human Papillomavirus Infection

Clinical Features

- The sexually transmitted human papillomavirus (HPV), usually HPV-6 or less common HPV-11, is the causative agent of the common condyloma acuminatum. The incidence of condylomas in the United States increased fourfold to fivefold between 1966 and 1981.
- Condylomas vary from those visible only colposcopically to large, sessile or pedunculated, white to red excrescences that are often multiple and occasionally confluent. They most commonly involve the vestibule and the medial aspects of the labia majora. Flat condylomas (see Chapter 5) are rare on the vulva, although they may occur on the fourchette.
- Vulvar condylomas are often associated with condylomas of the perineal and perianal skin and the anal and urethral mucosa, and in up to 50% of cases, they occur on other sites in the female genital tract (e.g., vagina, cervix). The lesions may be associated with precancerous changes or invasive squamous neoplasia of the lower genital tract.
- The clinical course of the lesions is typically protracted unless they are ablated or removed. The lesions may enlarge and increase in number during pregnancy but can regress postpartum. Condylomas may progress to vulvar intraepithelial neoplasia (VIN) or invasive squamous cell carcinoma, especially in immunosuppressed women.

Histologic Features

- Condylomas are characterized by complex branching papillae composed of acanthotic squamous epithelium and fibrovascular cores, and an endophytic or downward proliferation of rete pegs.

- The pathognomonic feature of condylomas is the presence of koilocytes in the superficial layers. They are usually prominent but occasionally may be focal or absent in a single section. In such cases, deeper or additional sections may be required to demonstrate their presence.
- Koilocytes are HPV-infected keratinocytes that are variable in size and have a perinuclear zone (halo) of clear cytoplasm that is of variable size and shape. The halo is surrounded by a peripheral zone of condensed amphophilic cytoplasm.
- Koilocytes have hyperchromatic, granular or smudgy, enlarged to shrunken nuclei with an irregular contour (i.e., koilocytotic atypia). Binucleated or multinucleated koilocytes are common. A few mitotic figures may be seen but are usually confined to the lower one third of the epithelium. MIB-1 expression in the upper two thirds of the epithelium is typical and may aid the diagnosis when the findings are only suggestive of condyloma.
- Nonspecific features include parakeratosis or orthokeratosis, hypergranulosis, parabasalar hyperplasia, and an underlying superficial chronic inflammatory infiltrate.
- Typical condylomas are considered by some authorities to be equivalent to VIN I. The occasional focal presence of more severe degrees of atypia (VIN II or III) (see Chapter 2) should be noted in the pathology report.
- A pseudobowenoid change rarely occurs in untreated condylomas consisting of apoptotic superficial keratinocytes in which a perichromatin halo is delineated by a rim of dense cytoplasm, beyond which a second zone of clearing is observed (see Fig. 2–5). In contrast to VIN, nuclear atypia and mitotic activity in the lower layers are absent.
- Podophyllin treatment of condylomas results in mitotic arrest in the lower epidermis, karyorrhexis, and cellular swelling, but in contrast to VIN, nuclear atypia is mild and confined to the upper layers. The history of recent podyphyllin treatment in such cases is helpful.

Differential Diagnosis

■ Warty VIN and warty invasive squamous cell carcinoma (ISCC). These lesions (see pages 22 and 27), in contrast to a typical condyloma, have significant degrees of nuclear atypicality and mitotic figures, often abnormal, that extend into the middle and upper layers. Warty ISCCs have a similar appearance but with the additional finding of invasion.

■ Verrucous carcinoma (page 30). Sometimes referred to as "giant condylomas" in the older literature, the tumors are usually large, solitary tumors in older women that lack the fine branching papillae and koilocytosis of condylomas. Their deep borders are formed by broad bulbous pegs.

■ Vestibular papillomatosis (see page 11). The squamous papillomas of this lesion are typically confined to the vestibular area, are usually much smaller than the condylomas, and typically lack koilocytosis and hyperkeratosis.

■ Condyloma lata (see Syphilis, page 4).

■ Epidermolytic hyperkeratosis. This lesion, characterized by acanthosis, compact papillomatous hyperkeratosis, and dissolution of the suprabasilar epithelium resulting in perinuclear clear zones, can simulate HPV infection. Distinctive findings, including keratohyaline clumping and dyskeratosis resulting in intracellular eosinophilic globules, facilitate its distinction from condyloma.

References

Lynch PJ. Condylomata acuminata (anogenital warts). Clin Obstet Gynecol 28:142–151, 1985.

McLachlin CM, Kozakewich H, Craighill M, et al. Histologic correlates of vulvar human papillomavirus infection in children and young adults. Am J Surg Pathol 18:728–735, 1994.

Nucci MR, Genest DR, Tate JE, et al. Pseudobowenoid change of the vulva: a histologic variant of untreated condyloma. Mod Pathol 9:375–379, 1996.

Pirog EC, Chen Y-T, Isacson C. MIB-1 immunostaining is a beneficial addition for the accurate diagnosis vulvar condyloma acuminatum [Abstract]. Mod Pathol 12:122A, 1999.

Quinn TR, Young RH. Epidermolytic hyperkeratosis in the lower female genital tract: an uncommon simulant of mucocutaneous papillomavirus infection—a report of two cases. Int J Gynecol Pathol 16:163–168, 1997.

Herpesvirus Infection

■ Most cases of herpetic vulvitis are caused by sexual transmission of herpes simplex virus (HSV) type 2 (HSV-2); less commonly, HSV type 1 is the agent.

■ The typical presentation is vulvar pain, inguinal lymphadenopathy, malaise, and fever. Vesicles, pustules, and painful ulcers appear sequentially. The perineum, perianal skin, cervix, vagina, and urinary tract are often synchronously involved. The lesions persist for 2 to 6 weeks (mean, 19 days) and then heal without scarring.

■ The most sensitive way to confirm HSV infection is by detection of HSV-2–specific antibodies. The presence of these antibodies in many women with no history of infection indicates that subclinical infections are common.

■ Cytologic smears or biopsy of the base or edges of a newly formed vesicle or ulcer reveal the characteristic ground-glass nuclei or the subsequent eosinophilic intranuclear inclusions. Cells infected by HSV type 1 or herpes zoster have a similar appearance.

■ Recurrent episodes are common after primary infection, although they are usually much milder and often inconspicuous and eventually tend to become less common.

■ Vulvitis secondary to herpes zoster (varicella) infection is rare, usually occurring in postmenopausal women who present with vulvar pain that precedes the appearance of vesicles and ulcers that are usually unilateral. Recurrent episodes of pain and new crops of vesicles are common.

References

Brown D. Herpes zoster of the vulva. Clin Obstet Gynecol 15:1010–1014, 1972.

Corey L, Adams HG, Brown ZA, Holmes KK. Genital herpes simplex virus infections: clinical manifestations, course, and complications. Ann Intern Med 98:958–972, 1983.

Kaufman RH, Faro S. Herpes genitalis: clinical features and treatment. Clin Obstet Gynecol 28:152–163, 1985.

Koutsky L, Stevens CE, Holmes KK, et al. Underdiagnosis of genital herpes by current clinical and viral-isolation procedures. N Engl J Med 326:1533–1539, 1992.

Human Immunodeficiency Virus

■ Human immunodeficiency virus (HIV) has been occasionally cultured from genital ulcers in infected women.

■ In one study of vulvar ulcers in HIV-infected women, however, no etiologic agent was found in 60%, HSV-2 was found in 28%, and unusual or mixed bacterial infections were identified in 12%, with single cases related to cytomegalovirus, *Chlamydia trachomatis,* and *Gardnerella vaginalis.* It was concluded that HIV might play a role in the causation or exacerbation of genital ulcers in HIV-infected women.

Reference

LaGuardia KD, White MH, Saigo PE, et al. Genital ulcer disease in women infected with human immunodeficiency virus. Am J Obstet Gynecol 172:553–562, 1995.

Other Viral Infections

■ Cytomegalovirus (CVM) can cause an ulcerative vulvovaginitis resembling a herpetic infection; HIV-positive women appear to be most susceptible.

  • Diagnosis rests on the demonstration of the characteristic CMV-inclusion bodies in epithelial and endothelial cells with routine and immunohistochemical stains, culture, or identification of the virus by the polymerase chain reaction.

■ Molluscum contagiosum, which can be venereally transmitted, causes vulvar and perineal lesions. The lesions are often asymptomatic and overlooked by patients and physicians. The histologic features are similar to those of lesions occurring in other sites.

■ Epstein-Barr virus is a rare cause of painful genital ulcers in women.

References

Friedmann W, Schafer A, Kretschmer R. CM virus infection of vulva and vagina. Geburtshilfe Frauenheilkd 50:729–730, 1990.

Hudson LB, Perlman SE. Necrotizing genital ulcerations in a premenarcheal female with mononucleosis. Obstet Gynecol 92:642–644, 1998.

Wilkin JK. Molluscum contagiosum venereum in a women's outpatient clinic: a venereally transmitted disease. Am J Obstet Gynecol 128: 531–535, 1977.

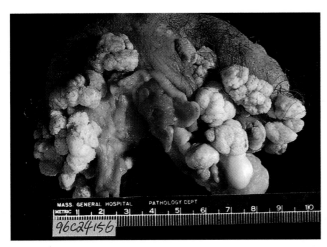

Figure 1–1. Condyloma acuminatum. Multiple condylomas are seen in this partial vulvectomy specimen.

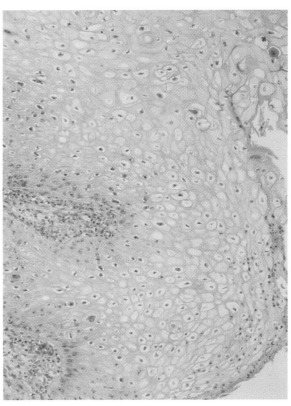

Figure 1–3. Condyloma acuminatum. Notice the koilocytotic atypia.

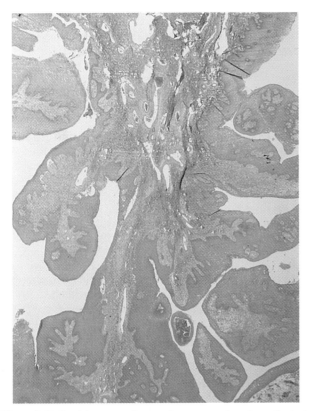

Figure 1–2. Condyloma acuminatum. Low-power view shows the typical papillary pattern.

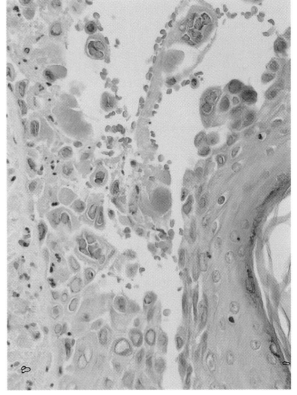

Figure 1–4. Herpetic ulcer of vulva. Notice the multinucleation and typical ground-glass nuclei.

Other Infections

Syphilis

- Syphilis is caused by the sexually transmitted spirochete *Treponema pallidum*. The primary lesion, or chancre, forms within days or several months of initial contact. The secondary phase becomes evident by 6 months as a mucocutaneous rash and papules (condyloma lata) that can involve the vulva. Gummas of tertiary syphilis only rarely involve the vulva.
- Chancres are superficial ulcers whereas the lesions of condyloma lata are nonulcerated with marked acanthosis and papillomatosis, often accompanied by intraepidermal neutrophilic infiltration. In both lesions, a perivascular plasmacellular infiltrate with endothelial proliferation provides a clue to the diagnosis, which can be confirmed by a Warthin-Starry stain to demonstrate the spirochetes.
- Dark-field examination or immunofluorescent staining of serum expressed from the lesions and serologic studies can facilitate the diagnosis.

Granuloma Inguinale

- This disorder is caused by the gram-negative bacteria *Calymmatobacterium granulomatis*. The primary vulvar, vaginal, or cervical lesions are painless papules or ulcers and appear within a month of exposure (sexual contact or fecal contamination).
- The ulcers may persist for years and may mimic a variety of other lesions, including squamous cell carcinoma. In later stages, lymphatic spread can result in brawny edema of the vulva or parametrial or retroperitoneal involvement.
- Unlike lymphogranuloma venereum, inguinal node lymphadenopathy is uncommon, but the latter may be mimicked by inguinal subcutaneous abscesses that often ulcerate.
- Granulation tissue is infiltrated by neutrophils, plasma cells, and vacuolated histiocytes containing the coccoid to bacillary organisms (i.e., Donovan bodies). The latter can be demonstrated within the vacuoles by Giemsa or Warthin-Starry staining of the tissue sections, similarly stained touch imprints of the lesion, or by culture.

Lymphogranuloma Venereum

- This sexually transmitted disease is caused by *Chlamydia*. An initial ulcer is followed by painful inguinal lymphadenitis (i.e., buboes) that may rupture and drain through the overlying skin. Later in the disease, chronic lymphatic obstruction can result in vaginal and rectal fibrosis (sometimes with strictures) and nonpitting vulvar edema.
- Because the inflammatory infiltrate is nonspecific (lymphocytes, plasma cells, histiocytes including giant cells), diagnosis rests on the characteristic clinical findings, culture, immunohistochemical staining, and complement fixation tests.

Chancroid

- This sexually transmitted disease, which is caused by the gram-negative bacillus *Haemophilus ducreyi*, presents with single or multiple, painful, often purulent, vulvar ulcers and tender, inguinal lymphadenopathy.
- The ulcer consists of a superficial zone, a middle zone with characteristic vascular changes, and a deep zone with a lymphoplasmacellular infiltrate. Gram stains of tissue sections or smears may reveal the organisms in the superficial zone, but definite diagnosis requires culture identification of the organism.

Tuberculosis

- Vulvar tuberculosis is rare and usually results from direct or lymphatic spread from other sites in the female genital tract, involvement of which is usually a result of blood-borne spread from pulmonary tuberculosis.
- The lesion begins as a nodule that later ulcerates and may drain caseous material and pus through multiple sinuses. In rare cases, epidermal hyperplasia results in a large, warty mass (i.e., hypertrophic tuberculosis) that may mimic a neoplasm.
- The typical granulomatous inflammation with caseation resembles that seen in tuberculosis of other sites. Diagnosis requires identification of the organisms (*Mycobacterium tuberculosis* or occasionally atypical mycobacteria) with acid-fast tissue stains or culture.
- The differential diagnosis includes noninfectious forms of granulomatous vulvitis (see page 6) and a foreign-body granulomatous reaction.

Necrotizing Fasciitis and Progressive Bacterial Synergistic Gangrene

- Necrotizing disorders, which represent mixed, synergistic bacterial infections, occasionally involve the vulva. They are frequently associated with diabetes mellitus and atherosclerosis.
- The initial presentation of necrotizing fasciitis is that of vulvar erythema, edema, and pain, which is followed by rapidly progressive dark discoloration, bullae, and necrosis of the skin, subcutaneous tissue, and fascia. Rare vulvar cases have been associated with the toxic shock syndrome. The infection can be fatal without prompt excision of involved tissues and antibiotic therapy.
- Progressive synergistic gangrene differs from necrotizing fasciitis in that it is a slowly progressive process that may extend to the fascia and has less severe systemic manifestations. It is more likely to develop in postoperative wounds, whereas necrotizing fasciits is more likely to develop at sites of minor injury.

Miscellaneous Infections

- Chronic infections of the vulvar and perianal skin are commonly caused by fungi (*Candida*, dermatophytes) and occasionally by the bacterium *Corynebacterium minutissimum* that causes erythrasma. These lesions are not usually biopsied because the fungi are identified by microscopic examination of skin scrapings or by culture; erythrasma is usually diagnosed by Wood lamp examination.

■ Bacterial infection of the Bartholin glands is usually caused by the sexually transmitted organisms *Neisseria gonorrhoeae* or *C. trachomatis;* occasional cases follow vulvovaginal operations. A Bartholin gland abscess, often associated with secondary infection by anaerobic bacteria, is a common complication. Toxic shock syndrome also has been a complication in rare cases.

■ Hidradenitis suppurativa is a chronic suppurative inflammatory disease of the apocrine sweat glands, including those in the vulva and groins, that frequently results in scarring and draining sinuses. Microscopic examination of the excised tisssues reveals acute and chronic inflammation and apocrine glands dilated with keratinaceous material. Squamous cell carcinoma has arisen in rare, long-standing cases.

■ A case of bacillary angiomatosis manifested as red-purple vulvar and cervical papules and nodules in a 32-year-old woman with acquired immunodeficiency syndrome (AIDS). Microscopic examination revealed a lobular epithelioid vascular proliferation and hazy clumps of bacteria (*Bartonella henselae*) that stained with the Warthin-Starry method.

■ Rare parasitic infestations of the vulva include enterobiasis, schistosomiasis, and myiasis; the latter is caused by infestation of the larva of the muscoid fly and sarcophaga.

References

Barnes R, Mahood S, Lammert N, Young RH. Extragenital granuloma inguinale mimicking a soft-tissue neoplasm: a case report and review of the literature. Hum Pathol 21:559–561, 1990.

Bhattacharya P. Hypertrophic tuberculosis of the vulva. Obstet Gynecol 51:21S–22S, 1978.

Farley DE, Katz VL, Dotters DJ. Toxic shock syndrome associated wtih vulvar necrotizing fasciitis. Obstet Gynecol 82:660–602, 1993.

Freinkel AL. Histological aspects of sexually transmitted genital lesions. Histopathology 11:819–831, 1987.

Long SR, Whitfeld MJ, Eades C, et al. Bacillary angiomatosis of the cervix and vulva in a patient with AIDS. Obstet Gynecol 88:709–711, 1996.

Mattox TF, Rutgers J, Yoshimori RN, Bhatia NN. Nonfluorescent erythrasma of the vulva. Obstet Gynecol 81:862–864, 1993.

McKee PH, Wright E, Hutt MSR. Vulvar schistosomiasis. Clin Exp Dermatol 8:189, 1983.

Meltzer RM. Necrotizing fasciitis and progressive bacterial synergistic gangrene of the vulva. Obstet Gynecol 61:757–760, 1983.

Peters WA III. Bartholinitis after vulvovaginal surgery. Am J Obstet Gynecol 178:1143–1144, 1998.

Roberts DB. Necrotizing fasciitis of the vulva. Am J Obstet Gynecol 157:568–571, 1987.

Shearin RS, Boehike J, Karanth S. Toxic shock–like syndrome associated with Bartholin's gland abscess: case report. Am J Obstet Gynecol 160:1073–1074, 1989.

Sobel JD, Faro S, Force RW, et al. Vulvovaginal candidiasis: epidemiologic, diagnostic, and therapeutic considerations. Am J Obstet Gynecol 178:203–211, 1998.

Thomas R, Barnhill D, Bibro M, Hoskins W. Hidradenitis suppurativa: a case presentation and review of the literature. Obstet Gynecol 66: 592–595, 1985.

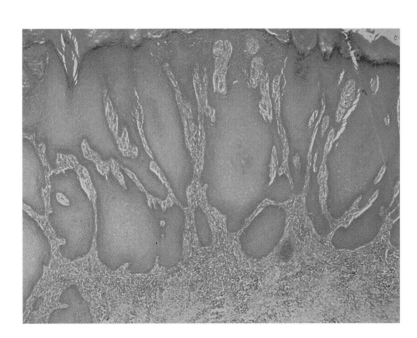

Figure 1–5. Condyloma lata (syphilis).

Inflammatory Lesions

Vulvar Vestibulitis

Clinical Features

- Vulvar vestibulitis, which affects up to 15% of patients in a general gynecologic practice, typically occurs in the reproductive age group, with an age range of 19 to 53 years (mean, 31 years) in one study.
- The characteristic clinical features are severe pain on attempted vaginal entry, point tenderness localized to the vulvar vestibule, and variable vulvar erythema.
- The cause is unknown. In most studies, human papillomavirus has been absent or identified with a frequency similar to that of control patients. An increased number of vulvar nerve fibers per square unit was found in one study.

Pathologic Features

- A mild to severe chronic inflammatory infiltrate (T lymphocytes, plasma cells, and occasional B lymphocytes, mast cells, and monocytes) involves the lamina propria of the squamous mucosa and, to a lesser extent, the fibrous tissue surrounding the vestibular glands and ducts. Lymphoid follicles are present in a few cases.
- Squamous metaplasia of the vestibular ducts and glands is found in a variable number of patients, although whether this finding is an inherent feature of the disorder is not certain.
- Complete replacement of the vestibular glands and ducts by squamous epithelium producing an invagination or cleft was considered a constant and diagnostic feature in one study. Two other studies, however, found clefts to be less common and difficult to distinguish from infoldings of surface epithelium.

References

Chadha S, Gianotten WL, Drogendijk AC, et al. Histopathologic features of vulvar vestibulitis. Int J Gynecol Pathol 17:7–11, 1998.

Prayson RA, Stoler MH, Hart WR. Vulvar vestibulitis: a histopathologic study of 36 cases, including human papillomavirus in situ hybridization analysis. Am J Surg Pathol 19:154–160, 1995.

Pyka RE, Wilkinson EJ, Friedrick EG Jr, Croker BP. The histopathology of vulvar vestibulitis syndrome. Int J Gynecol Pathol 7:249–257, 1988.

Westrom LV, Willen R. Vestibular nerve fiber proliferation in vulvar vestibulitis syndrome. Obstet Gynecol 91:572–576, 1998.

Plasma Cell Vulvitis

- The lesion, also known as Zoon's vulvitis, has typical presenting features of pruritis, burning, and red, sometimes multiple macules. The cause is unknown.
- There is a lichenoid infiltrate predominantly composed of plasma cells, a thinned epidermis, flattened rete ridges, absence of the granular or keratin layers, spongiotic parabasal ketatinocytes with spindled nuclei oriented horizontally (i.e., lozenge keratinocytes), and prominent dermal blood vessels with dermal hemorrhage and hemosiderin.
- The differential diagnosis includes syphilis, lichen planus, and other chronic dermatoses.

Reference

Souteyrand P, Wong E, MacDonald DM. Zoon's balanitis (balanitis circumscripta plasmacellularis). Br J Dermatol 105:195–199, 1981.

Granulomatous Vulvitis and Vulvar Involvement by Crohn's Disease

- Granulomatous vulvitis (vulvitis granulomatosa) refers to an idiopathic granulomatous inflammation of the vulva that appears to be the vulvar counterpart of granulomatous cheilitis; some patients have both lesions.
- The lesion, which occurs over a wide age range, usually manifests as a labial mass or as labial hypertrophy. Histologic examination reveals edema, fibrosis, lymphangiectasia, a mononuclear infiltrate, and nonnecrotizing granulomas with giant cells.
- More common than isolated granulomatous vulvitis, but identical histologically, is vulvar involvement by Crohn's disease. These patients usually have a history of or synchronous onset of intestinal Crohn's disease; in rare cases, the vulvar involvement precedes bowel involvement. Patients presenting with granulomatous vulvitis therefore need to be monitored for the possible development of Crohn's disease.

Reference

Guerrieri C, Ohlsson E, Ryden G, Westermark P. Vulvitis granulomatosa: a cryptogenic chronic inflammatory hypertrophy of vulvar labia related to cheilitis granulomatosa and Crohn's disease. Int J Gynecol Pathol 14:352–359, 1995.

Behçet's Disease

- Behçet's disease is a systemic vasculopathy that is most common in Japan and eastern Mediterranean countries. The mean age at onset is in the third decade; there is a slight male predominance.
- Behçet's disease is diagnosed by the presence of oral ulceration and any two of the following: genital ulceration, skin lesions (i.e., pustules or erythema nodosa–like lesions), and eye lesions (uveitis or retinal vasculitis). Synovitis and meningoencephalitis occur in some patients.
- The vulvar and oral ulcers are of the minor or major aphthous or herpetiform type. Major apthous ulcers, which may lead to gangrene, heal by scarring. Healing is often followed by new ulcers.
- Microscopic examination reveals a necrotizing vasculitis that may involve all calibers and types of dermal and subcutaneous vessels. The vasculitis may be lymphocytic or neutrophilic, and it can be associated with mural fibrin deposits, mural necrosis, and thrombosis.

References

Magro CM, Crowson AN. Cutaneous manifestations of Behçet's disease. Int J Dermatol 34:159–165, 1995.

Mangelsdorf HC, White WL, Jorizzo JL. Behçet's disease: report of twenty-five patients from the United States with prominent mucocutaneous involvement. J Am Acad Dermatol 34:745–750, 1996.

Lymphoma-like Lesion

■ Lymphoma-like lesions are rare in the vulva; their clinical and pathologic features resemble those occurring in the cervix (see page 76).

Reference

Young RH, Harris NL, Scully RE. Lymphoma-like lesions of the lower female genital tract: a report of 16 cases. Int J Gynecol Pathol 4:289–299, 1985.

Ligneous Vulvitis (see Chapter 4)

Nonneoplastic Epithelial Disorders

■ Classification of these disorders has been provided by the International Society for the Study of Vulvar Disease (ISSVD) and the International Society of Gynecological Pathologists (ISGP):
   • Lichen sclerosus (lichen sclerosus et atrophicus)
   • Squamous cell hyperplasia (formerly hyperplastic dystrophy)
   • Other dermatoses

Lichen Sclerosus

Clinical and Gross Features

■ Lichen sclerosus (LS) accounts for 30% to 40% of nonneoplastic epithelial vulvar lesions. It may occur at any age, including childhood, but is most common after menopause.

■ The cause is unknown. Autoimmune factors are suggested by the presence of autoantibodies and autoimmune diseases in some patients. A hormonal cause is suggested by the low serum levels of dihydrotestosterone, free testosterone, and androstenedione in untreated patients and a frequent response to topical testosterone. Genetic factors are suggested by a familial occurrence in some cases.

■ The lesions, which are often pruritic, may involve any part of the vulva. Hart and colleagues found involvement of the labia minora in 68% of their patients, the labia majora in 60%, the clitoris in 51%, the perineum in 41%, and the posterior fourchette in 36%. Extragenital lesions occur in two thirds of children with LS but in only 5% of affected adults.

■ Vulvar LS is characterized by irregular, ill-defined, white patches; telangiectatic vessels and melanin incontinence can result in focal red and brown areas, respectively. Almost 90% of the lesions are multiple; bilateral, sometimes symmetric lesions occur in 80% of patients.

■ In the late stages in adult women, the affected skin is shiny and wrinkled ("cigarette paper"), the labia are atrophic, and the introitus is narrowed. Agglutination and scarring of the prepuce and frenulum may obscure the clitoris. Complications, especially in children, include anal fissures and perianal and genital ulcers.

Microscopic Features

■ The diagnostic microscopic feature is a subepithelial homogenized zone that varies from edematous to hy-

alinized. Elastic staining reveals a marked loss or absence of elastic fibers in this zone, which is usually subtended by a band of lymphocytes and a few plasma cells. Vacuolar alteration at the dermal-epidermal interface is typical.

■ Carlson and coworkers found that, compared with extravulvar LS, vulvar LS less often shows epidermal atrophy and more commonly shows compact orthohyperkeratosis, parakeratosis, hypergranulosis, irregular psoriasiform hyperplasia, spongiosis, necrotic keratinocytes, subepidermal clefting, edema of the papillary dermis, and eosinophils.

■ Fung and LeBoit identified what they consider findings of early LS (i.e., inflammatory phase) adjacent to pathognomonic LS: a psoriasiform lichenoid pattern, basilar epidermotropism, loss of papillary dermal elastic fibers, basement membrane thickening, and epidermal atrophy.

Differential Diagnosis

■ Genital involvement by lichen planus (LP) can sometimes be difficult to distinguish from early LS. Features found by Fung and LeBoit in most or all cases of LP (but absent or uncommon in LS) included cytoid bodies, wedge-shaped hypergranulosis, basal squamatization, and pointed rete ridges.

Behavior

■ LS may undergo spontaneous remission at puberty or postpartum. LS responds in some cases to topical testosterone or corticosteroids.

■ Although in situ or invasive vulvar squamous cell carcinoma is associated with adjacent LS in as many as 60% of cases, LS has been considered to have no premalignant potential, and the association is attributed to the coincidental occurrence of two common diseases in the same patient. Challenging this view are the findings of several studies:
   • Tate and colleagues found that rare cases of LS are monoclonal.
   • Matias-Guiu and associates observed basal nuclear atypicality and marked elongation of the rete ridges in cases of LS before the appearance of a squamous cell carcinoma, findings that they interpreted as premalignant.
   • Carlson and coworkers found that 11% of uncomplicated cases of LS were aneuploid, compared with 52% of cases of LS associated with squamous carcinoma. Cases of aneuploid LS had an increased expression of p53 compared with their diploid counterparts. These investigators postulated that LS may act as an initiator and promoter of carcinogenesis.

Squamous Cell Hyperplasia

■ The term *squamous cell hyperplasia* (SCH) was proposed by the ISSVD in 1987 to replace the term *hyperplastic dystrophy*.

- These terms designate a nonspecific change of the vulvar skin consisting of variable degrees of acanthosis and hyperkeratosis or parakeratosis. Atypia, dermal inflammation, and fibrosis are absent. There may be a striking gross abnormality with "leukoplakia."
- Some lesions considered SCH are monoclonal, suggesting that SCH may be premalignant in some cases.
- The designation SCH has been criticized as too nonspecific and of little clinical value. According to Ambros and colleagues, its inappropriate use by pathologists often results in a failure to identify and treat specific vulvar dermatoses.

Other Dermatoses

- Almost any dermatosis can involve the vulva. The most common vulvar dermatoses, many of which may be inappropriately designated SCH, include lichen simplex chronicus, spongiotic dermatitis consistent with contact dermatitis, psoriasis, and LP (page 7).
- Some vulvar dermatoses occur with LS or VIN. In such cases, the surgical pathology report should indicate all the lesions that are present.
- Ambros and coworkers state that "careful histories and physical examinations aid in identifying less common vulvar dermatoses. Referral to a dermatologist/dermatopathologist is indicated when the diagnosis is in doubt or if the response to treatment is poor."

References

Ambros RA, Malfetano JH, Carlson JA, Mihm MC Jr. Non-neoplastic epithelial alterations of the vulva: recognition assessment and comparisons of terminologies used among various specialties. Mod Pathol 10:401–408, 1997.

Carlson JA, Ambros R, Malfetano J, et al. Vulvar lichen sclerosus and squamous cell carcinoma: a cohort, case control, and investigational study with historical perspective: implications for chronic inflammation and sclerosis in the development of neoplasia. Hum Pathol 29: 932–938, 1998.

Carlson JA, Lamb P, Malfetano J, et al. Clinicopathologic comparison of vulvar and extravulvar lichen sclerosus: histologic variants, evolving lesions, and etiology of 141 cases. Mod Pathol 11:844–854, 1998.

Friedrich EG Jr, Kalra PS. Serum levels of sex hormones in vulvar lichen sclerosus and the effect of topical testosterone. N Engl J Med 310:488–491, 1984.

Friedrich EG Jr, MacLaren NK. Genetic aspects of vulvar lichen sclerosus. Am J Obstet Gynecol 150:161, 1984.

Fung MA, LeBoit PE. Light microscopic criteria for the diagnosis of early vulvar lichen slcerosus: a comparison with lichen planus. Am J Surg Pathol 22:473–478, 1998.

Hart WR, Norris HJ, Helwig EB. Relation of lichen sclerosus et atrophicus of the vulva to development of carcinoma. Obstet Gynecol 45: 369, 1975.

Lawrence WD. Non-neoplastic epithelial disorders of the vulva (vulvar dystrophies): historical and current perspectives. Pathol Annu 28(2): 23–51, 1993.

Matias-Guiu X, Lerma E, Prat J. Current topics in pathology of gynecologic tumors. Int J Surg Pathol 6:121–134, 1998.

O'Keefe RJ, Scurry JP, Dennerstein G, et al. Audit of 114 non-neoplastic vulvar biopsies. Br J Obstet Gynaecol 102:780–786, 1995.

Tate JE, Mutter GL, Boynton KA, Crum CP. Monoclonal origin of vulvar intraepithelial neoplasia and some vulvar hyperplasias. Am J Pathol 150:315–322, 1997.

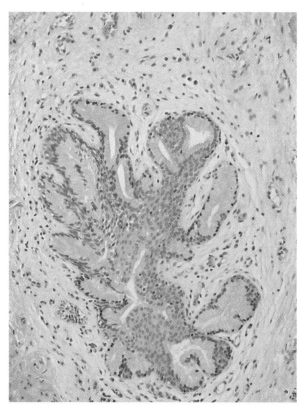

Figure 1–6. Vulvar vestibulitis. A minor vestibular gland exhibits squamous metaplasia, and chronic inflammatory cells are in the surrounding stroma.

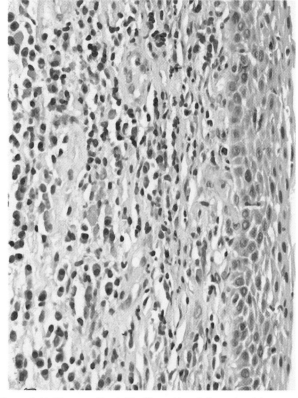

Figure 1–7. Plasma cell vulvitis. The epidermis is on the right.

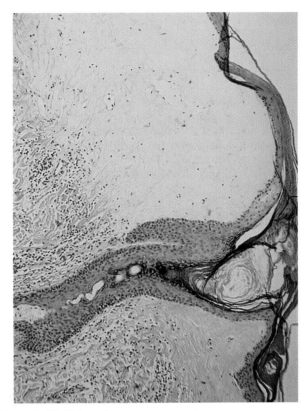

Figure 1–8. Granulomatous vulvitis.

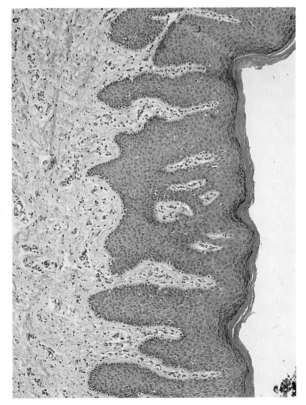

Figure 1–10. Lichen sclerosus.

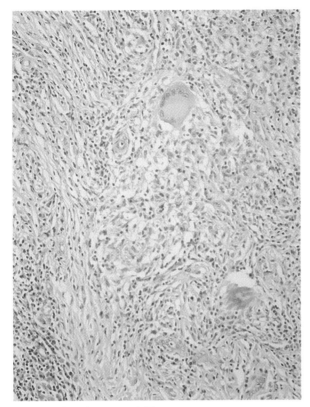

Figure 1–9. Lichen sclerosus.

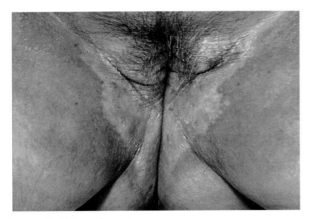

Figure 1–11. Lichen simplex chronicus with acanthosis and hyperkeratosis.

Cysts

Bartholin's Duct Cyst

■ Obstruction of the vestibular orifice of Bartholin's ducts results in accumulation of secretions from the gland with cystic dilatation.

■ The cysts are lined by squamous, transitional, mucinous, ciliated, or flattened, nonspecific epithelium.

■ A location consistent with Bartholin's origin and the presence of normal Bartholin's gland acini adjacent to the cyst facilitate distinction from cysts arising from minor vestibular glands.

Mucinous and Ciliated Vestibular Cysts

■ These cysts typically present as a solitary, sometimes painful, subcutaneous mass in the vulvar vestibule in women of reproductive age.

■ The cysts are usually less than 3 cm in maximal dimension. They are lined by a single layer of columnar mucinous epithelium, ciliated nonmucinous epithelium, or an admixture of the two. Focal squamous metaplasia may be present.

■ The cysts most likely arise from the minor vestibular glands, which are of presumed urogenital sinus origin.

Other Cysts

■ Epidermal inclusion cysts are commonly encountered in the vulva, usually the labia majora. They are lined by stratified squamous epithelium and filled with keratinaceous debris.

■ Rare mesothelial cysts derived from the canal of Nuck (the incompletely obliterated processus vaginalis) are usually found in the superior aspect of the labia majora or the inguinal canal. They may be associated with, and should be distinguished from, an inguinal hernia.

■ Rare mesonephric cysts occur in the lateral aspects of the vulva and have a histologic appearance similar to that of mesonephric cysts of the vagina (see Chapter 3).

■ Rare vulvar cysts may arise from the mammary-like glands in this site (see page 13).

References

Kucera PR, Glazer J. Hydrocele of the canal of Nuck: a report of four cases. J Reprod Med 30:439–442, 1985.

Robboy SJ, Ross JS, Prat J, et al. Urogenital sinus origin of mucinous and ciliated cysts of the vulva. Obstet Gynecol 51:347–351, 1978.

Rorat E, Ferenczy A, Richart RM. Human Bartholin gland, duct, and duct cyst: histochemical and ultrastructural Study. Arch Pathol 99:367–374, 1975.

van der Putte SCJ, van Gorp LHM. Cysts of mammary-like glands in the vulva. Int J Gynecol Pathol 14:184–188, 1995.

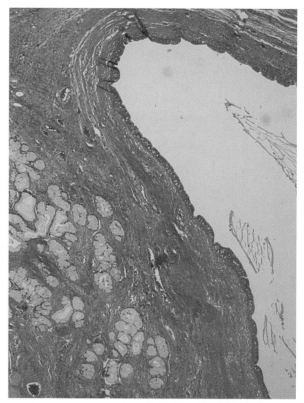

Figure 1–12. Bartholin's gland cyst. Notice the normal Bartholin's gland tissue (*lower left*).

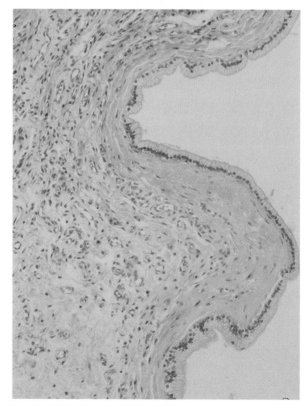

Figure 1–13. Mucinous vestibular cyst.

Pigmented Lesions

∎ Benign pigmented lesions of the vulva occur in about 10% of women. These lesions often have atypical clinical or histological features that may raise a concern about malignant melanoma.

Lentigo Simplex and Melanosis

∎ Lentigo simplex refers to a lesion consisting of benign epidermal hyperplasia, hyperpigmentation, and benign melanocytic hyperplasia. The term *melanosis* is most commonly used to refer to similar hyperpigmented lesions, with or without melanocytic hyperplasia, that lack epidermal hyperplasia.

∎ The lesions typically occur in white women of reproductive age. In some cases, they have been present for years.

∎ The typical appearance is that of melanotic macules on the labia, introital area, or perineum. Lentigines are usually less than 5 mm in diameter, whereas areas of melanosis may reach 2 cm. Some lesions have features suggestive of or indistinguishable from lentigo maligna or malignant melanoma, including multifocality, irregularity of outline, and variegated pigmentation.

∎ Microscopic examination typically reveals basal layer hyperpigmentation and slight basalar melanocytic hyperplasia without nesting or atypia. Some lesions desigated *melanosis* have lacked melanocytic hyperplasia. Acanthosis with elongation of rete pegs is present in lentigines; dermal melanophages also may be present.

∎ The differential diagnosis includes malignant melanoma in situ. This lesion, in contrast to lentigo or melanosis, is characterized by atypical melanocytes that are often in nests and in all layers of the epidermis. Mitotic figures may be seen in the melanocytes.

References

Barnhill RL, Albert LS, Shama SK, et al. Genital lentiginosis: a clinical and histopathologic study. J Am Acad Dermatol 22:453–460, 1990.

Rock B, Hood AF, Rock JA. Prospective study of vulvar nevi. J Am Acad Dermatol 22:104–106, 1990.

Sison-Torre EQ, Ackerman AB. Melanosis of the vulva: a clinical simulator of malignant melanoma. Am J Dermatopathol 7(Suppl):51–60, 1985.

Melanocytic Nevi

∎ Vulvar nevi are only one third as common as the lesions discussed in the preceding section; they were found in only 2.3% of women in one study. Most vulvar nevi resemble their extravulvar counterparts.

∎ A minority of vulvar nevi exhibit distinctive, atypical features that differ from those of the usual dysplastic nevus and have been designated *atypical melanocytic nevi of genital type* (AMNGT) by Clark and associates. Their features include:
  - Enlarged junctional melanocytic nests with variability in the size, shape, and position of the nests and, in some cases, a confluent band-like arrangement of the nests

  - Origin of nests from the sides of rete, between rete, and from adnexal structures, in addition to origin from the usual location at the rete tips
  - Lesional cells that may be dyshesive, with larger nuclei with more prominent nucleoli compared with those of nevus cells within the underlying dermal component
  - Pagetoid involvement of the upper epidermis that, in contrast to this finding in melanomas, lacks cytologic atypia and lateral extension and is usually focal or multifocal rather than extensive or diffuse
  - In about 50% of the cases, an underlying, usually large, common dermal nevus that is diffusely or focally covered by the distinctive junctional component
  - A stromal component that is often ill-defined, nondescript, and inconspicuous compared with the distinctive stromal patterns encountered in dysplastic nevi and superficial spreading melanomas

∎ The differential diagnosis of AMNGT includes vulvar dysplastic nevi and superficial spreading melanoma (see Clark et al. for a comprehensive discussion).

References

Blickstein I, Feldberg E, Dgani R, et al. Dysplastic vulvar nevi. Obstet Gynecol 78:968–970, 1991.

Christensen WN, Friedmann KJ, Woodruff JD, Hood AF. Histologic characteristics of vulvar nevocellular nevi. J Cutan Pathol 14:87–91, 1987.

Clark WH Jr, Hood AF, Tucker MA, Jampel RM. Atypical melanocytic nevi of the genital type with a discussion of reciprocal parenchymal-stromal interactions in the biology of neoplasia. Hum Pathol 29:S1–S24, 1998.

Haupt HM, Stern JB. Pagetoid melanocytosis: histologic features in benign and malignant lesions. Am J Surg Pathol 19:792–797, 1995.

Rock B, Hood AF, Rock JA. Prospective study of vulvar nevi. J Am Acad Dermatol 22:104–106, 1990.

Squamous Papillomatosis

∎ Squamous papillomatosis (squamous micropapillomatosis or vestibular papillomatosis) refers to multiple, often countless, squamous papillomas that typically involve the medial aspect of the labia minora, vulvar vestibule, hymen, introitus, and urethral meatus. Some physicians consider the finding of one or several vestibular papillomas to be normal.

∎ Squamous papillomatosis usually occurs in women of reproductive age, most of whom are asymptomatic, although some patients have pruritus, burning, and dyspareunia. The lesions typically regress without treatment.

∎ The cause is unknown. Most studies have shown no association with HPV. One study recording a high frequency of HPV included koilocytotic lesions that would be considered condylomas by others.

∎ Each papilloma is about 1 mm in diameter and 1 to 8 mm long. Microscopically, they consist of papillary fronds of bland, nonkeratotic, glycogenated squamous epithelium with an underlying proliferation of capillaries in the dermal papillae. Absence of koilocytosis is a definitional feature in most studies, allowing histologic distinction from condyloma.

References

De Deus JM, Focchi J, Stavale JN, De Lima GR. Histologic and biomolecular aspects of papillomatosis of the vulvar vestibule in relation to human papillomavirus. Obstet Gynecol 86:758–763, 1995.

Growdon WA, Fu YS, Lebherz TB, et al. Pruritic vulvar squamous papillomatosis: evidence for human papillomavirus etiology. Obstet Gynecol 66:564–568, 1985.

Moyal-Barracco M, Leibowitch M, Orth G. Vestibular papillae of the vulva: lack of evidence for human papillomavirus etiology. Arch Dermatol 126:1594–1598, 1990.

Potkul RK, Lancaster WD, Kurman RJ, et al. Vulvar condylomas and squamous vestibular micropapilloma: differences in appearance and response to treatment. J Reprod Med 35:1019–1022, 1990.

Wang AC, Hsu JJ, Hsueh S, et al. Evidence of human papillomavirus deoxyribonucleic acid in vulvar squamous papillomatosis. Int J Gynecol Pathol 10:44–50, 1991.

Welch JM, Nayagam M, Parry G, et al. What is vestibular papillomatosis? A study of its prevalence, aetiology and natural history. Br J Obstet Gynaecol 100:939–942, 1993.

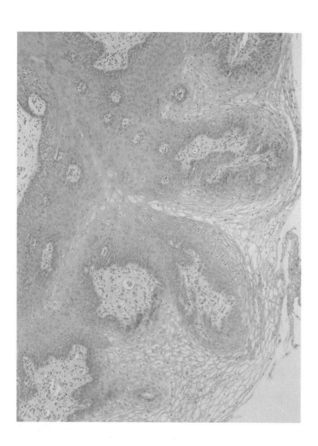

Figure 1–14. Vestibular papillomatosis. The squamous cells have clear cytoplasm because of their glycogen content but are not koilocytotic.

Ectopic Tissues

Ectopic Breast Tissue

- Ectopic breast tissue and lesions derived therefrom can theoretically occur anywhere along the embryonic milk line, including the vulva. Van der Putte, however, has proposed that vulvar mammary-type tissue arises from mammary-like glands, normally occurring glands of the anogenital skin that may also exhibit eccrine or apocrine features.
- Most cases of ectopic breast tissue occur on the labia majora and form unilateral or bilateral, solid to cystic subcutaneous masses that may reach 8 cm in diameter. Rare cases are associated with an ectopic nipple, but none has had an associated areola.
- The lesions may be first recognized at puberty but more commonly are found during pregnancy. Postpartum regression has occurred in some cases.
- In a few patients, usually women in the fifth or sixth decade, the lesions are first recognized because of the development of a cyst, a benign tumor (page 16), or malignant tumor (page 36) arising in the ectopic breast tissue. Some of these patients may have noticed a vulvar mass years earlier.
- Diagnosis and treatment of uncomplicated cases can be achieved by excisional biopsy, which yields normal or lactating breast tissue.

Other Ectopic Tissues

- A 6.0-cm tumor-like vulvar mass composed mainly of ectopic salivary gland tissue with a minor component of cartilage and respiratory epithelium was reported in a 38-year-old woman. The lesion was considered a choristoma.
- A lesion interpreted as "intestinal heterotopia" manifested as a vulvar ulcer in a 31-year-old woman. Excisional biopsy revealed that the epidermis was replaced by inflamed colonic mucosa with underlying smooth muscle and ganglion cells.

References

Garcia JJ, Verkauf BS, Hochberg CJ, Ingram JM. Aberrant breast tissue of the vulva: a case report and review of the literature. Obstet Gynecol 52:225–228, 1978.

Marwah S, Berman ML. Ectopic salivary gland in the vulva (choristoma): report of a case and review of the literature. Obstet Gynecol 56:389–391, 1980.

van der Putte SCJ. Mammary-like glands of the vulva and their disorders. Int J Gynecol Pathol 13:150–160, 1994.

Yeoh G, Bannatyne P, Kossard S, Russell P. Intestinal heterotopia: an unusual cause of vulval ulceration. Case report. Br J Obstet Gynaecol 94:600–602, 1987.

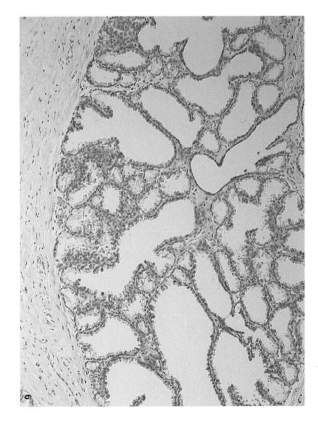

Figure 1–15. Ectopic breast tissue in the vulva of a pregnant woman. Lactational changes are striking.

Miscellaneous Tumor-like Lesions

Adenosis

■ Rare cases of introital adenosis have been described following CO_2 laser treatment and vulvar involvement in the Stevens-Johnson syndrome, but not, in contrast to vaginal adenosis, after in utero exposure to diethylstilbestrol. The adenosis in these cases was of the tuboendometrioid type.

■ One case of vulvar adenosis, reported as "mucinous metaplasia," presented as a 1.0-cm, depressed, red area near the clitoris in a 60-year-old woman. Histologic examination revealed that columnar mucinous cells had replaced the normal squamous epithelium.

References

Coghill SB, Tyler X, Shaxted EJ. Benign mucinous metaplasia of the vulva. Histopathology 17:373–375, 1990.

Marquette GP, Su B, Woodruff JD. Introital adenosis associated with Stevens-Johnson syndrome. Obstet Gynecol 66:243–245, 1985.

Sedlacek TV, Riva JM, Magen AB, et al. Vaginal and vulvar adenosis: an unsuspected side effect of CO_2 laser vaporization. J Reprod Med 35:995–1001, 1990.

Nodular Hyperplasia of Bartholin's Gland

■ This lesion occurs at an average age of 35 years (range, 19 to 56 years) and manifests as a solid or solid and cystic mass usually less than 4 cm in its maximal dimension. In some cases, it may be related to duct obstruction.

■ The proliferation has an irregular, lobulated contour and is composed of cytogically bland mucinous acini with maintenance of the normal duct-to-acinar relationship. Inflammation, cysts, and squamous metaplasia of the ducts are often present.

Reference

Koenig C, Tavassoli FA. Nodular hyperplasia, adenoma, and adenomyoma of Bartholin's gland. Int J Gynecol Pathol 17:289–294, 1998.

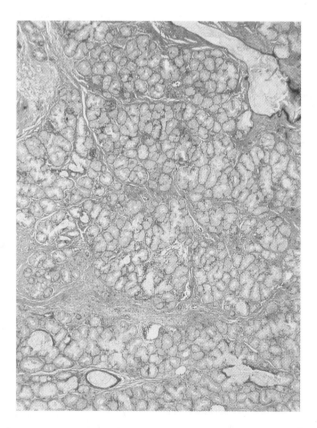

Figure 1–16. Nodular hyperplasia of Bartholin's gland.

Nodular Fasciitis

- Nodular fasciitis of the vulva occurs over a wide age range (7 to 51 years), although most of the women have been of reproductive age. The lesion typically manifests as a painless, subcutaneous labial mass, which in all the reported cases has been less than 3.5 cm in diameter. Except for a local recurrence in one case, all of the lesions were adequately treated by local excision.
- The histologic features are similar to these lesions in other sites.
- The wide differential diagnosis includes other reactive lesions, such as the postoperative spindle cell nodule (page 46), and many benign and malignant soft tissue tumors, including aggressive angiomyxoma (page 18), angiomyofibroblastoma (page 20), and leiomyosarcoma (page 39).

Reference

O'Connell JX, Young RH, Nielsen GP, et al. Nodular fasciitis of the vulva: a study of six cases and literature review. Int J Gynecol Pathol 16:117–123, 1997.

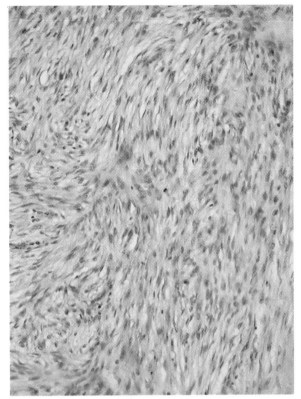

Figure 1–17. Nodular fasciitis of the vulva.

Other Tumor-like Lesions

- Rare examples of vulvar calcinosis, lymphoid hamartoma, and amyloidosis have been reported. In two cases of the latter, the vulvar lesions were the presenting manifestation of systemic amyloidosis; in one case, the vulvar lesions clinically mimicked an invasive squamous cell carcinoma.
- Fibroepithelial polyps are discussed in Chapter 3.

References

Balfour PJT, Vincenti AC. Idiopathic vulvar calcinosis. Histopathology 18:183–184, 1991.

Kernen JA, Morgan ML. Benign lymphoid hamartoma of the vulva. Obstet Gynecol 35:290–292, 1970.

Persoons JHA, Sutorius FJM, Koopman RJJ, et al. Vulvar paraneoplastic amyloidosis with the appearance of vulvar carcinoma. Am J Obstet Gynecol 180:1041–1044, 1999.

Taylor SC, Baker E, Grossman ME. Nodular vulvar amyloid as a presentation of systemic amyloidosis. J Am Acad Dermatol 24:139, 1991.

BENIGN TUMORS

Papillary Hidradenoma

- Papillary hidradenomas (hidradenoma papilliferum) are benign tumors of apocrine origin that usually present as painless vulvar nodules in women of reproductive or postmenopausal age. Two thirds of the tumors occur on the labia majora or minora.
- Almost all of the tumors are less than 2 cm, but exceptional tumors reach 8 cm in diameter; rare tumors are multiple. In one study, 55% of tumors were cystic, and 17% were ulcerated.
- Microscopic examination reveals a well-circumscribed to slightly infiltrative, complex proliferation of papillae, tubules, and cysts lined by an inner layer of cuboidal epithelial cells and an outer layer of myoepithelial cells. The epithelial cells, which may have an apocrine appearance, may exhibit mild atypia and stratification and have occasional mitotic figures.

■ Unusual features include sebaceous differentiation, numerous mitotic figures, inflammation, and calcification.

■ Two examples of malignant transformation have been reported. In one, an intraductal apocrine carcinoma arose in a papillary hidradenoma. In the other, a rapidly fatal adenosquamous carcinoma arose in a papillary hidradenoma that had been present for many years.

■ The differential diagnosis is with intraductal papillomas arising in ectopic breast tissue.

References

Bannatyne P, Elliott P, Russell P. Vulvar adenosquamous carcinoma arising in a hidiradenoma papilliferum, with rapidly fatal outcome: case report. Gynecol Oncol 35:395–398, 1989.

Woodworth H, Dockerty MB, Wilson RB, Pratt JH. Papillary hidradenoma of the vulva: a clinicopathologic study of 69 cases. Am J Obstet Gynecol 110:501–508, 1971.

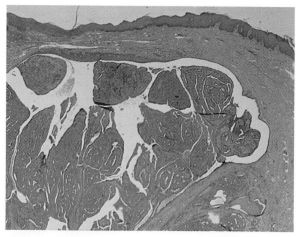

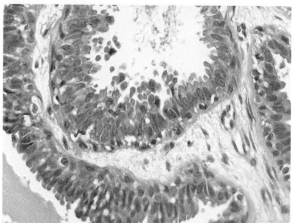

Figure 1–18. Low and high-power views of hidradenoma papilliferum.

Benign Mammary-type Tumors

■ Benign tumors of mammary type can arise within ectopic breast tissue. Intraductal papillomas of mammary type can be distinguished from papillary hidradenomas (discussed earlier) only by the presence of surrounding breast tissue.

■ Tumors resembling mammary fibroadenomas, often with apocrine differentiation, have been described in the vulva, and there have been rare examples of fibroadenoma phyllodes. One hamartoma arising in ectopic breast tissue arising in the inguinal region has been reported.

References

Dworak O, Reck T, Greskotter KR, Kockerling F. Hamartoma of an ectopic breast arising in the inguinal region. Histopathology 24:169–171, 1994.

Higgins CM, Strutton GM. Papillary apocrine fibroadenoma of the vulva. J Cutan Pathol 23:256–260, 1997.

Rickert RR. Intraductal papilloma arising in supernumerary vulvar breast tissue. Obstet Gynecol 55:84S–87S, 1980.

Tresserra F, Grases PJ, Izquierdo M, et al. Fibroadenoma phyllodes arising in vulvar supernumerary breast tissue: report of two cases. Int J Gynecol Pathol 17:171–173, 1998.

Woodworth H, Dockerty MB, Wilson RB, Pratt JH. Papillary hidradenoma of the vulva: a clinicopathologic study of 69 cases. Am J Obstet Gynecol 110:501–508, 1971.

Benign Tumors of Skin Appendage Origin

■ A variety of benign vulvar tumors can arise from skin appendages and resemble such tumors in extravulvar sites.

■ Tumors of sweat gland origin include syringoma, clear cell hidradenoma, and benign mixed tumors (i.e., pleomorphic adenomas). The latter may also arise from

Bartholin's gland (discussed later) or ectopic breast tissue.

■ Tumors of hair follicle origin include pilar tumor (i.e., proliferating trichilemmal tumor or trichilemmoma), trichoepithelioma, trichoblastic fibroma, and keratoacanthoma.

References

Avinoach I, Zirkin HJ, Glezerman M. Proliferating trichilemmal tumor of the vulva: case report of review of the literature. Int J Gynecol Pathol 8:163–168, 1989.

Belardi MC, Maglione MA, Vighi S, di Paola GR. Syringoma of the vulva: a case report. J Reprod Med 39:957–959, 1994.

Cho D, Woodruff JD. Trichoepithelioma of the vulva: a report of two cases. J Reprod Med 33:317–319, 1988.

Gilks CB, Clement PB, Wood WS. Trichoblastic fibroma—a report of three cases. Am J Dermatopathol 11:397–402, 1989.

Gilbey S, Moore DH, Look K, Sutton GP. Vulvar keratoacanthoma. Obstet Gynecol 89:848–850, 1997.

Rorat E, Wallach RC. Mixed tumors of the vulva: clinical outcome and pathology. Int J Gynecol Pathol 3:323–328, 1984.

Benign Tumors of Bartholin's Gland and Minor Vestibular Glands

■ Rare cases of adenoma and adenomyoma of the Bartholin's gland have been reported. These, in contrast to nodular hyperplasia, have a haphazard proliferation of acini and tubules with loss of the normal duct to acinar relationship. A small adenoid cystic carcinoma arose from one Bartholin's gland adenoma.

■ Two benign vulvar mixed tumors were probably of Bartholin's gland origin. Another report described a papilloma arising in a Bartholin's cyst.

■ Rare adenomas (or nodular hyperplasias) of minor vestibular glands have been reported, typically as an incidental finding in tissue removed for vestibulitis (page 6). Proliferations of small glands lined by mucinous columnar cells are seen on microscopic examination.

References

Axe S, Parmley T, Woodruff JD, Hlopak B. Adenomas in minor vestibular glands. Obstet Gynecol 68:16–18, 1986.

Enghardt MH, Valente PT, Day DH. Papilloma of Bartholin's gland duct cyst: first report of a case. Int J Gynecol Pathol 12:86–92, 1993.

Koenig C, Tavassoli FA. Nodular hyperplasia, adenoma, and adenomyoma of Bartholin's gland. Int J Gynecol Pathol 17:289–294, 1998.

Ordonez NG, Manning JT, Luna MA. Mixed tumor of the vulva: a report of two cases probably arising in Bartholin's gland. Cancer 48:181–186, 1981.

Granular Cell Tumor

■ Between 5% and 15% of granular cell tumors, which are probably of peripheral nerve sheath origin, arise in the vulva. Some patients with vulvar granular cell tumors have similar tumors in extravulvar sites.

■ The patients are usually of reproductive or postmenopausal age. They present with solitary or occasionally with multiple subcutaneous nodules that typically involve the labia majora and less commonly involve the clitoris or perineum. Most tumors are less than 4 cm in maximal dimension.

■ The tumors are composed of nests and sheets of eosinophilic, periodic acid–Schiff–positive, S-100–positive, granular cells with bland nuclei, intermingled with strands of collagen and occasional chronic inflammatory cells.

■ The overlying epidermis or squamous epithelium often shows striking degrees of pseudocarcinomatous hyperplasia, which can be confused with a well-differentiated squamous cell carcinoma, especially in a superficial biopsy specimen in which the granular cells are sparse or absent.

■ The tumors are almost always clinically benign. There are no microscopic features that can reliably identify the rare tumors that are clinically malignant.

References

Horowitz IR, Copas P, Majmudar B. Granular cell tumors of the vulva. Am J Obstet Gynecol 173:1710–1714, 1995.

Majmudar B, Castellano PZ, Wilson RW, Siegel RJ. Granular cell tumors of the vulva. J Reprod Med 35:1008–1014, 1990.

Wolber R, Wilkinson E, Talerman A, Clement PB. Granular cell tumors of the vulva with pseudocarcinomatous hyperplasia: a comparative morphological analysis with squamous cell carcinoma. Int J Gynecol Pathol 10:59–66, 1991.

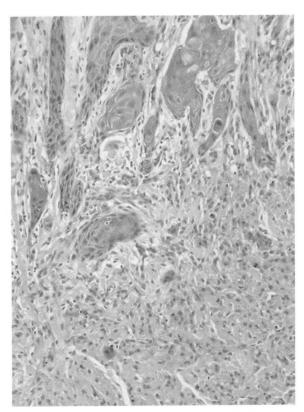

Figure 1–19. Granular cell tumor (*bottom*) associated with prominent pseudocarcinomatous hyperplasia (*top*).

Cellular Angiofibroma

■ The term cellular angiofibroma has been applied to an uncommon, distinctive soft tissue tumor of the vulva. The six examples occurred in women between 39 and 50 years of age who presented with a small (<3 cm) vulvar or perineal (one case) mass.

■ The tumors were well circumscribed, except in one case, and composed of a cellular proliferation of uniform, bland fibroblasts; numerous, thick-walled, and often hyalinized blood vessels; short bundles of wispy collagen; and a sparse component of mature fat. One tumor was diffusely myxoid. Most of the tumors were mitotically active (up to 11 mitoses/10 high-power fields).

■ The stromal cells are immunoreactive for vimentin and in some cases for CD34, but they are negative for actin, desmin, and epithelial membrane antigen.

■ Differentiation from angiomyofibroblastoma is discussed under that heading. Other tumors in the differential diagnosis include spindle cell lipoma, solitary fibrous tumor, pereineuroma, and leiomyoma.

Reference

Nucci MR, Granter SR, Fletcher CDM. Cellular angiofibroma: a benign neoplasm distinct from angiomyofibroblastoma and spindle cell lipoma. Am J Surg Pathol 21:636–644, 1997.

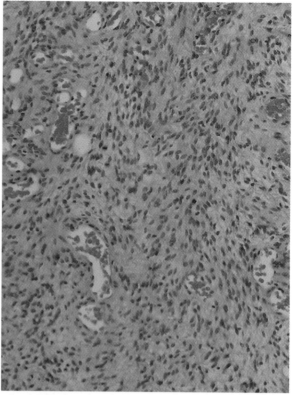

Figure 1–20. Cellular angiofibroma. (Courtesy of Dr. Marisa Nucci.)

Aggressive Angiomyxoma of Pelvic and Perineal Soft Tissues

Clinical Features

■ More than 90% of these tumors occur in women, who are usually in the reproductive age group (mean age, 32 years; range, 11 to 70 years).

■ The typical manifestation is that of a mass or an ill-defined swelling that may be vulvar, perineal, vaginal, inguinal, gluteal, ischiorectal, retroperitoneal, or combinations thereof. The initial clinical impression is often that of a Bartholin cyst or hernia.

■ The tumors are often much larger and extend more deeply than initially appreciated on pelvic examination. Large tumors may fill the pelvis, tending to displace rather than invade pelvic viscera.

Pathologic Features

■ The tumors are typically bulky, soft to rubbery, solid masses with a lobulated contour that appears partially or completely encapsulated. The sectioned surface has a glistening, gelatinous, relatively homogeneous appearance, although small cysts or areas of hemorrhage may be present.

■ Sparsely distributed, small, spindle and stellate cells are separated by a loose stroma that contains a dense network of delicate collagen fibrils and numerous thin- and thick-walled blood vessels of various sizes. Perivascular condensation of the collagen is a common finding.

■ The nuclei of the spindle and stellate cells are small and uniform, with small, indistinct nucleoli; rare multinucleated cells may be present. Mitotic figures have not been observed.

■ Smooth muscle differentiation, typically adjacent to blood vessels, was identified in all tumors in one study. In the same study, foci resembling angiomyofibroblastoma were found in several tumors.

■ The stroma shows only weak positivity with alcian blue at pH 1.0 and 2.5 and with colloidal iron, suggesting that edema fluid rather than mucosubstances is the predominant substance between the collagen fibrils. Extravasated erythrocytes and sparsely distributed mast cells are common within the stroma.

- The tumors lack a capsule and infiltrate the surrounding soft tissue that often includes fat and skeletal muscle; small nerves are commonly entrapped.
- The tumor cells are typically immunoreactive for vimentin, smooth muscle actin, muscle specific actin, estrogen and progesterone receptors, and in some studies, desmin and, less commonly, CD34.
- Ultrastructural studies of the spindle cells have shown fibroblastic, myofibroblastic, or both types of differentiation.

Behavior

- The tumors are typically indolent, with a tendency to recur locally because complete excision of the tumor is usually not technically feasible. The recurrences occur at postoperative intervals ranging from 8 months to 14 years.
- Distant metastases or death from tumor has not been described.

Differential Diagnosis

- Angiomyofibroblastoma is described later. Granter and colleagues consider this tumor and the aggressive angiomyxoma to be part of a spectrum of tumors showing myofibroblastic differentiation.
- Superficial angiomyxoma (cutaneous myxomas) differ from aggressive angiomyxomas by their occasional association with Carney's complex, superficial location, small size, abundant acid mucin, and nonreactivity for desmin and estrogen and progesterone receptors.
- Myxoma, spindle cell lipoma, myxoid neurofibroma, fibroepithelial polyp, fibromatosis, myxoid liposarcoma, myxoid smooth muscle tumors, embryonal rhabdomyosarcoma (i.e., sarcoma botryoides), and myxoid malignant fibrous histiocytoma are included in the differential diagnosis.
  - Aside from a myxoid stroma, all of these tumors lack the characteristic histologic appearance, including the distinctive vascular component, of the aggressive angiomyxoma.
  - Myxoid sarcomas usually contain nonmyxoid areas and cells with greater degrees of nuclear pleomorphism and mitotic activity than seen in the aggressive angiomyxoma.

References

Begin LR, Clement PB, Kirk ME, et al. Aggressive angiomyxoma of pelvic soft parts: a clinicopathological study of nine cases. Hum Pathol 16:621–628, 1985.

Fetsch JF, Laskin WB, Lefkowitz M, et al. Aggressive angiomyxoma: a clinicopathologic study of 29 female patients. Cancer 78:79–90, 1996.

Fetsch JF, Laskin WB, Tavassoli FA. Superficial angiomyxoma (cutaneous myxoma): a clinicopathologic study of 17 cases arising in the genital region. Int J Gynecol Pathol 16:325–334, 1997.

Granter SR, Nucci MR, Fletcher CDM. Aggressive angiomyxoma: reappraisal of its relationship to angiomyofibroblastoma in a series of 16 cases. Histopathology 30:3–10, 1997.

Steeper TA, Rosai J. Aggressive angiomyxoma of the female pelvis and perineum: report of nine cases of a distinctive type of gynecologic soft-tissue neoplasm. Am J Surg Pathol 7:463–475, 1983.

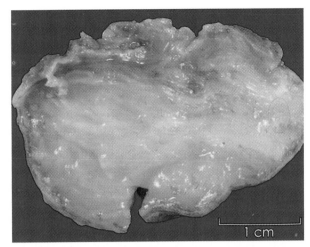

Figure 1–21. Sectioned surface of an aggressive angiomyxoma. The tumor is poorly circumscribed and glistening.

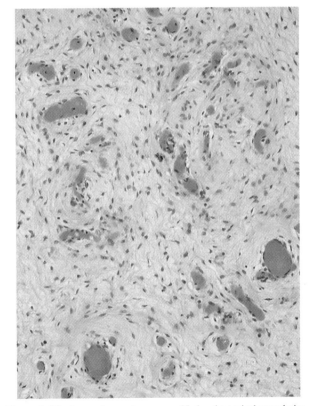

Figure 1–22. Aggressive angiomyxoma. Notice the typical vascularity.

Angiomyofibroblastoma

- These tumors occur in women of reproductive and postmenopausal ages (mean, 42 years) who present with a vulvar mass up to 12 cm in diameter, although most are less than 5 cm.
- Angiomyofibroblastomas are well-circumscribed grossly and microscopically and are characterized by alternating hypercellular and hypocellular edematous zones in which numerous small to medium, thin-walled, arborizing vessels (predominantly capillaries) are irregularly distributed.
- Spindled, oval, plasmacytoid, and epithelioid cells with eosinophilic cytoplasm, separated by wavy strands or thick bundles of collagen, are aggregated around blood vessels, sometimes forming solid, compact foci, or are loosely dispersed in the hypocellular areas. Fat has been present in rare cases. Scattered lymphocytes and mast cells are common.
- The nuclei of the tumor cells are typically bland, but in 40% of cases, rare nuclei are enlarged and hyperchromatic. Occasional cells are binucleated or multinucleated. The plasmacytoid cells have eccentrically placed nuclei. Mitotic figures are absent or rare.
- The cells are immunoreactive for vimentin and desmin, occasionally for actin and CD34, but not for cytokeratin or S-100. The cells have the ultrastructural features of myofibroblasts.
- Only one of the reported tumors has recurred after local excision. In that case, an otherwise typical angiomyofibroblastoma contained focal areas of sarcoma resembling malignant fibrous histiocytoma. The recurrent tumor, removed 2 years later, was purely sarcomatous.

Differential Diagnosis

- In contrast to aggressive angiomyxomas, angiomyofibroblastomas have circumscribed borders, are focally more cellular, have more blood vessels (that usually lack thick walls), and have plump to epithelioid stromal cells that often exhibit perivascular condensation.
- Features favoring a diagnosis of cellular angiofibroma include numerous vessels with hyalinized walls and an absence of perivascular epithelioid cells.

References

Fletcher CDM, Tsang WYW, Lee KC, Chang JKC. Angiomyofibroblastoma of the vulva: a benign neoplasm distinct from aggressive angiomyxoma. Am J Surg Pathol 16:373–382, 1992.

Fukunaga M, Nomura K, Matsumoto K, et al. Vulval angiomyofibroblastoma: clinicopathologic analysis of six cases. Am J Clin Pathol 107:45–51, 1997.

Granter SR, Nucci MR, Fletcher CDM. Aggressive angiomyxoma: reappraisal of its relationship to angiomyofibroblastoma in a series of 16 cases. Histopathology 30:3–10, 1997.

Nielsen GP, Rosenberg AE, Young RH, et al. Angiomyofibroblastoma of the vulva and vagina. Mod Pathol 9:284–291, 1996.

Nielsen GP, Young RH, Dickersin GR, Rosenberg AE. Angiomyofibroblastoma of the vulva with sarcomatous transformation ("angiomyofibrosarcoma"). Am J Surg Pathol 21:1104–1108, 1997.

Ockner DM, Sayadi H, Swanson PE, et al. Genital angiomyofibroblastoma: comparison with aggressive angiomyxoma and other myxoid neoplasms of skin and soft tissue. Am J Clin Pathol 107:36–44, 1997.

Vasquez MD, Ro JY, Park YW, et al. Angiomyofibroblastoma: a clinicopathologic study of eight cases and review of the literature. Int J Surg Pathol 7:161–169, 1999.

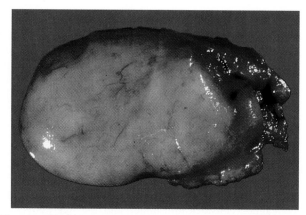

Figure 1–23. Sectioned surface of an angiomyofibroblastoma. The tumor is well circumscribed.

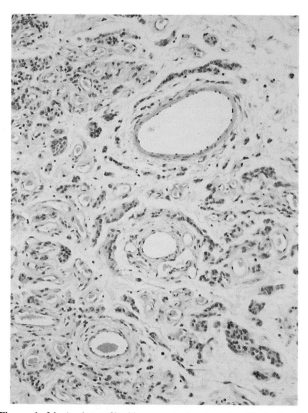

Figure 1–24. Angiomyofibroblastoma, with nests of epithelioid cells, some of which are perivascular.

Nonspecific Benign (or Locally Aggressive) Mesenchymal Tumors

- Within this category are leiomyomas (page 39), rhabdomyomas (page 51), lipomas and lipoma variants, and rare examples of desmoid tumor and fibromatosis of the soft tissue type.
- Vascular tumors of the vulva have included examples of glomus tumor, capillary and cavernous hemangioma, angiokeratoma, and lymphangioma (including lymphangioma circumscriptum). In some cases, the vulvar hemangiomas have been part of the blue rubber bleb nevus syndrome or the congenital dysplastic angiopathy (Klippel-Trénaunay-Weber) syndrome.
- Vulvar examples of solitary (sometimes giant) neurofibromas, neurofibromatosis, and schwannomas have been reported. Vulvar involvement is rarely the presenting manifestation of neurofibromatosis.
- One paraganglioma of the vulva has been reported. It occurred in a 58-year-old woman who presented with a 1-cm nodule of the labium minus.

References

Allen MV, Novotny DB. Desmoid tumor of the vulva associated with pregnancy. Arch Pathol Lab Med 121:512–514, 1997.

Brown JV, Stenchever MA. Cavernous lymphangioma of the vulva. Obstet Gynecol 73:877–879, 1989.

Busand B, Stray-Pedersen S, Iversen OH, Austad J. Blue rubber bleb nevus syndrome with manifestations in the vulva. Acta Obstet Gynecol Scand 72:310–313, 1993.

Colgan TJ, Dardick I, O'Connell G. Paraganglioma of the vulva. Int J Gynecol Pathol 10:203–208, 1991.

Cook CL, Sanfilippo JS, Verdi GD, Pietsch JB. Capillary hemangioma of the vagina and urethra in a child: response to short-term steroid therapy. Obstet Gynecol 73:883–884, 1989.

Haraoka M, Naito S, Kumazawa J. Clitoral involvement by neurofibromatosis: a case report and review of the literature. J Urol 139:95–96, 1988.

Huang HJ, Yamabe T, Tagawa H. A solitary neurilemmoma of the clitoris. Gynecol Oncol 15:103–110, 1983.

Johnson TL, Kennedy AW, Segal GH. Lymphangioma circumscriptum of the vulva: a report of two cases. J Reprod Med 36:808–812, 1991.

Lewis FM, Lewis-Jones MS, Toon PG, Rollason TP. Neurofibromatosis of the vulva. Br J Dermatol 127:540–541, 1992.

McNeely TBD. Angiokeratoma of the clitoris. Arch Pathol Lab Med 116:880–881, 1992.

Nielsen GP, Young RH. Fibromatosis of soft tissue type involving the female genital tract. Int J Gynecol Pathol 16:383–386, 1997.

Sonobe H, Ro JY, Ramos M, et al. Glomus tumor of the female external genitali: a report of two cases. Int J Gynecol Pathol 13:359–364, 1994.

Tjaden BL, Buscema J, Haller JA Jr, Rock JA. Vulvar congenital dysplastic angiopathy. Obstet Gynecol 75:553–554, 1990.

CHAPTER 2

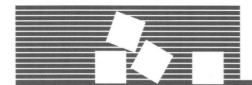

Malignant Tumors of the Vulva

SQUAMOUS CELL CARCINOMA AND ITS PRECURSORS

Vulvar Intraepithelial Neoplasia

Clinical Features

- Vulvar intraepithelial neoplasia (VIN), which refers to all preinvasive dysplastic squamous lesions, has almost doubled in incidence over the past several decades, with a striking decrease in the age of the affected patients, so that most of the latter are younger than 40 years of age.
- Risk factors for the most common types of VIN include human papillomavirus (HPV) and herpesvirus infection, smoking, human immunodeficiency virus (HIV) seropositivity, and sexual factors identical to those for cervical cancer (page 90).
- The typical presentation is a pruritic, burning, or asymptomatic, white, pink, red, or pigmented, maculopapular or plaquelike labial lesion that is multifocal in 50% to 80% of cases. Involved sites, in decreasing order of frequency, in one large study were labia minora, posterior forchette, labia majora, perianal skin, and periclitoral skin.
- The term *bowenoid papulosis* (BP) has been used to refer to usually multiple, red to brown papules occurring typically in young, often pregnant women that microscopically do not differ from typical VIN.
  - BP may spontaneously regress but is rarely associated with or progresses to invasive carcinoma.
  - Because BP has neither a predictable behavior nor a distinctive microscopic appearance, most authorities discourage use of the term, at least as a microscopic diagnosis.
- Between 50% and 65% of women with VIN, who are usually young and exhibit evidence of HPV infection, have similar synchronous or metachronous lesions in sites that may include the cervix, vagina, urethra, perineum, and anus ("lower genital tract neoplasia syndrome").
- About 50% of patients have a history or synchronous evidence of a sexually transmitted disease, most commonly condyloma acuminatum.

Pathologic Features

- VIN is characterized by various degrees of loss of normal maturation of the epidermis caused by the presence of keratinocytes with an increased nuclear to cytoplasmic ratio and various degrees of nuclear pleomorphism, hyperchromasia, chromatin clumping, multinucleation, individual cell keratinization, and mitotic activity. The affected epithelium may be thickened, and the skin appendages are commonly involved.
- Subtypes of VIN are basaloid (undifferentiated), warty (condylomatous), and well differentiated (simplex VIN). Basaloid and warty subtypes often occur together and may overlap in appearance.
- Basaloid VIN and warty VIN are usually encountered in young women, are commonly multifocal, are often associated with cervical intraepithelial neoplasia (CIN), have a strong association with HPV (usually HPV-16 or -33), occasionally regress, and are often not associated with an invasive component. When these types of VIN occasionally occur in older women, the same features pertain.
  - Basaloid VIN has a flat, sometimes keratotic surface and is composed of small, uniform basaloid cells with scanty cytoplasm, ill-defined cell membranes, large hyperchromatic nuclei, clumped chromatin, inapparent nucleoli, and numerous mitoses, with the appearance resembling typical CIN. Koilocytosis is less common and, if present, less striking than in warty VIN.
  - Warty VIN is typically acanthotic with a spiky or warty surface and large cells with copious eosinophilic cytoplasm, well-defined membranes, evidence of keratinization (dyskeratosis, corps ronds), marked nuclear pleomorphism, multinucleation, coarsely clumped chromatin, and numerous mitoses. There is superficial maturation, koilocytosis, and parakeratosis or hyperkeratosis. Wide rete pegs extend into the stroma.
- Well-differentiated VIN usually occurs in postmenopausal women, is usually unifocal, is typically HPV negative, and is commonly associated with lichen sclerosus (page 7) and with a prior, synchronous, or subsequent invasive squamous cell carcinoma of the vulva.

- Large basal keratinocytes have abundant eosinophilic cytoplasm, abnormal nuclei, and prominent nucleoli. The bases of the rete may contain keratin pearls. In the superficial layers, atypia in minimal and maturation is maintained. Elongated branching rete ridges are common.
  - p53 immunostaining, present in most cases, occurs in 20% to 100% of the basal cells and one third or more of the epithelial thickness. Positive p53 staining may be helpful in diagnosis.
- Basaloid and warty VIN is graded as I when only the lower third of the epithelium is involved, II when the process involves the lower two thirds of the epithelium, and III when more than two thirds of the epithelium (excluding the keratin layer) is involved. Most cases are VIN III. Well-differentiated VIN is considered VIN III. VIN I is rare if flat condylomas (which are considered equivalent to VIN I by some physicians) are excluded.
- Foci of unsuspected invasion can occur in up to 20% of women with VIN. Tangential sectioning of VIN and appendiceal involvement by VIN is common and should not be confused with invasion. Evidence of a residual appendage, the well-circumscribed border of the focus, and a lack of a desmoplastic stromal response facilitate the diagnosis. Invasive foci in cases of basaloid VIN often exhibit cytoplasm maturation.

Differential Diagnosis

- Condylomas (compared with warty VIN) (page 1), condylomas with pseudobowenoid change (page 1), condylomas with podophyllin effect (page 1).
- Inflammatory or reactive atypia. Prominent inflammation, spongiosis, lack of mitotic activity, and prominent nucleoli in the keratinocytes favor a reactive lesion over VIN.
- Multinucleated epithelial atypia. This is a common change occurring in vulvar and extravulvar skin characterized by multinucleation of keratinocytes. LeBoit has concluded that the change is an expression of a defect in nuclear division that occurs in persistently rubbed skin.
- Paget's disease and radial growth of malignant melanoma. In both disorders, the malignant cells are usually individually disposed and surrounded by benign keratinocytes. Glands may be seen in Paget's disease. Spe-

cial stains demonstrate mucin, carcinoembryonic antigen (CEA), and cytokeratin 7 (CK7) in Paget's cells, and S-100 protein and HMB-45 in melanoma cells.

Behavior

- Between 35% and 50% cases of VIN recur after local treatment, usually within the first 4 postoperative years. Recurrence is more common with multiple lesions, positive resection margins, and laser compared with surgical treatment.
- Progression to invasive carcinoma occurs in 4% to 7% of patients after local treatment. In contrast, invasive tumor developed in 7 (87.5%) of 8 untreated women with VIN over an 8-year period in one study. Invasion is more likely to occur in postmenopausal women and in immunocompromised (e.g., HIV-positive) patients.
- Spontaneous regression of VIN may occur, particularly in young, postpartum women.

References

Chafe W, Richards A, Morgan L, Wilkinson EJ. Unrecognized invasive carcinoma in vulvar intraepithelial neoplasia (VIN). Gynecol Oncol 31:154–165, 1988.
Crum CP, McLachlin CM, Tate JE, Mutter GL. Pathobiology of vulvar squamous neoplasia. Curr Opin Obstet Gynecol 9:63–69, 1997.
Haefner HK, Tate JE, McLachlin CM, Crum CP. Vulvar intraepithelial neoplasia: age, morphological phenotype, papillomavirus DNA, and coexisting invasive carcinoma. Hum Pathol 26:147–154, 1995.
Herod JJO, Shafi MI, Rollason TP, et al. Vulvar intraepithelial neoplasia: long term follow up of treated and untreated women. Br J Obstet Gynaecol 103:446–452, 1996.
Hording U, Daugaard S, Junge J, Lundvall F. Human papillomaviruses and multifocal genital neoplasia. Int J Gynecol Pathol 15:230–234, 1996.
Jones RW, Rowan DM. Vulvar intraepithelial neoplasia III: a clinical study of the outcome in 113 cases with relation to the later development of invasive vulvar carcinoma. Obstet Gynecol 84:741–745, 1994.
Kurman RJ, Toki T, Schiffman MH. Basaloid and warty carcinomas of the vulva: distinctive types of squamous cell carcinoma frequently associated with human papillomaviruses. Am J Surg Pathol 17:133–145, 1993.
LeBoit PE. Multinucleated atypia [Letter]. Am J Surg Pathol 20:507, 1996.
McLaughlin CM, Mutter GL, Crum CP. Multinucleated atypia of the vulva: report of a distinct entity not associated with human papillomavirus. Am J Surg Pathol 18:1233–1239, 1994.
Yang B, Hart WR, Vulvar intraepithelial neoplasia of the simplex type: a clinicopathologic study including analysis of HPV and p53 expression. Am J Surg Pathol (in press).

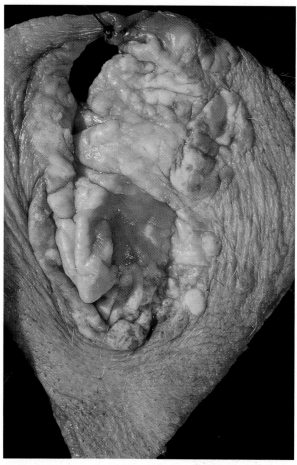

Figure 2–1. Vulvar intraepithelial neoplasia grade III. White, focally erythematous, plaque-like, and polypoid lesions are seen.

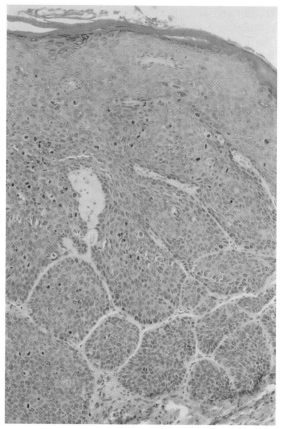

Figure 2–2. Vulvar intraepithelial neoplasia grade III, basaloid type. There is acanthosis and rounded projections into the dermis, a finding that should not be misinterpreted as invasion.

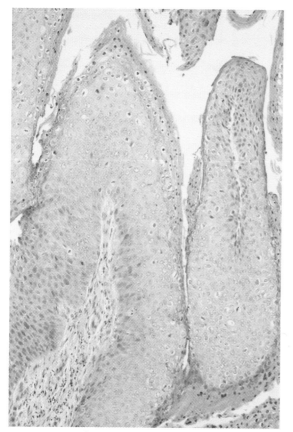

Figure 2–3. Vulvar intraepithelial neoplasia grade III, warty type.

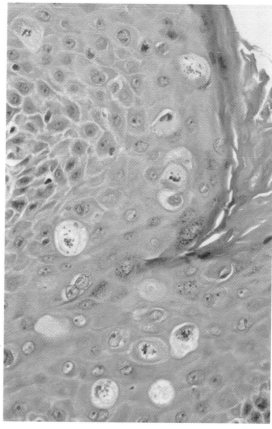

Figure 2–5. Pseudobowenoid change, a potential mimic of vulvar intra-epithelial neoplasia.

Figure 2–4. Vulvar intraepithelial neoplasia grade III, well-differentiated (simplex) type.

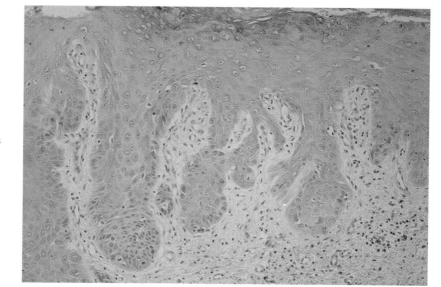

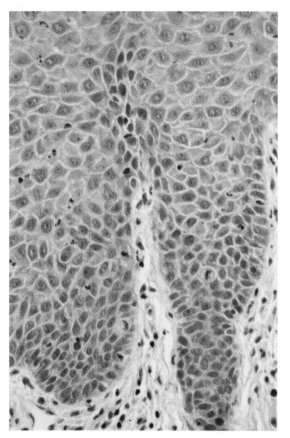

Figure 2–6. Reactive atypia. There is lack of maturation but no significant atypia, and mitotic figures are confined to the lower layers. Notice the spongiosis and sprinkling of stromal and intraepithelial inflammatory cells.

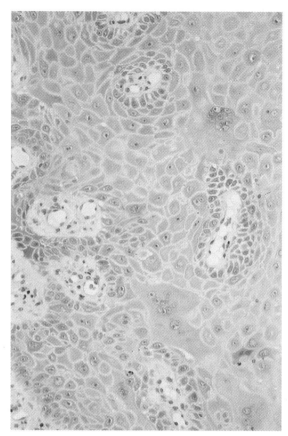

Figure 2–7. Multinucleated epithelial atypia.

Invasive Squamous Cell Carcinoma of Usual Type

Clinical Features

■ Invasive squamous cell carcinomas (ISCCs) account for about 90% of all vulvar cancers and about 5% of gynecologic cancers. The incidence of ISCCs, unlike VIN, has not increased over the past 20 years.

■ The average age (seventh to eighth decades of life) has remained unchanged in most studies. One study, however, found an increase of ISCCs in women under 50 years of age; most tumors arose in a field of warty or basaloid VIN. Exceptionally rare tumors arise in women younger than 30 years of age, especially those who are immunosuppressed.

■ Patients usually present with a vulvar or groin mass, which may be pruritic or painful or be associated with bleeding. Because patient and physician delays are common, 30% to 40% of vulvar ISCCs are not treated until they are stage III or IV (Table 2–1).

■ Two pathogenetic pathways appear to exist for vulvar ISCC:

　• One, usually occurring in younger women (38% younger than 55 years) and leading to warty (WISCC) or basaloid ISCC (BISCC), is usually associated with the presence of HPV (including a history of genital warts), warty and basaloid VIN, smoking, cervical cancer risk factors, and a high risk of in situ or ISCC of the cervix or, less commonly, the vagina. BISCCs and WISCCs accounted for 28% and 7% of vulvar ISCCS, respectively, in one series (Kurman and coworkers).

Table 2–1
FIGO STAGING OF CARCINOMA OF THE VULVA

Stage 0 Tis	Carcinoma in situ; intraepithelial carcinoma
Stage I T1 N0 M0	Tumor confined to the vulva and/or perineum, ≤2 cm in greatest dimension
Ia*	Depth of invasion not exceeding 1 mm
Stage II T2 N0 M0	Tumor confined to the vulva and/or perineum, >2 cm in greatest dimension
Stage III T3 N0 M0 T3 N1 M0 T1 N1 M0 T2 N1 M0	Tumor of any size with 1. Adjacent spread to the lower urethra, and/or vagina, and/or the anus (T3) and/or 2. Unilateral regional lymph node metastasis (N1)
Stage IVa T1 N2 M0 T2 N2 M0 T3 N2 M0 T4 Any N M0	Tumor invades any of the following: upper urethra, bladder mucosa, rectal mucosa, pelvic bone (T4) and/or bilateral regional lymph node metastasis (N2)
Stage IVb Any T Any N M1	Any distant metastasis including pelvic lymph nodes

* Proposed modification by International Society for the Study of Vulvar Diseases. Lymphatic invasion does not increase the stage.

- The other pathway, usually in older women (17% younger than 55 years), leading to keratinizing ISCC (KISCC), is usually unrelated to HPV infection but associated with lichen sclerosus, squamous cell hyperplasia, and well-differentiated VIN, alone or in combination. KISCCs accounted for 65% of vulvar ISCCs in the Kurman series.
- The two pathways may sometimes act in synchrony: 38% of lichen sclerosus–associated ISCCs were HPV positive in one study. Some ISCCs may be related to other causes, such as an association with chronic vulvar granulomatous diseases.

Pathologic Features

- Clinical and gross examination reveals a raised, white, sometimes warty, sometimes ulcerated mass that, in descending order of frequency, involves the labia majora, the labia minora, the perineal body, and the posterior fourchette, and the clitoris. About 10% are multifocal.
- The three main histologic subtypes of ISCC are KISCCs, BISCCs, and WISCCs. When mixtures of the subtypes occur, classification is by the predominant type.
- KISCCs resemble typical ISCCs in other sites, with various degrees of squamous maturation and keratin formation and an absence of koilocytosis. There is usually adjacent lichen sclerosus, squamous hyperplasia, well-differentiated VIN, or combinations thereof.
- The cells of BISCCs, which resemble basaloid VIN (page 22), typically grow in bands, sheets, or nests within a desmoplastic stroma. Focal cytoplasmic maturation and keratinization can occur, but there is an abrupt transition between the latter and the basaloid cells. Contiguous basaloid or warty VIN is present in about 80% of cases.
- WISCCs resemble warty VIN except for obvious invasion as irregular jagged nests, often with prominent keratinization. The koilocytotic tumor cells have pleomorphic to bizarre, often multiple nuclei with irregular contours that vary from hyperchromatic and shrunken (raisin-like) to those with clumped or smudged chromatin. Contiguous basaloid or warty VIN is present in about 80% of cases.
- There is no widely accepted grading system for vulvar ISCCs.
  - Kurman and colleagues do not grade BISCCs or WISCCs but grade KISCCs as well-differentiated (i.e., discrete nests with central keratinization and cells with low-grade nuclear features), poorly differentiated (i.e., diffuse stromal infiltration as small nests and cords, little or no keratinization, and high-grade nuclear features), and moderately differentiated (i.e., features intermediate between the well and poorly differentiated tumors).
  - The Gynecology Oncology Group (GOG) grading scheme for KISCCs is based on the proportion of the tumor that is undifferentiated (i.e., small cells with scanty cytoplasm infiltrating as small nests or cords): grade 1, no undifferentiated cells (UC); grade 2, 1% to 30% UC; grade 3, 31% to 50% UC; grade 4, more than 50% UC.
- Other definite or potential prognostic features of the primary tumor other than tumor diameter, subtype, and grade to note in the pathology report include pattern of invasion (pushing versus "spray"), intensity of mononuclear inflammatory infiltrate, a fibromyxoid stromal response, and lymphatic invasion.

Differential Diagnosis

- Amelanotic malignant melanoma (compared with poorly differentiated KISCC). The presence of a junctional component, keratinization, and immunoreactivity for S-100 and HMB-45 facilitate the diagnosis of melanoma.
- Epithelioid sarcoma (compared with poorly differentiated KISCC). The deep location, absence of VIN, zonal necrosis, absence of keratinization, presence of rhabdoid cells in some cases, and immunoreactivity for mesenchymal antigens facilitate the diagnosis of epithelioid sarcoma. This sarcoma can be cytokeratin positive.
- Basal cell carcinoma (compared with BISCC). Features favoring basal cell carcinoma include a lobular, well-circumscribed contour, peripheral palisading, and an absence of VIN.
- Metastatic small cell carcinoma and Merkel cell tumor (compared with BISCC). These tumors tend to have a highly infiltrative pattern (often with single cell invasion), smaller cells with scanty cytoplasm, and immunohistochemical evidence of neuroendocrine differentiation.
- Verrucous carcinoma (compared with WISCCs). Differential features indicating verrucous carcinoma include absent or minimal cytologic atypia, absence of koilocytosis, and a well-circumscribed, deep border formed by rounded bulbous masses.

Behavior and Prognostic Factors

■ The tumors can spread directly to adjacent structures (vagina, urethra, anus), through lymphatics to lymph nodes, and rarely by hematogenous spread. Many of the prognostic factors related to the primary tumor affect prognosis by increasing the risk of nodal spread.

■ The inguinofemoral nodes are involved in about 30% to 40% of cases; bilateral involvement is present in about one third of these. The pelvic lymph nodes are involved in about 5% of cases overall and in about 25% of cases in which the inguinofemoral nodes are involved. The pelvic nodes are rarely involved in the absence of inguinal node involvement.

■ Clinical factors that have adverse prognostic significance include increasing stage (see Table 2–1) with 5-year survival rates of 85% to 98%, 60% to 85%, 40% to 74%, and 10% to 30% for stages I through IV, respectively; older age; smoking; and "suspicious," fixed, or ulcerated groin nodes.

■ The most important adverse prognostic features of the primary tumor are increasing tumor diameter, increasing depth of invasion, increasing grade, and lymphovascular space invasion.

• Tumors invading 1 mm or less (measured from point of origin of invasive cells, or if this is not possibile, from the most superficial dermal papilla adjacent to tumor's deepest focus of invasion) are stage Ia (Table 2–1) and have a negligible risk of nodal spread.

• Tumors invading to a depth of 1.1 to 5 mm have a risk of nodal metastases of 10% to 20%.

■ Other features that are of less certain prognostic significance are histologic type, infiltrative (spray) compared with a pushing pattern, intensity of mononuclear inflammatory infiltrate, a fibromyxoid stromal response, and p53 expression.

■ Recurrences develop in about 50% of patients with positive inguinofemoral nodes; these women have a 40% 5-year survival, compared with 85% for those with negative nodes. Involvement of three or more inguinofemoral nodes, bilateral nodes, extranodal tissue, or pelvic nodes result in an even worse prognosis.

■ The site of recurrence was the only significant predictor of survival in one study (Piura and colleagues). Recurrences confined to the vulva were associated with a 62% survival, whereas the corresponding figure for tumors associated with extravulvar recurrence was 12%.

References

Ambros RA, Malfetano JH, Mihm MC Jr. Cinicopathologic features of vulvar squamous cell carcinomas exhibiting prominent fibromyxoid stromal response. Int J Gynecol Pathol 15:137–145, 1996.

Ansink AC, Krul MRL, De Weger RA, et al. Human papillomavirus, lichen sclerosus, and squamous cell carcinoma of the vulva: detection and prognostic signficance. Gynecol Oncol 52:180–184, 1994.

Carter J, Carlson J, Fowler J, et al. Invasive vulvar tumors in young women—a disease of the immunosuppressed? Gynecol Oncol 51:307–310, 1993.

Crum CP, McLachlin CM, Tate JE, Mutter GL. Pathobiology of vulvar squamous neoplasia. Curr Opin Obstet Gynecol 9:63–69, 1997.

Drew PA, Al-Abbadi MA, Orlando CA, et al. Prognostic factors in carcinoma of the vulva: a clinicopathologic and DNA flow cytometric study. Int J Gynecol Pathol 15:235–241, 1996.

Herod JJO, Shafi MI, Rollason TP, et al. Vulvar intraepithelial neoplasia with superficially invasive carcinoma of the vulva. Br J Obstet Gynaecol 103:453–456, 1996.

Homesley HD, Bundy BN, Sedlis A, et al. Assessment of current International Federation of Gynecology and Obstetrics staging of vulvar carcinoma relative to prognostic factors for survival (a Gynecologic Oncology Group study). Am J Obstet Gynecol 164:997–1004, 1991.

Homesley HD, Bundy BN, Sedlis A, et al. Prognostic factors for groin node metastasis in squamous cell carcinoma of the vulva (a Gynecologic Oncology Group study). Gynecol Oncol 49:279–283, 1993.

Hording U, Daugaard S, Junge J, Lundvall F. Human papillomaviruses and multifocal genital neoplasia. Int J Gynecol Pathol 15:230–234, 1996.

Jones RW, Baranyai J, Stables S. Trends in squamous cell carcinoma of the vulva: the influence of vulvar intraepithelial neoplasia. Obstet Gynecol 90:448–452, 1997.

Kirschner CV, Yordan EL, De Geest K, Wilbanks GD. Smoking, obesity, and survival in squamous cell carcinoma of the vulva. Gynecol Oncol 56:79–84, 1995.

Kurman RJ, Toki T, Schiffman MH. Basaloid and warty carcinomas of the vulva: distinctive types of squamous cell carcinoma frequently associated with human papillomaviruses. Am J Surg Pathol 17:133–145, 1993.

Leibowitch M, Neill S, Pelisse M, Moyal-Baracco M. The epithelial changes associated wtih squamous cell carcinoma of the vulva: a review of the clinical, histological and viral findings in 78 women. Br J Obstet Gynaecol 97:1135–1139, 1990.

Pinto AP, Signorello L, Crum CP, et al. Prognostic factors in invasive squamous cell carcinoma of the vulva: potential significance of histologic type [Abstract]. Mod Pathol 11:111A, 1998.

Piura B, Masotina A, Murdoch J, et al. Recurrent squamous cell carcinoma of the vulva: a study of 73 cases. Gynecol Oncol 48:189–195, 1993.

Price JH, Heath AB, Sunter JP, et al. Inflammmatory cell infiltration and survival in squamous cell carcinoma of the vulva. Br J Obstet Gynaecol 95:808–813, 1988.

Rosen C, Malmstrom H. Invasive cancer of the vulva. Gynecol Oncol 65:213–217, 1997.

Sedlis A, Homesley H, Bundy BN, et al. Positive groin nodes in superficial squamous cell vulvar cancer: a Gynecologic Group study. Am J Obstet Gynecol 156:1159–1164, 1987.

Trimble CL, Hildesheim A, Brinton LA, et al. Heterogeneous etiology of squamous carcinoma of the vulva. Obstet Gynecol 87:59–64, 1996.

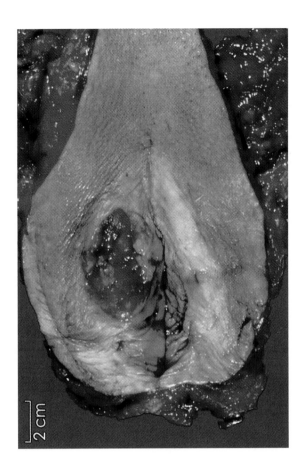

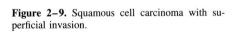

Figure 2–8. Invasive squamous cell carcinoma (*left*) associated with lichen sclerosus (*bottom left and right*).

Figure 2–9. Squamous cell carcinoma with superficial invasion.

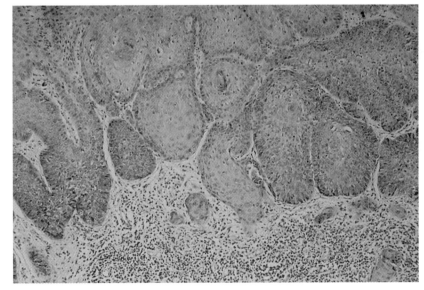

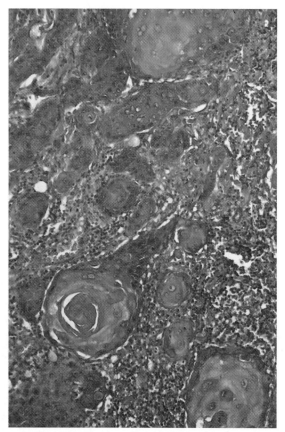

Figure 2–10. Invasive keratinizing squamous cell carcinoma.

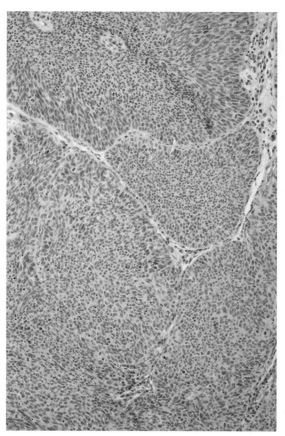

Figure 2–11. Invasive squamous cell carcinoma, basaloid type.

Verrucous Carcinoma

- Verrucous carcinomas (VCs) are uncommon, highly differentiated squamous cell carcinomas. Many of the lesions in the older literature referred to as *giant condylomas* of *Buschke-Löwenstein* would be considered warty carcinomas or VCs by current criteria.
- VCs typically occur in women in the late reproductive and postmenopausal age groups who present with pain, pruritis, and a large, gray-white, fungating mass on the labia majora.
- A delay in diagnosis may occur if previous biopsies of the tumor are misdiagnosed as squamous papilloma or condyloma. In the largest series, two thirds of the tumors were stage II or higher.
- The tumors have a papillary architecture with prominent acanthosis, hyperkeratosis, and a deep pushing invasive border composed of broad bulbous pegs. Koilocytosis is usually absent.
- The neoplastic squamous cells have abundant eosinophilic cytoplasm and absent to mild nuclear atypia.

Mitoses, if present, are confined to the basal layers. HPV has been identified in some tumors.

- VCs should be distinguished from condyloma (page 1) and warty carcinoma (page 27). Conventional squamous cell carcinomas with a verrucoid architecture can be distinguished from VCs by the presence of more than mild nuclear atypia and an infiltrative border.
- VCs may invade local structures, and tumors presenting at an advanced stage may occasionally be fatal. However, the tumors rarely metastasize. Metastases should prompt thorough sampling of the primary tumor to exclude a component of conventional invasive squamous cell carcinoma that rarely may arise in an otherwise typical VC.

References

Japaze H, Van Dinh T, Woodruff JD. Verrucous carcinoma of the vulva: study of 24 cases. Obstet Gynecol 60:462–466, 1982.

Pilotti S, Donghi R, D'Amato L, et al. HPV detection and p53 alteration in squamous cell verrucous malignancies of the lower genital tract. Diagn Mol Pathol 2:248–256, 1993.

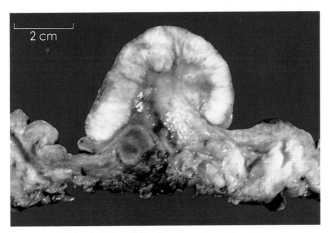

Figure 2–12. Sectioned surface of a verrucous carcinoma.

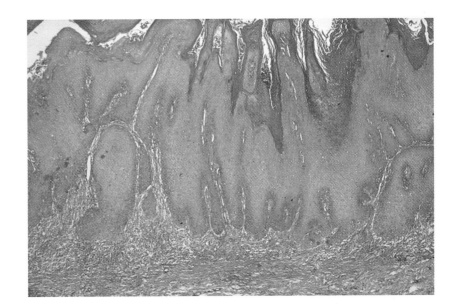

Figure 2–13. Verrucous carcinoma.

Rare Variants of Squamous Cell Carcinoma

- Three vulvar sarcomatoid ISSCs and one ISCC with numerous giant cells have been reported, all in postmenopausal women; two of the former and the latter were ultimately fatal. Merging of the spindle cells and giant cells with typical ISCC and their focal immunoreactivity for cytokeratin facilitate the diagnosis.
- Occasional vulvar ISCCs are acantholytic with prominent spaces within the tumor that can be confused with glands (i.e., adenoid squamous cell carcinoma) or vascular spaces (i.e., pseudoangiosarcomatous carcinoma).
- A unique vulvar tumor (considered a carcinosarcoma) in a 54-year-old woman was initially composed almost exclusively of osteosarcoma and a single microscopic focus of ISCC. Subsequent recurrences consisted of ISCC and spindle cell sarcoma (first, third, and fourth recurrences) and ISCC and osteosarcoma (second recurrence).
- One lymphoepithelioma-like carcinoma has been described involving the perineum of a 47-year-old woman who was clinically free of disease 9 months after vulvectomy. The tumor was Epstein-Barr virus negative.

References

Axelsen SM, Stamp IM. Lymphoepithelioma-like carcinoma of the vulvar region. Histopathology 27:281–283, 1995.

Lasser A, Cornog JL, Morris JM. Adenoid squamous cell carcinoma of the vulva. Cancer 33:224–227, 1974.

Parham DM, Morton K, Robertson AJ, Philip WDP. The changing phenotypic appearance of a malignant vulval neoplasm containing both carcinomatous and sarcomatous elements. Histopathology 19: 263–268, 1991.

Pitt MA, Morphopoulos G, Wells S, Bisset DL. Pseudoangiosarcomatous carcinoma of the genitourinary tract. J Clin Pathol 48:1059–1061, 1995.

Santeusanio G, Schiaroli S, Anemona L, et al. Carcinoma of the vulva with sarcomatoid features: a case report with immunohistochemical study. Gynecol Oncol 40:160–163, 1991.

Wilkinson EJ, Croker BP, Friedrich EG Jr, Franzini DA. Two distinct pathologic types of giant cell carcinoma of the vulva: a report of two cases. J Reprod Med 33:519–522, 1988.

PAGET'S DISEASE

Clinical Features

■ Paget's disease (PD), which accounts for about 1% of vulvar cancers, occurs in the late reproductive and postmenopausal age groups; the median age and mean ages in most series are in the seventh decade. PD may be present for years before diagnosis, in some cases because of patient-related delay and in other cases related to physician failure to perform a biopsy promptly.

■ The usual clinical presentation is that of pruritic or burning, eczematoid, erythematous, weeping patches interspersed with white (hyperkeratotic) or ulcerated areas. Early lesions are usually confined to the labia, but long-standing lesions may involve the labia, mons, clitoris, urethra, perianal area, and medial aspect of the thighs.

■ About 30% of patients have a synchronous or metachronous internal carcinoma, most commonly of the breast or genitourinary system (uterine cervix, urinary bladder). With rare exceptions, these tumors are unrelated to the vulvar PD.

Histogenesis

■ About 95% of cases of vulvar PD begin as a primary cutaneous in situ carcinoma, probably originating from an intraepidermal stem cell or the cells of the poral portion of the sweat ducts. Associated in situ involvement of skin appendages reflects pagetoid spread of the tumor cells or multifocal PD, not an underlying sweat gland carcinoma.

■ Rare cases (<5%) of vulvar PD represent secondary vulvar involvement by a regional internal cancer, such as those arising in the urinary bladder or rectum. A primary rectal adenocarcinoma should be excluded in cases of vulvar PD associated with prominent perianal PD.

Microscopic Features

■ Large, malignant epithelial cells are disposed singly, in clusters, and occasionally as glands within the epidermis. The concentration of tumor cells is usually greatest in the basal layer, but in most cases, all epidermal layers are involved. The pilosebaceous units and the poral and dermal portions of sweat ducts are involved in almost all cases.

■ The typical Paget's cell contains a vesicular nucleus, a prominent nucleolus, and abundant pale, amphophilic cytoplasm. In some cases, signet-ring cells with abundant cytoplasmic mucin are present, usually admixed with the typical cells. In one study, intraepidermal signet-ring cells were more common in cases associated with invasion.

■ The disease is typically much more extensive and more multifocal than appreciable on clinical or gross examination; positive resection margins are therefore a frequent finding.

■ The tumor cells typically contain mucin demonstrable with mucin stains, although the mucin may be focal and difficult to find in a small biopsy specimen.

■ Paget cells are diffusely and strongly immunoreactive for CK7; CK7 is considered the marker of choice for Paget's disease in several studies.
  • Paget's cells are also usually immunoreactive for CEA, CAM 5.2, and gross cystic disease fluid protein (GCDFP), but they are typically nonreactive for CK20.
  • Goldblum and Hart found that the rare cases of vulvar PD secondary to spread from an internal cancer will have the immunoprofile of the primary tumor rather than the typical CK7$^+$/CK20$^-$/GCDFP$^+$ immunoprofile of usual vulvar PD. Vulvar PD with a CK20$^+$/GCDFP$^-$ phenotype should therefore suggest spread from an associated internal cancer.

■ In about 30% of cases, dermal invasion (that is usually unsuspected clinically) is found microscopically. The detection of rare invasive cells in the superficial dermis can be facilitated by staining for CK 7.

■ The depth of invasion in millimeters (measured from the basement membrane) and the presence or absence of lymphatic invasion should be included in the pathology report.

■ Invasion should be differentiated from rare cases of noninvasive vulvar PD associated with marked and complex epidermal hyperplasia with deep invaginations into the reticular dermis (see Billings and Roth).

■ Brainard and Hart found proliferative squamous lesions in 33% of cases of vulvar Paget's disease, which they categorized as squamous cell hyperplasia (SCH) not otherwise specified, fibroepithelioma-like SCH, and papillomatous SCH. Single cases of Bowenoid carcinoma in situ and invasive squamous cell carcinoma were also found.

Differential Diagnosis

■ Pagetoid VIN is indicated by single-cell keratinization, intercellular bridges, cytoplasmic keratohyaline granules, association with typical VIN, absence of cytoplasmic mucin, and nonreactivity for CEA, cytokeratin 7 (CK7), and GCDFP.

■ Superficial spreading malignant melanoma (SSMM). In contrast to Paget cells, the cells of SSMM lack mucin and are immunoreactive for S-100 and HMB-45 but not CK7. Cytoplasmic melanin can occur in both SSMM and Paget's cells and is therefore not a differential feature.

- Rarer lesions in the differential (see Kohler et al.) include pagetoid Spitz nevus, clear cells of Toker, pagetoid dyskeratosis, clear cell papulosis, epidermal involvement by sebaceous carcinoma, Merkel cell carcinoma, eccrine porocarcinoma, cutaneous T-cell lymphoma, and lesions of Langerhans' cells (histiocytosis X, Langerhans' cell microabscesses).

Behavior

- Because of the high frequency of incomplete excision, intraepidermal recurrence is common. In one review, recurrences occurred in 34% of patients at a median postoperative interval of 3 years. The frequency of recurrence, however, correlates poorly with resection margin status.
- Some patients have multiple recurrences, often over a period of many years. Rarely, there is progression to invasive PD during the follow-up period.
- Minimal dermal invasion (<1 mm), except in very rare cases, does not appear to affect prognosis, whereas tumors with deeper invasion are associated with a risk of metastases to inguinal lymph nodes and other sites and a potentially fatal outcome.

References

Battle OE, Page DL, Johnson JE. Cytokeratins, CEA, and mucin histochemistry in the diagnosis and characterization of extramammary Paget's disease. Am J Clin Pathol 108:6–12, 1997.

Billings SD, Roth LM. Pseudoinvasive, nodular extramammary Paget's disease of the vulva. Arch Pathol Lab Med 122:471–474, 1998.

Brainard JA, Hart WR. Proliferative squamous cell lesions in anogenital Paget's disease [Abstract]. Mod Pathol 12:113A, 1999.

Crawford D, Nimmo M, Clement PB, et al. Vulvar Paget's disease: prognostic factors. Int J Gynecol Pathol 18:351–359, 1999.

Fanning J, Lambert L, Hale TM, et al. Paget's disease of the vulva: prevalence of associated vulvar adenocarcinoma, invasive Paget's disease, and recurrence after surgical excision. Am J Obstet Gynecol 180:24–27, 1999.

Goldblum JR, Hart WR. Vulvar Paget's disease: a clinicopathologic and immunohistochemical study of 19 cases. Am J Surg Pathol 21:1178–1187, 1997.

Gunn RA, Gallagher HS. Vulvar Paget's disease: a topographic study. Cancer 46:590–594, 1980.

Kohler S, Rouse RV, Smoller BR. The differential diagnosis of Pagetoid cells in the epidermis. Mod Pathol 11:79–82, 1998.

Scheistroen M, Trope C, Kaern J, et al. DNA ploidy and expression of p53 and C-erb-2 in extramammary Paget's disease of the vulva. Gynecol Oncol 64:88–92, 1997.

Smith KJ, Corvette D, Lupton GP, Skelton HG. Cytokeratin 7 staining in mammary and extramammary Paget's disease. Mod Pathol 10:1069–1074, 1997.

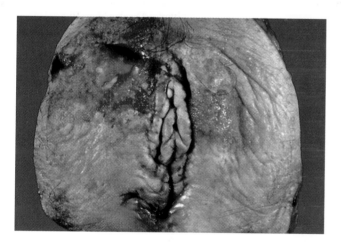

Figure 2–14. Paget's disease with extensive involvement of the vulva.

Figure 2–15. Paget's disease.

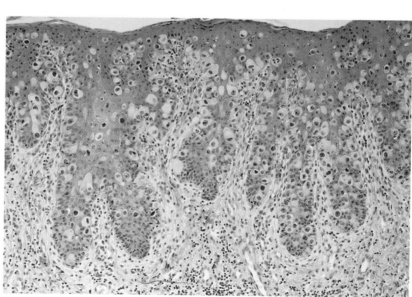

CARCINOMA OF BARTHOLIN'S GLAND

■ These tumors, which account for less than 5% of vulvar carcinomas, occur in the reproductive and postmenopausal age groups; the median age in the largest series was 50 years. HPV has been found in Bartholin's gland carcinomas of squamous and transitional type.

■ Criteria proposed by Chamlian and Taylor for the diagnosis are
  • Areas of transition occur between the normal gland and tumor.
  • The tumor involves the area of Bartholin's gland, is histologically compatible with Bartholin's origin, and there is no evidence of a primary tumor elsewhere.

■ The presentation may include a mass, pain, pruritus, bleeding, discharge, or combinations thereof. In as many as 50% of patients, the lesion is initially misdiagnosed as a Bartholin's gland cyst or abscess, resulting in diagnostic delay. In the most recent large series, the International Federation of Gynecology and Obstetrics (FIGO) stages were I in 25%, II in 42%, III in 28%, and IV in 5%.

■ On microscopic examination, the approximate frequencies of the most frequent histologic subtypes are squamous cell carcinoma, 40%; adenocarcinoma not otherwise specified, 25%; and adenoid cystic carcinoma (ACC), 12%; the rest are composed of adenosquamous carcinoma, transitional cell carcinoma, and undifferentiated carcinoma, including one example of a small cell neuroendocrine carcinoma.

■ In the most recent large series, about 40% of patients had nodal spread. Distant metastases (e.g., lungs, bone) may also occur, particularly in ACCs.

■ In the study just indicated, the 5-year survival rate (after wide local excision, inguinal lymphadenectomy, and in some cases, irradiation) was 84% for all histologic subtypes. Patients with ACCs may have multiple local recurrences and distant metastases and survive for many years. The 10-year survival rate for these patients in one review was 60%.

References

Chamlian DL, Taylor HB. Primary carcinoma of Bartholin's gland: a report of 24 patients. Obstet Gynecol 39:489–494, 1972.

Copeland LJ, Sneige N, Gershenson DM, et al. Adenoid cystic carcinoma of Bartholin gland. Obstet Gynecol 67:115–120, 1986.

Copeland LJ, Sneige N, Gershenson DM, et al. Bartholin gland carcinoma. Obstet Gynecol 67:794–801, 1986.

Felix JC, Cote RJ, Kramer EEW, et al. Carcinoma of Bartholin's gland: histogenesis and the etiological role of humanpapillomavirus. Am J Pathol 142:925–933, 1993.

Flam F, Larson B. Adenoid cystic carcinoma of Bartholin's gland: a review of the literature and report of a patient with widespread metastases to bone. Int J Gynecol Cancer 7:458–460, 1997.

Jones MA, Mann EW, Caldwell CL, et al. Small cell neuroendocrine carcinoma of Bartholin's gland. Am J Clin Pathol 94:439–442, 1990.

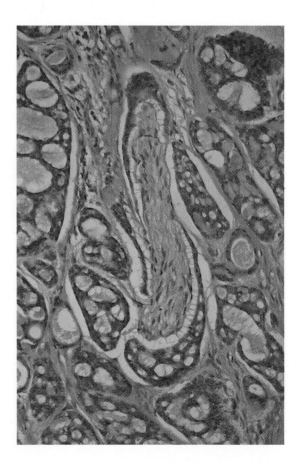

Figure 2–16. Adenoid cystic carcinoma of Bartholin's gland. Notice the perineural invasion.

BASAL CELL CARCINOMA

- Basal cell carcinomas (BCCs) account for only 2% to 3% of vulvar carcinomas. They typically occur in elderly women; the mean age in the largest series was 76 years. About one third of women in one series had synchronous or metachronous extravulvar BCCs.
- The typical presentation is that of a localized irritation, soreness, or pruritis and a nodular, polypoid, ulcerated, pigmented or nonpigmented lesion on the labia majora.
- The histologic features are identical to those of typical cutaneous BCCs and can include those of superficial, solid, and adenoid types. No morphic BCCs were encountered in the largest series.

- Vulvar BCCs are usually cured by wide local excision. Occasional tumors have recurred locally, and rare tumors have metastasized to inguinal or other lymph nodes. Only rarely have tumors been fatal.

References

Benedet JL, Miller DM, Ehlen TG, Bertrand MA. Basal cell carcinoma of the vulva: clinical features and treatment results in 28 patients. Obstet Gynecol 90:765–768, 1997.

Feakins RM, Lowe DG. Basal cell carcinoma of the vulva: a clinicopathologic study of 45 cases. Int J Gynecol Pathol 16:319–324, 1997.

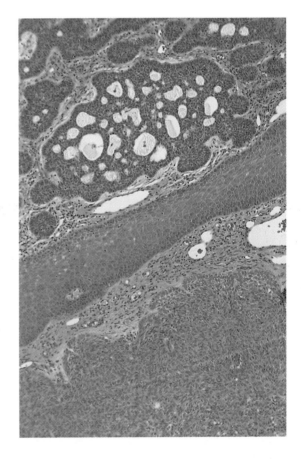

Figure 2–17. Basal cell carcinoma has solid (*bottom*) and adenoidal (*top*) patterns.

OTHER CARCINOMAS

Adenocarcinoma of Mammary Type

■ Rare primary vulvar adenocarcinomas resemble primary carcinomas of the breast; such tumors are believed to arise from ectopic breast tissue or mammary-like glands in this site (page 13).

■ The tumors usually arise in women in the late reproductive and postmenopasual age groups and often pursue a malignant clinical course, including inguinal lymph node involvement.

■ All tumors have resembled mammary ductal carcinomas, including immunoreactivity for estrogen and progesterone receptors and gross cystic disease fluid protein.

■ The differential diagnosis is with primary vulvar carcinomas of apocrine origin, some of which resemble mammary carcinomas, and with metastatic carcinoma from the breast. A negative history of a primary breast carcinoma and demonstration of origin from ectopic breast tissue facilitate the diagnosis. Steroid receptor immunoreactivity favors a breast-type carcinoma over one of cutaneous adnexal origin.

References

Carcangiu ML. Letters to the case. Pathol Res Pract 188:211–214, 1992.

Levin M, Pakarakas RM, Chang HA, et al. Primary breast carcinoma of the vulva: a case report of review of the literature. Gynecol Oncol 56: 448–451, 1995.

van der Putte SCJ, van Gorp LHM. Adenocarcinoma of the mammary-like glands of the vulva: a concept unifying sweat gland carcinoma of the vulva, carcinoma of the supernumerary mammary glands and extramammary Paget's disease. J Cutan Pathol 21:157–163, 1994.

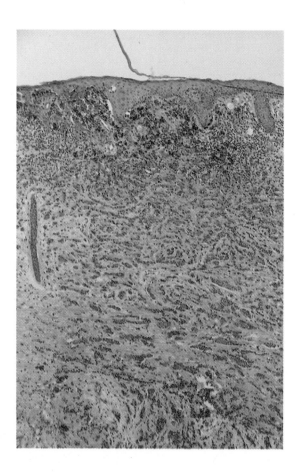

Figure 2–18. Mammary-type adenocarcinoma arising in the vulva.

Adenocarcinomas of Skin Appendage Origin

- Vulvar adenocarcinomas of suspected or proven eccrine origin have included mucinous adenocarcinomas with abundant intracellular and extracellular mucin and, in one case, neuroendocrine differentiation, clear cell hidradenocarcinoma, and eccrine porocarcinoma. Some of these tmors have been associated with alpha or beta human chorionic gonadotropin production.
- Some vulvar carcinomas resembling mammary carcinomas may arise from vulvar apocrine sweat glands.
- Underwood and colleagues reported a series of vulvar adenosquamous carcinomas that were similar to extravulvar tumors of presumed sweat gland or hair sheath origin. The tumors were aggressive, with 15 of 18 patients dying of the tumor.
- Rare vulvar sebaceous carcinomas have been reported.

References

Carcangiu ML. Letters to the case. Pathol Res Pract 188:211–214, 1992.

Carlson JW, McGlennen RC, Gomez R, et al. Sebaceous carcinoma of the vulva: a case report and review of the literature. Gynecol Oncol 60:489–491, 1996.

Fukuma K, Inoue S, Tanaka N, et al. Eccrine adenocarcinoma of the vulva producing isolated alpha-subunit of gycoprotein hormones. Obstet Gynecol 67:293–296, 1986.

Ghamande SA, Kasnzica J, Griffiths T, et al. Mucinous adenocarcinomas of the vulva. Gynecol Oncol 57:117–120, 1995.

Katsanis WA, Doering DL, Bosscher JR, O'Connor DM. Vulvar eccrine porocarcinoma. Gynecol Oncol 62:396–399, 1996.

Messing MJ, Richardson MS, Smith MT, et al. Metastatic clear-cell hidradenocarcinoma. Gynecol Oncol 48:264–268, 1993.

Rahilly MA, Beattie GJ, Lessells AM. Mucinous eccrine carcinoma of the vulva with neuroendocrine differentiation. Histopathology 27:82–86, 1995.

Underwood JW, Adcock LL, Okagaki T. Adenosquamous carcinoma of skin appendages (adenoid squamous cell carcinoma, pseudoglandular squamous cell carcinoma, adenoacanthoma of sweat gland of Lever) of the vulva: a clinical and ultrastructural study. Cancer 42:1851–1858, 1978.

Wick MR, Goellner JR, Wolfe JT III, Su WPD. Vulvar sweat gland carcinomas. Arch Pathol Lab Med 109:43–47, 1985.

Rare Adenocarcinomas

- Rare vulvar adenocarcinomas or adenosquamous carcinomas have been postulated to be of cloacogenic origin.

References

Kennedy JC, Majmudar B. Primary adenocarcinoma of the vulva, possibly cloacogenic: a report of two cases. J Reprod Med 38:113–116, 1993.

Rhatigan RM, Mojadidi Q. Adenosquamous carcinomas of the vulva and vagina. Am J Clin Pathol 59:208–217, 1973.

Merkel Cell Tumor

- About 10 Merkel cell tumors of the vulva have been reported in women 28 to 73 years of age who usually presented with a labial mass.
- The tumors pathologically resemble Merkel cell tumors in other sites. One otherwise typical tumor showed squamous and glandular differentiation.
- The tumors appear to more aggressive than their extravulvar counterparts. Almost all of the tumors have been associated with widespread metastases and a fatal clinical course.

Reference

Cliby W, Soisson AP, Berchuk A, Clarke-Pearson DL. Stage I small cell carcinoma of the vulva treated with vulvectomy, lymphadenectomy, and adjuvant chemotherapy. Cancer 67:2415–2157, 1991.

Gil-Moreno A, Garcia-Jimenez A, Gonzalez-Bosquet J, et al. Merkel cell carcinoma of the vulva. Gynecol Oncol 64:526–532, 1997.

Scurry J, Brand A, Planner R, et al. Vulvar Merkel cell tumor with glandular and squamous differentiation. Gynecol Oncol 62:292–297, 1996.

MALIGNANT MELANOMA

Clinical Features

- These tumors, which account for 5% to 10% of vulvar cancers, may occur as early as the second decade of life, but the majority of patients are older than 50 years of age; the mean and median ages in most series are in the sixth or seventh decades.
- The presence of a vulvar or inguinal mass, pruritis, bleeding, or a change in a preexisting lesion are the most common presenting manifestations. The usual locations, in descending order of frequency, are the labia majora, the labia minora, the clitoris, and the perineum. Multifocal lesions are present in about one third of cases.
- The lesion is usually a plaque or nodule, often with a serpiginous border, that may be diffusely pigmented, focally pigmented, or nonpigmented. Almost half of the tumors are ulcerated. The clinical appearance occasionally can be mimicked by a benign pigmented lesion (page 11).

Microscopic Features

- Most vulvar melanomas are of the superficial spreading or acral lentiginous type; nodular (including nodular polypoidal) melanomas occur less frequently.
- The invasive component is of spindle cell type, epithelioid type, or mixed spindle-epithelioid type in approximately equal proportions. Cytoplasmic melanin can vary from copious to absent. Striking neurotropism was found in 50% of the lentiginous tumors in one study. Prominent desmoplasia is present in some tumors, especially lentiginous melanomas.
- Microscopic evidence of a preexisting nevus or melanosis is present in some cases.
- The depth of invasion should be assessed by at least one of the following:
  - Breslow's method. Raber and colleagues found that 14.6% of tumors were 0.75 mm or less, 14.6% were 0.76 to 1.5 mm, 25.6% were 1.51 to 3 mm, 11% were 3.01 to 4 mm, and 34.2% were deeper than 4 mm.

- Clark's levels. Raber and coworkers found that 2.4% were level I, 12.2% were level II, 17.1% were level III, 51.2 % were level IV, and 17.1% were level V.
- The modification of Clark's levels proposed by Chung and associates for vulvar malignant melanomas: level II, invasion less than 1 mm; level III, 1 to 2 mm of invasion; level IV, more than 2 mm of invasion; levels I and V are as described by Clark. The study by Chung and colleagues found that 24% of tumors were level II, 15% were level III, 46% were level IV, and 15% were level V.

■ The American Joint Committee on Cancer staging (AJCC) for melanomas incorporates depth: stage I, less than 1.5 mm deep or Clark's level III and no metastases; stage II, more than 1.5 but less than 4 mm or Clark's level IV and no metastases; stage III, more than 4 mm or Clark's level V or nodal metastases; stage IV, distant metastases.

Differential Diagnosis

■ The radial growth phase may be confused with Paget's disease (see page 32) or pagetoid VIN. Because the tumor cells of both these lesions can occasionally contain melanin pigment, its presence does not aid in the differential diagnosis.

■ The invasive component of an epithelioid melanoma can occasionally be confused with a poorly differentiated squamous cell carcinoma or adenocarcinoma, and the invasive component of a spindle cell melanoma can be confused with a sarcoma. The presence of a malignant junctional component, cytoplasmic melanin pigment, and imunoreactivity for S-100 and HMB-45 facilitate the diagnosis in these cases.

■ The diagnosis of melanoma should always be considered when a poorly differentiated malignant vulvar tumor proves difficult to classify on microscopic examination.

Behavior and Prognostic Factors

■ Local recurrences affect as many as one third of patients because of the persistence of the radial growth phase. Spread to the urethra is a frequent source of recurrence.

■ Lymph node and hematogenous spread is common. The

5-year survival rate in most studies has varied from 28% to 50%.

■ Prognostic factors, many of which are interrelated, include
- Depth of invasion (which correlates highly with lymph node spread). Raber and colleagues found 5-year survival rates for tumors more than 1.5 mm deep to be 20%, compared with 69% for tumors 1.5 mm or less deep. The 10-year survival rates by Clark's levels in a Mayo Clinic study were 100% (level II), 83% (level III), 65% (level IV), and 23% (level V).
- Between 90% and 100% of patients with inguinal node involvement die of the disease.
- AJCC staging was the only independent prognostic factor in a large GOG study of vulvar melanomas.
- Other factors in some studies that have correlated with poor prognosis or lymph node spread included older patient age, black race, FIGO stage, ulceration, a clitoral or bilateral location, multifocality, tumor size, epithelioid cell type, mitotic rate, lymphovascular space invasion, and DNA nondiploidy.

References

Benda JA, Platz CE, Anderson B. Malignant melanoma of the vulva: a clinical-pathologic review of 16 cases. Int J Gynecol Pathol 5:202–216, 1986.

Bradgate MG, Rollason TP, McConkey CC, Powell J. Malignant melanoma of the vulva: a clinicopathological study of 50 women. Br J Obstet Gynaecol 97:124–133, 1990.

Chung AF, Woodruff JM, Lewis JL Jr. Malignant melanomas of the vulva: a report of 44 cases. Obstet Gynecol 45:638–646, 1975.

Look KY, Roth LM, Sutton GP. Vulvar melanoma reconsidered. Cancer 72:143–146, 1993.

Lynn AAA, Elder DE. Local recurrence and urethral involvement in vulvar melanoma [Abstract]. Mod Pathol 11:108A, 1998.

Phillips GL, Bundy BN, Okagaki T, et al. Malignant melanoma of the vulva treated by radical hemivulvectomy: a prospective study of the Gynecologic Oncology Group. Cancer 73:2626–2632, 1994.

Podratz KC, Gaffey TA, Symmonds RE, et al. Melanoma of the vulva: an update. Gynecol Oncol 16:153–168, 1983.

Raber G, Mempel V, Jackisch C, et al. Malignant melanoma of the vulva: report of 89 patients. Cancer 78:2353–2358, 1996.

Scheistroen M, Trope C, Kaern J, et al. Malignant melanoma of the vulva: evaluation of prognostic factors with emphasis on DNA ploidy in 75 patients. Cancer 75:72–80, 1995.

Trimble EL, Lewis JL Jr, Williams LL, et al. Management of vulvar melanoma. Gynecol Oncol 45:254–258, 1992.

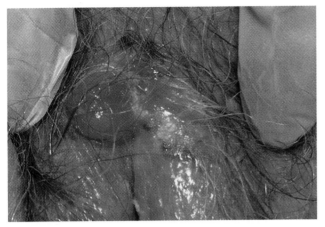

Figure 2–19. Malignant melanoma is focally pigmented.

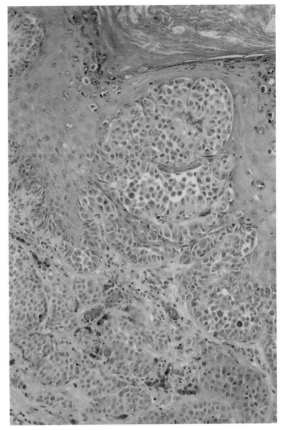

Figure 2–20. Malignant melanoma has a prominent in situ component (*top*) and an invasive component (*bottom*), both composed of epithelioid cells, some of which are pigmented.

BENIGN AND MALIGNANT SMOOTH MUSCLE TUMORS AND OTHER SARCOMAS

Smooth Muscle Tumors

Clinical Features

- Vulvar smooth muscle tumors (VSMTs) are uncommon, occur over a wide age range, and usually manifest as a painless mass. Some tumors clinically mimic a Bartholin cyst, although only rarely do such tumors arise in Bartholin's gland.
- Tumors occurring in pregnant women may noticeably enlarge during pregnancy, consistent with their typical content of estrogen and progesterone receptors.
- In occasional cases, a vulvar mass present for years has rapidly enlarged; the histologic findings in some of these tumors suggested transformation of a leiomyoma to a leiomyosarcoma.

- Rare VSMTs, some of which are familial, are associated with esophageal leiomyomas. The vulvar tumors in these cases are multiple and ill defined.

Pathologic Features

- Most VSMTs are composed of spindle cells growing in intersecting fascicles. In a few cases, there is a prominent component of eosinophilic or clear epithelioid cells in a plexiform pattern with a hyalinized or myxoid stroma. Myxoid change, which also occurs in spindle cell tumors, is more common in VSMTs in pregnant women.
- VSMTs that have three or all four of the following features are considered leiomyosarcomas by Nielsen and coworkers: 5 cm or larger in the maximal dimension, infiltrative margins, at least 5 mitotic figures per 10 high-power-fields, and moderate to severe atypia.
- Usual leiomyomas have none or one of the described

features, and atypical leiomyomas have only two features. Atypical leiomyomas are considered benign but should be excised with a narrow margin and receive long-term follow-up.

■ Only about 25% of vulvar leiomyosarcomas are clinically malignant, usually manifested by one or more local recurrences followed by metastases and death.

■ The differential diagnosis of VSMTs includes aggressive angiomyxoma, angiomyofibroblastoma, myxoid malignant fibrous histiocytoma, nerve sheath tumors, glomus tumors, and malignant melanoma (see Nielsen and colleagues).

References

Fred-Oginski W, Lovecchio JL, Farahani G, Smilari T. Malignant myxoid sarcoma of the Bartholin gland in pregnancy. Am J Obstet Gynecol 175:1633–1635, 1995.

Newman PL, Fletcher CDM. Smooth muscle tumours of the external genitalia: clinicopathological analysis of a series. Histopathology 18:532–539, 1991.

Nielsen GP, Rosenberg AE, Koerner FC, et al. Smooth-muscle tumors of the vulva: a clinicopathological study of 25 cases and review of the literature. Am J Surg Pathol 20:779–793, 1996.

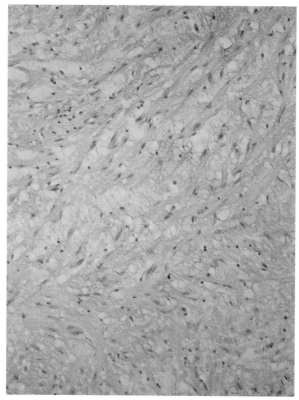

Figure 2–21. Myxoid leiomyoma.

Rhabdomyosarcoma

■ The vulva is the least common site of rhabdomyosarcomas in the lower female genital tract; the most common site is the vagina (page 56), followed by the uterus. The tumors almost always occur in the first 2 decades of life.

■ The tumors may be of the embryonal type (i.e., sarcoma botryoides) or of the alveolar type. In one study of tumors involving the female genitalia, five of eight tumors arose from the perineum.

■ Affected patients have a good prognosis when treated by chemotherapy and excision. In one study, eight of nine patients were disease-free at 4 to 10 years, and one was alive with probable disease at 2.5 years.

References

Andrassy RJ, Hays DM, Raney RB, et al. Conservative surgical management of vaginal and vulvar pediatric rhabdomyosarcoma: a report from the Intergroup Rhabdomyosarcoma Study III. J Pediatr Surg 30:1034–1037, 1995.

Copeland LJ, Sneige N, Stringer A, et al. Alveolar rhabdomyosarcoma of the female genitalia. Cancer 56:849–855, 1985.

Hays DM, Shimada H, Raney RB Jr, et al. Clinical staging and treatment results in rhabdomyosarcoma of the female genital tract among children and adolescents. Cancer 61:1893–1903, 1988.

Liposarcoma

■ About 12 vulvar liposarcomas have been reported, usually in middle-aged women who present with a painless vulvar mass. In four of six cases in the only series of vulvar liposarcomas, five were more than 3 cm in maximal dimension and three were well demarcated on gross examination.

■ In the same series, four tumors were classified as well-differentiated liposarcoma or atypical lipoma, with variation in adipocyte size, adipocyte nuclear atypia, and occasional lipoblasts.

■ In the other two cases, the tumors had an unusual appearance, with an admixture of neoplastic bland spindle and round cells, adipocytes showing variation in size, and numerous bivacuolated lipoblasts.

■ None of the six tumors recurred after local excision, although the follow-up was limited.

■ One example of a myxoid liposarcoma of the vulva has been reported in a 15-year-old girl. The tumor recurred as a poorly differentiated round cell liposarcoma that was fatal.

References

Brooks JJ, LiVolsi VA. Liposarcoma presenting on the vulva. Am J Obstet Gynecol 156:73–75, 1987.

Nucci MR, Fletcher CDM. Liposarcoma (atypical lipomatous tumors) of the vulva: a clinicopathologic study of six cases. Int J Gynecol Pathol 17:17–23, 1998.

Epithelioid Sarcoma

■ Most epithelioid sarcomas of the vulva (including Bartholin's gland), perineum, and pelvic soft tissues are of the proximal type. They share some of the morphologic, immunohistochemical, and ultrastructural features of typical epithelioid sarcoma, extrarenal rhabdoid tumor, and undifferentiated carcinoma. Most vulvar tumors reported as malignant rhabdoid tumor probably fall into this category.

■ The patients are usually in the reproductive age group and present with a mass involving the subcutis or deep soft tissues.

■ The tumor cells have prominent epithelioid or rhabdoid features, marked cytologic atypia, and in one half of the cases, grow in a multinodular pattern. Necrosis is common, but the granuloma-like pattern of typical epithelioid sarcoma is present only rarely.

■ The tumors are typically immunoreactive for cytokeratin, epithelial membrane antigen, and vimentin; less commonly for desmin and CD34; and occasionally for smooth-muscle actin.

■ Ultrastructural findings include prominent aggregates of paranuclear intermediate filaments and epithelial differentiation.

■ These tumors as a group appear to be somewhat more aggressive than typical (distal) epithelioid sarcomas, with a tendency for early metastasis.

References

Guillou L, Wadden C, Coindre J-M, et al. "Proximal-type" epithelioid sarcoma, a distinctive aggressive neoplasm showing rhabdoid features: clinicopathologic, immunohistochemical, and ultrastructural study of a series. Am J Surg Pathol 21:130–146, 1997.

Konefka T, Senkus E, Emerich J, Dudziak M. Epithelioid sarcoma of the Bartholin's gland primarily diagnosed as vulvar carcinoma. Gynecol Oncol 54:393–395, 1994.

Perrone T, Swanson PE, Twiggs L, et al. Malignant rhabdoid tumor of the vulva: is distinction from epithelioid sarcoma possible? A pathologic and immunohistochemical study. Am J Surg Pathol 13:848–858, 1989.

Other Sarcomas

■ Vulvar examples of dermatofibrosarcoma protuberans, malignant fibrous histiocytoma, malignant schwannoma, fibrosarcoma, vascular tumors (angiosarcoma, Kaposi's sarcoma, hemangioendothelioma, hemangiopericytoma), synovial sarcoma, alveolar soft part sarcoma, Ewing's sarcoma, and mesenchymal chondrosarcoma have been reported.

References

Ghorbani RP, Malpica A, Ayala AG. Dermatofibrosarcoma protuberans of the vulva: clinicopathologic and immunohistochemical analysis of four cases, one with fibrosarcomatous change, and review of the literature. Int J Gynecol Pathol 18:366–373, 1999.

Lin J, Yip KMH, Maffulli N, Chow LTC. Extraskeletal mesenchymal chondrosarcoma of the labium majus. Gynecol Oncol 60:492–493, 1996.

Macasaet MA, Duerr A, Thelmo W, et al. Kaposi sarcoma presenting as a vulva mass. Obstet Gynecol 86:695–697, 1995.

Nielsen GP, Shaw PA, Rosenberg AE, et al. Synovial sarcoma of the vulva: a report of two cases. Mod Pathol 9:970–974, 1996.

Nirenberg A, Östör AG, Slavin J, et al. Primary vulvar sarcomas. Int J Gynecol Pathol 14:55–62, 1995.

Santala M, Suonio S, Syrjanen K, et al. Malignant fibrous histiocytoma of the vulva. Gynecol Oncol 27:121–126, 1987.

Shen JT, d'Ablaing G, Morrow CP. Alveolar soft part sarcoma of the vulva: report of a first case and review of literature. Gynecol Oncol 13:120–128, 1982.

Strayer SA, Yum MN, Sutton GP. Epithelioid hemangioendothelioma of the clitoris: a case report with immunohistochemical and ultrastructural findings. Int J Gynecol Pathol 11:234–239, 1992.

Terada KY, Schmidt RW, Roberts JA. Malignant schwannoma of the vulva: a case report. J Reprod Med 33:969–972, 1988.

Zakut H, Lotan M, Lipnitzky M. Vulvar hemangiopericytoma: a case report and review of previous cases. Acta Obstet Gynecol Scand 64:619–621, 1985.

YOLK SAC TUMOR

■ Eight vulvar yolk sac tumors (YSTs) have been reported. The tumors presented as a labial or clitoral mass in females 1 to 26 years of age. The tumors resembled YSTs of the ovary on histologic examination.

■ Of six patients with follow-up information, three died of disease within a year despite excision and combination chemotherapy, although in none of these cases was the chemotherapy platinum based.

Reference

Flanagan CW, Parker JR, Mannel RS, et al. Primary endodermal sinus tumor of the vulva: a case report and review of the literature. Gynecol Oncol 66:515–518, 1997.

HEMATOPOETIC TUMORS

■ Thirteen women with primary vulvar lymphoma and who were 25 to 79 years of age presented with a vulvar nodule, swelling, or induration, sometimes accompanied by vaginal discharge or dyspareunia. Nine lymphomas were classified as diffuse large cell type and one each as lymphoplasmacytic, angiocentric, "lymphosarcoma," and Hodgkin's disease. Four patients died of tumor despite treatment.

■ The vulva was the initial site of involvement in two women with widespread lymphoma. One was a 13-year-old Nigerian girl with Burkitt's lymphoma and the other an 89-year-old woman with a diffuse large cell lymphoma.

■ Bartholin's gland involvement by a diffuse large cell immunoblastic lymphoma has been reported.

■ The vulva is rarely the presenting site of involvement by an acute or chronic myeloblastic leukemia. Women with chronic lymphocytic leukemia occasionally have vulvar involvement.

References

Ferry JA, Young RH. Malignant lymphoma of the genitourinary tract. Curr Diagn Pathol 4:145–169, 1997.

Macleod C, Palmer A, Findlay M. Primary non-Hodgkin's lymphoma of the vulva: a case report. Int J Gynecol Cancer 8:504–508, 1998.

Van den Broecke R, Van Droogenbroek J, Dhont M. Vulvovaginal manifestation of acute myeloblastic leukemia. Obstet Gynecol 88:735, 1996.

HISTIOCYTOSIS X

■ This lesion can occasionally involve the vulva, and in some such cases, the vulvar involvement is the initial manifestation of the disease. Most patients with vulvar involvement are found to have or subsequently develop systemic manifestations.

References

Axiotis CA, Merino MJ, Duray PH. Langerhans cell histiocytosis of the female genital tract. Cancer 67:1650–1660, 1991.

Otis CN, Fischer RA, Johnson N, et al. Histiocytosis of the vulva: a case report and review of the literature. Obstet Gynecol 75:555–558, 1990.

SECONDARY TUMORS

■ These tumors accounted for 8% of malignant vulvar tumors in one hospital-based series. The labium majus is most commonly involved; less commmonly the labium minus, the clitoris, an episiotomy scar, or Bartholin's gland is involved.

■ In most cases in which vulvar metastases appear after discovery of the primary tumor, the latter is at an advanced stage when initially diagnosed. In the series previously mentioned, the primary tumor and the vulvar metastases were diagnosed synchronously in about 25% of the cases. Ninety percent of the patients died of tumor within 1 year of the diagnosis of the vulvar metastasis.

■ The most common primary tumor to spread to the vulva in the series was squamous cell carcinoma of the cervix (which accounted for almost one half of the cases), followed by carcinomas of the endometrium, kidney, and urethra. Other studies have documented vulvar involvement by metastatic adenocarcinomas of the breast and endocervix and transitional cell carcinomas of the urinary bladder.

References

Dehner LP. Metastatic and secondary tumors of the vulva. Obstet Gynecol 42:47–57, 1973.

Menzin AW, De Risi D, Smilari TF, et al. Lobular breast carcinoma metastatic to the vulva: a case report and literature review. Gynecol Oncol 69:84–88, 1998.

van Dam PA, Irvine L, Lowe DG, et al. Carcinoma in episiotomy scars. Gynecol Oncol 44:96–100, 1992.

CHAPTER 3

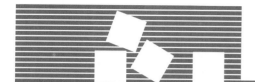

The Vagina

TUMOR-LIKE LESIONS

Condyloma Acuminata

- Vaginal condylomas are similar to those arising in the vulva (see Chapter 1), although flat condylomas are more common in the vagina than in the vulva.
- Roy and colleagues described vaginal condylomas with a "spiked" surface caused by asperities or minute surface projections that contain capillaries and scanty stroma. Diffuse vaginal involvement by such lesions has been referred to as *condylomatous vaginitis*.

Reference

Roy M, Meisels A, Fortier M, et al. Vaginal condylomata: a human papilloma virus infection. Clin Obstet Gynecol 24:461–483, 1981.

Cysts

- These are uncommon lesions that occur in the reproductive and postmenopausal age groups. The usual symptom is awareness of a mass in the vagina; small cysts may be an incidental finding on pelvic examination.
- The cysts are of the following types:
  - Müllerian cysts, which are most commonly lined by endocervical-type epithelium and less commonly by tubal or endometrioid epithelium; some may arise from adenosis
  - Epithelial inclusion cysts, lined by squamous epithelium and filled with keratin; most arise in sites of a previous episiotomy or laceration
  - Mesonephric (Gartner's duct) cysts, lined by cuboidal to flattened epithelial cells that are devoid of cytoplasmic mucin; these cysts are presumed to arise from mesonephric remnants that are found in the lateral vaginal walls
  - Endometriotic cysts (see Chapter 19) or cysts of Bartholin's duct origin (see Chapter 1)

References

Deppisch LM. Cysts of the vagina: classification and clinical correlations. Obstet Gynecol 45:632–637, 1975.

Pradham S, Tobon H. Vaginal cysts: a clinicopathologic study of 41 cases. Int J Gynecol Pathol 5:35–46, 1986.

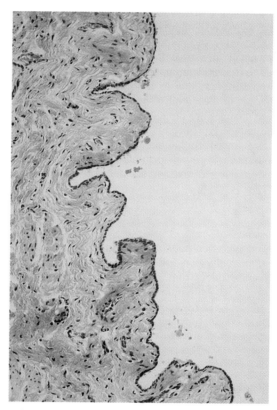

Figure 3–1. Gartner's duct cyst that was in the lateral wall of the vagina. Notice the cuboidal to flattened lining cells devoid of cilia and intracellular mucin.

Vaginal Adenosis

■ Before the use of diethylstilbestrol (DES), vaginal adenosis was a rare lesion that typically was encountered in the reproductive and postmenopausal age groups (median, 44 years in one study). In contrast, adenosis is found in about one third of asymptomatic girls or young women exposed in utero to DES. Rare cases of adenosis may be caused by CO_2 laser vaporization or topical 5-fluorouracil treatment of condylomata.

■ Macroscopically, the vaginal mucosa is red and granular and fails to stain with iodine. The upper one third of the vagina is almost always affected; the middle one third is involved in about 10% of cases and the lower third in only 2% of cases.

■ In about 20% of DES-exposed patients, grossly evident congenital malformations of the cervix and vagina accompany the adenosis.

■ Adenosis is characterized by the presence of benign-appearing glandular epithelium that replaces the normal squamous epithelium or forms glands within the superficial stroma. The epithelium is of the endocervical-type or, less commonly, of tuboendometrioid type. The latter type of epithelium is disproportionately common in the lower vagina and is much more common within glands than on the vaginal surface.

■ Rare findings in adenosis include papillae (i.e., papillary adenosis), microglandular hyperplasia from oral contraceptive use or pregnancy; Arias-Stella reaction in pregnancy; intestinal metaplasia; and atypical changes (cellular stratification, nuclear pleomorphism, hyperchromasia), usually in tuboendometrioid adenosis and adjacent to clear cell adenocarcinomas, suggesting that these changes are premalignant.

■ The glands typically undergo replacement by metaplastic squamous epithelium with the formation of squamous pegs. Striking examples of this process may be misconstrued as invasive squamous cell carcinoma.

• The pegs and small mucin-filled spaces (mucin "droplets") within the pegs or surface squamous epithelium may be the only clues to the diagnosis of adenosis.

• The glycogen-poor metaplastic squamous epithelium is gradually converted to an epithelium that is indistinguishable from normal glycogen-rich, vaginal squamous epithelium.

• Adenosis is rarely complicated by the development of a vaginal or cervical clear cell adenocarcinoma (page 54) or by vaginal intraepithelial neoplasia (page 52).

References

Bornstein J, Kaufman RH, Adam E, Adler-Storthz K. Human papillomavirus associated with vaginal intraepithelial neoplasia in women exposed to diethylstilbestrol in utero. Obstet Gynecol 70:75–80, 1987.

Bornstein J, Sova Y, Atad J, et al. Development of vaginal adenosis following combined 5-fluorouracil and carbon dioxide laser treatments for diffuse vaginal condylomatosis. Obstet Gynecol 81:896–898, 1993.

Merchant WJ, Gale J. Intestinal metaplasia in stilbestrol-induced vaginal adenosis. Histopathology 23:373–376, 1993.

Robboy SJ, Hill EC, Sandberg EC, Czernobilsky B. Vaginal adenosis in women born prior to the diethlystilbestrol era. Hum Pathol 17:488–492, 1986.

Robboy SJ, Kaufman RH, Prat J, et al. Pathologic findings in young women enrolled in the National Cooperative Diethystilbestrol Adenosis (DESAD) Project. Obstet Gynecol 53:309–317, 1979.

Robboy SJ, Scully RE, Welch WR, Herbst AL. Intrauterine diethylstilbestrol exposure and its consequences. Arch Pathol Lab Med 101:1–5, 1977.

Robboy SJ, Welch WR. Microglandular hyperplasia in vaginal adenosis associated with oral contraceptives and prenatal diethylstilbestrol exposure. Obstet Gynecol 49:430–434, 1977.

Robboy SJ, Young RH, Welch WR, et al. Atypical vaginal adenosis and cervical ectropion: association with clear cell adenocarcinoma in diethylstilbestrol-exposed offspring. Cancer 54:869–875, 1984.

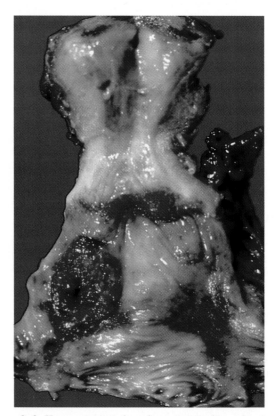

Figure 3–2. Hysterectomy and vaginectomy specimen demonstrates vaginal adenosis (*flat red areas, bottom right*) and clear cell adenocarcinoma (*polypoid red mass, bottom left*).

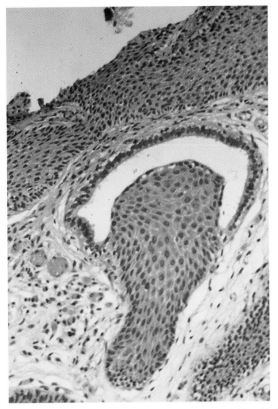

Figure 3–3. Adenosis. A gland lined by tuboendometrioid epithelium and partly replaced by metaplastic squamous epithelium lies in the superficial stroma.

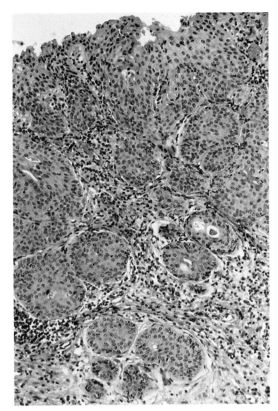

Figure 3–4. Adenosis with florid squamous metaplasia.

Prolapse of Fallopian Tube

- Tubal prolapse occasionally occurs after a hysterectomy, which in about 80% of cases has been a vaginal hysterectomy. On clinical examination, a lesion simulating granulation tissue is visible at the vaginal apex.
- An erroneous microscopic diagnosis of papillary adenocarcinoma may occur if the tubal plicae and their lining of bland tubal epithelium are not recognized.

References

Ellsworth HS, Harris JW, McQuarrie HG, et al. Prolapse of the fallopian tube following vaginal hysterectomy. JAMA 224:891–892, 1973.

Sapan IP, Solberg NS. Prolapse of the uterine tube after abdominal hysterectomy. Obstet Gynecol 42:26–32, 1973.

Silverberg SG, Frable WJ. Prolapse of fallopian tube into vaginal vault after hysterectomy. Arch Pathol 97:100–103, 1974.

Wheelock JB, Schneider V, Goplerud DR. Prolapsed fallopian tube masquerading as adenocarcinoma of the vagina in a postmenopausal woman. Gynecol Oncol 21:369–375, 1985.

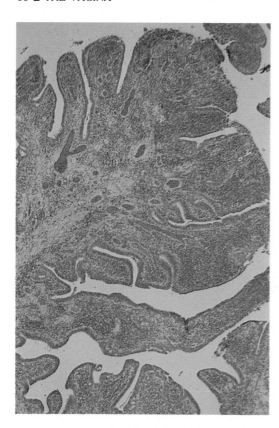

Figure 3–5. Prolapsed fallopian tube.

Postoperative Spindle Cell Nodule of the Female Genital Tract

Clinical Features

- Postoperative spindle cell nodule (PSCN) refers to a proliferative, reactive, pseudosarcomatous spindle cell lesion that develops shortly after an operation in the lower genitourinary tract.
- In women, PSCNs typically involve the vagina, but occasionally involve the vulva and rarely the endocervix or endometrium.
- PSCNs are detected in the operative site 1 to 12 weeks after a surgical procedure. PSCNs in the upper vagina have usually followed a vaginal hysterectomy, whereas those in the lower vagina or vulva have usually followed an episiotomy.
- PSCNs have a benign clinical follow-up after their excision. Rare lesions that have recurred have been successfully treated by re-excision.

Pathologic Features

- Vaginal PSCNs are soft polypoid masses that are less than 4 cm in maximal size. The endocervical and endometrial lesions have been incidental microscopic findings in repeated curettage specimens or in a hysterectomy specimen that followed a curettage.
- Microscopically, spindle cells are arranged in intersecting fascicles often with a network of small blood vessels. The cells have plump, vesicular nuclei with one or two prominent nucleoli but lack significant cytologic atypia.
- Mitotic figures are often numerous: as many as 25 mitotic figures (MFs) per 10 high-power-fields (HPFs) have been reported, and we have seen cases with as many as 50 MFs per 10 HPFs.
- The lesion may infiltrate the surrounding normal tissue to a limited degree. There is frequently overlying ulceration with a superficial infiltrate of neutrophils, a chronic inflammatory cell infiltrate in the deeper por-

tion of the lesion, and small foci of hemorrhage and mild to moderate edema.

■ PSCNs are usually immunoreactive for vimentin, desmin, muscle-specific actin, and surprisingly, cytokeratin.

Differential Diagnosis With Well-Differentiated Leiomyosarcoma

■ This distinction may be difficult on microscopic examination, because a leiomyosarcoma may exhibit no more cytologic atypia and may be less mitotically active than a PSCN.

■ Sarcomas with mitotic rates as high as those in PSCNs, however, usually exhibit greater degrees of nuclear atypicality than present in PSCNs.

■ The prominent delicate network of small blood vessels typical of PSCNs is usually not a feature of leiomyosarcoma.

■ History of a recent operation in the site of the lesion strongly favors a diagnosis of PSCN over that of leiomyosarcoma.

References

Clement PB. Postoperative spindle-cell nodule of the endometrium. Arch Pathol Lab Med 112:566–568, 1988.

Kay S, Schneider V. Reactive spindle cell nodule of the endocervix simulating uterine sarcoma. Int J Gynecol Pathol 4:255–257, 1985.

Manson CM, Hirsch PJ, Coyne JD. Post-operative spindle cell nodule of the vulva. Histopathology 26:571–574, 1995.

Proppe KH, Scully RE, Rosai J. Postoperative spindle cell nodules of genitourinary tract resembling sarcomas. Am J Surg Pathol 8:101–108, 1984.

Wick MR, Brown BA, Young RH, et al. Spindle-cell proliferations of the urinary tract. An immunohistochemical study. Am J Surg Pathol 12:379–389, 1988.

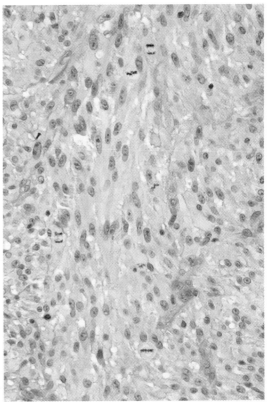

Figure 3–6. Postoperative spindle cell nodule of the vagina within an episiotomy scar. Notice the spindle cells with bland nuclei and mitotic figures.

Fibroepithelial Polyps of the Lower Female Genital Tract

Clinical Features

■ Fibroepithelial polyps are most commonly found in the vagina; the vulva and the cervix are much less common sites. The polyps usually occur in women of reproductive and postmenopausal age (rarely in newborn infants) who may be asymptomatic, have postcoital bleeding, or a mass.

■ About 20% of the patients are pregnant at the time of diagnosis, and an additional 10% have given a history of hormonal treatment with estrogen, oral contraceptives, or a hormonal agent of unspecified type, suggesting a possible hormonal cause in some cases.

■ Laskin and coworkers have referred to similar or identical lesions as "superficial myofibroblastomas."

Pathologic Features

■ The polyps are usually single but occasionally multiple and numerous, are sessile to pedunculated to villiform, soft to rubbery, and gray-pink. Occasional vaginal lesions have a botryoid appearance. The polyps are usually 4 cm or less in greatest dimension, but examples up to 12 cm have been reported.

■ The polyps are usually covered by unremarkable squamous epithelium, but occasionally the latter is koilocytotic or dysplastic.

■ The typically edematous or myxoid stroma of the polyps usually contains dilated, thin-walled vessels, a sprinkling of inflammatory cells, and widely scattered stromal cells. Occasionally, the stroma is intensely cellular.

- The polygonal to stellate to spindle-shaped, benign-appearing stromal cells have pale cytoplasm and tapering cytoplasmic processes. Multiple nuclei (or multilobed nuclei) are often present and may be disposed in a wreathlike arrangement.

- Occasionally, especially in pregnant patients, the stroma of the polyp contains cells with eosinophilic cytoplasm and bizarre, hyperchromatic, multiple or multilobed nuclei that may contain prominent nucleoli ("pseudosarcoma botryoides"). In such cases, mitotic figures (usually less than 3 but rarely more than 5 MFs per 10 HPFs) and abnormal MFs may be present.

- The stromal cells are typically immunoreactive for vimentin, less commonly for desmin and muscle-specific actin, and in some cases, for estrogen and progesterone receptors.

- Ultrastructural studies have indicated that the stromal cells are fibroblasts and myofibroblasts.

Behavior

- Local excision has been almost always curative; in the rare cases in which the lesions have recurred, re-excision has been successful.

- In pregnant patients, the polyps may regress during the puerperium.

Differential Diagnosis

- Multinucleated stromal giant cells. These cells, identical to those occurring in fibroepithelial polyps, are a common incidental microscopic finding in the loose subepithelial stroma of the lower female genital tract, including the cervix, vagina, and vulva.

- Aggressive angiomyxoma. These tumors, in contrast to usual fibroepithelial polyps, typically form a bulky mass, contain numerous blood vessels of various sizes (including thick-walled vessels), have infiltrative borders, and have only rare multinucleated cells. The distinction between the two lesions sometimes may be difficult in a small biopsy specimen.

- Sarcoma botryoides (page 56). Features favoring this diagnosis over a fibroepithelial polyp with stromal atypia include an age younger than 5 years; a history of rapid growth; small, mitotically active cells with scanty cytoplasm and hyperchromatic nuclei within a cambium layer (or similar cells elsewhere in the lesion); tumor invading the squamous epithelium; and cells with cytoplasmic cross striations or immunoreactive for myoglobin.

References

Abdul-Karim FW, Cohen RE. Atypical stromal cells of lower female genital tract. Histopathology 17:249–253, 1990.

Al-Nafussi AI, Rebello G, Hughes D, Blessing K. Benign vaginal polyp: a histological, histochemical and immunohistochemical study of 20 polyps with comparison to normal vaginal subepithelial layer. Histopathology 20:145–150, 1992.

Chirayil SJ, Tobon H. Polyps of the vagina: a clinicopathologic study of 18 cases. Cancer 47:2904–2907, 1981.

Elliot GB, Elliot JDA. Superficial stromal reactions of lower genital tract. Arch Pathol 95:100–101, 1973.

Hartman C, Sperling M, Stein H. So-called fibroepithelial polyps of the vagina exhibiting an unusual but uniform antigen profile characterized by expression of desmin and steroid hormone receptors but no muscle-specific actin or macrophage markers. Am J Clin Pathol 93:604–608, 1990.

Laskin WB, Fetsch JF, Michal M, Tavassoli FA. Superficial myofibroblastoma: nine cases of a newly characterized mesenchymal tumor of the specialized subepithelial cervical and vaginal stroma [Abstract]. Mod Pathol 12:119A, 1999.

Miettinen M, Wahlstrom T, Vesterinen E, Saksela E. Vaginal polyps with pseudosarcomatous features: a clinicopathologic study of seven cases. Cancer 51:1148–1151, 1983.

Mucitelli DR, Charles EZ, Kraus FT. Vulvovaginal polyps: histologic appearance, ultrastructure, immunocytochemical characteristics, and clinicopathologic correlations. Int J Gynecol Pathol 9:20–40, 1990.

Norris HJ, Taylor HB. Polyps of the vagina: a benign lesion resembling sarcoma botryoides. Cancer 19:227–232, 1966.

Nucci MR, Young RH, Fletcher CDM. Cellular pseudosarcomatous fibroepithelial polyps of the lower female genital tract: an underrecognized lesion often misdiagnosed as sarcoma [Abstract]. Mod Pathol 12:121A, 1999.

Östör AG, Fortune DW, Riley CB. Fibroepithelial polyps with atypical stromal cells (pseudosarcoma botryoides) of vulva and vagina: a report of 13 cases. Int J Gynecol Pathol 7:351–360, 1988.

Pitt MA, Roberts ISD, Agbamu DA, Eyden BP. The nature of atypical multinucleated stromal cells: a study of 37 cases from different sites. Histopathology 23:137–145, 1993.

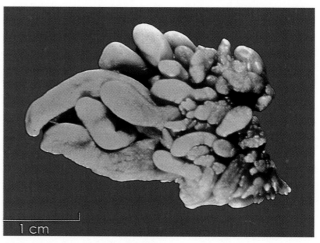

Figure 3–7. Fibroepithelial polyps.

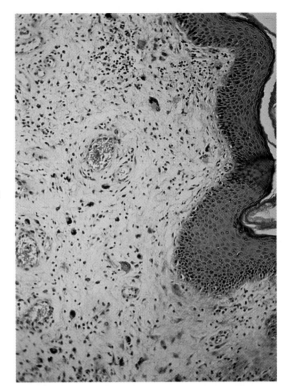

Figure 3–8. Fibroepithelial polyp in a pregnant woman. Notice the giant cells with hyperchromatic bizarre nuclei.

Rare Tumor-like Lesions

■ Tuberculosis, nonspecific xanthogranulomatous inflammation, typical malakoplakia, ligneous inflammation (see Chapter 4), and a fibrohistiocytic reaction have been documented in the vagina. The latter lesion had a storiform pattern and mimicked a fibrous histiocytoma except for the presence of a foreign-body reaction to polarizable material.

■ Emphysematous vaginitis is a self-limiting lesion that occurs in the reproductive and postmenopausal age groups. Gas-filled cystic spaces beneath the squamous epithelium are focally lined by foreign-body giant cells and chronic inflammatory cells. The cervix, vulva, or both can be also involved. The pathogenesis is obscure; at least some cases appear to be caused by gas-forming bacteria.

■ Ectopic decidua within the vagina in pregnant women has clinically mimicked carcinoma in some cases. The histologic features are similar to those of eutopic decidua (see Chapter 7) and ectopic decidua in other sites (see Chapters 4 and 19).

■ Benign pigmented lesions of the vaginal mucosa include melanosis, blue nevus of the usual and cellular type, and atypical melanocytic hyperplasia.

■ Rare vaginal examples of ectopic skin (including cutaneous appendages) and thyroid or parathyroid tissue have been documented.

■ Single cases of vaginal endocervicosis and vaginal involvement by retroperitoneal fibrosis have been reported.

References

Bottles K, Lacey CG, Miller TR. Atypical melanocytic hyperplasia of the vagina. Gynecol Oncol 19:226–230, 1984.

Fishman A, Ortega E, Girtanner RE, Kaplan AL. Malacoplakia of the vagina presenting as a pelvic mass. Gynecol Oncol 49:380–382, 1993.

Heah JTC. Idiopathic retroperitoneal fibrosis involving the vagina: case report. Br J Obstet Gynaecol 86:407–410, 1979.

Kramer K, Tobon H. Vaginitis emphysematosa. Arch Pathol Lab Med 111:746–749, 1987.

Kurman RJ, Prabha AC. Thyroid and parathyroid glands in the vaginal wall: report of a case. Am J Clin Pathol 59:503–507, 1973.

Ladefoged C, Lorentzen M. Xanthogranulomatous inflammation of the female genital tract. Histopathology 13:541–551, 1988.

Martinka M, Allaire C, Clement PB. Endocervicosis presenting as a painful vaginal mass: A case report. Int J Gynecol Pathol 18:274–276, 1999.

Mathie JG. Vaginal deciduosis simulating carcinoma. J Obstet Gynaecol Br Empire 64:720–721, 1957.

Nicholson GW. An epidermal heteromorphosis of the vaginal vault. J Pathol Bacteriol 43:209–221, 1936.

Nogales-Ortiz F, Tarancon I, Nogales F. The pathology of female genital tract tuberculosis. Obstet Gynecol 53:422–428, 1979.

Snover DC, Phillips G, Dehner LP. Reactive fibrohistiocytic proliferation simulating fibrous histiocytoma. Am J Clin Pathol 76:232–235, 1981.

Strate SM, Taylor WE, Forney JP, Silva FG. Xanthogranulomatous pseudotumor of the vagina: evidence of a local response to an unuusal bacterium (mucoid *Escherichia coli*). Am J Clin Pathol 79:637–643, 1983.

Tobon H, Murphy AI. Benign blue nevus of the vagina. Cancer 40:3174–3176, 1977.

Tsukuda Y. Benign melanosis of the vagina and cervix. Am J Obstet Gynecol 124:211–212, 1976.

BENIGN TUMORS

Epithelial Tumors

■ Most benign papillary squamous lesions of the vagina are condylomas with the same histologic features as condylomas in the vulva (see Chapter 1). Noncondylomatous squamous papillomas are rare in the vagina and are similar to those occurring in the cervix (see Chapter 4). Vestibular squamous papillomatosis is discussed in Chapter 1.

■ Rare papillomas, similar to the müllerian papillomas of the cervix (see Chapter 4), may arise from the vaginal mucosa, usually in children.

• Two otherwise similar papillomas *within* the vaginal wall, one in a 5-year-old girl and the other in a 24-year-old woman, consisted of fibrous-cored papillae, occasional glands, and solid areas lined by or composed of eosinophilic cells with bland nuclei. In both cases, the physicians favored a müllerian origin based on the immunohistochemical and ultrastructural features.

■ Several vaginal tubulovillous adenomas of enteric type, which closely resembled colonic tubulovillous adenomas, have been reported. The tumors contained goblet cells and Paneth cells, and they stained for enteric mucin.

■ Ovarian-type epithelial-stromal tumors occurring in the vagina have included rare Brenner tumors and an endometrioid papillary cystadenofibroma. The latter presented as a 2-cm mass submucosal mass in the lower vagina of a 41-year-old woman.

References

Fox H, Wells M, Harris M, et al. Enteric tumours of the lower female genital tract: a report of three cases. Histopathology 12:167–176, 1988.

Kerner H, Munichor M. Papillary müllerian cystadenofibroma of the vagina. Histopathology 30:84–86, 1997.

Luttges JE, Lubke M. Recurrent benign müllerian papilloma of the vagina. Immunohistochemical findings and histogenesis. Arch Gyneol Obstet 255:157–160, 1994.

McCluggage WG, Nirmala V, Radhakumari K. Intramural mullerian papilloma of the vagina. Int J Gynecol Pathol 18:94–95, 1999.

Mortensen BB, Nielsen K. Tubulo-villous adenoma of the female genital tract: a case report and review of the literature. Acta Obstet Gynecol Scand 70:161–163, 1991.

Ben-Izhak O, Munichor M, Malkin L, Kerner H. Brenner tumor of the vagina. Int J Gynecol Pathol 17:79–82, 1998.

Ulbright TM, Alexander RW, Kraus FT. Intramural papilloma of the vagina: evidence of a mullerian histogenesis. Cancer 48:2260–2266, 1981.

Benign Mixed Tumor

■ Benign mixed tumors ("spindle cell epitheliomas") are uncommon and almost always occur near the hymenal ring in women who are in the reproductive or postmenopausal age groups. The tumors are typically discovered incidentally during a pelvic examination, or the patients are aware of a slowly enlarging, painless mass.

■ The tumors are benign. The rare tumors that have recurred have been successfully managed with re-excision.

■ The tumors range from 1 to 6 cm in diameter and are typically well circumscribed with a solid, gray to white, sometimes myxoid sectioned surface.

■ The tumors usually lie just beneath but are only rarely in contact with an intact squamous mucosa. Microscopically, their borders are usually well circumscribed but nonencapsulated, and they are characterized by a major component of stromal-type cells and a minor component of well-differentiated epithelial elements.

■ The stromal-type cells have scanty cytoplasm, round to spindled nuclei, fine chromatin, indistinct nucleoli, and rare to absent mitoses, and they are arranged in cords, nests, whorls, and intersecting fascicles, or they surround hyalinized spherules. The cellularity varies with the amount of alcianophilic material and collagen between the stromal cells. The stromal cells are typically immunoreactive for cytokeratin, smooth muscle actin, and progesterone receptor.

■ The sparse epithelial component consists of benign glands lined by mucinous or nonspecific epithelium that undergoes variable degrees of replacement by metaplastic squamous epithelium, resulting in the formation of squamous nests. Some of the latter may contain stainable mucin.

■ The cytokeratin immunoreactivity of the spindle cells and their apparent epithelial nature on ultrastructural examination have led one group of investigators to prefer the designation "spindle cell epithelioma" for these tumors.

References

Branton PA, Tavassoli FA. Spindle cell epithelioma, the so-called mixed tumor of the vagina: a clinicopathologic, immunohistochemical, and ultrastructural analysis of 28 cases. Am J Surg Pathol 17:509–515, 1993.

Sirota RL, Dickersin GR, Scully RE. Mixed tumors of the vagina: a clinicopathologic analysis of eight cases. Am J Surg Pathol 5:413–422, 1981.

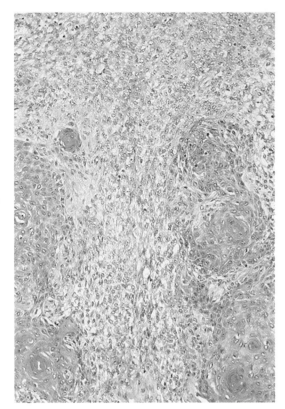

Figure 3–9. Benign mixed tumor (spindle cell epithelioma). Notice the nests of squamous epithelium that merge with the spindled stromal cells.

Aggressive Angiomyxoma and Angiomyofibroblastoma (see Chapter 1)

Leiomyoma

- Leiomyomas are the most common mesenchymal tumor of the vagina; about 300 cases have been reported. They typically occur in the reproductive and postmenopausal age groups. The smaller tumors are often unassociated with symptoms, whereas larger tumors may cause pain, dyspareunia, dystocia, or urinary tract symptoms.
- The gross and microscopic features are similar to those occurring in the uterus (see Chapter 9). Tumors occurring in pregnant women may show increased mitotic activity.
- Rare tumors may recur in one or more pregnancies, suggesting hormone dependency in some cases.
- The differential diagnosis is with leiomyosarcoma. Tumors with moderate to marked atypia and at least 5 MFs per 10 HPFs should be considered leiomyosarcomas; such tumors only rarely metastasize, but may recur locally.

References

Liu M. Fibromyoma of the vagina. Eur J Obstet Gynaecol Reprod Biol 29:321–328, 1988.

Rywlin AM, Simmons RJ, Robinson MJ. Leiomyoma of vagina recurrent in pregnancy: a case with apparent hormone dependency. South Med J 62:1449–1451, 1969.

Tavassoli FA, Norris HJ. Smooth muscle tumors of the vagina. Obstet Gynecol 53:689–693, 1979.

Vaginal, Vulvar, and Cervical Rhabdomyomas

- These rare benign tumors of the female genital tract are most common in the vagina but also occur in the vulva and rarely the cervix. The tumors typically present in women in the reproductive or postmenopausal age groups as a smooth, solitary, submucosal or subcutaneous mass and range up to 11 cm but are usually <3 cm. They are cured by local excision.
- Most tumors are covered by intact squamous epithelium and composed of variable numbers of benign, amitotic, skeletal muscle cells (eosinophilic cytoplasm, cross striations, immunoreactivity for myoglobin) that

appear round or strap-shaped depending on the plane of section. The neoplastic cells are separated by variable amounts of a vascular, fibromyxoid stroma.

■ Rare tumors have had an admixed component of rhabdomyosarcoma or had an appearance intermediate between the two lesions.

■ Differential dignosis:
  • Fibroepithelial polyps (page 47). These lesions, unlike rhabdomyomas, lack skeletal muscle differentiation.
  • Embryonal rhabdomyosarcoma (page 56). These tumors, in contrast to rhabdomyomas, are characterized by occurrence in infants or children, a history of rapid growth, a cambium layer, mitotic activity, and an infiltrative border.

References

Chabrel CM, Beilby JOW. Vaginal rhabdomyoma. Histopathology 4: 645–651, 1980.

Iversen UM. Two cases of benign vaginal rhabdomyoma. Case reports. APMIS 104:575–578, 1996.

Jacques SM, Lawrence WD, Malviya VK. Uterine mixed embryonal rhabdomyosarcoma and fetal rhabdomyoma. Gynecol Oncol 48:272–276, 1993.

Wertheim RA, Krebs H-B, Frable WJ. Intermediate form of cervical fetal rhabdomyoma? A case report. Diagn Gynecol Pathol 4:57–62, 1982.

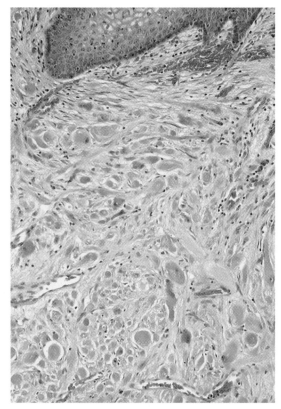

Figure 3–10. Rhabdomyoma.

Miscellaneous Benign Tumors

■ Rare cases of dermoid cyst, adenomatoid tumor, myxoma, angiomyolipoma, mesenchymoma (containing skeletal and smooth muscle and fat), hemangioma, glomus tumor, neurofibroma, schwannoma, cellular schwannoma, granular cell tumor, and paraganglioma have been documented in the vagina.

References

Chen KTK. Angiomyolipoma of the vagina. Gynecol Oncol 37:302–304, 1990.

Dekel A, Avidan D, Bar-Ziv J, et al. Neurofibroma of the vagina presenting with urinary retention: review of the literature and report of a case. Obstet Gynecol Surv 43:325–327, 1988.

Egley CC, Fox JS. Vaginal myxoma presenting as acute urinary retention. Obstet Gynecol 73:882–883, 1989.

Ellison DW, MacKenzie IZ, McGee JO'D. Cellular schwannoma of the vagina. Gynecol Oncol 46:119–121, 1992.

Hirose R, Imai A, Kondo H, et al. A dermoid cyst of the paravaginal space. Arch Gynecol Obstet 249:39–41, 1991.

Koskela O. Granular-cell myoblastoma of the vagina. Ann Chir Gynaecol Fenn 53:270–273, 1964.

Lorenz G. Adenomatoid tumor of the ovary and vagina. Zent Gynakkol 100:1412–1416, 1978.

Mann S, Russell P, Wills EJ, et al. Benign vaginal mesenchymoma showing mature skeletal muscle, smooth muscle, and fatty differentiation. Int J Surg Pathol 4:49–54, 1996.

Pezeshkpour G. Solitary paraganglioma of the vagina—report of a case. Am J Obstet Gynecol 139:219–221, 1981.

Rezvani FF. Vaginal cavernous hemangioma in pregnancy. Obstet Gynecol 89:824–825, 1997.

Moldavsky M, Stayerman C, Turani H. Vaginal glomus tumor presented as as painless cystic mass. Gynecol Oncol 69:172–174, 1998.

Terada S, Suzuki N, Tomimatsu N, Akasofu K. Vaginal schwannoma. Arch Gynecol Obstet 251:203–206, 1992.

MALIGNANT TUMORS

Vaginal Intraepithelial Neoplasia

■ Vaginal intraepithelial neoplasia (VaIN) is only about 1% as common as its cervical counterpart (CIN) and tends to occur in women who are a decade older (mean age, 50 to 55 years) than women with CIN. The patients are typically asymptomatic and present with an abnormal Pap smear.

■ In 50% to 80% of cases, there is prior or synchronous preinvasive or invasive squamous neoplasia elsewhere in the lower anogenital tract. Less common risk factors include immunosupppression, prior pelvic irradiation, and adenosis.

- The affected area, which is in the upper third of the vagina in about 90% of cases, may be macroscopically abnormal (raised, roughened, white, pink) but is often only appreciable colposcopically. VaIN is multifocal in about 50% of cases.
- The microscopic features and the differential diagnosis are the same as those for CIN (see Chapter 5).
- VaIN 1 (mild dysplasia) is now designated by some authorities as low-grade squamous intraepithelial lesion and VaIN 2 (moderate dysplasia) and VaIN 3 (severe dysplasia; carcinoma in situ) are collectively termed high-grade squamous intraepithelial lesion.
- A substantial proportion of cases (20% to 78%) undergo postbiopsy remission, and most others are cured by one or two local treatment procedures (i.e., resection, chemosurgery, laser, irradiation, or combinations thereof). In 3% to 10% of cases, there is progression to invasive squamous carcinoma despite close follow-up.

References

Aho M, Vesterinen E, Meyer B, et al. Natural history of vaginal intra-epithelial neoplasia. Cancer 68:195–197, 1991.

Benedet JL, Sanders BH. Carcinoma in situ of the vagina. Am J Obstet Gynecol 148:695–700, 1984.

Lenehan PM, Meffe F, Lickrish GM. Vaginal intraepithelial neoplasia: biologic aspects and management. Obstet Gynecol 68:333–337, 1986.

Sillman FH, Fruchter RG, Chen Y-S, et al. Vaginal intraepithelial neoplasia: risk factors for persistence, recurrence, and invasion and its management. Am J Obstet Gynecol 176:93–99, 1997.

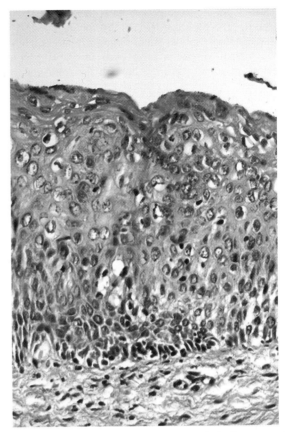

Figure 3–11. Grade 3 vaginal intraepithelial neoplasia (i.e., severe dysplasia, high-grade intraepithelial lesion).

Squamous Cell Carcinoma

- Squamous cell carcinomas (SCCs) account for about 90% of primary vaginal cancers and about 1% of cancers of the female genital tract. The ratio of vaginal to cervical SCCs is about 1:50. The risk factors are the same as for VaIN (discussed earlier). As many as 50% of patients have had a previous hysterectomy for benign disease or squamous neoplasia of the cervix.
- The patients are usually in the late reproductive or postmenopausal age groups (mean age, 58 to 64 years), but 10% of tumors occur in women younger than 40. The typical presentation includes vaginal bleeding or discharge, urinary symptoms, abnormal cytologic findings, a mass, or combinations thereof. The tumors, most of which arise in the upper third of the vagina, vary from polypoid to ulcerating.
- Microscopically, vaginal SCCs resemble those arising in the cervix (see Chapter 5). Most are typical keratinizing or nonkeratinizing SCCs. Uncommon variants include verrucous SCCs (see Chapter 2), warty SCCs

(see Chapter 5), and sarcomatoid SCCs (see Chapter 5). A single example of lymphoepithelioma-like carcinoma of the vagina has been recently reported.
- The most important prognostic factor is stage (Table 3–1). Survival figures from a Stanford study of patients

Table 3–1
FIGO STAGING OF CARCINOMA OF THE VAGINA

Stage I	The carcinoma is limited to the vaginal wall.
Stage II	The carcinoma has involved the subvaginal tissue, but tumor has not extended to the pelvic wall.
IIa*	Paravaginal submucosal extension only
IIb*	Parametrial extension
Stage III	The carcinoma has extended to the pelvic wall.
Stage IV	The carcinoma has extended beyond the true pelvis or has involved the mucosa of the bladder or rectum. A bullous edema does not allow designation of this stage.
IVa	Spread of tumor to adjacent organs and/or direct extension beyond the true pelvis
IVb	Spread of tumor to distant organs

* Modification suggested by Perez et al. Cancer 31:36–44, 1973.

treated with irradiation were 94% for stage I, 80% for stage II, 50% for stage III, and 0% for stage IV.

■ Low histologic grade, small tumor size, and an absence of lymphatic invasion have been favorable prognostic factors in some studies. Although the term *microinvasive SCC* has been suggested for tumors that infiltrate to a depth of less than 2.5 mm, such tumors are occasionally fatal, and this term has not been adopted.

References

Di Domenico A. Primary vaginal squamous cell carcinoma in the young patient. Gynecol Oncol 35:181–187, 1989.

Dietl J, Horny H-P, Kaiserling E. Lymphoepithelioma-like carcinoma of the vagina: a case report with special reference to the immunophenotype of the tumors cells and tumor-infiltrating lymphoreticular cells. Int J Gynecol Pathol 13:186–189, 1994.

Gallup DG, Talledo OE, Shah KJ, Hayes C. Invasive squamous cell carcinoma of the vagina: a 14-year study. Obstet Gynecol 69:782–785, 1987.

Eddy GL, Singh KP, Gansler TS. Superficially invasive carcinoma of the vagina following treatment for cervical cancer: a report of six cases. Gynecol Oncol 36:376–379, 1990.

Kirkbride P, Fyles A, Rawlings GA, et al. Carcinoma of the vagina— experience at the Princess Margaret Hospital (1974–1989). Gynecol Oncol 56:435–443, 1995.

Davis DP, Stanhope SR, Garton GR, et al. Invasive vaginal carcinoma: analysis of early-stage disease. Gynecol Oncol 42:131–136, 1991.

Peters WA III, Kumar NB, Morley GW. Microinvasive carcinoma of the vagina: a distinct clinical entity? Am J Obstet Gynecol 153:505–507, 1985.

Jones MJ, Levin HS, Ballard LA Jr. Verrucous squamous cell carcinoma of the vagina: report of a case and review of the literature. Cleve Clin Q 48:305–313, 1981.

Raptis S, Haber G, Ferenczy A. Vaginal squamous cell carcinoma with sarcomatoid spindle cell features. Gynecol Oncol 49:100–106, 1993.

Spirtos NM, Doshi BP, Kapp DS, Teng N. Radiation therapy for primary squamous carcinoma of the vagina: Stanford University experience. Gynecol Oncol 35:20–26, 1989.

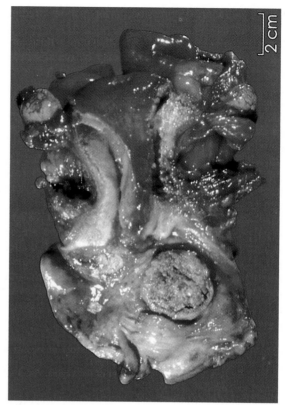

Figure 3–12. Vaginal squamous cell carcinoma in a hysterectomy-vaginectomy specimen. Notice the polypoid mass in the upper vagina.

Clear Cell Adenocarcinoma

■ Vaginal clear cell carcinomas (CCCs) were rare before the use of DES in the early 1950s; since then, about 400 vaginal CCCs have been reported by 1994, mostly in adolescents and young adults (median age, 19 years). About 80% of these patients were exposed in utero to DES, a related synthetic estrogen, or an unknown medication.

■ Larger CCCs may be associated with bleeding, but many small tumors are asymptomatic and are found during an examination performed because of a history of DES exposure. The tumors usually occur in the upper third of the vagina on the anterior wall (the most common site of adenosis); rare tumors are multicentric.

■ CCCs range from microscopic to large; the latter are polypoid (see Fig. 3–2), nodular, flat, or ulcerated. Small tumors may not be seen colposcopically if covered by intact mucosa, but some of these may be palpable. The depth of invasion varies from a few millimeters to transmural invasion.

■ The microscopic features are identical to CCCs in other sites of the female genital tract (see Chapters 6, 8, and 14). Adenosis, which may be atypical (see Adenosis, page 44), usually abuts the tumor.

■ The differential diagnosis includes microglandular hyperplasia and Arias-Stella reaction, both of which may occur in vaginal adenosis (see Differential Diagnosis under these headings in Chapter 4).

■ About 15% of stage I tumors and about 40% of stage

II tumors have spread to lymph nodes at the time of presentation. Approximately one third of the recurrences are extraabdominal; the corresponding figure for vaginal squamous cell carcinomas is only 10%.

- The survival rates are approximately 90% for stage I tumors and almost 100% for small, incidentally discovered tumors. DES-related CCCs have a better prognosis than DES-unrelated CCCs, a difference which appears to be unrelated to tumor stage or size.

References

Robboy SJ, Scully RE, Welch WR, Herbst AL. Intrauterine diethylstilbestrol exposure and its consequences. Arch Pathol Lab Med 101:1–5, 1977.

Robboy SJ, Young RH, Welch WR, et al. Atypical vaginal adenosis and cervical ectropion: association with clear cell adenocarcinoma in diethylstilbestrol-exposed offspring. Cancer 54:869–875, 1984.

Waggoner SE, Mittendorf R, Biney N, et al. Influence of in utero diethylstilbestrol on the prognosis and biological behavior of vaginal clear-cell adenocarcinoma. Gynecol Oncol 55:238–244, 1994.

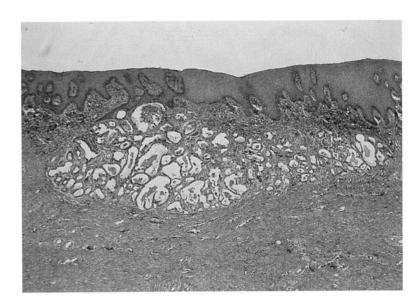

Figure 3–13. Clear cell carcinoma of the vagina with tubulocystic pattern.

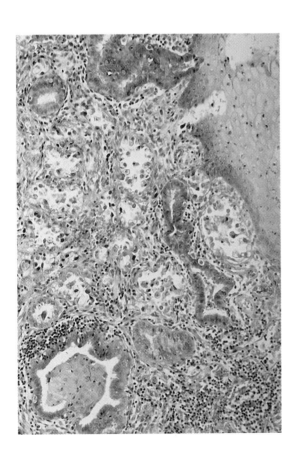

Figure 3–14. Clear cell carcinoma admixed with adenosis. Notice the clear and hobnail cells within the tumor.

Other Adenocarcinomas and Adenosquamous Carcinomas

■ Two cases of adenocarcinoma in situ (AIS) of the vagina have occurred in women who had previously been treated for typical AIS of the uterine cervix. In one of the cases, adenocarcinomatous cells of signet-ring type exhibited pagetoid invasion into the surrounding squamous epithelium.
■ Invasive vaginal adenocarcinomas other than clear cell carcinomas include endometrioid adenocarcinomas (most of which arose from endometriosis or, less commonly, adenosis); adenocarcinomas of mucinous or intestinal type (two were DES related; another two were admixed with small cell carcinoma) (see below, Small Cell Carcinoma); adenosquamous carcinomas; paravaginal mesonephric adenocarcinomas and adnexal (wolffian) tumors (see Chapter 11); serous papillary adenocarcinoma; and adenoid cystic carcinoma.

References

Clement PB, Benedet JL. Adenocarcinoma in situ of the vagina. Cancer 43:2479–2485, 1979.
Cullimore JE, Luesley DM, Rollason TP, et al. A case of glandular intraepithelial neoplasia involving the cervix and vagina. Gynecol Oncol 34:249–252, 1989.
Daya D, Murphy J, Simon G. Paravaginal female adnexal tumor of probable wolffian origin. Am J Clin Pathol 101:275–278, 1994.
Demars LR, Van Le L, Huang I, Fowler WC. Primary non-clear-cell adenocarcinomas of the vagina in older DES-exposed women. Gynecol Oncol 58:389–392, 1995.
Fukushima M, Twiggs LB, Okagaki T. Mixed intestinal adenocarcinoma-argentaffin carcinoma of the vagina. Gynecol Oncol 23:387–394, 1986.
Haskel S, Chen SS, Spiegel G. Vaginal endometrioid adenocarcinoma arising in vaginal endometriosis: a case report and literature review. Gynecol Oncol 34:232–236, 1989.
Hinchey WM, Silva EG, Guarda LA, et al. Paravaginal wolffian duct (mesonephros) adenocarcinoma: a light and electron microscopic study. Am J Clin Pathol 80:539–544, 1983.
Riva C, Fabbri A, Facco C, et al. Primary serous papillary adenocarcinoma of the vagina: a case report. Int J Gynecol Pathol 16:286–290, 1997.
Rhatigan RM, Mojadidi Q. Adenosquamous carcinomas of the vulva and vagina. Am J Clin Pathol 59:208–217, 1973.
Yaghsezian H, Palazzo JP, Finkel GC, et al. Primary vaginal adenocarcinoma of the intestinal type associated with adenosis. Gynecol Oncol 45:62–65, 1992.

Small Cell Carcinoma

■ About 15 cases of primary small cell carcinoma of the vagina have been reported, most of which occurred in postmenopausal women. Most patients died of the disease, usually within 2 years of presentation.
■ Unusual clinical features included a presentation mimicking a Bartholin's gland abscess in one case and associated Cushing's syndrome related to corticotropin production by the tumor in another case. One tumor arose on a background of vaginal adenosis, and another had preceding vaginal intraepithelial neoplasia (VaIN).
■ On pathologic examination, the tumors were identical to their more common counterparts in the uterine cervix (see Chapter 6). Two tumors were associated with

an adenocarcinoma that were both of the intestinal type; one of these cases also had synchronous VaIN.

References

Colleran KM, Burge MR, Crooks LA, Dorin RI. Small cell carcinoma of the vagina causing Cushing's syndrome by ectopic production and secretion of ACTH: a case report. Gynecol Oncol 65:526–529, 1997.
Mirhashemi R, Kratz A, Weir MM, et al. Vaginal small cell carcinoma mimicking a Bartholin's gland abscess: a case report. Gynecol Oncol 68:297–300, 1998.

Transitional Cell Carcinoma

■ Three examples of transitional cell carcinomas (TCCs) and one squamotransitional cell carcinoma of the vagina have been reported in postmenopausal women. The three women with pure TCCs had had prior TCCs removed from the urinary tract.
■ The vaginal TCCs were all low grade and noninvasive and were multiple in two cases. One was associated with pagetoid spread of tumor cells into the surrounding benign epithelium. Two were associated with transitional cell metaplasia of the vaginal squamous epithelium.
■ Two tumors recurred, but there was no evidence of malignant behavior in any of the cases.

References

Bass PS, Birch B, Smart C, et al. Low-grade transitional cell carcinoma of the vagina—an unusual cause of vaginal bleeding. Histopathology 24:581–583, 1994.
Fetissof F, Haillot O, Lanson Y, et al. Papillary tumour of the vagina resembling transitional cell carcinoma. Pathol Res Pract 186:358–364, 1990.
Rose PG, Stoler MH, Abdul-Karim FW. Papillary squamotransitional cell carcinoma of the vagina. Int J Gynecol Pathol 17:372–375, 1998.
Singer G, Hohl MK, Hering F, Anabitarte M. Transitional cell carcinoma of the vagina with pagetoid spread pattern. Hum Pathol 29:299–301, 1998.

Embryonal Rhabdomyosarcoma

■ Embryonal rhabdomyosarcoma represents the most common type of vaginal cancer in infants and young children. About 90% are diagnosed in girls younger than 5 years of age (mean, 1.8 years); rare examples occur in young adults or even postmenopausal women.
■ The presenting features are vaginal bleeding and a vaginal mass that on clinical and gross examination is typically soft, edematous, and nodular, papillary, or polypoid (i.e., sarcoma botryoides), often with protrusion through the introitus.
■ On microscopic examination, a densely cellular zone (i.e., cambium layer) of primitive, small, mitotic cells subtends the squamous epithelium, which may be invaded by the tumor cells. Beneath the cambium layer lies a more sparsely cellular edematous zone in which similar small cells and rhabdomyoblasts are identified. Small islands of hyaline cartilage may also be present.
■ The rhabdomyoblasts, which vary from round to strap shaped, have eosinophilic cytoplasm in which cross

striations are usually evident. The rhabdomyoblasts may be sparse, and their identification can be facilitated with desmin and myoglobin stains, although only the latter is specific for skeletal muscle differentiation.

- The differential diagnosis includes fibroepithelial polyps with atypical cells (page 47) and rhabdomyomas (page 51). The latter lack the cambium layer and the primitive, small mitotic cells of rhabdomyosarcomas.
- The tumors can invade local structures and metastasize to regional lymph nodes or hematogenously to distant sites. Combinations of chemotherapy, irradiation, and surgery have resulted in cure rates of 90% to 95% in the Intergroup Rhabdomyosarcoma Studies.

References

Andrassy RJ, Hays DM, Raney RB, et al. Conservative surgical management of vaginal and vulvar pediatric rhabdomyosarcoma: a report from the Intergroup Rhabdomyosarcoma Study III. J Pediatr Surg 30: 1034–1037, 1995.

Hays DM, Shimada H, Raney B Jr, et al. Sarcomas of the vagina and uterus: the Intergroup Rhabdomyosarcoma Study. J Pediatr Surg 20: 718–724, 1985.

Hays DM, Shimada H, Raney B Jr, et al. Clinical staging and treatment results in rhabdomyosarcoma of the female genital tract among children and adolescents. Cancer 61:1893–1903, 1988.

Shy S-W, Lee W-H, Chen D, Ho S-Y. Rhabdomyosarcoma of the vagina in a postmenopausal woman: report of a case and review of the literature. Gynecol Oncol 58:395–399, 1995.

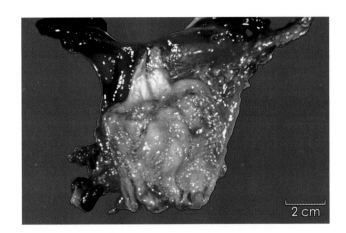

Figure 3–15. Embryonal rhabdomyosarcoma (sarcoma botryoides). A polypoid mass fills the vagina.

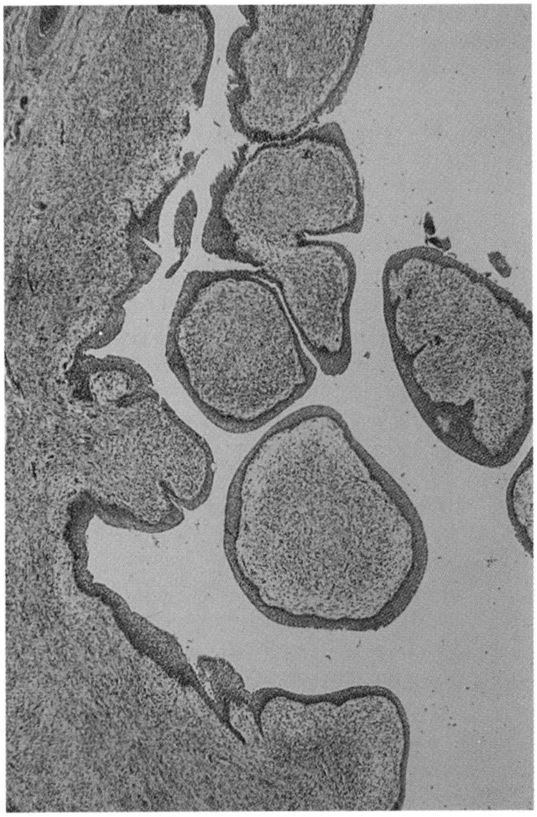

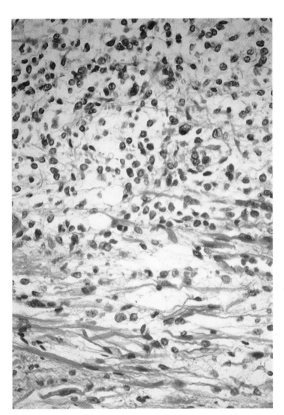

Figure 3–16. Embryonal rhabdomyosarcoma. The surface of the tumor is papillary. Notice the subepithelial cellular zone (cambium layer).

Figure 3–17. Embryonal rhabdomyosarcoma. Notice the admixture of small, round tumor cells with scanty cytoplasm and strap-shaped cells with eosinophilic cytoplasm.

Leiomyosarcoma

■ Leiomyosarcoma accounted for only 5 of 60 cases in the only large series of vaginal smooth muscle tumors. The patients with leiomyosarcoma were 32 to 72 years of age, and each presented with a vaginal mass. One patient was pregnant.

■ The leiomyosarcomas were 3 to 4 cm in the maximal dimension, and none was obviously malignant on gross examination. Mitotic rates ranged from 5 to 16 MFs per 10 HPFs, and the tumors had atypia that ranged from mild (one), to moderate (three), to severe (one). Only one had an infiltrative border.

■ The five tumors recurred locally after local excision. Only one tumor metastasized, and that patient died of the disease 10 months after diagnosis; it was the only tumor with infiltrating borders.

■ The foregoing findings contrast with those of two other studies (published in 1963 and 1984), in which most patients presented with larger, more advanced stage tumors. Ten of of the 13 tumors in these two series were fatal.

■ One paravaginal leiomyosarcoma in a 43-year-old woman was composed of epithelioid cells, some with a signet-ring appearance, separated by a myxoid stroma. Ultrastructural examination revealed smooth muscle differentiation. The patient died of the disease 22 months after presentation.

References

Chen KTK, Hafez GR, Gilbert EF. Myxoid variant of epithelioid smooth muscle tumor. Am J Clin Pathol 74:350–353, 1980.

Malkasian GD Jr, Welch JS, Soule EH. Primary leiomyosarcoma of the vagina: report of 8 cases. Am J Obstet Gynecol 86:730–736, 1963.

Rastogi BL, Bergman B, Angervall L. Primary leiomyosarcoma of the vagina: a study of five cases. Gynecol Oncol 18:77–86, 1984.

Tavassoli FA, Norris HJ. Smooth muscle tumors of the vagina. Obstet Gynecol 53:689–693, 1979.

Miscellaneous Sarcomas

■ Rare vaginal malignant müllerian mixed tumors (MMMTs), adenosarcomas, endometrial stromal sarcomas, alveolar soft part sarcomas, angiosarcomas (some after irradiation), malignant fibrous histocytomas, neurofibrosarcomas, and malignant schwannomas have been reported.

■ Two vaginal malignant mixed tumors that differed from the usual MMMT have been reported in women who were 24 and 33 years of age. Both of the tumors arose in the upper lateral vaginal wall. One tumor was thought to represent a synovial sarcoma, whereas light microscopic and ultrastructural findings in the other tumor suggested a mesonephric derivation.

■ Two "hemangiopericytomas" of the vagina have been reported, although the histologic features of these tumors could also be interpreted as extrauterine lowgrade endometrial stromal sarcomas.

References

Buscema J, Rosenshein NB, Taqi F, Woodruff JD. Vaginal hemangiopericytoma: a histopathologic and ultrastructural evaluation. Obstet Gynecol 66:82S–85S, 1985.

Curtin JP, Saigo P, Slucher B, et al. Soft-tissue sarcoma of the vagina and vulva: a clinicopathologic study. Obstet Gynecol 86:269–272, 1995.

Davis I, Abell MR. Sarcoma of the vagina. Obstet Gynecol 47:342–350, 1976.

McAdam JA, Stewart F, Reid R. Vaginal epithelioid angiosarcoma. J Clin Pathol 51:928–930, 1998.

Neesham D, Kerdemelidis P, Scurry J. Primary malignant mixed mullerian tumor of the vagina. Gynecol Oncol 70:303–307, 1999.

Nielsen GP, Oliva E, Young RH, et al. Alveolar soft-part sarcoma of the female genital tract. Int J Gynecol Pathol 14:283–292, 1995.

Okagaki T, Ishida T, Hilgers RD. A malignant tumor of the vagina resembling synovial sarcoma: a light and electron microscopic study. Cancer 37:2306–2320, 1976.

Peters WA III, Kumar NB, Andersen WA, Morley GW. Primary sarcoma of the adult vagina: a clinicopathologic study. Obstet Gynecol 65:699–704, 1985.

Shevchuk MM, Fenoglio CM, Lattes R, et al. Malignant mixed tumor of the vagina probably arising in mesonephric rests. Cancer 42:214–223, 1978.

Webb MJ, Symmonds RE, Weiland LH. Malignant fibrous histocytoma of the vagina. Am J Obstet Gynecol 119:190–192, 1974.

Malignant Melanoma

■ About 150 cases of vaginal melanoma have been reported, which represent 0.3% to 1% of all melanomas and 3% to 5% of vaginal cancers.

■ The tumors occur from the third to the ninth decades, but about 75% occur in women older than 50 years of age. The patients typically present with vaginal bleeding and, occasionally, a mass. Some tumors have been preceded by melanocytic hyperplasia (melanosis).

■ About 40% of the tumors occur in the lower third of the vagina. Some tumors also involve the vulva (i.e., vulvovaginal melanoma). The tumors are usually large, nodular to polypoid, and often ulcerated. Their typical pigmentation usually suggests the diagnosis; some tumors, however, are nonpigmented.

■ Vaginal melanomas resemble mucosal melanomas in other sites, including the usual presence of a junctional in situ component typically of lentiginous type with epidermal nests of atypical spindled melanocytes. The presence of the in situ component is helpful in establishing the diagnosis of melanoma and its primary nature. The invasive component may be spindled, epithelioid, or mixed.

■ In the differential diagnosis, the presence of an in situ component excludes metastatic melanoma and aids in the distinction of an amelanotic spindle cell melanoma from a sarcoma or a spindle cell carcinoma. Immunoreactivity for HMB-45 and S-100 and cytokeratin negativity help to confirm the diagnosis of melanoma. Benign pigmented lesions (page 49) lack the atypia, mitotic activity, and invasion of melanomas.

■ The prognosis is poor because of the usual presence of deep invasion (>3 mm) and often advanced stage of the disease, including involved local lymph nodes. A literature review up to 1985 found a 5-year survival rate of only 8.4%, although the corresponding figure from a more recent review was 21%. In the same study, 43% of patients with tumors 3 cm or smaller survived 5 years, compared with 0% of those with tumors larger than 3 cm.

References

Brand E, Fu YS, Lagasse LD, Berek JS. Vulvovaginal melanoma: report of seven cases and literature review. Gynecol Oncol 33:54–60, 1989.

Chung AF, Casey MJ, Flannery JT, et al. Malignant melanoma of the vagina—report of 19 cases. Obstet Gynecol 55:720–727, 1980.

Kerley SW, Blute ML, Keeney GL. Multifocal malignant melanoma arising in vesicovaginal melanosis. Arch Pathol Lab Med 115:950–952, 1991.

Petru E, Nagele F, Czerwenka K, et al. Primary malignant melanoma of the vagina: long-term remission following radiation therapy. Gynecol Oncol 70:23–26, 1998.

Van Nostrand KM, Lucci JA III, Schell M, et al. Primary vaginal melanoma: improved survival with radical pelvic surgery. Gynecol Oncol 55:234–237, 1994.

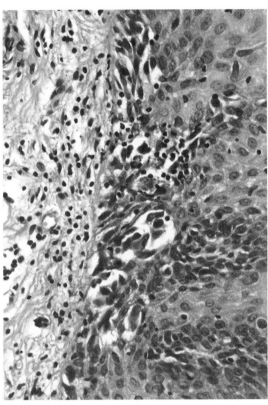

Figure 3–18. Malignant melanoma. The in situ lentiginous component was associated with invasive melanoma.

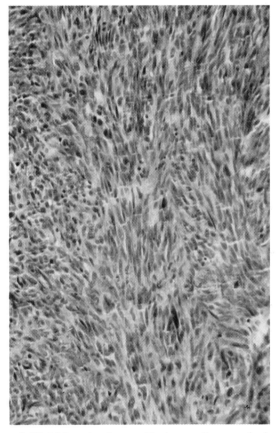

Figure 3–19. Malignant melanoma. The tumor cells are predominantly spindled, potentially mimicking a sarcoma. No pigment is seen in this field.

Yolk Sac Tumors of Vagina and Cervix

■ About 75 yolk sac tumors (YSTs) have been reported in the vagina, which account for 90% of extragonadal yolk sac tumors in the female genital tract. Much less common, but otherwise similar in age and presentation, are cases of YST involving both the vagina and cervix or the cervix alone.

■ Vaginal YSTs occur in children younger than 3 years of age who typically present with vaginal bleeding or discharge and a vaginal mass. The serum alpha-fetoprotein level is usually elevated.

■ On gross examination, the vaginal mucosa is involved by a polypoid or sessile, sometimes ulcerated, tumor that is usually smaller than 5 cm. The sectioned surfaces are typically soft, friable, and white to gray-tan and have areas of hemorrhage and necrosis. One vaginal YST was a 6-cm paravaginal mass without mucosal involvement.

■ The microscopic features are identical to ovarian YSTs (see Chapter 15).

■ More than 50% of patients with vaginal YSTs in the older literature died of their disease despite radical surgical therapy. Current combination chemotherapy, with or without conservative surgical removal, achieves a cure in most cases.

References

Copeland LJ, Sneige N, Ordonez NG, et al. Endodermal sinus tumor of the vagina and cervix. Cancer 55:2558–2565, 1985.

Liebhart M. Histopathological diagnosis of vaginal endodermal sinus tumors in infants. Int J Gynecol Pathol 5:217–222, 1986.

Young RH, Scully RE. Endodermal sinus tumor of the vagina: a report of nine cases and review of the literature. Gynecol Oncol 18:380–392, 1984.

Hematopoietic Tumors

■ Secondary involvement of the vagina is much more common than primary vaginal lymphoma. Patients with the latter have been 19 to 79 years old (mean, about 50 years) and presented with vaginal bleeding or discharge, pain or dyspareunia, or a mass. Clinical and gross examination reveals an ill-defined, rubbery to firm, gray-white thickening or induration of the vaginal wall.

■ Most of the lymphomas are of the diffuse large cell type, but rare cases of follicular mixed small and large cell, diffuse mixed, Burkitt's, and angiocentric T-cell lymphoma have been reported. Sclerosis, as in cervical lymphomas, is often prominent. Rare vaginal plasmacytomas have been documented.

■ Vaginal lymphomas are often misdiagnosed. The differential diagnosis is the same as for cervical lymphomas (see Chapter 10).

■ Vaginal lymphomas that are Ann Arbor stage I have a favorable prognosis after treatment with radiation therapy, chemotherapy, or both. In one review of seven patients, all were free of disease at last follow-up, although one patient had had a relapse at 5 years.

References

Doss LL. Simultaneous extramedullary plasmacytomas of the vagina and vulva: a case report and review of the literature. Cancer 41:2468–2474, 1978.

Ferry JA, Young RH. Malignant lymphoma of the genitourinary tract. Curr Diagn Pathol 4:145–169, 1997.

Harris NL, Scully RE. Malignant lymphoma and granulocytic sarcoma of the uterus and vagina: a clinicopathologic analysis of 27 cases. Cancer 53:2530–2545, 1984

Perren T, Farrant M, McCarthy K, et al. Lymphomas of the cervix and upper vagina: a report of five cases and a review of the literature. Gynecol Oncol 44:87–95, 1992.

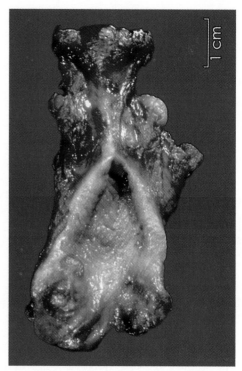

Figure 3–20. Yolk sac tumor in a hysterectomy-vaginectomy specimen. A polypoid mass is in the lower vagina (*lower left*).

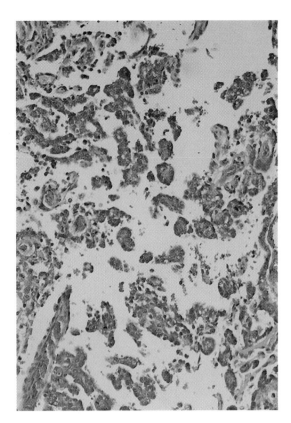

Figure 3–21. Yolk sac tumor of the vagina. The tumor has an unusually florid papillary pattern.

Histiocytosis X

- Rare cases of vaginal involvement by histiocytosis X have been documented. In some of these cases, the vaginal involvement was the presenting manifestation of subsequent progressive disease. In other cases, the vaginal lesions followed oral or cutaneous lesions or diabetes insipidus.

References

Axiotis CA, Merino MJ, Duray PH. Langerhans cell histiocytosis of the female genital tract. Cancer 67:1650–1660, 1991.

Secondary Tumors

- Fu and Reagan found that only 16% of invasive carcinomas involving the vagina were primary. The remainder were secondary from tumors primary in other pelvic sites that included, in order of frequency, the cervix, endometrium, colon and rectum, ovary, vulva, and urinary bladder or urethra. Even 75% of vaginal squamous cell carcinomas were secondary, usually from the cervix or vulva.

- In most such cases, the spread is by direct invasion or through lymphatics, the primary tumor is clinically evident or has already been treated, and the diagnosis is straightforward. In contrast, carcinomas in distant sites, particularly the kidney and breast, can rarely metastasize to the vagina and may be the presenting manifestation of the tumor.

- Metastatic renal cell carcinoma may be confused with a primary vaginal clear cell carcinoma. The latter diagnosis should be favored in the presence of vaginal adenosis or endometriosis, a tubulocystic pattern, hobnail cells, and mucin, as well as an absence of the characteristic sinusoidal vascular pattern of renal cell carcinomas.

- Spread of trophoblast to the vagina can occur in patients with gestational trophoblastic disease. Vaginal spread of choriocarcinoma occurs in as many as 50% of patients with uterine chorocarcinoma. In molar gestations, vaginal nodules can consist of typical molar villi or avillous trophoblast. Vaginal nodules of intermediate trophoblast have also been described in normal pregnancies.

References

Fu YS, Reagan JW. Nonepithelial and metastatic tumors of the lower genital tract. In Fu YS, Reagan JW (eds): Pathology of the Uterine Cervix, Vagina, and Vulva. Major Problems in Pathology, vol 21. Philadelphia: WB Saunders, 1989.

Haines M. Hydatidiform mole and vaginal nodules. J Obstet Gynaecol Br Emp 62:6–11, 1955.

Tarraza HM Jr, Meltzer SE, DeCain M, Jones MA. Vaginal metastases from renal cell carcinoma: report of four cases and review of the literature. Eur J Gynecol Oncol 19:14–18, 1998.

CHAPTER 4

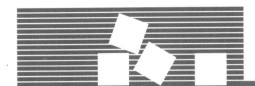

Tumor-like Lesions and Benign Epithelial Tumors of the Uterine Cervix

METAPLASIAS

Typical Squamous Metaplasia

- Squamous metaplasia results in the replacement of endocervical surface and glandular epithelium by squamous epithelium. Florid squamous metaplasia within the endocervical glands can simulate invasive squamous cell carcinoma.
- Features favoring squamous metaplasia include a superficial location, nests of cells with smooth contours consistent with replaced endocervical glands, bland nuclear features, absence of a stromal response, the presence of residual mucinous epithelial cells, gland lumens, or luminal mucin, and absence of dysplasia in the adjacent squamous epithelium.

Transitional Cell Metaplasia of the Cervix and Vagina

General Features

- Transitional cell metaplasia (TCM) is usually an incidental microscopic finding in postmenopausal women. An abnormal Pap smear is occasionally the presenting feature in premenopausal or postmenopausal women. The appearance of the cells of TCM on Pap smears is distinctive, allowing their separation from cervical intraepithelial neoplasia (CIN), atrophy, and tubal metaplasia.
- The occurrence in postmenopausal women and in transsexual women receiving androgen therapy suggests hypoestrinism as a cause in some cases.

Microscopic Features

- The surface or glandular epithelium of the endocervix and transformation zone, native ectocervix, and vagina

may be involved. Occasionally, the involved epithelium may invaginate into the underlying stroma, or nests of transitional cells are isolated in the stroma.
- The epithelium is replaced by 6 to 30 layers of cells with pale, uniform, oval to spindle nuclei that are usually oriented vertically in the deeper layers and horizontally with a streaming or whorled pattern superficially. Perinuclear halos may be present. A superficial layer of "umbrella" cells is seen in some cases.
- The nuclear to cytoplasmic ratio varies, and the nuclei have finely stippled chromatin, inconspicuous nucleoli, and occasional longitudinal nuclear grooves; mitotic figures are rare or absent.
- Rarely, cells with features of TCM have superimposed dysplastic changes.

Differential Diagnosis

- The lack of normal maturation may result in confusion with high-grade CIN, but the bland nuclear features and absent or rare mitotic figures distinguish typical TCM from CIN.
- The numerous layers of cells and nuclear grooves distinguish TCM from atrophic squamous epithelium.

References

Egan AJM, Russell P. Transitional (urothelial) cell metaplasia of the uterine cervix: morphological assessment of 31 cases. Int J Gynecol Pathol 16:89–98, 1997.

Miller N, Bedard YC, Cooter NB, Shaul DL. Histological changes in the genital tract in transsexual women following androgen therapy. Histopathology 10:661–669, 1986.

Weir MM, Bell DA. Transitional cell metaplasia of the cervix: a newly described entity in cervicovaginal smears. Diagn Cytopathol 18:222–226, 1998.

Weir MM, Bell DA, Young RH. Transitional cell metaplasia of the uterine cervix and vagina: An underecognized lesion that may be confused with high-grade dysplasia. Am J Surg Pathol 21:510–517, 1997.

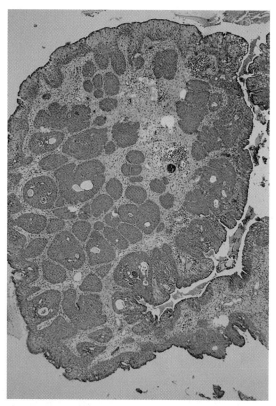

Figure 4–1. Florid squamous metaplasia in a cervical polyp. This appearance may be misdiagnosed as invasive squamous carcinoma.

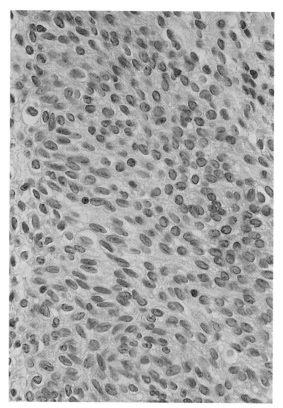

Figure 4–2. Transitional cell metaplasia. The nuclei are elongated and appear to be "streaming."

Tubal, Tuboendometrioid, and Endometrioid Metaplasia

General Features

■ Tubal metaplasia (TM) refers to the replacement of the endocervical columnar epithelium by tubal-type epithelium. Less commonly, the epithelium is intermediate in appearance between tubal and endometrioid epithelium (i.e., tuboendometrioid metaplasia [TEM]), or rarely, it is purely endometrioid in appearance (i.e., endometrioid metaplasia).

■ These metaplasias are almost always an incidental microscopic finding. The initial manifestation of TM is often the presence of abnormal cells in a Pap smear.

■ TM was found in 21% of cone biopsy and 62% of hysterectomy specimens in one study. TEM was found in 26% of post–cone biopsy hysterectomy specimens in one series, suggesting that it may be a reparative response in some cases.

Microscopic Features

■ In TM, the endocervical surface or glandular epithelium is replaced by a single layer composed of admixed ciliated, nonciliated, and peg cells. TEM is similar to TM, except that ciliated cells are less common. The nonciliated columnar cells of TEM may have apical snouts.

■ The glands involved by TM and TEM are usually similar to normal endocervical glands in size, shape, and distribution. Unusual findings in TM and TEM include variability in gland size and shape, cystic dilatation, focal crowding, a deep location (see Deep Glands and Cysts, page 70), and periglandular stromal hypercellularity or edema.

■ TM and TEM are distinguished from adenocarcinoma in situ by an admixture of cell types, an absence of atypia, and an absence or paucity of mitotic figures and from invasive adenocarcinoma by the absence of an infiltrative pattern.

■ Rarely, TM may merge with atypical TM and ciliated adenocarcinoma in situ (see Chapter 6).

Differential Diagnosis

■ Typical endometriosis of the cervix (page 72). The finding that differentiates this lesion from tuboendometrioid or endometrioid metaplasia is the presence of endometrial-type periglandular stroma. The latter, however, may be sparse and partly obscured by inflammatory cells.

■ Ciliated adenocarcinoma in situ (see Chapter 6). This lesion is distinguished from tubal and tuboendometrioid metaplasia by the presence of malignant nuclear features.

■ Mesonephric hyperplasia (page 73). This lesion can contain glands with an endometrioid-like appearance. The usual deep location of the process and admixture of more typical mesonephric tubules with their characteristic colloid-like luminal secretions facilitate the diagnosis.

References

Babkowski RC, Wilbur DC, Rutkowski MA, et al. The effects of endocervical canal topography, tubal metaplasia, and high canal sampling on the cytologic presentation of nonneoplastic endocervical cells. Am J Clin Pathol 105:403–410, 1996.

Jonasson JG, Wang HH, Antonioli DA, Ducatman BS. Tubal metaplasia of the uterine cervix: a prevalence study in patients with gynecologic pathologic findings. Int J Gynecol Pathol 11:89–95, 1992.

Ismail SM. Cone biopsy causes cervical endometriosis and tubo-endometrioid metaplasia. Histopathology 18:107–114, 1991.

Oliva E, Clement PB, Young RH. Tubal and tubo-endometrioid metaplasia of the uterine cervix: unemphasized features that may cause problems in differential diagnosis. A report of 25 cases. Am J Clin Pathol 103:618–623, 1995.

Schlesinger C, Silverberg SG. Endocervical adenocarcinoma in situ of tubal type and its relation to atypical tubal metaplasia. Int J Gynecol Pathol 18:1–4, 1999.

Suh K, Silverberg SG. Tubal metaplasia of the uterine cervix. Int J Gynecol Pathol 9:122–128, 1990.

Yeh I, Bronner M, LiVolsi VA. Endometrial metaplasia of the uterine cervix. Arch Pathol Lab Med 117:734–735, 1993.

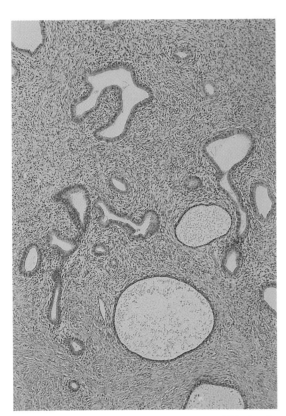

Figure 4–3. Tubal metaplasia. The glands are variable in size and shape, and some are cystic. The periglandular stroma is more cellular than normal endocervical stroma.

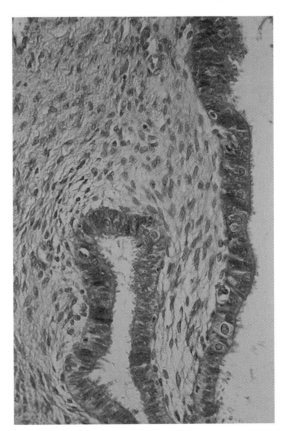

Figure 4–4. Tubal metaplasia.

Intestinal Metaplasia

■ Intestinal metaplasia is characterized by the presence of goblet and argentaffin cells within the endocervical glands.

■ The finding is rare in a pure (nondysplastic) form as it is usually associated with nuclear features of adenocarcinoma in situ (i.e., intestinal type of adenocarcinoma in situ) (see Chapter 6).

Reference

Trowell JE. Intestinal metaplasia with argentaffin cells in the uterine cervix. Histopathology 9:551–559, 1985.

Oxyphilic Metaplasia

■ Oxyphilic metaplasia, which is an incidental microscopic finding of no apparent clinical significance, is characterized by replacement of the endocervical glandular or surface epithelium by a single layer of large, often cuboidal cells with dense, eosinophilic, focally vacuolated cytoplasm with enlarged hyperchromatic nuclei but usually no mitotic activity.

■ A lack of cellular stratification, marked atypicality, and mitotic activity facilitates distinction from endocervical glandular dysplasia and adenocarcinoma in situ.

Reference

Jones MA, Young RH. Atypical oxyphilic metaplasia of the endocervical epithelium: a report of six cases. Int J Gynecol Pathol 16:99–102, 1997.

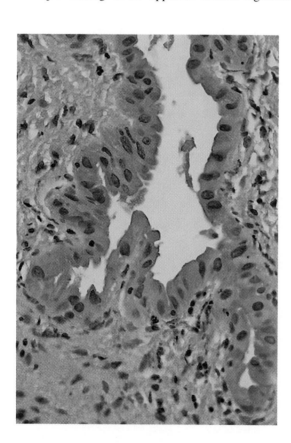

Figure 4–5. Atypical oxyphilic metaplasia.

ENDOCERVICAL GLANDULAR HYPERPLASIAS

Microglandular Hyperplasia

- Microglandular hyperplasia (MGH) is a distinctive proliferation of endocervical glands, often related to estrogen and progesterone stimulation (e.g., oral contraceptives, pregnancy). Occasional examples occur in women receiving only estrogen, only progesterone, or those with no apparent hormonal intake.
- MGH usually occurs in the reproductive age group; fewer than 5% of cases are postmenopausal. The patients are usually asymptomatic; vaginal bleeding or discharge are rare symptoms. There is usually no grossly visible lesion, but occasionally MGH appears as an erosion or polyp.
- Microscopically, closely packed glands range from small and round to larger and cystic with a variable shape. Their lumens often contain inspissated mucin and inflammatory cells. Scanty stroma is usually infiltrated with acute and chronic inflammatory cells.
- The glands are lined by low columnar, cuboidal, or flattened cells, frequently with subnuclear vacuoles and small, regular nuclei with inconspicuous nucleoli and absent to rare mitotic figures. Focal squamous metaplasia is often present.
- Unusual microscopic features include:
  - Solid, reticular, and trabecular patterns
  - An edematous, myxoid, or hyalinized stroma, sometimes containing irregularly disposed epithelial aggregates, resulting in a pseudoinfiltrative pattern
  - Unusual cell types including spindle-shaped cells, polygonal cells with abundant eosinophilic cytoplasm, and cells with intracellular mucin vacuoles resembling signet-ring cells
  - Mild to moderate degrees of nuclear pleomorphism
- The differential diagnosis is usually with clear cell adenocarcinoma or rare cervical adenocarcinomas of the endocervical type with a microglandular pattern. Features indicating or favoring adenocarcinoma include symptoms, a mass, cells with abundant clear (glycogen-rich) cytoplasm (in clear cell carcinoma), marked nuclear atypicality, more than rare mitotic figures, strong cytoplasmic immunoreactivity for carcinoembryonic antigen (CEA), and obvious invasion.

References

Nichols TM, Fidler HK. Microglandular hyperplasia in cervical cone biopsies taken for suspicious and positive cytology. Am J Clin Pathol 56:424–429, 1971.

Leslie KO, Silverberg SG. Microglandular hyperplasia of the cervix: unusual clinical and pathological presentations and their differential diagnosis. Prog Surg Pathol 5:95–114, 1984.

Chumas JC, Nelson B, Mann WJ, et al. Microglandular hyperplasia of the uterine cervix. Obstet Gynecol 66:406–409, 1985.

Greeley C, Schroeder S, Silverberg SG. Microglandular hyperplasia of the cervix: a true "pill" lesion? Int J Gynecol Pathol 14:50–54, 1995.

Steeper TA, Wick MR. Minimal deviation adenocarcinoma of the uterine cervix ("adenoma malignum"): an immunohistochemical comparison with microglandular endocervical hyperplasia and conventional endocervical adenocarcinoma. Cancer 58:1131–1138, 1986.

Wilkinson E, Dufour DR. Pathogenesis of microglandular hyperplasia of the cervix uteri. Obstet Gynecol 47:189–195, 1976.

Young RH, Scully RE. Atypical forms of microglandular hyperplasia of the cervix simulating carcinoma: a report of five cases and review of the literature. Am J Surg Pathol 13:50–56, 1989.

Young RH, Scully RE. Uterine carcinomas simulating microglandular hyperplasia: a report of six cases. Am J Surg Pathol 16:1092–1097, 1992.

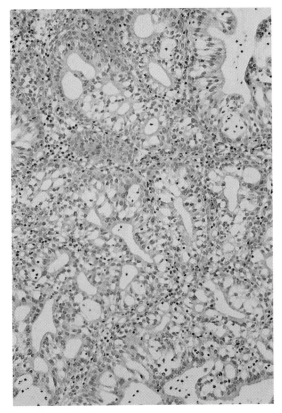

Figure 4–6. Microglandular hyperplasia.

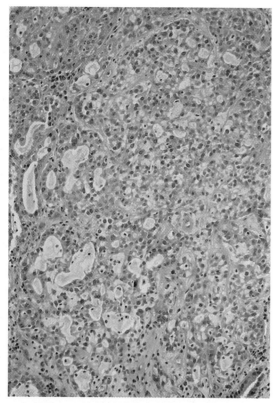

Figure 4–7. Microglandular hyperplasia. The proliferation is unusually cellular, and there is mild nuclear atypia.

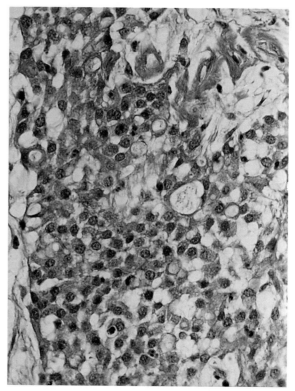

Figure 4–8. Microglandular hyperplasia. There is a solid proliferation of cells with mild nuclear atypicality and occasional signet-ring–like cells.

Diffuse Laminar Endocervical Glandular Hyperplasia

- Diffuse laminar endocervical glandular hyperplasia is a rare, incidental microscopic finding, which occurs in women of reproductive age and is characterized by a circumferential, bandlike proliferation of closely packed endocervical glands that is sharply circumscribed from the underlying cervical stroma.
- The usually moderately sized glands are lined by endocervical columnar cells, sometimes with mild reactive cytologic atypia. Marked stromal chronic inflammation is common.
- Distinguishing features from adenoma malignum (see Chapter 6) include a sharply circumscribed border, absence of invasion, and lack of focally malignant cytologic features or a desmoplastic stroma.

Reference

Jones MA, Young RH, Scully RE. Diffuse laminar endocervical glandular hyperplasia: a report of seven cases. Am J Surg Pathol 15:1123–1129, 1991.

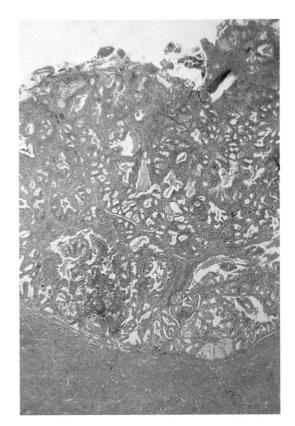

Figure 4–9. Diffuse laminar endocervical glandular hyperplasia. Notice the sharp margin with the subjacent stroma.

Lobular and Generalized Glandular Hyperplasia

- These endocervical glandular proliferations are usually an incidental histologic finding in women in the reproductive and postmenopausal age groups. Rare cases have been associated with a mucoid discharge, abnormal glandular cells on Pap smear, or a gross abnormality.
- There is a spectrum of changes ranging from distinctinctly lobular proliferations of small to moderate sized glands that often are centered on a larger central gland to more generalized proliferations of more variably sized glands. Cystic glands are prominent in some cases and may be grossly visible.
- The glands are lined by benign-appearing endocervical columnar mucinous cells with focally mild atypia and rare mitotic figures in occasional cases. Intraglandular

bridging, including a cribriform pattern, may be seen in some cases.
- The stroma immediately surrounding the glands varies from normal to thin cuffs of slightly to moderately cellular fibroblastic stroma.
- Distinguishing features from minimal-deviation adenocarcinoma include a superficial location, a lobular pattern in some cases, no more than mild atypia and occasional mitoses, and absence of a desmoplastic stromal response.

Reference

Nucci MR, Clement PB, Young RH. Lobular endocervical glandular hyperplasia, a clinicopathologic analysis of thirteen cases of a distinctive pseudoneoplastic lesion and comparison with fourteen cases of adenoma malignum. Am J Surg Pathol 23:886–891, 1999.

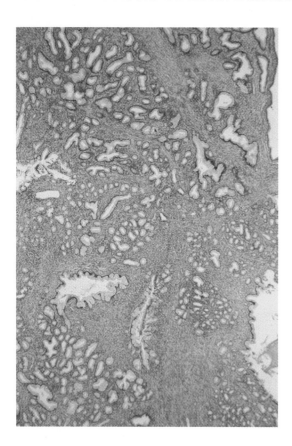

Figure 4–10. Lobular endocervical glandular hyperplasia.

MISCELLANEOUS ENDOCERVICAL GLANDULAR LESIONS

Deep Glands and Cysts

- Otherwise typical endocervical glands or their cystic counterparts (i.e., nabothian cysts) uncommonly extend into the outer third of the cervical wall. Deep glands are an incidental microscopic finding, but deep nabothian cysts may result in a striking gross appearance.
- In contrast to the glands of adenocarcinoma (see Chapter 6), deep glands and cysts are usually widely spaced, relatively uniform in size and shape, and lack cytologic atypia and a periglandular stromal response.

References

Clement PB, Young RH. Deep Nabothian cysts of the endocervix: a possible source of confusion with minimal-deviation adenocarcinoma (adenoma malignum). Int J Gynecol Pathol 8:340–348, 1989.
Daya D, Young RH. Florid deep glands of the uterine cervix: another mimic of adenoma malignum. Am J Clin Pathol 103:614–617, 1995.

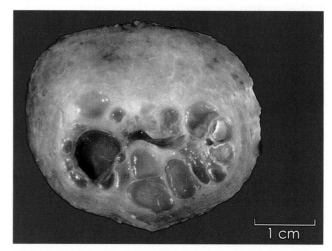

Figure 4–11. Deep nabothian cysts.

Tunnel Clusters

- Tumor clusters (TCs), first described by Fluhmann, who recognized cystic (type B) and noncystic (type A) forms, are almost always an incidental pathologic finding that occur in about 10% of adult women. Rare cases may be associated with a mucoid discharge. Cystic TCs are grossly visible in 40% of cases.
- TCs are multiple in 80% of cases, and in such cases are occasionally confluent. They are usually superficial but occasionally extend deeply, and are surrounded by normal endocervical stroma.
- A TC is a discrete, rounded aggregate of 20 to 50 oval, round or irregular, closely packed tubules of various sizes. The tubules are lined by a single layer of flattened to cuboidal cells when cystic or by cuboidal to columnar cells when noncystic.
- The nuclear features are usually bland, and mitotic figures are usually absent. Mild to moderate nuclear atypia and rare mitoses are present in some cases, particularly in noncystic TCs.
- The lobular arrangment, lack of an infiltrative pattern, and a lack of a stromal response facilitate distinction from adenoma malignum (see Chapter 6).
- The appearance of TCs and their strong association with multiparity suggests that TCs are involutional in nature and should not be referred to as "adenomatous hyperplasia."

References

Fluhmann CF. Focal hyperplasia (tunnel clusters) of the cervix uteri. Obstet Gynecol 17:206–214, 1961.

Jones MA, Young RH. Endocervical type A (noncystic) tunnel clusters with cytologic atypia: a report of 14 cases. Am J Surg Pathol 20: 1312–1318, 1996.

Segal GH, Hart WR. Cystic endocervical tunnel clusters: a clinicopathologic study of 29 cases of so-called adenomatous hyperplasia. Am J Surg Pathol 14:895–903, 1990.

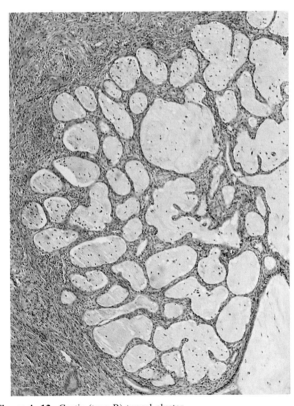

Figure 4–12. Cystic (type B) tunnel cluster.

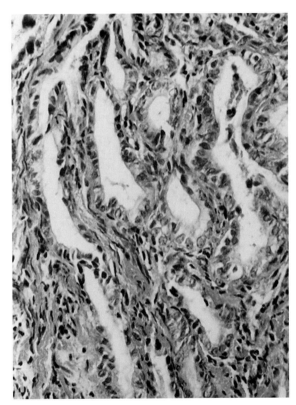

Figure 4–13. Noncystic (type A) tunnel cluster. Notice the degenerative-type nuclear atypia.

ENDOMETRIOSIS AND ENDOCERVICOSIS

Typical Endometriosis

■ Cervical endometriosis may be superficial (mucosal) or deep. Superficial cervical endometriosis is frequently localized to areas of prior biopsy or cautery, suggesting implantation of menstrual endometrium as a causative factor. Deep cervical endometriosis is usually an extension of cul-de-sac involvement in women with more widespread pelvic endometriosis.

■ The microscopic diagnosis of superficial endometriosis can be missed when hemorrhage or inflammation obscures the sometimes sparse endometriotic stroma. In such cases, atypia or mitotic activity in the endometriotic glands can be misinterpreted as endocervical glandular dysplasia or adenocarcinoma in situ.

Stromal Endometriosis

■ Stromal endometriosis, an uncommon variant of endometriosis characterized by an exclusive or almost exclusive component of endometriotic stroma, is most common in the cervix and ovary. The term should not be used (as in the older literature) to refer to low-grade endometrial stromal sarcoma (LGESS).

■ In stromal endometriosis, well-circumscribed foci within the superficial cervical stroma are composed of endometrial stromal cells, small blood vessels, and extravasated erythrocytes.

■ Rare endometriotic glands are identifiable in some cases. The characteristic permeative growth pattern and vascular invasion of LGESS are absent.

References

Baker PM, Clement PB, Bell DA, Young RH. Superficial endometriosis of the uterine cervix: a report of 20 cases of a process that may be confused with endocervical glandular dysplasia or adenocarcinoma in situ. Int J Gynecol Pathol 18:198–205, 1999.

Clement PB, Young RH, Scully RE. Stromal endometriosis of the uterine cervix: a variant of endometriosis that may simulate a sarcoma. Am J Surg Pathol 14:449–455, 1990.

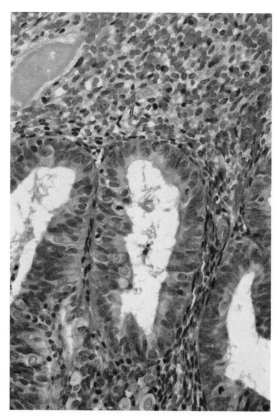

Figure 4–14. Superficial endometriosis. The endometriotic stroma is partly obscured by stromal hemorrhage. Notice the mitotic figures in the endometriotic glands.

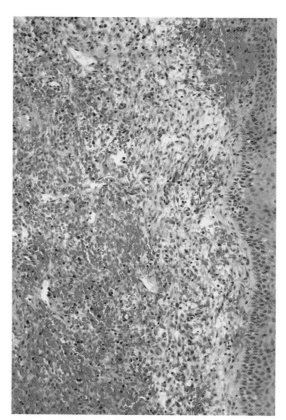

Figure 4–15. Stromal endometriosis. Notice the extensive extravasation of erythrocytes that partially obscure the endometrial stromal cells.

Endocervicosis

- Endocervicosis refers to the presence of ectopic, benign-appearing endocervical-like glands (see Chapter 19). Involvement of the outer wall of the cervix is encountered in rare cases of endocervicosis of the urinary bladder, a finding that may simulate adenoma malignum (minimal-deviation adenocarcinoma) of the endocervix.
- Features distinguishing endocervicosis from adenoma malignum include a mass in the posterior wall of the urinary bladder and an absence of a mucosa-based endocervical tumor.

Reference

Clement PB, Young RH. Endocervicosis of the urinary bladder: a report of six cases of a benign müllerian lesion that may mimic adenocarcinoma. Am J Surg Pathol 16:533–542, 1992.

MESONEPHRIC LESIONS

Mesonephric Remnants

- Mesonephric remnants, which occur in the walls of the cervix in as many as 10% of women, are an incidental microscopic finding in reproductive and postmenopausal age groups.
- The remnants consist of one to several small, well-circumscribed, lobular aggregates of mesonephric tubules, with or without a central mesonephric duct. The cells lining the tubules exhibit no atypia or mitotic activity.

Mesonephric Hyperplasia

- Mesonephric hyperplasia usually occurs in reproductive and postmenopausal age groups. It is almost always an incidental microscopic finding, but it is rarely associated with induration, nodularity, or an "erosion."
- Remnants of the mesonephric duct are present in most cases. The proliferation may extend to the overlying endocervical mucosa or margins of a cone biopsy specimen. Extension into the deep cervical stroma or the lower uterine segment may be seen in some hysterectomy specimens.
- Tubules in a lobular (80% of cases) or diffuse (nonlobular) pattern range from small and uniform to variably sized and shaped and cystic. The tubules usually contain a characteristic eosinophilic, colloid-like, periodic acid–Schiff (PAS) positive luminal secretion. There is usually no stromal response.
- The tubules and cysts are usually lined by a single layer of mucin-free cuboidal and flattened cells, respectively. The nuclei are usually uniform but occasionally mildly atypical. Mitotic figures are rare (less than 1 mitotic figure per 10 high-power fields) or absent.
- Unusual features include the focal presence of columnar cells that impart a pseudoendometrioid appearance. Cellular stratification and bridging are rare.
- The postoperative clinical course is uneventful, including cases in which the lesion extends to the margin of the specimen. Rare mesonephric neoplasms (see Chapter 6) have been contiguous with mesonephric hyperplasia.
- The differential diagnosis is with adenocarcinoma, especially adenoma malignum (see Chapter 6) and clear cell carcinoma (see Chapter 6). Features favoring mesonephric hyperplasia over adenoma malignum include an absence of mucosal involvement, mucin-free cytoplasm, absence of a periglandular stromal response, and nonreactivity for CEA.
- Features favoring or establishing a diagnosis of clear cell adenocarcinoma over that of mesonephric hyperplasia include papillary and solid growth patterns; cells with clear, glycogen-rich cytoplasm; hobnail cells; marked nuclear atypia; and frequent mitotic figures.

Mesonephric Ductal Hyperplasia

- This finding, in which the mesonephric duct is lined by hyperplastic epithelium, typically in the form of micropapillary tufts, is most commonly associated with mesonephric hyperplasia but rarely is an isolated finding.
- Misdiagnosis as a premalignant or malignant glandular lesion may occur, particularly when it is an isolated finding. Features favoring mesonephric ductal hyperplasia include an elongated duct, micropapillae, an absence of nuclear atypia, and lack of association with endocervical glands.

References

Clement PB, Young RH, Keh P, et al. Malignant mesonephric neoplasms of the uterine cervix: a report of eight cases, including four with a malignant spindle cell component. Am J Surg Pathol 19:1158–1171, 1995.

Ferry JA, Scully RE. Mesonephric remnants, hyperplasia and neoplasia in the uterine cervix: a study of 49 cases. Am J Surg Pathol 14:1100–1111, 1990.

Jones MA, Andrews J, Tarraza H. Mesonephric remnant hyperplasia of the cervix: a clinicopathologic analysis of 14 cases. Gynecol Oncol 49:41–47, 1993.

Seidman JD, Tavassoli FA. Mesonephric hyperplasia of the uterine cervix: a clinicopathologic study of 51 cases. Int J Gynecol Pathol 14:293–299, 1995.

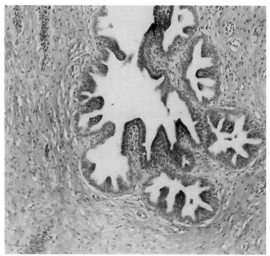

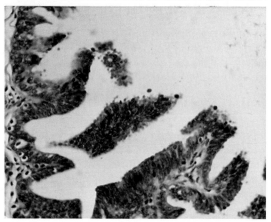

Figure 4–16. Mesonephric duct remnant (*top*) shows ductal hyperplasia with stratified cells and cellular papillae (*bottom*).

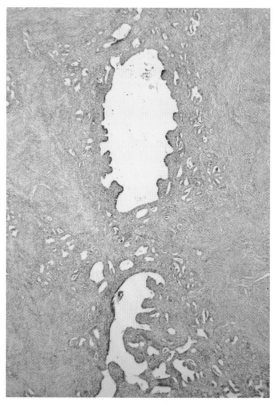

Figure 4–17. Mesonephric hyperplasia. The mesonephric duct remnants are surrounded by lobular clusters of mesonephric tubules.

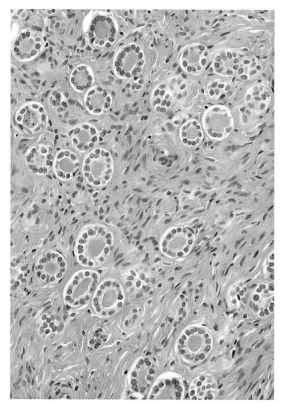

Figure 4–18. Mesonephric hyperplasia. Notice the uniform, small tubules with eosinophilic luminal secretion.

INFLAMMATORY, INFECTIOUS, REACTIVE, AND REPARATIVE LESIONS

Postbiopsy Pseudoinvasion of Squamous Epithelium

- This finding, which results from implantation of squamous epithelium at the time of a previous biopsy, may be confused with squamous carcinoma because of a deep location, a lack of nearby endocervical glands, irregularity of the squamous nests, associated fibrotic stroma, and the presence of preneoplastic changes in the previous biopsy.
- The correct diagnosis is suggested by the presence of only a few nests, presence of bland nuclear features, absence of abnormal epithelium between the deep nests and surface epithelium, and absence of associated dysplasia of the surface epithelium.
- A similar finding was exemplified by a case in which there was artifactual displacement of CIN epithelium into blood vessels caused by lidocaine injection before loop diathermy.

References

McLachlin CM, Devine P, Muto M, Genest DR. Pseudoinvasion of vascular spaces: report of an artifact caused by cervical lidocaine injection prior to loop diathermy. Hum Pathol 25:208–211, 1994.

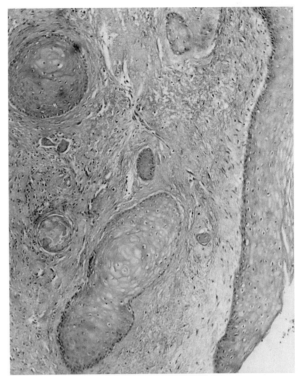

Figure 4–19. Postbiopsy pseudoinvasion of squamous epithelium. Irregular nests of benign squamous epithelium lie within a fibrotic stroma.

Reactive and Reparative Atypia

- Squamous atypia is discussed in Chapter 5.
- Glandular atypia may occur in otherwise normal endocervical surface or glandular epithelium, metaplastic epithelium (e.g., tubal metaplasia), or the glands of non-neoplastic cervical lesions (e.g., tunnel clusters).
  - The cytoplasm may be mucin depleted and variably eosinophilic; the appearance may merge with that of atypical oxyphilic metaplasia (page 79). The nuclei are variable in size and shape and variably hyperchromatic with a "smudgy" appearance. There are usually associated chronic inflammatory cells in the superficial stroma.
  - Differences from adenocarcinoma in situ include atypical cells separated by normal-appearing cells, lack of cellular stratification, absence or rarity of mitotic figures, and lack of apoptotic bodies. Similar changes may be seen after irradiation to the cervix (see page 79).

Papillary Endocervicitis

- Papillary endocervicitis is usually an incidental microscopic finding that is of no apparent clinical significance. Generally regular stromal papillae contain chronic inflammatory cells covered by a single layer of benign-appearing endocervical columnar epithelium.
- A lack of cellular stratification and atypia facilitates distinction from villoglandular endocervical adenocarcinoma.

Follicular Cervicitis

- Follicular cerviticis refers to inflammation of the endocervical mucosa with striking numbers of subepithelial and periglandular lymphoid follicles, typically with germinal centers. The causative organism in most cases is *Chlamydia trachomatis,* the presence of which can be confirmed with culture or immunohistochemical staining.

- Other frequent findings include a marked periglandular plasmacellular infiltrate and neutrophilic infiltration of the columnar epithelium. Stromal lymphocytes and histiocytes may also be present. The surface epithelium may be lost, but deep necrotic ulcers characteristic of herpetic cervicitis are absent.
- Distinguishing features from nodular lymphoma include an absence of a mass, the presence of follicles with germinal centers, and a mixed inflammatory infiltrate.

References

Kiviat NB, Paavonen JA, Wolner-Hanssen P, et al. Histopathology of endocervical infection caused by *Chlamydia trachomatis,* herpes simplex virus, *Trichomonas vaginalis,* and *Neisseria gonorrhoeae.* Hum Pathol 21:831–837, 1990.

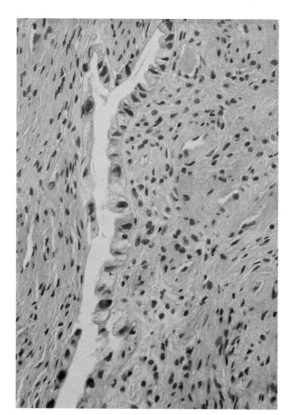

Figure 4–20. Endocervical gland with reactive atypia.

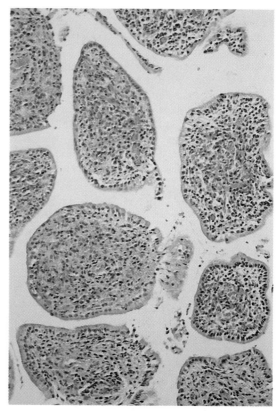

Figure 4–21. Papillary endocervicitis.

Lymphoma-like Lesions

- Lymphoma-like lesions are typically encountered in women of reproductive age. Rare cervical cases have been associated with infectious mononucleosis, cytomegalovirus infection, or Epstein-Barr virus infection. There is frequently an abnormal gross appearance (wich may include ulceration) but not, in contrast to lymphoma, cervical enlargement.
- The typical finding is that of a dense, superficial, band-like lymphoid infiltrate composed predominantly of large lymphoid cells with mitotic activity. An admixture of plasma cells, polymorphonuclear leukocytes,

and plasma cells is usually present. There are no helpful immunohistochemical findings.
- Features favoring this reactive lesion over lymphoma include an admixture of different cell types and an absence of the following: a large mass, cervical enlargement, deep invasion, perivascular involvement, and sclerosis.

References

Hachisuga T, Ookuma Y, Fukuda K, et al. Detection of Epstein-Barr virus DNA from a lymphoma-like lesion of the uterine cervix. Gynecol Oncol 46:69–73, 1992.

Young RH, Harris NL, Scully RE. Lymphoma-like lesions of the lower female genital tract: a report of 16 cases. Int J Gynecol Pathol 4:289–299, 1985.

Plasma Cell Cervicitis

∎ This lesion, which is characterized by dense plasma cell infiltrates in the endocervical stroma, is usually an incidental microscopic finding but rarely may simulate carcinoma on pelvic examination.

∎ The process may be mistaken for multiple myeloma on cytologic or histologic examination.

References

Doherty MG, Van Dinh T, Payne D, et al. Chronic plasma cell cervicitis simulating a cervical malignancy: a case report. Obstet Gynecol 82:646–650, 1993.

Qizilbash AH. Chronic plasma cell cervicitis: a rare pitfall in gynecologic cytology. Acta Cytol 18:198–200, 1974.

Eosinophilic Cervicitis

∎ Eosinophilic cervicitis is a rare form of cervicitis that is usually a response to biopsy or curettage performed within the preceding 2 weeks. One neonatal case with no obvious cause has been reported.

∎ The eosinophils are most numerous within the perivascular connective tissue within the cervical stroma.

References

Bjersing L, Borglin NE. Eosinophilia in the myometrium of the human uterus. Acta Pathol Microbiol Scand 54:353–364, 1962.

Divack DM, Janovski NA. Eosinophilia encountered in female genital organs. Am J Obstet Gynecol 84:761–763, 1962.

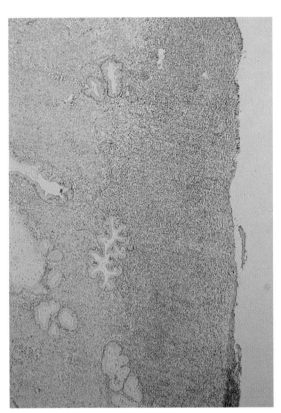

Figure 4–22. Lymphoma-like lesion. Notice the superficial bandlike distribution.

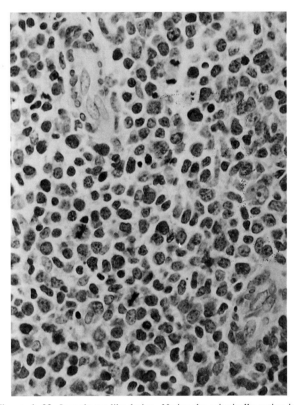

Figure 4–23. Lymphoma-like lesion. Notice the mitotically active immunoblasts.

Histiocytic Cervicitis, Xanthogranulomatous Cervicitis, and Malacoplakia

■ These lesions have in common an inflammatory infiltrate of histiocytes within the cervical stroma. The histiocytes occasionally contain ceroid (i.e., ceroid granuloma).

■ Xanthogranulomatous cervicitis is characterized by numerous histiocytes with foamy, lipid-rich cytoplasm, whereas malacoplakia is characterized by histiocytes with adundant eosinophilic cytoplasm and Michaelis-Gutmann bodies.

References

Al-Nafussi, Hughes D, Rebello G. Ceroid granuloma of the uterine cervix. Histopathology 21:282–284, 1992.

Falcón-Escobedo R, Mora-Tiscareno A, Pueblitz-Peredo S. Malacoplakia of the uterine cervix. Acta Cytol 30:281–284, 1986.

Young RH, Clement PB. Tumorlike lesions of the uterine cervix. In Clement PB, Young RH (eds): Tumors and Tumorlike Lesions of the Uterine Corpus and Cervix. New York: Churchill Livingstone, 1993: 1–50.

Necrobiotic Granulomas

■ Necrobiotic granulomas within the cervical stroma resembling rheumatoid nodules are usually a response to a prior local operation.

Reference

Evans CS, Goldblum RL, Klein HZ, Kohout ND. Necrobiotic granulomas of the uterine cervix: a probable postoperative reaction. Am J Surg Pathol 8:841–844, 1984.

Ligneous Cervicitis

■ Ligneous inflammation of the cervix occurs in women who almost always have or eventually develop ligneous conjunctivitis. Other sites in the female genital tract that may be involved include the vulva, vagina, endometrium, and fallopian tubes.

■ The clinical manifestations include vaginal discharge, dysmenorrhea, and a necrotic cervical lesion on clinical examination. Infertility in some cases may be caused by endometrial or tubal involvement.

■ Microscopic examination reveals loss of the surface epithelium and massive deposition of amorphous, eosinophilic, hyaline, or necrotic material, some of which is fibrin.

References

Rubin A, Buck D, Macdonald MR. Ligneous conjunctivitis involving the cervix: case report. Br J Obstet Gynaecol 96:1228–1230, 1989.

Scurry J, Planner R, Fortune DW, et al. Ligneous (pseudomembranous) inflammation of the female genital tract: a report of two cases. J Reprod Med 38:407–412, 1993.

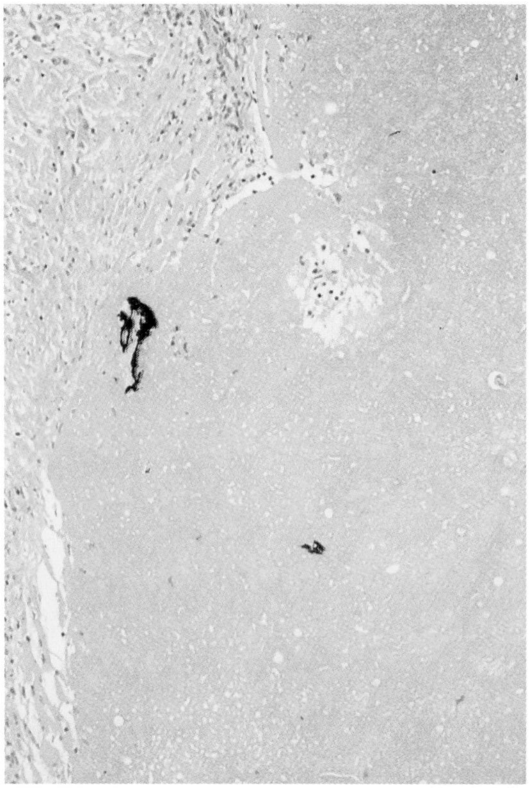

Figure 4–24. Ligneous cervicitis with massive deposition of amorphous eosinophilic material.

Cytomegalovirus Cervicitis

- Cytomegalovirus (CMV) cervicitis may be diagnosed by biopsy or Pap smear as an incidental finding in women not known to be immunocompromised or in immunocompromised women. In the latter population, other sites in the female genital tract may be affected.
- Epithelial cells, endothelial cells, or both contain characteristic intranuclear and intracytoplasmic inclusions. We have seen a case associated with a dense lymphoid and plasmacellular inflammatory reaction (lymphoma-like lesion, page 76).

References

Byard RW, Mikhael NZ, Orlando G, et al. The clinicopathological significance of cytomegalovirus inclusions demonstrated by endocervical biopsy. Pathology 23:318–321, 1991.
Friedmann W, Schafer A, Kretschmer R, Lobeck H. Disseminated cytomegalovirus infection of the female genital tract. Gynecol Obstet Invest 31:56–57, 1991.
Huang JC, Naylor B. Cytomegalovirus infection of the cervix detected by cytology and histology: a report of five cases. Cytopathology 4: 237–241, 1993.

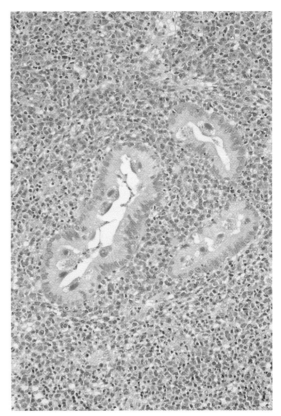

Figure 4–25. Cytomegaloviral endocervicitis. Several glands are lined by cells containing characteristic inclusion bodies. Notice the dense chronic inflammatory cell infiltrate within the stroma.

Herpetic Cervicitis

- Herpetic cervicitis typically appears as a necrotic ulcer that extends more deeply than endocervical glands. The ulcer is subtended by granulation tissue and an infiltrate that contains lymphocytes (which usually predominate), neutrophils, and histiocytes. Intraepithelial and intraluminal neutrophils are common.
- Characteristic herpetic inclusions may be present but were absent in all nine cases of culture-proven herpetic cervicitis in the series of Kiviat and colleagues.

References

Kiviat NB, Paavonen JA, Wolner-Hanssen P, et al. Histopathology of endocervical infection caused by *Chlamydia trachomatis,* herpes simplex virus, *Trichomonas vaginalis,* and *Neisseria gonorrhoeae.* Hum Pathol 21:831–837, 1990.

Radiation-Induced Atypia

- Atypia of squamous or endocervical glandular epithelium may occur weeks to years after irradiation. Gross examination may occasionally show mucosal irregularity, fibrosis, induration, or stenosis.
- Squamous and glandular cells contain abundant cytoplasm and hyperchromatic nuclei that are variable in size and shape, but with a low nuclear to cytoplasmic ratio, uniform nuclear spacing, and smudged, indistinct chromatin. Cellular degeneration, cytoplasmic vacuoles, and cell necrosis may be seen. Mitotic figures are typically absent.
- Radiation-induced changes in the stroma and blood vessels are common, but radiation fibroblasts are present in only occasional cases.
- Attention to these features and knowledge of the patient's history facilitate distinction from premalignant glandular or squamous changes.

Reference

Lesack D, Wahab I, Gilks CB. Radiation-induced atypia of endocervical epithelium: a histological, immunohistochemical and cytometric study. Int J Gynecol Pathol 15:242–247, 1996.

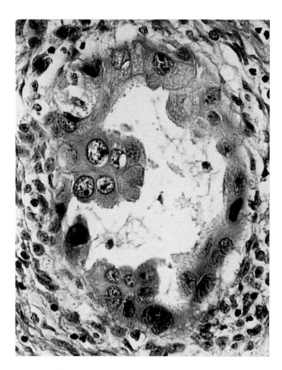

Figure 4–26. Radiation-induced atypia.

Effects of Extravasation of Mucin

■ Mucin extravasation from a ruptured gland may result in periglandular edema and inflammatory cells, including foamy histiocytes and foreign-body–type giant cells. Rarely, extravasated mucin is found within the cervical lymphatics.

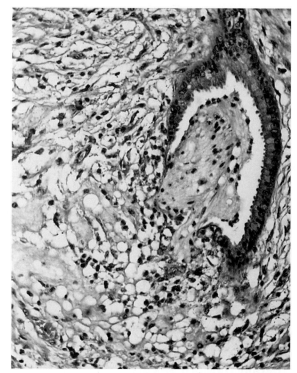

Figure 4–27. Ruptured endocervical gland with inflammatory response to the mucin.

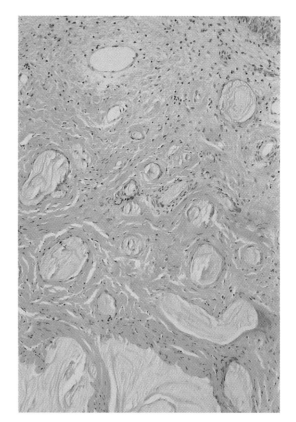

Figure 4–28. Mucin dissection into endocervical stroma and lymphatics from a ruptured endocervical gland (gland not illustrated).

Cautery Artifact

- Changes are commonly seen with the widespread use of the large loop electrosurgical excision procedure of the cervix. The cautery-induced nuclear alterations in the endocervical glands and squamous epithelium may be interpreted as dysplasia.
- The epithelial nuclei are stratified, compressed, and often markedly elongated, and they have hyperchromatic nuclei with smudged chromatin. Cautery changes may be seen in the adjacent stroma.

Postoperative Spindle Cell Nodule (see Chapter 3)

Bacillary Angiomatosis (see Chapter 1)

PREGNANCY-RELATED CHANGES

Cervical Pregnancy

- A cervical pregnancy resulting in a hemorrhagic mass can occasionally be mistaken on macroscopic examina-

tion for a malignant tumor, although the diagnosis is typically straightforward on microscopic examination.
- Distinction between ectopic pregnancy and the rare examples of primary gestational trophoblastic disease in the cervix is made by applying criteria similar to those used for the uterine corpus.

Reference

Renade V, Palmerino DA, Tronik B. Cervical pregnancy. Obstet Gynecol 51:502–505, 1978.

Ectopic Decidua

- Decidua is found in approximately one third of cervical biopsy or hysterectomy specimens from pregnant women at term and typically disappears by 8 weeks postpartum. The same finding has been rarely documented in the cervix of newborns. The decidua is almost always an incidental histologic finding; rare manifestations have included hemorrhage and a tumor-like mass.

- The process may be confused with early invasive squamous cell carcinoma when contiguous with CIN. The presence of bland nuclear features, an absence of mitotic figures, and negative immunoreactivity for cytokeratin facilitate this differential diagnosis.

References

Armenia CS, Shaver DN, Modisher MW. Decidual transformation of the cervical stroma simulating reticulum cell sarcoma. Am J Obstet Gynecol 89:808–816, 1964.

Schneider V, Barnes LA. Ectopic decidual reaction of the uterine cervix: frequency and cytologic presentation. Acta Cytol 25:616–622, 1981.

Arias-Stella Reaction

- The Arias-Stella reaction (ASR) is an incidental microscopic finding in endocervical glands in approximately 10% of gravid hysterectomy specimens. The finding is typically limited to only one or two glands; occasionally endocervical polyps are involved.
- The ASR may be confused with adenocarcinoma in situ (AIS) or clear cell adenocarcinoma, especially in a small biopsy or curettage specimen and if the pathologist is unaware that the patient is pregnant.
- Features distinguishing the ASR from AIS include the presence of clear and hobnail cells, an absence of uniformly atypical nuclei, rare or absent mitotic figures, and an absence of apoptotic bodies.
- Features favoring or indicating the ASR over clear cell adenocarcinoma include a young age, an absence of symptoms or a mass, an absence of invasion, an absence of tubulocystic and solid patterns, and an absence of papillae with hyalinized cores.

References

Cariani DJ, Guderian AM. Gestational atypia in endocervical polyps—the Arias-Stella reaction. Am J Obstet Gynecol 95:589–590, 1966.

Cove H. The Arias-Stella reaction occurring in the endocervix in pregnancy: recognition and comparison with an adenocarcinoma of the endocervix. Am J Surg Pathol 3:567–568, 1979.

Schneider V. Arias-Stella reaction of the endocervix: frequency and location. Acta Cytol 25:224–228, 1981.

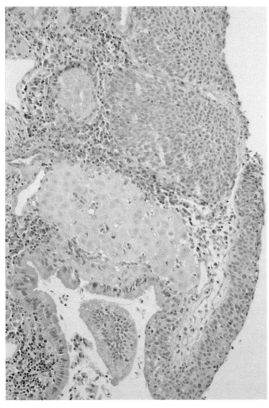

Figure 4–29. Ectopic decidua abuts high-grade cervical intraepithelial neoplasia, an appearance that should not be mistaken for early stromal invasion.

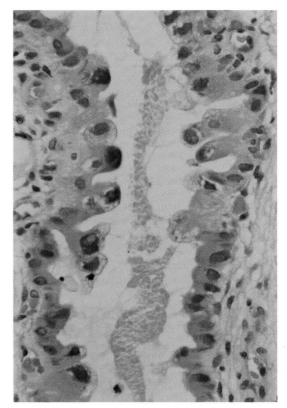

Figure 4–30. Arias-Stella reaction within an endocervical gland.

Placental Site Nodules and Plaques (see Chapter 10)

MELANOTIC LESIONS

Blue Nevus

- A blue nevus in the uterine cervix is usually an incidental microscopic finding but occasionally is grossly visible as an area of mucosal pigmentation.
- The lesions, which are typically less than 4 mm in the maximal dimension, consist of a cluster of melanin-laden polygonal and spindle cells within the superficial endocervical stroma. The pigmented cells are argyrophilic, argentaffinic, and immunoreactive for S-100 protein.
- Malignant melanoma can be excluded by using criteria applied to cutaneous lesions.

Mucosal Melanosis

- Mucosal melanosis appears as an irregular area of mucosal pigmentation on clinical or gross examination.
- Microscopic examination reveals a pigmentation of the basal epithelium, with or without the presence of benign basal melanocytes. A lentigo-like pattern is seen in some cases.

References

Dundore W, Lamas C. Benign nevus (ephelis) of the uterine cervix. Am J Obstet Gynecol 152:881–882, 1985.
Patel DS, Bhagavan BS. Blue nevus of the uterine cervix. Hum Pathol 16:79–86, 1985.
Uehara T, Isumo T, Kishi K, et. al. Stromal melanocytic foci ("blue nevus") in step sections of the uterine cevix. Acta Pathol Jpn 41:751–756, 1991.
Yilmaz AG, Chandler P, Hahm GK, et al. Melanosis of the uterine cervix: a report of two cases and discussion of pigmented cervical lesions. Int J Gynecol Pathol 18:73–76, 1999.

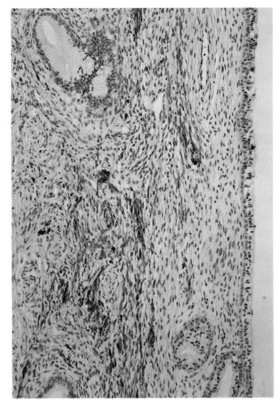

Figure 4–31. Blue nevus of the endocervix.

MISCELLANEOUS TUMOR-LIKE LESIONS

Amyloidosis

- Localized amyloidosis in the cervix is rare and usually associated with primary squamous cell carcinomas in this site, in which the amyloid is composed of cytokeratin, presumably derived from degenerating tumor cells.
- A single case of tumor-like amyloidosis of the cervix has been reported as a 1-cm nodule in a 28-year-old woman in the absence of a cervical neoplasm or systemic amyloidosis.

Reference

Gibbons D, Lindberg GM, Ashfaq R, Saboorian MH. Localized amyloidosis of the uterine cervix. Int J Gynecol Pathol 17:368–371, 1998.

Ectopias

- Rare examples of ectopic prostatic tissue have been described in the cervix, usually as an incidental microscopic finding, but in one case, the ectopic tissue formed a 4.0-cm mural mass grossly resembling a leiomyoma. The ectopic glands microscopically resemble normal prostatic glands, including immuoreactivity for PSA and prostatic acid phosphatase (PAP).

■ Rare examples of sebaceous glands, hair follicles, or both have been described as incidental microscopic findings in the cervix.

References

Larraza-Hernandez O, Molberg KH, Lindberg G, Albores-Saavedra J. Ectopic prostatic tissue in the uterine cervix. Int J Gynecol Pathol 16: 291–293, 1997.

Nucci MR, Ferry JA, Young RH. Ectopic prostate in uterine cervix: a report of 2 cases and review of ectopic prostate tissue. (submitted).

Robledo MC, Vazquez JJ, Contreras-Mejuto F, Lopez-Garcia G. Sebaceous glands and hair follicles in the cervix uteri. Histopathology 21: 278–280, 1992.

Multinucleated Stromal Giant Cells (see Chapter 3)

BENIGN TUMORS

■ Benign tumors in the cervix are rare, with the exception of leiomyomas, although even these tumors are uncommon in the cervix. Most benign tumors in the cervix are mesenchymal or mixed epithelial-mesenchymal tumors and are discussed with their much more common counterparts involving the uterine corpus in Chapter 9.

Reference

Tiltman AJ, Leiomyomas of the uterine cervix: a study of frequency. Int J Gynecol Pathol 17:231–234, 1998.

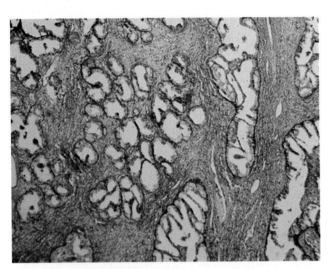

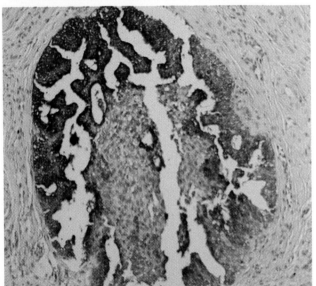

Figure 4–32. Ectopic prostatic glands within the endocervix. The glands are immunoreactive for prostatic-specific antigen (*bottom*).

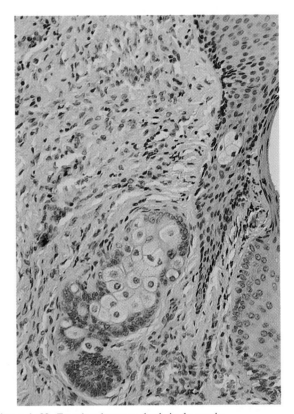

Figure 4–33. Ectopic sebaceous glands in the cervix.

Endocervical Polyps

- These very common lesions occasionally may cause concern for a malignant tumor on clinical examination, but the diagnosis is usually straightforward on pathologic examination.
- Endocervical polyps occur over a wide age range, but 90% of patients are 40 years or older. In 75% of patients, the polyp is an incidental finding in an asymptomatic woman; the most common symptom is abnormal vaginal bleeding. Between 80% and 90% of polyps are less than 1 cm in diameter and single.
- The typical or "adenomatous" polyp accounts for 90% of endocervical polyps; the remainder in the study by Aaro and colleagues were classified as cystic, fibrous, vascular, inflammatory, and "fibromyomatous," the last type representing submucosal leiomyomas.
- Occasional endocervical polyps may harbor an in situ or invasive carcinoma, occasionally confined to the polyp but more commonly representing part of more widespread cervical involvement.
- Nonneoplastic findings found within polyps that may be mistaken for a neoplasm include florid squamous metaplasia, papillary hyperplasia, microglandular hyperplasia (page 67), and decidua (page 81).
- Fibroepithelial polyps with stromal atypia may rarely occur in the cervix (see Chapter 3).

Reference

Aaro LA, Jacobson LJ, Soule EH. Endocervical polyps. Obstet Gynecol 21:659–665, 1963.

Squamous Papilloma

- Noncondylomatous, nondysplastic squamous papillomas of the cervix in our experience are rare. They lack the koilocytosis and the complex arborizing architecture of condylomas.
- Most papillary squamous lesions are more appropriately classified as typical or dysplastic condyloma acuminatum, papillary squamous cell carcinoma in situ (see Chapter 5), or verrucous carcinoma (see Chapter 5).
- The diagnosis is appropriate only after the lesion has been completely examined microscopically to exclude the lesions in the differential diagnosis previously described.

Reference

Qizilbash AH. Papillary squamous tumors of the uterine cervix: a clinical and pathological study of 21 cases. Am J Clin Pathol 61:508–520, 1974.

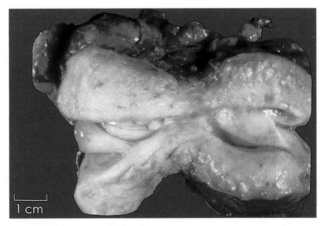

Figure 4–34. Endocervical polyp.

Inverted Transitional Cell Papilloma

- Five cases of inverted transitional cell papilloma (ITCP) have been reported in women 25 to 71 years of age. Four patients presented with abnormal cytology; a cervical lesion was seen on pelvic examination in the fifth case. A synchronous vaginal ITCP was found in one patient. The lesions were polypoid and ranged from 0.6 to 2.0 cm in the maximal dimension.
- On microscopic examination, the lesions resembled ITCP of the urinary bladder, with transitional cells forming anastomosing trabeculae with peripheral palisading. Microcysts were present in four cases. Cytologic atypia was minimal, and no mitotic figures were seen.
- Three patients had subsequent hysterectomies that re-vealed no residual tumor. None of the lesions recurred, although follow-up was limited.
- ITCP should be distinguished from transitional cell carcinoma (which may have a growth pattern resembling that of ITCP) and papillary squamotransitional cell carcinoma of the cervix (see Chapter 5). Both tumors, in contrast to ITCP, exhibit obvious cytologic atypia, mitotic activity, and in many cases, stromal invasion.

Reference

Albores-Saavedra J, Young RH. Transitional cell neoplasms (carcinomas and inverted papillomas) of the uterine cervix: a report of five cases. Am J Surg Pathol 19:1138–1145, 1995.

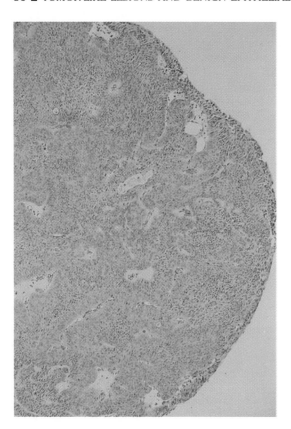

Figure 4–35. Inverted transitional cell papilloma.

Müllerian Papillomas

- These papillomas are rare lesions once thought to be of mesonephric origin and now considered müllerian.
- The papillomas occur almost exclusively in children who are typically between 2 and 5 years of age (range, 14 months to 9 years) and who present with vaginal bleeding or discharge and a friable, polypoid to papillary cervical lesion, usually less than 2 cm.
- Fine branching papillae are typically lined by a single layer of benign epithelial cells that vary from flattened to cuboidal to columnar. A focal lining of stratified squamous epithelium has been identified in some cases.
- Edema and inflammatory cells typically occupy the stroma of the papillae. Psammoma bodies or osseous metaplasia have been seen in rare cases.
- The follow-up has been uneventful in most cases. Occasionally, a local "recurrence" (possibly from incomplete primary excision) has been treated successfully by re-excision.
- The differential diagnosis includes papillary endocervicitis (page 75), villous and villoglandular papillary adenomas (see Villous and Villoglandular Adenomas), and villoglandular carcinomas (see Chapter 6).

Reference

Smith YR, Quint EH, Hinton EL. Recurrent benign mullerian papilloma of of the cervix. J Pediatr Adolesc Gynecol 11:29–31, 1998.

Villous and Villoglandular Adenomas

- Rare cervical adenomas have a villoglandular architecture similar to that of a villoglandular adenocarcinomas (see Chapter 6). The adenomas, in contrast, have uniformly well-differentiated cells. Thorough sampling is important.
- Two cervical "villous adenomas" have reported, but both were associated with an underlying invasive adenocarcinoma.

References

Alvaro T, Nogales F. Villous adenoma and invasive adenocarcinoma of the cervix [Letter]. Int J Gynecol Pathol 7:96, 1988.

Michael H, Sutton G, Hull MT, Roth LM. Villous adenoma of the uterine cervix associated with invasive adenocarcinoma: a histologic, ultrastructural, and immunohistochemical study. Int J Gynecol Pathol 5:163–169, 1986.

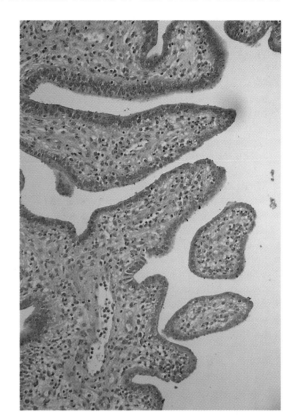

Figure 4–36. Müllerian papilloma.

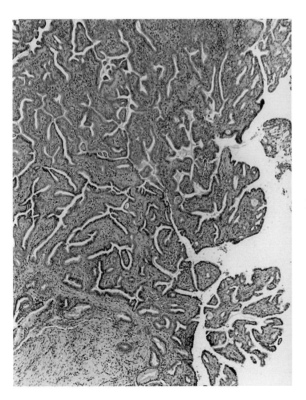

Figure 4–37. Villoglandular adenoma.

Adenomyomas of Endocervical Type

■ These lesions are usually an incidental finding in women of reproductive or postmenopausal age (mean, 40 years). A polypoid mucosal mass, typically less than 8 cm, is present in most cases. Less commonly, there is cervical enlargement by a mural mass without mucosal involvement.

■ Gross examination reveals a grey-white to tan, well-circumscribed tumor with, in half the cases, mucin-filled cysts.

■ Microscopically, a well-circumscribed tumor is composed of benign endocervical-type glands, often in a lobular arrangement, admixed with smooth muscle. Tubal-type or endometrioid glands are present in some cases.

■ Follow-up reveals a benign course. The tumors occasionally persist or recur after incomplete excision. No cases of extracervical spread have been reported.

■ Adenoma malignum (minimal-deviation adenocarcinoma) can be excluded by the noninvasive borders, the lobular arrangement of the glands, a background of myomatous smooth muscle, an absence of invasive glands with a desmoplastic reaction, and a lack of even focal atypia.

Reference

Gilks CB, Young RH, Clement PB, et al. Adenomyomas of the uterine cervix of endocervical type: a report of 10 cases of a benign cervical tumor that may be confused with adenoma malignum. Mod Pathol 9: 220–224, 1996.

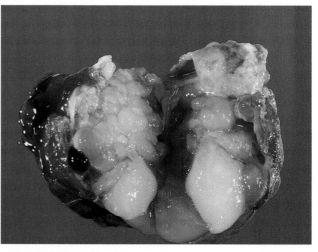

Figure 4–38. Sectioned surface of an endocervical-type adenomyoma. The tumor formed a mural mass within the cervix. Notice the multiple cysts filled with gelatinous contents.

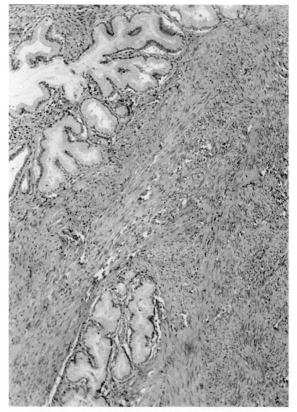

Figure 4–39. Adenomyoma of endocervical type. Clusters of benign endocervical glands are surrounded by smooth muscle.

Glomus Tumor

- Two examples of glomus tumor of the uterine cervix were incidental findings in women 39 and 52 years of age.
- The tumors were 0.4 and 0.8 cm in the maximal dimension; only the large tumor was recognized on gross examination. The tumors histologically resembled glomus tumors in other sites.

Reference

Albores-Saavedra J, Gilcrease M. Glomus tumor of the uterine cervix. Int J Gynecol Pathol 18:69–72, 1999.

CHAPTER 5

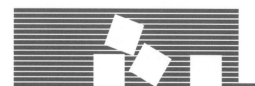

Invasive Squamous Cell Carcinoma of the Cervix and Its Precursors

PRECURSOR LESIONS

Classification

- The classification systems for lesions that are considered precursors of cervical invasive squamous cell carcinoma (ISCC), in order of their historical development, are dysplasia/carcinoma in situ (CIS); cervical intraepithelial neoplasia (CIN); and squamous intraepithelial lesions (SILs) (Bethesda system). The World Health Organization (WHO) favors the first system but includes the second parenthetically and describes the Bethesda system in a footnote. The three systems are compared in Table 5–1.
- The Bethesda terminology is used in this chapter because it is widely used in North America, but we continue to use in our daily practice the traditional dysplasia/CIS or CIN terminology, with a separate comment indicating the presence or absence of koilocytosis (described later).
- A diagnosis of condyloma acuminatum is made when the distinctive features of that lesion are seen (see Chapter 1). Foci of dysplasia or even carcinoma in situ, if present within the condyloma, should be documented. The typical condyloma is exophytic, but the terms *flat* or *endophytic* condyloma are used by some observers when a flat or endophytic lesion exhibits koilocytotic atypia.
- SILs often are accompanied by light microscopic evidence of human papillomavirus (HPV) infection in the form of koilocytosis, and all or almost all of them can be shown to contain HPV DNA using the polymerase chain reaction.
- Condyloma acuminata and low-grade SILs (LSILs) are usually associated with low-risk HPVs (types 6 or 11) or occasionally intermediate-risk HPVs (types 31, 33, or 35), or rarely HPV 18. They are typically nonaneuploid and are associated with a low risk of eventual development of ISCC.
- High-grade SILs (HSILs) are usually associated with high-risk HPV (typically type 16 or sometimes 18) or

occasionally intermediate-risk HPVs. They are typically aneuploid and have a significant risk of progression to ISCC (described later).

Risk Factors

- The primary risk factor for the development of SILs is HPV infection. Other risk factors (most of which are cofactors that increase the risk of HPV infection) include first coitus before 17 years, increased number of sexual partners, long-term oral contraceptive use, early first pregnancy, high parity, lower socioeconomic status, other sexually transmitted diseases (e.g., herpes simplex, gonorrhea, chlamydial infection), prior abnormal Pap smear, smoking, and immunosuppression, including human immunodeficiency virus (HIV) seropositivity.
- Characteristics of the male sexual partner that are considered risk factors include a history of one or more of the following: penile warts, multiple sexual partners, and cervical cancer in a previous partner.

Clinical Features

- The prevalence of HPV DNA detection in the cervix and LSILs peaks among women at the initiation of their sexual activity in their teens and early twenties. HSILs peak about 5 to 10 years later (age 25 to 29 years). SILs increased 10-fold between 1978 and 1988 in one study.
- The presenting clinical feature is almost always an abnormal Pap smear. The clinical evaluation of the lesion requires a colposcopic examination; a variety of colposcopic patterns can be correlated with the grade of the SIL.

Microscopic Features of Low-Grade Intraepithelial Lesions

- We diagnose lesions with dysplastic nuclear features (as described for HSILs) but confined to the lower one

Table 5–1

COMPARISON OF CLASSIFICATION SYSTEMS
FOR PRECURSORS OF SQUAMOUS CELL
CARCINOMA OF THE UTERINE CERVIX

Dysplasia, Carcinoma In Situ	Cervical Intraepithelial Neoplasia	Squamous Intraepithelial Lesions (Bethesda System)
Mild dysplasia	CIN 1	LSIL
Moderate dysplasia	CIN 2	HSIL
Severe dysplasia	CIN 3	HSIL
Carcinoma in situ	CIN 3	HSIL

CIN, cervical intraepithelial neoplasia; LSIL, low-grade squamous intraepithelial lesion; HSIL, high-grade squamous intraepithelial lesion.

third of the epithelium as mild dysplasia (CIN 1 or LSIL). Koilocytosis is often present in the upper layers. Some investigators consider lesions with dysplastic atypia confined to the basal layers as HSILs, provided that the cytologic features are sufficiently striking.

- Koilocytosis is characterized by variation of cell size and shape, thickened cell membranes, a perinuclear cytoplasmic clear zone (i.e., halo) of variable size and shape surrounded by a rim of dense cytoplasm, and nuclear atypia (i.e., koilocytotic atypia).
- The central to eccentric nuclei of koilocytes are of variable size (enlarged or small and pyknotic) and shape, have wrinkled contours, and are hyperchromatic; binucleated and multinucleated cells are common. The nuclei, however, are more uniform in shape and in the intensity of their hyperchromasia than the koilocytes in some HSILs.
- Mitotic figures are common in LSILs, with or without koilocytotic change, and may be occasionally tripolar. Ki-67 staining in cases of CIN 1 shows positivity mostly within the lower one third of the epithelium and occasional scattered positive cells within the middle third of the epithelium.

Microscopic Features of High-Grade Intraepithelial Lesions

- The cardinal feature is nuclear atypia in all epithelial layers, usually with loss of maturation. HSILs with some maturation or koilocytotic atypia correspond to CIN 2, whereas those lacking these features correspond to CIN 3. The surface is often parakeratotic.
- The atypical nuclear features include enlargement, variation in size, pleomorphism (including irregular nuclear contours), hyperchromasia, and irregularly distributed coarse chromatin. Prominent nucleoli and chromocenters are uncommon. The parabasal cells are typically crowded and have indistinct cell membranes and overlapping nuclei.
- Koilocytes, if present, may be identical to those in LSILs but often have smaller halos, and more densely hyperchromatic and more pleomorphic nuclei.
- Rare HSILs contain intracellular mucin droplets (i.e.,

squamomucinous intraepithelial lesion), representing an in situ counterpart of invasive squamous cell carcinomas with intracellular mucin (page 101).
- Mitotic figures, normal and abnormal, are common in all layers. Ki-67 staining shows positivity ranging from two thirds to the full thickness of the epithelium.
- About 15% of HSILs coexist with an LSIL, although this figure is higher with intermediate-risk HPV subtypes, such as HPV 31.

Topography of Squamous Intraepithelial Lesions

- SILs usually begin at the squamocolumnar junction (transformation zone); the anterior lip is involved twice as frequently as the posterior lip. About 10% of SILs involve the endocervical canal without involvement of the squamocolumnar junction.
- SILs spread along the basement membrane by replacing the metaplastic and glandular epithelial cells. Involvement of endocervical glands is common, often with luminal obliteration, a finding that should not be confused with early invasion (see page 98). HSILs tend to involve a larger area and are more likely to extend into the endocervical canal than LSILs.
- HSILs can replace the transformation zone and extend for a variable distance up the endocervical canal. Rarely, HSILs extend into the endometrium and fallopian tube and on to the ovarian surfaces, and they exceptionally can be associated with an ISCC in these sites.

Microscopic Features of Nonpapillary Atypical Immature Squamous Metaplasia

- Atypical immature squamous metaplasias (AIMs) are characterized by absent or minimal maturation of the metaplastic squamous epithelium and mild to prominent hyperchromasia with absent to mild chromatin irregularities. Nuclear membrane irregularities and coarsely clumped chromatin are absent; mitotic figures are absent or scarce.
- Geng and associates found that 67% of AIMs harbored HPV DNA; the latter was always of the intermediate or high-risk subtype and occurred in 12 of the 14 AIMs for which a diagnosis of HSIL was a strong consideration.
  - The Ki-67 index in AIMs was similar to that of LSILs and lower than that of HSILs.
  - Eighty percent of HPV-positive cases were associated with a synchronous or subsequent typical HSIL, compared with only 16.7% of HPV-negative cases.
- AIMs appear to be a heterogeneous group of lesions that include bona fide HSILs (high-risk HPV positive, high Ki-67 index), possible precursors of HSILs (high-risk HPV positive, low to moderate Ki-67 index), and benign reactive lesions (HPV negative, variable Ki-67 index).

■ In the absence of HPV or Ki-67 evaluation, a diagnosis of AIM should include a comment indicating a preference for an HSIL or a reactive lesion, depending on the appearance of the lesion. If the pathologist is unsure of the diagnosis after appropriate consultation, a diagnosis of squamous atypia of uncertain nature is appropriate.

Microscopic Features of Papillary Immature Metaplasia

■ A distinct lesion of the cervix is designated *papillary immature metaplasia* (PIM). PIM often extends into the endocervical canal. Similar or perhaps identical lesions have also been reported as transitional cell papillomas.

■ PIM typically contains HPV type 6 and 11 but not high-risk HPV subtypes. Rare PIMs, however, are contiguous with an HSIL, presumably because of different, simultaneous HPV infections.

■ PIM is characterized by a proliferation of immature parabasal-type squamous cells with absent to mild cytologic atypia. The lesions have minimal cell crowding, well-defined cell membranes, an increased nuclear to cytoplasm (N:C) ratio, smooth nuclear contours, and uniformly distributed, fine chromatin with prominent chromocenters. Mitoses are uncommon but if present are typical.

■ PIM may replace the full thickness of the epithelium, although endocervical columnar cells may persist on the surface. Filiform papillae and superficial koilocytotic atypia are usually present focally, the latter feature placing PIM in the category of LSIL according to those who believe that koilocytosis equates with LSIL.

■ PIMs have a low index of Ki-67 staining in the mid and upper layers, in contrast to HSILs and papillary squamous carcinomas (PSCs, page 105), lesions with which PIM may be confused. Some PSCs, however, show focal surface maturation with an associated reduction in Ki-67 staining.

Features of Squamous Intraepithelial Lesions Suggesting the Presence of Early Invasion

■ HSILs associated with early stromal invasion often exhibit extensive involvement of the surface epithelium and deep, expansile glandular involvement, luminal necrosis, and intraepithelial squamous maturation (e.g., large keratinized cells, keratin pearls).

■ Other features include numerous mitoses and apoptotic bodies, periglandular concentric fibrosis and inflammation, severe nuclear pleomorphism, distinct nucleoli, chromatin clearing, and spindle cells oriented at right angles to the basement membrane.

■ Biopsy specimens of HSILs exhibiting these features should be serially sectioned to exclude early invasion. In the absence of the latter, a notation in the pathology report should indicate the possibility of invasion unsampled by the biopsy.

Differential Diagnosis of Squamous Intraepithelial Lesions

■ Typical immature squamous metaplasia

• Squamous metaplasia is a normal process in the cervix whereby the endocervical columnar epithelium is replaced by squamous epithelium. In the early phases of this process, the metaplastic squamous epithelium is often composed of a monotonous population of cells with a high N:C ratio that lack cytoplasmic maturation in the superficial layers.

• In contrast to SILs, the immature squamous cells have minimal cell crowding, no to mild cytologic atypia, uniformly distributed fine chromatin, and smooth nuclear contours. Mitoses are uncommon but if present are typical and confined to the basal layers. The papillarity and the koilocytosis of PIM are absent.

• Florid squamous metaplasia that can be mistaken for invasive squamous cell carcinoma is discussed on page 63.

■ Reactive and reparative changes

• Reactive nuclear atypia, which may include nucleomegaly, hyperchromasia, and binucleation or multinucleation, in contrast to SILs, is usually confined to the lower layers, with normal maturation and minimal nuclear enlargement in the upper layers. There may be a sharp demarcation between the atypical cells in the lower layers and the mature cells in the upper layers.

• Unlike typical SILs, reactive cells often show spongiosis, distinct cell borders, regular nuclear spacing, prominent nucleoli or chromocenters, and an absence of marked variation in nuclear size and contour and coarse hyperchromasia. Cytoplasmic halos, if present, are round and uniform with central nuclei.

• Intraepithelial neutrophils may be seen. Numerous neutrophils, ulceration, and necrotic cells should prompt a search for herpetic inclusions (page 79). Dense acute and chronic inflammation with lymphoid follicles (i.e., follicular cervicitis) suggests chlamydial infection (page 75).

• In one study, Ki-67 reactivity was significantly less in inflamed or metaplastic epithelum than in LSILs, occurring in fewer than 15% of the basal cells and almost never in the superficial one half of the epithelium.

• Nuclear atypia in the upper layers and cells with multiple enlarged nuclei, in the presence of the reactive changes described previously, may indicate the diagnosis of an SIL with reactive changes. It may not be possible to grade such lesions (i.e., "SIL with reactive changes").

• In some cases, a definite distinction between a benign reactive lesion and an SIL with or without reactive changes may not be possible (i.e., "atypical squamous epithelium of undetermined significance"). In such cases, the opinion of a second experienced pathologist and correlation with cytologic findings are important.

- Postmenopausal squamous atypia and other forms of pseudokoilocytosis
  - Postmenopausal squamous atypia (PSA), which usually occurs in women older than 50 years of age, is characterized by prominent perinuclear halos, no more than twofold nuclear enlargement, hyperchromasia, and multinucleation. The pseudokoilocytosis in PSA may be misdiagnosed as an LSIL, but PSA is negative for HPV. There may be associated atrophy or transitional cell metaplasia (TCM).
  - Compared with koilocytotic atypia, PSA has less variation in nuclear size (less than twofold compared with more than threefold) and staining intensity and more finely and evenly distributed nuclear chromatin. The nuclei are uniformly spaced and slightly elongated and lie centrally within a uniformly contoured halo. Some nuclear grooves may be present; mitoses are rare or absent.
  - An absence of binucleated or multinucleated cells favors PSA over koilocytotic atypia, whereas the presence of two or more binucleated cells in a high-power field strongly suggests koilocytotic atypia.
  - Other forms of pseudokoilocytosis include those in which perinuclear halos occur as an isolated finding with no nuclear atypia (as in normal glycogenated squamous epithelium) or perinuclear halos with mild reactive atypia.
- TCM (page 63) and atrophy. Both these processes result in loss of normal maturation and may be composed of cells with a high N:C ratio, but they typically lack the nuclear atypia and mitotic activity of SILs. The atrophic epithelium is thin and shows no Ki-67 staining.
  - Metaplastic transitional epithelium, however, can become dysplastic and should be diagnosed as LSIL or HSIL on a background of TCM.
  - Crum and associates recognize a category of "atypical atrophy" that may be difficult to distinguish from an SIL.
- ISCC. A study comparing the morphology of HSILs with that of ISCCs found that two or more of the following features suggest ISCC in a biopsy specimen, even when stroma is absent or too scanty to assess invasion: giant bizarre cells, large keratinized cells, keratin pearls, necrosis, and neovascularization.
- Radiation effect (page 79).
- Placental site nodules and plaques (page 220).

Natural History

- Follow-up studies of women with HSILs (CIN 3) and the observation that most ISCCs are contiguous with an HSIL indicate that the latter precedes most ISCCs. In more than 80% of cases, the first abnormal smear preceding a ISCC shows CIN 3, whereas CIN 1 in smears preceding ISCCs is rare (1% to 3% of cases). Some ISCCs occur without a previously documented precursor lesion.
- Östör reviewed the literature and calculated the approximate frequency of regression for CIN 1 to be 60%; persistence, 30%; progression to CIN 3, 10%; and progression to invasion, 1%. Most investigators, however, now believe that most cases of "progression" of LSILs represent the presence of a synchronous unsampled HSIL or the de novo development of the latter in a patient with an LSIL.
- The corresponding figures from the Östör study for CIN 2 were 40% for regression, 40% for persistence, 20% for progression to CIN 3, and 5% for progression to ISCC.
- The corresponding figures from the Östör study for CIN 3 were 33% for regression, "less than 56%" for persistence, and "more than 12%" for progression to ISCC; other studies have found as many as 70% of CIN 3 lesions progress to ISCC.
- These observations notwithstanding, the behavior of a precursor lesion, even a CIN 3 lesion or one harboring a high-risk HPV, cannot be predicted with certainty in an individual case.
- Rare SILs "recur" as SIL or ISCC after their conservative ablation or even after hysterectomy, although some of these recurrences may represent new lesions. The risk of posttreatment recurrences in some studies is higher with positive resection margins, but all women with treated SILs require long-term follow-up.

References

Al-Nafussi AI, Hughes DE. Histological features of CIN3 and their value in predicting invasive microinvasive squamous carcinoma. J Clin Pathol 47:799–804, 1994.

Crum CP. Genital papillomaviruses and related neoplasms: causation, diagnosis and classification (Bethesda). Mod Pathol 7:138–145, 1994.

Crum CP. Detecting every genital papilloma virus infection: what does it mean? [Editorial]. Am J Pathol 153:1667–1671, 1998.

Crum CP, Cibas ES, Lee KR. Pathology of early cervical neoplasia. In Contemporary Issues in Surgical Pathology, vol 22. New York: Churchill Livingstone, 1997.

Geng L, Connolly DC, Isacson C, et al. Atypical immature metaplasia (AIM) of the cervix: Is it related to high-grade squamous intraepithelial lesion (HSIL)? Hum Pathol 30:345–351, 1999.

Jovanovic AS, McLachlin CM, Shen L, et al. Postmenopausal squamous atypia: a spectrum including "pseudo-koilocytosis." Mod Pathol 8:408–412, 1995.

McCluggage WG, Buhidma M, Tang L, et al. Monoclonal antibody MIB1 in the assessment of cervical squamous intraepithelal lesions. Int J Gynecol Pathol 15:131–136, 1996.

Leung K, Chart W, Hui P. Invasive squamous cell carcinoma and cervical intraepithelial neoplasia III of uterine cervix: morphological differences other than stromal invasion. Am J Clin Pathol 101:508–513, 1994.

Mittal K, Palazzo J. Cervical condylomas show higher proliferation than do inflamed or metaplastic cervical epithelium. Mod Pathol 11:780–783, 1998.

Östör AG. Natural history of cervical intraepithelial neoplasia: a critical review. Int J Gynecol Pathol 12:186–192, 1993.

Park J, Sun D, Crum CP. Squamo-mucinous intraepithelial and invasive lesions of the cervix: a distinct pathologic entity [Abstract]. Mod Pathol 12:121A, 1999.

Pins MR, Young RH, Crum CP, et al. Cervical squamous cell carcinoma in situ with intraepithelial extension to the upper genital tract and invasion of tubes and ovaries: report of a case with human papilloma virus analysis. Int J Gynecol Pathol 16:272–278, 1997.

Prasad CJ, Genest DR, Crum CP. Nondiagnostic squamous atypia of the cervix (atypical squamous epithelium of undetermined significance): histologic and molecular correlates. Int J Gynecol Pathol 13:220–227, 1994.

Tam D, Demattia A, Pirog E, et al. Diagnostic accuracy of low grade cervical lesions is improved with MIB-1 [Abstract]. Mod Pathol 11: 115A, 1988.

Trivijitsilp P, Mosher R, Sheets EE, et al. Papillary immature metaplasia: a clinicopathologic analysis and comparison with papillary squamous carcinoma. Hum Pathol 29:641–648, 1998.

Yelverton CL, Bentley RC, Olenick S, et al. Epithelial repair of the uterine cervix: assessment of morphologic features and correlations with cytologic diagnosis. Int J Gynecol Pathol 15:338–344, 1996.

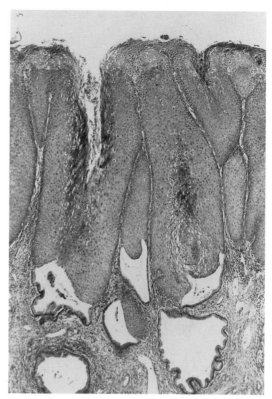

Figure 5–2. Endophytic growth pattern of condyloma acuminatum.

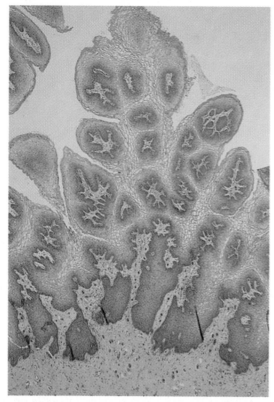

Figure 5–1. "Typical" or exophytic type condyloma acuminatum.

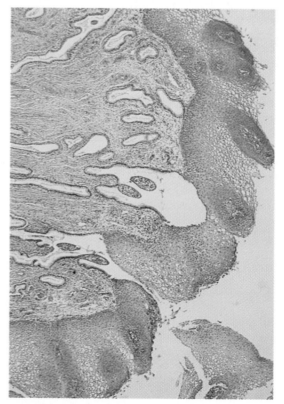

Figure 5–3. Condyloma acuminatum that is mainly flat but with focal early papillae.

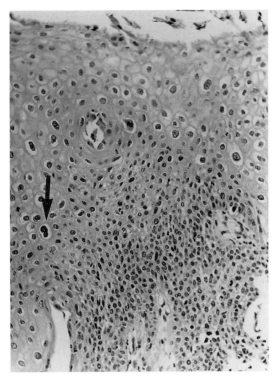

Figure 5–4. Koilocytotic atypia. Notice the binucleate cell (*arrow*).

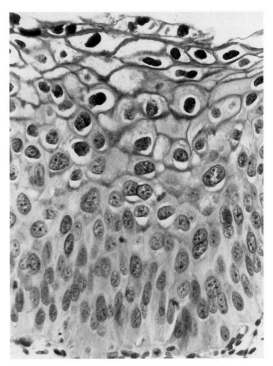

Figure 5–6. High-grade intraepithelial lesion (i.e., moderate dysplasia or CIN 2) with koilocytosis.

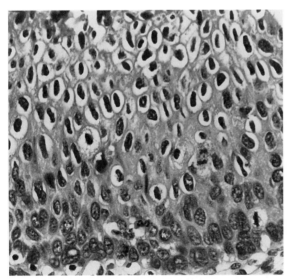

Figure 5–5. Low-grade intraepithelial lesion (i.e., mild dysplasia or CIN 1) with koilocytosis. Because of significant atypia in the basal and parabasal layers, some investigators would consider this a high-grade intraepithelial lesion.

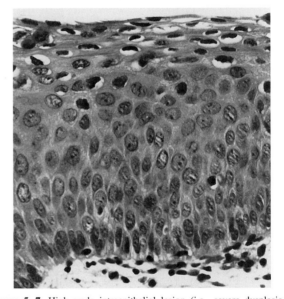

Figure 5–7. High-grade intraepithelial lesion (i.e., severe dysplasia or CIN 3) with koilocytosis.

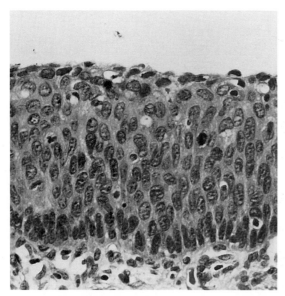

Figure 5–8. High-grade intraepithelial lesion (i.e., severe dysplasia or CIN 3).

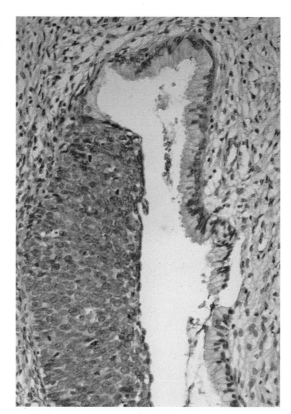

Figure 5–10. High-grade intraepithelial lesion with glandular involvement.

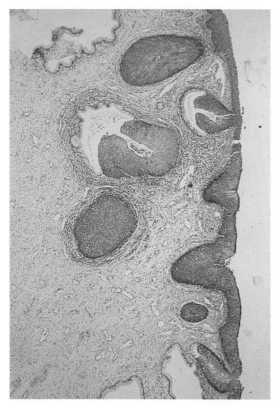

Figure 5–9. High-grade intraepithelial lesion with surface and glandular involvement.

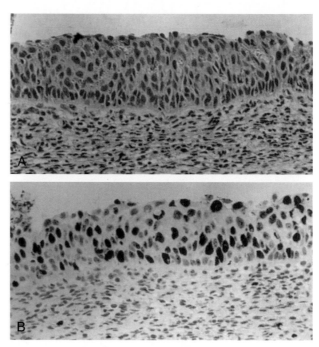

Figure 5–11. Atypical immature squamous metaplasia. *A,* The lesion exhibits loss of maturation anid enlarged hyperchromatic nuclei, but the epithelium is thin, and there are no evident mitotic figures. *B,* Immunostain for Ki-67 shows positive nuclei at all levels of the epithelium. The lesion contained human papillomavirus types 31 and 18 as determined by polymerase chain reaction. (From Geng L, Connolly DC, Isacson C, Ronnett BM, Cho KR. Atypical immature metaplasia [AIM] of the cervix: is it related to high-grade squamous intraepithelial lesion [HSIL]? Hum Pathol 30:345–351, 1999.)

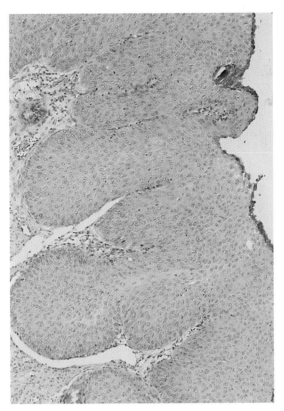

Figure 5–12. Papillary immature metaplasia. Residual columnar epithelium is on the surface (*extreme right*).

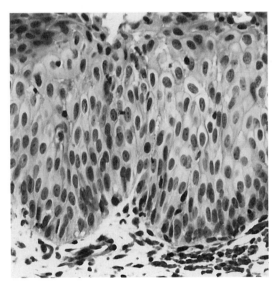

Figure 5–13. Typical immature squamous metaplasia.

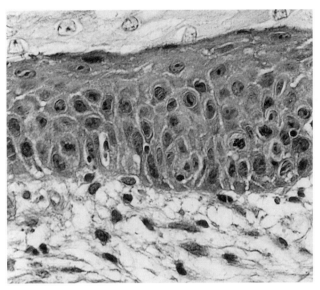

Figure 5–14. Reactive atypia. Notice the spongiosis and distinct cell borders. The nuclei are irregular and hyperchromatic but lack coarse hyperchromasia.

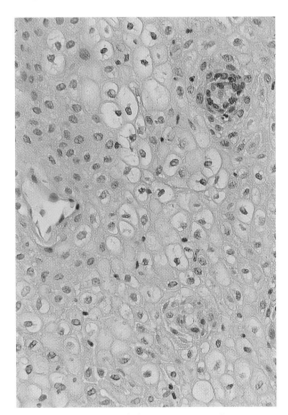

Figure 5–15. Pseudokoilocytosis in a postmenopausal woman.

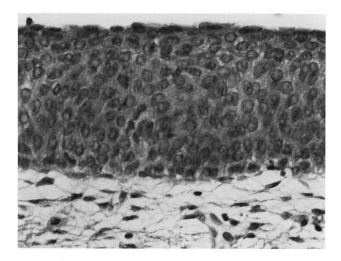

Figure 5–16. Atrophy. The cells have a high nucleus to cytoplasm ratio and show no maturation, but the nuclei lack dysplastic features and mitotic figures.

EARLY INVASIVE SQUAMOUS CELL CARCINOMAS

- These tumors are also referred to as ISCCs, stage Ia or microinvasive SCCs.
- The International Federation of Gynecology and Obstetrics (FIGO) definition for stage Ia ISCCs states that they are identified only microscopically and that measured stromal invasion does not exceed 5 mm deep and 7 mm wide (Table 5–2).
- Stage Ia ISCCs can only be diagnosed in conization or hysterectomy specimens that include the entire lesion. Clinically visible tumors are stage Ib, regardless of size.
  - Stage Ia1 ISCCs are those exhibiting measured stromal invasion no greater than 3 mm deep and no greater than 7 mm wide. Stage Ia2 lesions are those exhibiting measured stromal invasion greater than 3 mm but no deeper than 5 mm and no wider than 7 mm.
  - The depth of invasion is measured from the base of the epithelium from which it originates. The proximity of the invasive tumor (and any associated SIL) to the resection margins should be determined. Vascular space involvement (venous or lymphatic) does not alter the staging but should be recorded.
- The Society of Gynecologic Oncologists (SGO) defines microinvasive carcinoma as a lesion that invades the cervical stroma to a depth of 3.0 mm or less below the base of the epithelium and in which there is no evidence of lymphovascular space invasion.

Clinical Features

- Ia ISCCs are found in about 5% of serially sectioned cone biopsy specimens performed for HSILs. The mean

Table 5–2
FIGO STAGING OF CARCINOMA OF THE UTERINE CERVIX

Stage 0	Carcinoma in situ, intraepithelial carcinoma
Stage I	Carcinoma is confined to the cervix (extension to the corpus is disregarded).
Ia	Invasive cancer is identified only microscopically. Invasion is limited to measured stromal invasion with maximum depth of 5 mm and no wider than 7 mm. The depth of invasion is measured from the base of the epithelium from which it originates. Vascular space involvement (venous or lymphatic) does not alter the staging but should be recorded.
Ia1	Measured stroma invasion no deeper than 3 mm and no wider than 7 mm
Ia2	Measured stroma invasion deeper than 3 mm and no deeper than 5 mm and no wider than 7 mm
Ib	Clinical lesions confined to the cervix or preclinical lesions greater than stage IA
Ib1	Clinical lesions not greater than 4 cm in size
Ib2	Clinical lesions greater than 4 cm in size
Stage II	The carcinoma extends beyond the cervix but has not extended to the pelvic wall. The carcinoma involves the vagina but not the lower third.
IIa	No obvious parametrial involvement
IIb	Obvious parametrial involvement
Stage III	The carcinoma has extended to the pelvic wall. On rectal examination, there is no cancer-free space between the tumor and the pelvic wall. The tumor involves the lower third of the vagina.
IIIa	No extension to the pelvic wall
IIIb	Extension to the pelvic wall and/or hydronephrosis or nonfunctioning kidney
Stage IV	The carcinoma has extended beyond the true pelvis or has clinically involved the mucosa of the bladder or rectum. Bullous edema does not allow designation of this stage.
IVa	Spread of the growth to adjacent organs
IVb	Spread of tumor to distant organs

age of the patients is about 45 years, which is about 10 years younger than the mean age of women with ISCCs in general.

■ The presenting clinical features are similar to those of patients with SILs. In some cases, the diagnosis of early invasion may be suspected on the Pap smears. Some patients have a visible colposcopic abnormality that differs from the surrounding HSIL, allowing localization by a punch biopsy.

Microscopic Features

■ Early stromal invasion usually begins as one or more tongues of neoplastic cells that have broken through the basement membrane of the surface or glandular epithelium involved by an SIL, which is usually widespread, including extensive glandular involvement. More than 90% arise within the transformation zone, the remainder arising from the native ectocervical squamous epithelium.

■ Larger tumors may form solid masses (i.e., confluent pattern), numerous small nests widely separated by stroma (i.e., spray pattern), or both. Some early invasive ISCCs are multifocal.

■ The invasive tongues or nests of cells usually show greater differentiation than the overlying SIL, with more abundant eosinophilic cytoplasm and, in some cases, intercellular bridges or keratinization. Many investigators do not grade stage Ia ISCCs, because this feature has no prognostic significance.

■ There is almost always a stromal reaction to the invasive tumor that may include edema, fibrosis, chronic inflammatory cells, and occasionally, a granulomatous response to keratin.

■ Lymphovascular space invasion (LVSI) should be searched for, because its presence may affect treatment and prognosis (described later). The frequency of LVSI increases with the depth of invasion; frequencies of 4.4% in tumors less than 1 mm deep, 16.4% in tumors 1 to 2.9 mm, and 19.7% in tumors 3 to 5 mm were found in one study.

■ The status of the margins of the cone biopsy specimen should be determined. When the margins are positive for SIL or invasive tumor, the risk of invasive tumor in the hysterectomy specimen is about 70%, compared with about 5% when the margins are negative.

■ Findings within SILs that may indicate the presence of early invasion are discussed on page 92.

Differential Diagnosis

■ Nonneoplastic lesions, including florid squamous metaplasia (page 63), postbiopsy pseudoinvasion of squamous epithelium (page 75), ectopic decidua (page 81), and placental site nodule (page 220). Pseudoinvasion of vascular spaces by an SIL has been described as an artifact caused by cervical lidocaine injection before loop diathermy.

■ Endocervical gland involvement by SILs. Such glands maintain the location and configuration of normal endocervical glands and the involved glands have a well-circumscribed, smooth border with the endocervical stroma and lack the irregular contours and the maturational and stromal changes of early ISCCs.

Prognosis and Behavior of Stage Ia1 Lesions

■ Lymph node metastases occur with 1.7% of Ia1 lesions; the risk is higher for tumors with LVSI (8.2%) than in those without LVSI (0.8%). Recurrences develop in only 1.0% of women; the risk is higher for tumors with LVSI (3.1%) than those without LVSI (0.6%). Only 0.2% to 0.5% of patients die of disease.

■ These findings reflect the general consensus that Ia1 ISCCs without LVSI have a negligible risk of nodal involvement and can be treated by cone biopsy (if the resection margins are negative). The treatment of Ia1 ISCCs with lymphatic invasion is individualized, but in some centers, these lesions are treated like IA2 lesions.

Prognosis and Behavior of Stage Ia2 Lesions

■ Lymph node metastases occur in about 8.0% of cases. A literature review found that, surprisingly, the risk of nodal spread for tumors with LVSI (7.5%) was similar to that for tumors without LVSI (8.3%). Recurrences develop in 4% to 6% of women with Ia2 ISCCs; the risk is much higher for tumors with LVSI (15.7%) than those without LVSI (1.7%).

■ Buckley and colleagues found that lymphovascular space invasion by the primary tumor decreased the 5-year survival rate from 98% to 89%.

■ These observations indicate that patients with Ia2 ISCCs require pelvic lymphadenectomy, usually as part of a radical hysterectomy. Fertility-sparing treatment, consisting of cone biopsy (with negative margins) and pelvic lymphadenectomy, has been successful in some women.

References

Al-Nafussi AI, Hughes DE. Histological features of CIN3 and their value in predicting invasive microinvasive squamous carcinoma. J Clin Pathol 47:799–804, 1994.

Benedet JL, Anderson GH. Stage IA carcinoma of the cervix revisited. Obstet Gynecol 87:1052–1059, 1996.

Buckley SL, Tritz DM, Van Le L, et al. Lymph node metastases and prognosis in patients with stage Ia2 cervical cancer. Gynecol Oncol 63:4–9, 1996.

Burghardt E, Girardi F, Lahousen M, et al. Microinvasive carcinoma of the uterine cervix (International Federation of Gynecology and Obstetrics stage IA). Cancer 67:1037–1045, 1991.

Creasman WT, Zaino RJ, Major FJ, et al. Early invasive carcinoma of the cervix (3 to 5 mm invasion): risk factors and prognosis. A Gynecologic Oncology Group study. Am J Obstet Gynecol 178:62–65, 1998.

McLachlin CM, Devine P, Muto M, Genest DR. Pseudoinvasion of vascular spaces: report of an artifact caused by cervical lidocaine injection prior to loop diathermy. Hum Pathol 25:208–211, 1994.

Östör AG. Studies on 200 cases of early squamous cell carcinoma of the cervix. Int J Gynecol Pathol 12:193–207, 1993.

Östör AG. Pandora's box or Ariadne's thread? Definition and prognostic significance of microinvasion in the uterine cervix: squamous lesions. Pathol Annu 30(2):103–135, 1995.

Östör AG, Rome RM. Micro-invasive squamous cell carcinoma of the cervix: a clinico-pathologic study of 200 cases with long-term follow-up. Int J Gynecol Cancer 4:257–264, 1994.

Sevin B-U, Nadji M, Averette HE, et al. Microinvasive carcinoma of the cervix. Cancer 70:2121–2128, 1992.

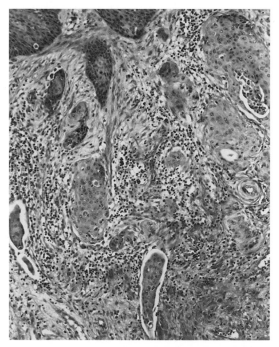

Figure 5–18. Early invasive squamous cell carcinoma, stage Ia1. The invasive nests are better differentiated than the overlying high-grade intraepithelial lesion. Notice the lymphatic invasion.

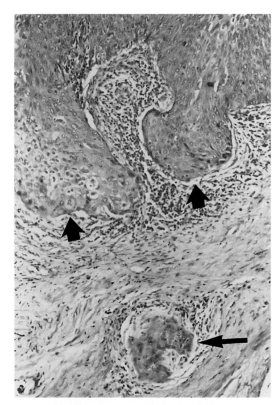

Figure 5–17. Early invasive squamous cell carcinoma, stage Ia1. Two tongues of invasive tumor (*arrows*) arise from the overlying high-grade intraepithelial lesion (HSIL). A detached nest of invasive tumor is seen at the bottom of the figure (*long arrow*). Notice the maturation of invasive foci (compared with the HSIL) and the stromal inflammatory response.

INVASIVE SQUAMOUS CELL CARCINOMA

Clinical Features

■ ISCCs account for 80% of invasive cervical carcinomas. The mean age is 55 years, which is about 20 years after that of HSILs. Approximately 30% of cervical ISCCs, however, occur in women younger than 35 years of age.

■ In contrast to the rising incidence of SILs, the incidence of ISCC and its associated mortality have decreased dramatically during the past 30 years in countries in which most women receive regular screening by Pap smears. Most ISCCs in these countries occur in women who have never had a Pap smear or who have not had a Pap smear for many years. ISCCs are still among the most common fatal cancers in women in countries that lack mass screening programs.

■ Between 2% and 10% of ISCCs are diagnosed in women within a year of a negative Pap smear. The previous negative smear on review in these cases is often found to be positive, but they occasionally are truly negative (i.e., rapidly progressive or rapid-onset ISCCs).

- The risk factors are the same as for SILs. The HPV subtypes that are found in all or almost all cervical ISCCs are the same as those associated with HSILs (page 90).
- Patients with small tumors are often asymptomatic, and the tumors are detected by an abnormal Pap smear, findings on pelvic or colposcopic examination, or combinations thereof.
- Women with symptomatic tumors usually have painless, intermittent (often postcoital) vaginal bleeding. More advanced tumors may cause continuous bleeding (or discharge), pain, or symptoms related to bowel or bladder or lymph node involvement.
- A mass is usually found on pelvic examination, and the diagnosis is usually made by a punch biopsy.
- The serum level of squamous cell carcinoma antigen is elevated in about 60% of patients. The elevated levels are often a reflection of metastatic disease and can be used to monitor response to treatment. The serum carcinoembryonic antigen (CEA) and CA-125 levels also correlate with the stage of the tumor, but they are less useful.

Gross Features

- The tumors, when small, are almost always localized to the transformation zone. They may be exophytic (polypoid or papillary), ulcerative, endophytic, or combinations thereof. A barrel-shaped cervix may result from diffuse cervical expansion by an endophytic tumor.
- Local extension to the parametrium, vagina, or corpus may be appreciable grossly in the hysterectomy specimen.

Usual Microscopic Features

- Most tumors are of conventional type and traditionally divided into nonkeratinizing and keratinizing subtypes, although there appears to be no prognostic differences between these subtypes. Rare squamous cell carcinomas are characterized by a predominant component of small cells, as discussed later. Warty and basaloid squamous carcinomas of the cervix, which resemble their vulvar counterparts (see Chapter 2), are so rare in the cervix that their clinicopathologic features in this site have not been defined.
- Nonkeratinizing ISCCs lack squamous pearls, but individual cell keratinization is often evident. The tumor cells, typically arranged in nests, tend to be uniform with indistinct cell borders, round to oval nuclei with coarse chromatin, and frequent mitotic figures.
- Keratinizing ISCCs, by definition, contain keratin pearls; individual cell keratinization is also usually present. The tumor cells, which are arranged in nests and cords that tend to be more irregular than those of the nonkeratinizing tumors, have eosinophilic cytoplasm, distinct cell borders, and variably sized nuclei. Mitotic figures are less numerous than in the nonkeratinizing tumors.
- Most tumors referred to as small cell carcinomas in the older literature are currently classified as small cell undifferentiated (neuroendocrine) carcinomas (page 128). Bona fide small cell squamous carcinomas (SCSCs) are rare. The only recent study (based on 13 cases) found that the prognosis of SCSCs is similar to that of other ISCCs.
  - SCSCs are composed of cohesive nests of predominantly small cells with scanty cytoplasm and small, round to oval nuclei, with the appearance resembling that of the cells within HSILs.
  - SCSCs usually lack individual cell keratinization or pearl formation, although in some tumors, the small cells merge with larger cells with more abundant eosinophilic cytoplasm that are more overtly squamous in nature. Occasionally, there is an abrupt transition from small cells to rounded foci of keratin.
- No widely accepted grading system exists for cervical ISCCs. None of those that have been applied has been consistently useful in predicting prognosis.

Unusual Microscopic Features

- Between 20% and 35% of otherwise typical ISCCs of the cervix contain intracellular mucin demonstrable with mucin stains (so-called mucoepidermoid carcinoma). In contrast to adenosquamous carcinomas (page 125), glandular differentiation is absent.
  - Although three studies concluded that these tumors are more commonly associated with lymph node spread or a worse prognosis than typical ISCCs, two other studies using multivariate analysis found no such differences.
- Rare, otherwise typical ISCCs contain cells with glycogen-rich clear cytoplasm. Such tumors may be confused with a clear cell adenocarcinoma (see Differential Diagnosis, page 102).
- Rare tumors have a deceptively benign pattern of invasion, growing as well-circumscribed, typically large, oval to round nests with smooth borders and little or no stromal response.
- Rare, otherwise typical ISCCs have distinctive stromal changes:
  - A massive inflammatory component of eosinophils; in such cases, eosinophils may also be found in the regional lymph nodes or within the blood.
  - Deposits of amyloid immunoreactive for cytokeratin, probably derived from cytokeratin intermediate filaments.
  - A prominent myxoid stroma or a prominent, densely hyalinized stroma.

Differential Diagnosis

- Nonneoplastic lesions including florid squamous metaplasia (page 63), postbiopsy pseudoinvasion of squamous epithelium (page 75), ectopic decidua (page 81), and placental site nodule (versus ISCC with hyalinized stroma) (page 220).
- HSIL with extensive endocervical gland involvement (versus ISCC with a deceptively benign pattern of invasion, as described previously). The distribution and

depth of the nests of ISCCs are usually inconsistent with even extensive endocervical glandular involvement by an HSIL; in the latter situation, glands that are only partially replaced by HISL are usually found. Some ISCCs with a deceptively benign invasive pattern may contain foci of conventional ISCC.

■ Epithelioid trophoblastic tumor (page 227).
■ Clear cell adenocarcinoma (versus ISCCs with clear cells). The presence of typical ISCC in other areas of the tumor and an absence of glandular and papillary areas and hobnail cells facilitate the diagnosis.
■ Small cell undifferentiated carcinoma (SCUC).
  • Histologic features favoring SCUC over SCSC include a highly infiltrative pattern as sheets, nests, ribbons, cords, and single cells; rosette-like spaces; hyperchromatic molded nuclei lacking nucleoli, often with smudged chromatin or crush artifact; a high mitotic rate; prominent lymphatic invasion; and an absence of merging of the small cells with more typical squamous cells.
  • Ambros and coworkers found other features favoring SCSC over SCUC, including an older age (mean of 50 versus 36 years for SCUC), associated CIN (62% versus 0%), cytokeratin-positive and neuroendocrine marker–negative immunoprofile (62% versus 0%), and nonreactivity for HPV 18 DNA (64% versus 40%). Because of overlap with respect to these features between the two groups, the distinction between SCSC and SCUC should be based primarily on the appearance of the tumor on hematoxylin and eosin–stained slides.

Prognostic Factors

■ Prognostic factors are numerous and interdependent. Those included here are significant by multivariate analysis.
■ Clinical stage (see Table 5–2). Stage is the most important prognostic factor. The 5-year survival rates are 90% to 95% for stage I; 50% to 70% for stage II; about 30% for stage III; and less than 20% for stage IV. Other factors are important in predicting prognosis within stage I and stage II tumors.
■ Size and depth. The 5-year disease-free survival rates by size in one series were 93% for 1 cm or less, 76% for 1.1 to 2 cm, 64% for 2.1 to 3 cm, and 60% for more than 3 cm. Survival by depth was 92% for 5 mm or less, 74% for 6 to 10 mm, and 60% for more than 10 mm.
■ LVSI. LVSI was documented in about 50% of stage Ib tumors in one study and about 70% of stage Ib and IIa tumors in another study.
  • LVSI is a significant predictor of lymph node metastases and disease-free survival. In one study, 25% of women with LVSI had positive nodes, compared with 8% of those without LVSI. In a different study, 5-year disease-free intervals were 85% (no LVSI) and 62% (LVSI).
  • In one study, the proportion of tissue sections that contained LVSI was a better predictor of lymph node metastases than simply the presence of LVSI.

■ Parametrial involvement. Zriek and colleagues found this to be significantly associated with a shorter disease-free interval, independent of lymph node involvement.
■ Pelvic lymph node status. The risk of nodal involvement increases with depth of invasion: about 15% in tumors 5.1 to 10 mm and about 25% in tumors 10.1 to 15 mm.
  • Five-year disease free intervals in one study were 77% with no positive pelvic nodes, 55% with one or two positive nodes, and 39% with more than two positive nodes.
  • Five-year survival rates from another study were 89% with no nodes involved, 70% with one positive node, and 38% with four or more positive nodes. In the latter study, the 5-year survival rate was 70% when the metastases were less than 2 mm but 39% when more than 20 mm in diameter.
  • Paraaortic node involvement is associated with a poor prognosis and recurrences at distant sites.
■ DNA ploidy. Ploidy has been an independent prognostic factor in only some studies. Nguyen and coworkers found that a DNA index of 1.7 or less was an adverse prognostic indicator by multivariate analysis (median survival of 39 versus 73.5 months).

References

Ambros RA, Park J, Shah KV, Kurman RJ. Evaluation of histologic, morphometric, and immunohistochemical criteria in the differential diagnosis of small cell carcinomas of the cervix with particular reference to human papillomavirus types 16 and 18. Mod Pathol 4:586–593, 1991.

Dallenbach-Hellweg G. On the origin and histological structure of adenocarcinoma of the endocervix in women under 50 years of age. Pathol Res Pract 179:38–50, 1984.

Delgado G, Bundy B, Zaino R, et al. Prospective surgical-pathologic study of disease-free interval in patients with stage Ib squamous carcinoma of the cervix: a Gynecologic Oncology Group study. Gynecol Oncol 38:352–357, 1990.

Foschini MP, Fulcheri E, Baracchini P, et al. Squamous cell carcinoma with prominent myxoid stroma. Hum Pathol 21:859–865, 1990.

Girardi F, Haas J. The importance of the histologic processing of pelvic lymph nodes in the treatment of cervical cancer. Int J Gynecol Oncol 3:12–17, 1993.

Kapp DS, LiVolsi VA. Intense eosinophilic stromal infiltration in carcinoma of the uterine cervix: a clinicopathologic study of 14 cases. Gynecol Oncol 16:19–30, 1983.

Langlois NEI, Ellul B, Miller ID. A study of the value and prognostic significance of mucin staining in squamous cell carcinoma of the uterine cervix. Histopathology 28:175–178, 1996.

Lovecchio JL, Averette HE, Donato D, Bell J. Five-year survival of patients with periaortic nodal metastases in clinical stage IB and IIA cervical carcinoma. Gynecol Oncol 34:43–45, 1989.

Nguyen HN, Sevin B, Averette HE, et al. The role of DNA index as a prognostic factor in early cervical carcinoma. Gynecol Oncol 50:54–59, 1993.

Roman LD, Felix JC, Muderspach LI, et al. Influence of quantity of lymph-vascular space invasion on the risk of nodal metastases in women with early-stage squamous cancer of the cervix. Gynecol Oncol 68:220–225, 1998.

Samlal RAK, Ten Kate FJW, Hart AAM, Lammes FB. Do mucin-secreting squamous cell carcinomas of the uterine cervix metastasize more frequently to pelvic lymph nodes? A case-control study. Int J Gynecol Pathol 17:201–204, 1998.

Sevin B, Nadji M, Lampe B, et al. Prognostic factors of early stage cervical cancer treated by radical hysterectomy. Cancer 76:1978–1986, 1995.

Sevin B, Lu Y, Bloch DA, et al. Surgically defined prognostic parameters in patients with early cervical carcinoma: a multivariate survival tree analysis. Cancer 78:1438–1446, 1996.

Thelmo WL, Nicastri AD, Fruchter R, et al. Mucoepidermoid carcinoma of uterine cervix stage Ib. Int J Gynecol Pathol 9:316–324, 1990.

Tsang WYW, Chart JKC. Amyloid-producing squamous cell carcinoma of the uterine cervix. Arch Pathol Lab Med 117:199–201, 1993.

Wain GV, Farnsworth A, Hacker NF. Cervical carcinoma after negative Pap smears: evidence against rapid-onset cancers. Int J Gynecol Cancer 2:318–322, 1992.

Zaino RJ, Ward S, Delgado G, et al. Histopathologic predictors of the behavior of surgically treated stage IB squamous cell carcinoma of the cervix: a Gynecologic Oncology Group Study. Cancer 69:1750–1758, 1992.

Zriek TG, Chambers JT, Chambers SK. Parametrial involvement, regardless of nodal status: a poor prognostic factor for cervical cancer. Obstet Gynecol 87:741–746, 1996.

Variants of Squamous Cell Carcinoma

Verrucous Carcinoma

- About 35 verrucous carcinomas in the cervix have been reported. Some of these tumors, however, do not meet the rigid microscopic criteria for verrucous carcinoma (page 30) as this term has sometimes been used loosely for any well differentiated papillary squamous cell carcinoma.
- Their clinicopathologic features and differential diagnosis resemble those of their more common counterparts in the vulva (page 30).
- About 50% of the tumors have involved local structures such as the vagina, lower uterine segment, endometrium, or parametrium. Rare tumors have been a composite of conventional ISCC and verrucous carcinoma.
- The differential diagnosis includes papillary squamous carcinoma (page 105) and warty carcinoma (page 101).

References

Benedet JL, Clement PB. Verrucous carcinoma of the cervix and endometrium. Diagn Gynecol Obstet 2:197–203, 1980.

Degefu S, O'Quinn G, Lacey CG, et al. Verrucous carcinoma of the cervix: a report of two cases and literature review. Gynecol Oncol 25:37–47, 1986.

De Jesus M, Tang W, Sadiadi M, et al. Carcinoma of the cervix with extensive endometrial and myometrial involvement. Gynecol Oncol 36:263–270, 1990.

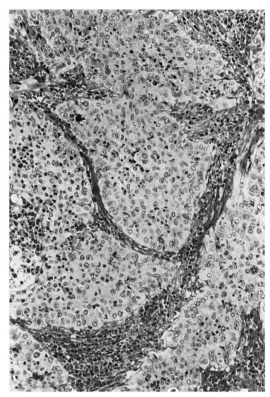

Figure 5–20. Invasive squamous cell carcinoma of the nonkeratinizing type. There is a prominent stromal inflammatory infiltrate between the nests of tumor.

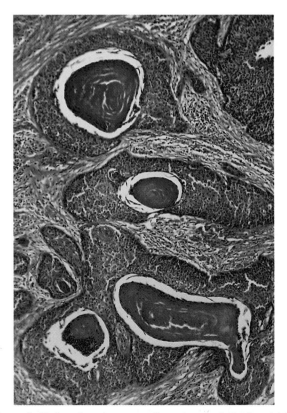

Figure 5–21. Invasive squamous cell carcinoma of the keratinizing type.

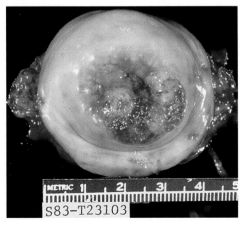

Figure 5–19. Invasive squamous cell carcinoma. A mass is present at the external os.

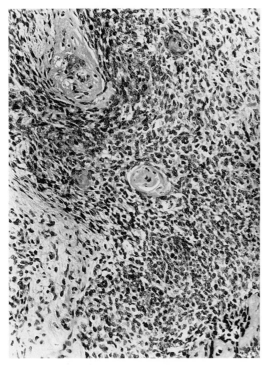

Figure 5–22. Invasive squamous cell carcinoma of the small cell type. Notice the keratin pearls.

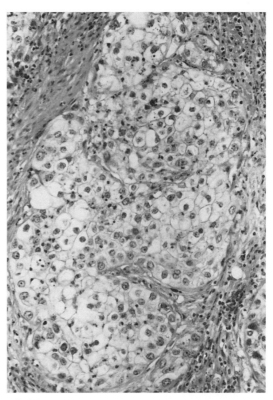

Figure 5–24. Invasive squamous cell carcinoma with clear (glycogen-rich) cytoplasm.

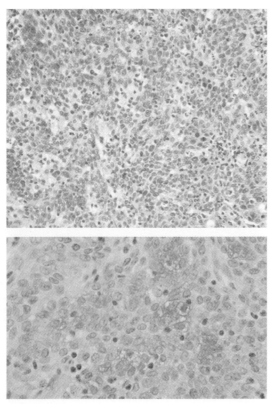

Figure 5–23. Invasive squamous cell carcinoma with intracellular mucin (*top*, hematoxylin and eosin stain; *bottom*, mucicarmine stain).

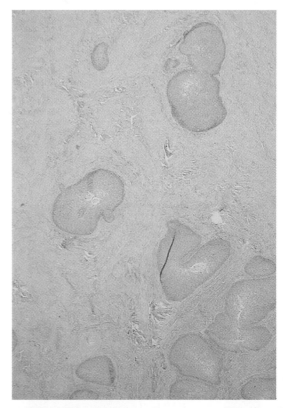

Figure 5–25. Invasive squamous cell carcinoma with a deceptively benign pattern of invasion. The invasive nests are very well circumscribed and elicit no stromal reaction.

Papillary Squamous Carcinoma

- In the only published series of papillary squamous carcinomas (PSCs), the patients were between 43 and 80 years old (mean, 57 years) and usually presented with vaginal bleeding. Large exophytic masses, some with papillary excrescences, were found on pelvic examination.
- On microscopic examination, thin to thick papillae with fibrovascular cores are covered by dysplastic squamous cells with mitotic figures throughout the epithelium, an appearance potentially mimicking that of HSIL.
- Invasive tumor, which occurs at the base of the papillae and may not be appreciated on a superficial biopsy specimen, typically exhibits maturation with cells containing more abundant eosinophilic cytoplasm compared to the cells in the papillae. Some PSCs lack definite invasion.
- PSCs have a high index of Ki-67 staining in the upper layers. One PSC tested for HPV was found to be positive for HPV-16.
- Four of nine patients in one series died of tumor (all were stage II or higher); two patients died after disease-free intervals of more than 7 years.

Differential Diagnosis

- Verrucous carcinoma. These tumors, in contrast to PSCs, have bland nuclear features and a pushing, rather than infiltrative, deep border.
- Warty carcinoma. These tumors are rare in the cervix and resemble their much more common vulvar counterparts (page 27). In contrast to PSCs, koilocytosis is a prominent feature.
- Papillary immature metaplasia (page 92). This lesion lacks the marked atypia, high mitotic rate, and the high Ki-67 index of PSCs.

References

Ollayos CW, Lichy J, Duncan BW, Ali IS. Papillary squamous cell carcinoma of the uterine cervix: report of a case with HPV 16 DNA and brief review. Gynecol Oncol 63:388–391, 1996.

Randall ME, Andersen WA, Mills SE, Kim JC. Papillary squamous cell carcinoma of the uterine cervix: a clinicopathologic study of nine cases. Int J Gynecol Pathol 5:1–10, 1986.

Trivijitsilp P, Mosher R, Sheets EE, et al. Papillary immature metaplasia: a clinicopathologic analysis and comparison with papillary squamous carcinoma. Hum Pathol 29:641–648, 1998.

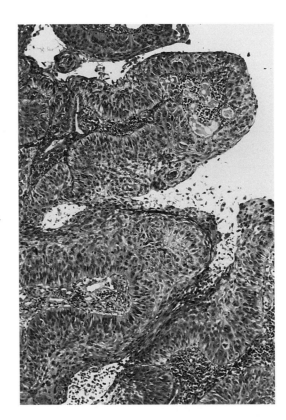

Figure 5–26. Papillary squamous carcinoma.

Papillary Transitional Cell Carcinoma and Squamotransitional Cell Carcinomas

- Rare cervical carcinomas resemble papillary transitional cell carcinomas (TCCs) of the urinary bladder. Such tumors may be pure TCCs or exhibit focal squamous differentiation (squamotransitional cell carcinoma) (STCC). One cervical TCC had a growth pattern resembling that of an inverted papilloma (page 85).
- These tumors overlap with and otherwise resemble papillary squamous cell carcinomas (PSCs) of the cervix. The classification of a papillary tumor as TCC, STCC, or PSC is subjective in some cases.
- Based on the small number of reported cases, the clinical and gross features and behavior of these tumors do not differ significantly from those of pure squamous cell carcinomas, including the presence of HPV-16 in four of six cervical TCCs in one study.

References

Albores-Saavedra J, Young RH. Transitional cell neoplasms (carcinomas and inverted papillomas) of the uterine cervix: a report of five cases. Am J Surg Pathol 19:1138–1145, 1995.

Fukunaga M. Inverted papilloma-like transitional cell carcinoma of the uterine cervix [Letter]. Histopathology 33:189–191, 1998.

Koenig C, Turnicky RP, Kankam CF, Tavassoli FA. Papillary squamo-transitional cell carcinoma of the cervix: report of 32 cases. Am J Surg Pathol 21:915–921, 1997.

Lininger RA, Wistuba I, Gazdar A, et al. Human papillomavirus type 16 is detected in transitional cell carcinomas and squamotransitional cell carcinomas of the cervix and endometrium. Cancer 83:521–527, 1998.

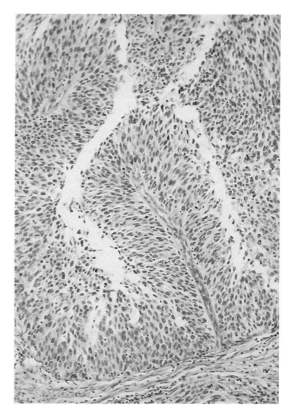

Figure 5–27. Transitional cell carcinoma.

Pseudosarcomatous Squamous Cell Carcinoma

- Five pseudosarcomatous squamous cell carcinomas have been reported in the uterine cervix, all in postmenopausal women. In each tumor, typical ISCC merged with malignant spindle cells.
- In the two most recently reported tumors, the spindle cells were immunoreactive for cytokeratin and each tumor had an additional component of osteoclastic-type giant cells.
- Of the three patients with follow-up, all died of tumor 7 to 14 weeks after presentation, one with intraabdominal carcinomatosis.
- Sarcomatoid ISCCs should be distinguished from malignant müllerian mixed tumors (MMMT) (carcinosarcoma) of the cervix (page 197).
  - A lack of merging of the two components and the presence of an admixed adenocarcinoma, heterologous elements, or both favor the diagnosis of MMMT.
- Strong, diffuse immunoreactivity of the sarcomatoid component for epithelial markers favors a diagnosis of ISCC. The immunostains, however, must be interpreted with caution, because the malignant spindle cells of sarcomatoid ISCCs may be only focally immunoreactive or nonreactive for cytokeratins, and the sarcomatous elements of MMMTs may focally immunoreact with antikeratin antibodies.

References

Clement PB, Zubovits JT, Young RH, Scully RE. Malignant müllerian mixed tumors of the uterine cervix: a clincopathological study of 9 cases. Int J Gynecol Pathol 17:211–222, 1998.

Pong L-C. Sarcomatoid squamous cell carcinoma of the uterine cervix with osteoclastic-like giant cells: report of two cases. Int J Gynecol Pathol 17:174–177, 1998.

Steeper TA, Piscioli F, Rosai J. Squamous cell carcinoma with sarcoma-like stroma of the female genital tract: clinicopathologic study of four cases. Cancer 52:890–898, 1983.

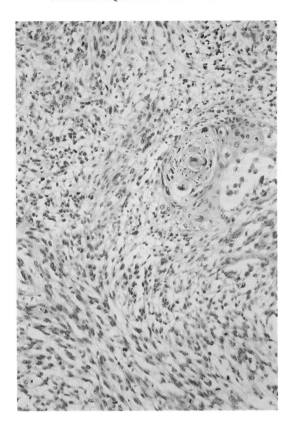

Figure 5–28. Pseudosarcomatous invasive squamous cell carcinoma. A nest of typical squamous cell carcinoma merges with malignant spindle cells.

Lymphoepithelioma-like Carcinoma

- Although only about 25 tumors designated lymphoepithelioma-like carcinoma have been reported in the literature, similar or identical tumors have been included in series of tumors labeled "inflammatory" carcinomas, "circumscribed carcinomas with marked lymphocytic infiltration," and "medullary carcinomas with lymphoid infiltration."
- The tumors occur over a wide age range (29 to 74 years); the median age in one series was 56 years. The presenting clinical features and the gross features do not differ significantly from usual ISCCs of the cervix.
- The tumors microscopically resemble their counterparts in the nasopharynx and other sites. Singly disposed or syncytial aggregates of epithelial cells with moderate amounts of pale cytoplasm; large, uniform, vesicular nuclei; and small nucleoli are dispersed within a dense lymphoplasmacytic infiltrate. Mitotic figures are usually present but are not numerous.
- Eosinophils and histiocytes may also be present; the former occasionally is the predominant cell type. The histiocytes may occur singly or as granulomatous aggregates.

- Tseng and associates found the Epstein-Barr virus gene sequence in 73.3% of cases (versus 26.7% in typical ISCCs) and HPV-16, HPV-18, or both in 20% (versus 80% in typical ISCCs).
- Based on a small number of cases, the prognosis appears to be better than that of typical ISCCs. All of the 15 patients in the largest series had a benign clinical course, although some tumors in other studies have been clinically malignant.

Differential Diagnosis

- Malignant lymphoma. Cytokeratin stains to highlight the neoplastic epithelial cells can facilitate the diagnosis in tumors in which the neoplastic epithelial cells are widely dispersed.
- Glassy cell carcinoma (page 125). Although these tumors can have a prominent inflammatory infiltrate, the tumor cells have ground-glass cytoplasm, distinct cell borders, macronucleoli, and a high mitotic rate.
- Conventional ISCCs with a prominent inflammatory infiltrate. These tumors usually have larger aggregates of tumor cells and tumor cells with more abundant cyto-

plasm, focally distinct cell borders, and more pleomorphic and hyperchromatic nuclei. Focal keratinization may be present.

References

Mills SE, Austin MB, Randall ME. Lymphoepithelioma-like carcinoma of the uterine cervix: a distinctive, undifferentiated carcinoma with inflammatory stroma. Am J Surg Pathol 9:883–889, 1985.
Tseng C, Pao C, Tseng L, et al. Lymphoepithelioma-like carcinoma of the uterine cervix: association with Epstein-Barr virus and human papillomavirus. Cancer 80:91–97, 1997.

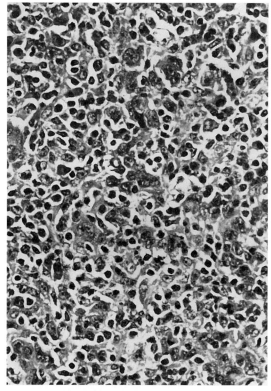

Figure 5–29. Lymphoepithelioma-like carcinoma. Single and small nests of epithelial cells are separated by a mononuclear inflammatory infiltrate of lymphocytes and plasma cells.

CHAPTER 6

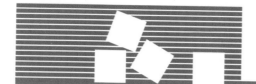

Glandular Carcinomas of the Cervix, Related Tumors, and Their Precursors

PREINVASIVE GLANDULAR LESIONS AND EARLY INVASIVE ADENOCARCINOMAS

Adenocarcinoma in Situ

Clinical Features

- Adenocarcinoma in situ (AIS), a precursor of invasive adenocarcinoma, accounts for only 10% of endocervical adenocarcinomas; this low frequency, which contrasts with that of most precursor lesions, partially results from underdiagnosis.
- Median and mean ages at diagnosis are in the fourth decade, 10 to 15 years lower than corresponding ages of patients with invasive adenocarcinoma. Twenty percent of patients have a history of squamous cervical intraepithelial neoplasia (CIN).
- The patients are usually asymptomatic, but almost all have abnormal Pap smears that may contain dysplastic glandular cells, dysplastic squamous cells, or both. The smears of 50% to 95% of patients contain atypical glandular cells; a review of previous smears from patients with AIS usually increases the frequency of smears positive for atypical glandular cells.
- A visible lesion is rare. AIS may be detectable colposcopically, but there is no diagnostic appearance, and in some cases, the colposcopic abnormality is related to synchronous squamous CIN.

Microscopic Features

- AIS typically occurs in the transformation zone and is multifocal in about 15% of cases. The surface columnar and glandular epithelia are typically involved, but AIS occasionally is confined to only one of these sites. The involved glands are typically admixed with normal glands, and the distribution and configuration of the involved glands is similar to those of normal glands, including glands with an abnormal contour or those that are cystic or clustered.

- AIS is characterized by pseudostratified or stratified columnar cells with malignant nuclear features that focally replace the normal endocervical epithelium and occasionally form intraluminal cribriform or solid patterns or line intraglandular or surface papillae. The involved epithelium is usually recognizable on low-power examination because it appears darker than the normal glandular epithelium, from which it is usually sharply demarcated.

- Enlarged, fusiform, variably hyperchromatic nuclei are oriented perpendicular to the lumen, with fine to coarse chromatin and prominent nucleoli. Numerous normal and abnormal mitotic figures, which are often juxtaluminal, are usually present, as are apoptotic bodies. The cytoplasm of the lesional cells is typically immunoreactive for carcinoembryonic antigen.

- The three major types of AIS are listed in order of frequency (the two less common subtypes are almost always admixed with the endocervical subtype):
  - Typical or endocervical type: lesional cells have moderate amounts of juxtaluminal cytoplasm that stains variably positive for mucin, although the latter is diminished compared with normal endocervical cells.
  - Intestinal type: mucin-rich goblet cells (and less commonly, argentaffin cells and Paneth cells) contain intestinal type sialomucins.
  - Endometrioid type: the cells lack stainable mucin.

- Uncommon to rare variants of AIS include ciliated AIS, adenosquamous carcinoma in situ, serous papillary carcinoma in situ, glassy cell carcinoma in situ, and clear cell adenocarcinoma in situ

- Associated lesions include squamous CIN in 50% to 95%; endocervical glandular dysplasia (EGD) (discussed later) in a variable proportion of cases; coexis-

Table 6–1

DIFFERENTIAL FEATURES OF ENDOCERVICAL GLANDULAR DYSPLASIA AND ADENOCARCINOMA IN SITU

Feature	EGD	AIS
Nuclear pseudostratification	Slight	Moderate to marked
Nuclear enlargement and hyperchromasia	Present	Present
Chromatin pattern	Finely to moderately granular	Finely to moderately granular
Nucleoli	Inconspicuous	Inconspicuous to macronucleoli
Nuclear shape	Oval to elongated	Oval or irregular
Apoptosis	Present	Present, often prominent
Mitoses	Occasional	Frequent, may be abnormal
Cribriform pattern	Absent	May be present

Adapted from Jaworski RC. Endocervical glandular dysplasia, adenocarcinoma in situ, and early invasive (microinvasive) adenocarcinoma of the cervix. Semin Diagn Pathol 7:190–204, 1990.

tent microinvasive or invasive squamous cell or adenosquamous carcinoma in occasional cases; and an early invasive adenocarcinoma in 10% to 45% of cases.

Evidence Supporting Precancerous Potential

- AIS typically occurs in women 10 to 15 years younger than those with invasive cervical adenocarcinoma of the cervix.
- AIS is commonly associated with microinvasive adenocarcinoma or invasive adenocarcinoma in the same cone biopsy or hysterectomy specimen.
- AIS may precede invasive adenocarcinoma in the same patient.
- AIS is associated with a high frequency of human papillomavirus (HPV)–related antigens (especially types 16 and 18), which are also present in invasive adenocarcinoma.
- AIS has a histologic similarity to invasive adenocarcinoma.

Differential Diagnosis

- The differential of AIS includes endocervical glandular dysplasia (see next section and Table 6–1) and a variety of nonneoplastic glandular lesions, the differential features of which are discussed in Chapter 4, including tubal and tuboendometrioid metaplasia, oxyphilic metaplasia, reactive atypia, Arias-Stella reaction, radiation-induced atypia, and cautery artifact.

References

Biscotti CV, Hart WR. Apoptotic bodies: a consistent morphological feature of endocervical adenocarcinoma in situ. Am J Surg Pathol 22: 434–439, 1998.

Boon ME, Baak JPA, Kurver PJH, et al. Adenocarcinoma in situ of the cervix: an underdiagnosed lesion. Cancer 48:768–773, 1981.

Christopherson WM, Nealon N, Gray LA Sr. Noninvasive precursor lesions of adenocarcinoma and mixed adenosquamous carcinoma of the cervix uteri. Cancer 44:975–983, 1979.

Colgan TJ, Lickrish GM. The topography and invasive potential of cervical adenocarcinoma in situ, with and without associated squamous dysplasia. Gynecol Oncol 36:246–249, 1990.

Duggan MA, Benoit JL, McGregor E, et al. Adenocarcinoma in situ of the endocervix: human papillomavirus determination by dot blot hybridization and polymerase chain reaction amplification. Int J Gynecol Pathol 13:143–149, 1994.

Gloor E, Hurlimann J. Cervical intraepithelial glandular neoplasia (adenocarcinoma in situ and glandular dysplasia): a correlative study of 23 cases with histologic grading, histochemical analysis of mucins, and immunohistochemical determination of the affinity for four lectins. Cancer 58:1272–1280, 1986.

Gloor E, Ruzicka J. Morphology of adenocarcinoma in situ of the uterine cervix: a study of 14 cases. Cancer 49:294–302, 1982.

Hasumi K, Ehrmann RL. Clear cell carcinoma of the uterine endocervix with an in situ component. Cancer 42:2435–2438, 1978.

Jaworski RC, Pacey NF, Greenberg ML, Osborn RA. The histologic diagnosis of adenocarcinoma in situ and related lesions of the cervix uteri: adenocarcinoma in situ. Cancer 61:1171–1181, 1988.

Lee KR, Minter LJ, Granter SR. Papanicolaou smear sensitivity for adenocarcinoma in situ of the cervix: a study of 34 cases. Am J Clin Pathol 107:30–35, 1997.

Östör AG, Pagano R, Davoren RAM, et al. Adenocarcinoma in situ of the cervix. Int J Gynecol Pathol 3:179–190, 1984.

Schlesinger C, Silverberg SG. Endocervical adenocarcinoma in situ of tubal type and its relation to atypical tubal metaplasia. Int J Gynecol Pathol 18:1–4, 1999.

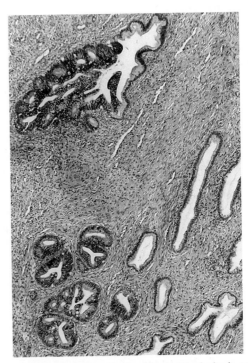

Figure 6–1. Adenocarcinoma in situ. The involved glands are darker than the normal glands. Notice the one gland (*upper left*) that is only partially replaced by the adenocarcinoma in situ.

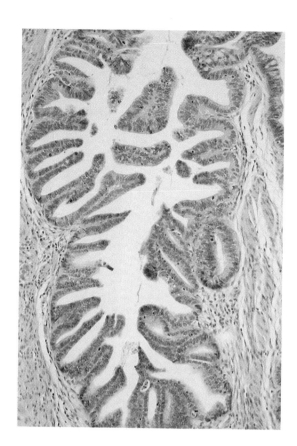

Figure 6–2. Adenocarcinoma in situ. The neoplastic cells line intraglandular papillae.

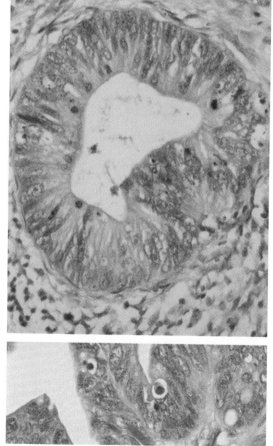

Figure 6–3. Adenocarcinoma in situ. Notice the malignant nuclear features, mitotic figures including juxtaluminal mitoses, and apoptotic bodies (bottom panel).

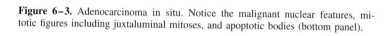

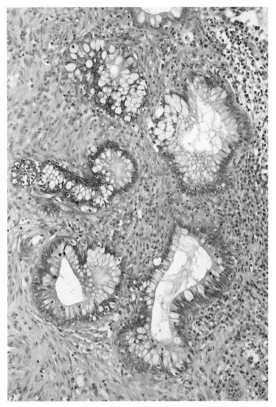

Figure 6–4. Intestinal-type adenocarcinoma in situ. Notice the numerous goblet cells.

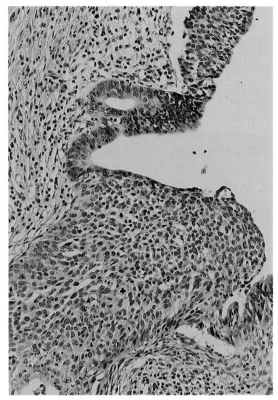

Figure 6–5. Adenocarcinoma in situ with grade 3 cervical intraepithelial neoplasia (i.e., high-grade intraepithelial squamous lesion).

Endocervical Glandular Dysplasia

- The clinical and pathologic features of this lesion are poorly characterized. Indeed, some investigators have cast doubt on the very existence of a precancerous glandular lesion of the endocervix that precedes or culminates in AIS.

- Most physicians use the term EGD to refer to a spectrum of dysplastic changes that are less severe than those of AIS. The mean age and age range of patients are similar to those of AIS patients. Atypical columnar cells in Pap smears were present in only 23% of cases in one study. EGD is most commonly found adjacent to AIS or squamous CIN III, but it is rarely an isolated finding.

- Gloor and coworkers subdivided EGD into cervical intraepithelial glandular neoplasia (CIGN) grades 1, 2, and 3, with CIGN 3 equivalent to AIS. Brown and Wells use a two-level classification of low-grade and high-grade EGD. However, the distinction between low-grade EGD from reactive atypias and the distinction between high-grade EGD and AIS are subjective and of unproven clinical utility.

- The minimal criteria for EGD (without subdivision into grades) proposed by Jaworski include evidence of cellular proliferation and turnover (i.e., occasional mitotic figures and apoptotic bodies) and nuclear atypia (see Table 6–1). The lesional cells are immunoreactive for HPV antigens in some cases.

Behavior

- The opportunity to study the behavior of EGD is limited because of its usual association with AIS or CIN III, lesions for which a cone biopsy or hysterectomy is usually performed. As a result, the premalignant potential of EGD is unknown, including the proportion of cases of AIS preceded by EGD, the proportion of cases of EGD that progress to AIS, and the time interval between the appearance of EGD and AIS.

- Several studies have shown no development of AIS in patients with EGD that extended to the margins of the cone biopsy.

References

Alva J, Lauchlan SC. The histogenesis of mixed cervical carcinomas: the concept of endocervical columnar-cell dysplasia. Am J Clin Pathol 64:20–25, 1975.

Anciaux D, Lawrence WD, Gregoire L. Glandular lesions of the uterine cervix: prognostic implications of human papillomavirus status. Int J Gynecol Pathol 16:103–110, 1997.

Brown LJR, Wells M. Cervical glandular atypia associated with squamous intraepithelial neoplasia: a premalignant lesion? J Clin Pathol 39:22–28, 1986.

Casper GR, Östör AG, Quinn MA. A clinicopathologic study of glandular dysplasia of the cervix. Gynecol Oncol 64:166–170, 1997.

Gloor E, Hurlimann J. Cervical intraepithelial glandular neoplasia (adenocarcinoma in situ and glandular dysplasia): a correlative study of 23 cases with histologic grading, histochemical analysis of mucins, and immunohistochemical determination of the affinity for four lectins. Cancer 58:1272–1280, 1986.

Goldstein NS, Ahmad E, Hussain M, et al. Endocervical glandular atypia: does a preneoplastic lesion of adenocarcinoma in situ exist? Am J Clin Pathol 110:200–209, 1998.

Hitchcock A, Johnson J, McDowell K, Johnson IR. A retrospective study into the occurrence of cervical glandular atypia in cone biopsy specimens from 1977–1978 with clinical follow-up. Int J Gynecol Cancer 3:164–168, 1993.

Jaworski RC. Endocervical glandular dysplasia, adenocarcinoma in situ, and early invasive (microinvasive) adenocarcinoma of the uterine cervix. Semin Diagn Pathol 7:190–204, 1990.

Leary J, Jaworski R, Houghton R. In-situ hybridization using biotinylated DNA probes to human papillomavirus in adenocarcinoma-in-situ and endocervical glandular dysplasia of the uterine cervix. Pathology 23:85–89, 1991.

Luesley DM, Jordan JA, Woodman CBJ, et al. A retrospective review of adenocarcinoma-in-situ and glandular atypia of the uterine cervix. Br J Obstet Gynaecol 94:699–703, 1987.

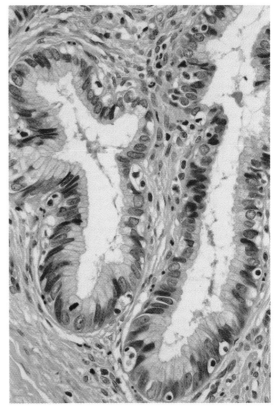

Figure 6–6. Endocervical glandular dysplasia.

Microinvasive Adenocarcinoma

- Early-invasive or microinvasive adenocarcinoma (MIA) is defined in most studies by depth of invasion (< 5 mm from base of surface epithelium) or by volume (<500 mm³).
- The mean age of 39 to 44 years is intermediate between that of patients with AIS and those with clinically invasive adenocarcinoma. The clinical manifestations are similar to those of AIS except that postcoital bleeding was a common presenting symptom in one series. The colposcopic changes suggest early invasion in a minority of patients. The findings in Pap smears are similar to those of patients with AIS.

Microscopic Features

- MIA is most commonly characterized by aggregates of malignant glands resembling those of AIS but that are more crowded (or even confluent) and haphazardly disposed within normal or reactive endocervical stroma. The distinction between early-invasive and extensive AIS may be very difficult in some cases. Architectural features are paramount for this distinction.
- MIA less commonly may appear as irregular budlike projections, small glands, or uncommonly, solid nests of cells arising from AIS, sometimes with a stromal reaction (i.e., desmoplasia or mononuclear inflammatory cells). The invasive cells resemble those of AIS or occasionally are squamoid with abundant eosinophilic cytoplasm and enlarged, rounded nuclei with chromatin clearing and prominent nucleoli.
- Lymphatic invasion occurs in a minority of cases.

Behavior

- MIA has an excellent prognosis when treated by radical hysterectomy. More conservative treatment (cone biopsy with or without pelvic lymphadenectomy) has also been successful in many patients.
- Teshima and colleagues found recurrences in only 1 of 22 cases with tumor less than 5 mm deep (i.e., vaginal recurrence, 2.3 years after radical hysterectomy; the primary tumor was 3 mm deep).

- Kaku and associates found a recurrence in only 1 of 25 patients with tumor less than 5 mm deep (i.e., vaginal recurrence, 1.5 years); the primary tumor was 4.1 mm deep but 1222 mm³).
- Berek and coworkers found pelvic node metastases in 2 of 18 patients with 2 to 5 mm of invasion. Pulmonary metastases occurred in one patient with a tumor that invaded to 5 mm, although the tumor was "poorly differentiated." There were no nodal metastases in six patients who had tumors less than 2 mm deep.
- Kaspar and coworkers found no lymph node spread or recurrence in 22 tumors that were less than 500 mm³. In contrast, 3 of 25 tumors larger than 500 mm³ but less than 5 mm deep metastasized to lymph nodes, recurred, or both.
- Östör and associates found only two recurrences in 77 tumors less than 5 mm deep, and there were no tumor-related deaths. One of the recurrences, both of which were at the vaginal vault, was a squamous cell carcinoma and therefore presumably unrelated to the original tumor.

References

Berek JS, Hacker NF, Fu Y-S, et al. Adenocarcinoma of the uterine cervix: histologic variables associated with lymph node metastasis and survival. Obstet Gynecol 65:46–52, 1985.

Jaworski RC. Endocervical glandular dysplasia, adenocarcinoma in situ, and early invasive (microinvasive) adenocarcinoma of the uterine cervix. Semin Diagn Pathol 7:190–204, 1990.

Kaku T, Kamura T, Sakai K, et al. Early adenocarcinoma of the uterine cervix [Abstract]. Int J Gynecol Cancer 5 (Suppl 1):56, 1995.

Kaspar HG, Dinh TV, Doherty MG, et al. Clinical implications of tumor volume measurement in stage I adenocarcinoma. Obstet Gynecol 81:296–300, 1993.

Östör AG, Rome R, Quinn M. Microinvasive adenocarcinoma of the cervix: a clinicopathologic study of 77 women. Obstet Gynecol 89:88–93, 1997.

Qizilbash AH. In-situ and microinvasive adenocarcinoma of the uterine cervix: a clinical, cytologic and histologic study of 14 cases. Am J Clin Pathol 64:155–170, 1975.

Rollason TP, Cullimore J, Bradgate MG. A suggested columnar cell morphological equivalent of squamous carcinoma in situ with early stromal invasion. Int J Gynecol Pathol 8:230–236, 1989.

Teshima S, Shimosato Y, Kishi K, et al. Early stage adenocarcinoma of the uterine cervix: histopathologic analysis with consideration of histogenesis. Cancer 56:167–172, 1985.

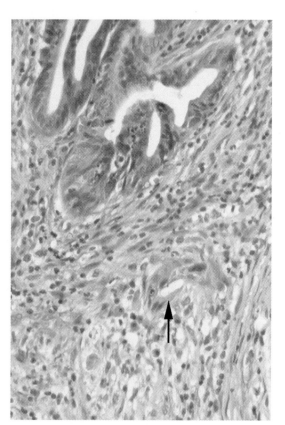

Figure 6–7. Early invasive adenocarcinoma. A small gland lined by eosinophilic cells lies within desmoplastic stroma (*arrow*). Adenocarcinoma in situ is seen at the top.

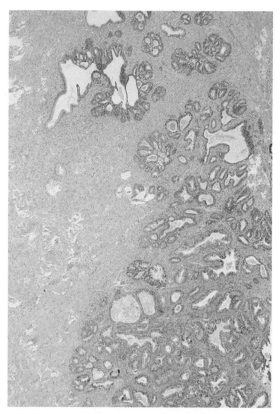

Figure 6–8. Invasive adenocarcinoma. Foci of adenocarcinoma in situ (*top*) merge with confluent malignant glands (*bottom*). The glands lack a stromal response, but their number and confluent and complex pattern indicate invasion. The endocervical canal is to the right of this field.

INVASIVE CARCINOMAS WITH GLANDULAR DIFFERENTIATION

General Features

- Invasive carcinomas with glandular differentiation account for 15% to 25% of cervical carcinomas. This proportion represents a marked increase over the past 30 years, an increase related to a true increased frequency of cervical adenocarcinomas and a decrease in invasive squamous cell carcinomas.
- HPV (particularly HPV types 16 and 18) is identified in most cases, and in more than 95% of those of endocervical type. There has been a suggested but not proven association with oral contraceptive use.
- Those affected are almost always adult women; the mean age in most series is between 44 and 54 years. The tumors are rare in the first decade and uncommon in the second. The proportion of tumors occurring in women younger than 35 years has increased.
- Abnormal uterine bleeding occurs in 80% of cases; some women complain of vaginal discharge or pain. An abnormal Pap smear is found in only a minority of cases in most studies.
- The gross appearance includes ulcerated lesions, elevated granular masses, or strikingly polypoid tumors. Some tumors produce little or no mucosal abnormality but manifest as a barrel-shaped cervix. The appearance of the cervix may be normal in 20% to 30% of cases.
- The tumors are subdivided by cell type in World Health Organization classification (Table 6–2); the various microscopic subtypes are discussed in the following sections. Tumors containing more than one subtype in which the minor component accounts for at least

10% of the neoplasm are categorized as mixed carcinomas.
- No concensus exists concerning the prognosis of the more common subtypes compared with that of squamous cell carcinoma. The behavior of less common types are discussed in the following sections.

References

Angel C, Dubeshter B, Lin JY. Clinical presentation and management of stage I cervical adenocarcinoma: a 25 year experience. Gynecol Oncol 44:71–78, 1992.

Berek JS, Hatcher NF, Fu YS, et al. Adenocarcinoma of the uterine cervix: histologic variables associated with lymph node metastasis and survival. Obstet Gynecol 65:46–52, 1985.

Eifel PJ, Burke TW, Morris M, Smith TL. Adenocarcinoma as an independent risk factor for disease recurrence in patients with stage IB cervical carcinoma. Cancer 59:38–44, 1995.

Fu YS, Reagan JW, Hsiu JG, et al. Adenocarcinoma and mixed carcinoma of the uterine cervix. 1. A clinicopathologic study. Cancer 49:2560–2570, 1982.

Goodman HM, Buttlar CA, Niloff JM, et al. Adenocarcinoma of the uterine cervix: prognostic factors and patterns of recurrence. Gynecol Oncol 33:241–247, 1989.

Hopkins MP, Schmidt RW, Roberts JA, Morley GW. The prognosis and treatment of stage I adenocarcinoma of the cervix. Obstet Gynecol 72:915–921, 1988.

Hopkins MP, Sutton P, Roberts JA. Prognostic features and treatment of endocervical adenocarcinoma of the cervix. Gynecol Oncol 27:69–75, 1987.

Horowitz IR, Jacobson LP, Zucker PK, et al. Epidemiology of adenocarcinoma of the cervix. Gynecol Oncol 31:25–31, 1988.

Jones MW, Silverberg SG. Cervical adenocarcinoma in young women: possible relationship to microglandular hyperplasia and use of oral contraceptives. Obstet Gynecol 73:984–989, 1989.

Kilgore LC, Soong S-J, Gore H, et al. Analysis of prognostic features in adenocarcinoma of the cervix. Gynecol Oncol 31:137–148, 1988.

Maier RC, Norris HJ. Coexistence of cervical intraepithelial neoplasia with primary adenocarcinoma of the endocervix. Obstet Gynecol 56:361–364, 1980.

Miller BE, Flax SD, Arheart K, Photopulos G. The presentation of adenocarcinoma of the uterine cervix. Cancer 72:1281–1285, 1993.

Saigo PE, Cain JM, Kim WS, et al. Prognostic factors in adenocarcinoma of the uterine cervix. Cancer 57:1584–1593, 1986.

Shingleton HM, Bell MC, Fremgen A, et al. Is there really a difference in survival of women with squamous cell carcinoma, adenocarcinoma, and adenosquamous carcinoma? Cancer 76:1948–1955, 1995.

Tenti P, Romagnoli S, Silini E, et al. Human papillomavirus types 16 and 18 infection in infiltrating adenocarcinoma of the cervix: PCR analysis of 138 cases and correlation with histologic type and grade. Am J Clin Pathol 106:52–56, 1996.

Vesterinen E, Forss M, Nieminen U. Increase of cervical adenocarcinoma: a report of 520 cases of cervical carcinoma including 112 tumors with glandular elements. Gynecol Oncol 33:49–53, 1989.

Table 6–2

CLASSIFICATION OF CERVICAL GLANDULAR CARCINOMAS AND RELATED TUMORS

1. Adenocarcinoma
   A. Endocervical type
      Variants
      i. Adenoma malignum (minimal-deviation adenocarcinoma)
      ii. Well-differentiated villoglandular
   B. Endometrioid
      Variant
      Minimal-deviation adenocarcinoma
   C. Clear cell
   D. Serous
   E. Mesonephric
   F. Intestinal-type
   G. Signet-ring cell
2. Adenosquamous carcinoma
   Variant
   Glassy cell carcinoma
3. Adenoid basal carcinoma
4. "Adenoid cystic" carcinoma
5. Neuroendocrine tumors
   A. Typical carcinoid tumor
   B. Atypical carcinoid tumor
   C. Small cell carcinoma
   D. Large cell neuroendocrine carcinoma
6. Carcinoma, mixed (specify subtypes)
7. Metastatic adenocarcinoma

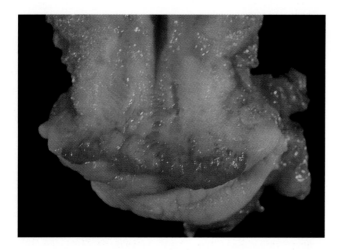

Figure 6–9. Invasive endocervical adenocarcinoma. A polypoid mass is associated with a deeply invasive component within the cervical wall.

Endocervical-Type Mucinous Adenocarcinoma

- Endocervical mucinous adenocarcinomas, which account for 70% of cervical adenocarcinomas, are mostly well to moderately differentiated mucinous adenocarcinomas with medium-sized glands lined by stratified, atypical columnar cells, some of which contain mucin.
- The gland pattern varies from widely spaced to closely packed, sometimes with a cribriform pattern. Uncommon patterns include macrocystic, solid, papillary, and microglandular; the latter pattern is associated with oral contraceptive use and may resemble microglandular hyperplasia. Rare, poorly differentiated tumors may contain signet-ring cells. The stroma varies from absent or scanty and from desmoplastic to fibromatous.
- Synchronous premalignant squamous lesions occur in as many as 43% of the cases. Synchronous mucinous tumors are found elsewhere in female genital tract (e.g., ovary, fallopian tube) in some cases.

Differential Diagnosis

- Mucinous adenocarcinoma of endometrium is discussed in Chapter 8.
- Endometrioid carcinoma of cervix (page 121).
- Microglandular hyperplasia (MGH). Endocervical adenocarcinomas with a microglandular pattern have at least focal nuclear atypicality that exceeds that allowable in MGH, and areas of more conventional adenocarcinoma.

Variant: Adenoma Malignum

- Adenoma malignum (i.e., minimal-deviation adenocarcinoma) accounts for 1% to 10% of cervical adenocarcinomas and occurs over a wide age range (mean, 42 years). The presenting symptom is usually abnormal vaginal bleeding or occasionally a mucoid vaginal discharge. Some patients have mucinous tumors elsewhere in the female genital tract (e.g., ovary, fallopian tube). About 20 patients have had the Peutz-Jeghers syndrome (PJS).
- The cervix is firm or indurated, with a hemorrhagic, friable, or mucoid mucosal surface and a yellow or tan-white sectioned surface. Cysts are occasionally prominent.
- Most or rarely all of the tumor is composed of glands lined by deceptively benign-appearing, mucin-rich columnar epithelial cells with basal nuclei. Some glands in most well-sampled tumors are lined by dysplastic to malignant epithelium, and in some cases, foci of less well-differentiated adenocarcinoma are found.
- The neoplastic glands are closely to widely spaced and highly variable in size and shape. Some glands may be cystic or exhibit papillary infolding. A periglandular desmoplastic stromal response occurs in most tumors but is often focal.
- Vascular and perineural invasion occurs in one half and one sixth of tumors, respectively. Deep invasion of the cervical wall is found in most cases. Transmural spread or spread to the parametrium is seen in 40% of cases, and the myometrium is involved in a similar proportion of cases.
- The tumor cells typically contain gastric-type mucin and are frequently argyrophilic with the Grimelius stain.
- Immunostains frequently show cytoplasmic carcinoembryonic antigen (CEA) immunoreactivity, although in some tumors, the staining is very focal or absent; focal serotonin positivity is demonstrated in some tumors. In contrast to normal endocervical epithelium, adenoma

malignum lacks immunoreactivity for estrogen and progesterone receptors and CA-125.

Differential Diagnosis

- Features favoring or establishing a diagnosis of adenoma malignum over a benign glandular lesion include the presence of symptoms or a mass; associated PJS; a periglandular stromal response; deep invasion; lymphatic, vascular, or perineural invasion; occasional glands lined by clearly malignant epithelium; and strong cytoplasmic immunoreactivity for CEA.
- The benign glandular lesions that may be confused with adenoma malignum (i.e., deep glands and cysts, tunnel clusters, diffuse laminar endocervical glandular hyperplasia, adenomyoma of endocervical type) are discussed in Chapter 4.

Prognosis

- Adenoma malignum has a worse prognosis than other well-differentiated endocervical adenocarcinomas. In a literature review, only 30% of patients (all stages) and only 50% of patients with stage I tumors were alive and free of disease at 2 years.

Variant: Well-Differentiated Villoglandular Adenocarcinoma

- Villoglandular adenocarcinomas (VGAs) usually occur at a younger age (average, 35 years) than cervical adenocarcinomas in general. Sixty-two percent of patients in one series had a history of oral contraceptive use.
- VGAs are characterized by a surface component of papillae that are usually tall and thin, but occasionally short and broad, and that have a fibromatous stromal core.
- The papillae and glands are usually lined by one or several layers of columnar cells, some of which contain mucin. If intracellular mucin is not demonstrable, the tumor should be considered a endometrioid VGA.
- Mild nuclear atypicality and scattered mitotic figures are characteristic. Marked cellular stratification and cellular buds are absent in pure tumors, and the presence of these features may indicate an admixed serous carcinoma.
- VGAs are usually well circumscribed, with absent or only superficial invasion; rare tumors, however, may invade deeply. The invasive portion is typically composed of elongated branching glands separated by a fibromatous stroma or, occasionally, a desmoplastic or myxoid stroma; lymphatic invasion is rare. Acute and chronic inflammatory cells are typical in the stroma of the papillae and within any invasive component.
- Adenocarcinoma in situ or squamous CIN within the adjacent epithelium is common. VGAs are occasionally admixed with another subtype, such as serous. The proportion of each type should be specified in the pathology report.
- Lymph node metastases have been reported in only two cases, both of which had lymphatic invasion in the primary tumors.
- The clinical follow-up has been uneventful in all cases except in the two cases with nodal metastases.
- Conservative management (cone biopsy and careful follow-up) has been successful in some cases. This treatment should probably be reserved for tumors that are pure VGA and that are noninvasive or superficially invasive, well differentiated, and without vascular space invasion or involvement of resection margins.

Differential Diagnosis

- Other papillary adenocarcinomas: typical endocervical adenocarcinoma with focal papillary pattern (admixed conventional glandular pattern and higher grade nuclear features), papillary serous adenocarcinoma (irregular, fine papillae with conspicuous cellular budding and high-grade atypia), and papillary clear cell carcinomas (papillae with hyalinized cores, clear and hobnail cells).
- Benign lesions: papillary endocervicitis (papillae lined by a single layer of bland-appearing mucinous cells), müllerian papilloma (usually children; absence of atypia, mitotic activity, and invasion), villoglandular adenoma (absence of atypia and invasion), and müllerian adenofibroma (typically broad, nonvillous, and polypoid fronds, with an absence of atypia)

References

Fetissof F, Heitzman A, Machet M-C, Lansac J. Unusual endocervical lesions with endocrine cells. Pathol Res Pract 189:928–939, 1993.

Gilks CB, Young RH, Aguirre P, et al. Adenoma malignum (minimal deviation adenocarcinoma) of the uterine cervix: a clinicopathological and immunohistochemical analysis of 26 cases. Am J Surg Pathol 13:717–729, 1989.

Jones MW, Silverberg SG, Kurman RJ. Well differentiated villoglandular adenocarcinoma of uterine cervix: a clinicopathological study of 24 cases. Int J Gynecol Pathol 12:1–7, 1993.

Kaku T, Kamura T, Shigematsu T, et al. Adenocarcinoma of the uterine cervix with predominantly villoglandular papillary growth pattern. Gynecol Oncol 64:147–152, 1997.

Kaminski PF, Norris HJ. Minimal deviation carcinoma (adenoma malignum) of the cervix. Int J Gynecol Pathol 2:141–153, 1983.

Mayorga M, Garcia-Valtuille A, Fernandez F, et al. Adenocarcinoma of the uterine cervix with massive signet-ring cell differentiation. Int J Surg Pathol 5:95–100, 1997.

Michael H, Grawe L, Kraus FT. Minimal deviation endocervical adenocarcinoma: clinical and histologic features, immunohistochemical staining for carcinoembryonic antigen, and differentiation from confusing benign lesions. Int J Gynecol Pathol 3:261–276, 1984.

Seidman JD. Mucinous lesions of the fallopian tube. Am J Surg Pathol 18:1205–1212, 1994.

Toki T, Shiozawa T, Hosaka N, et al. Minimal deviation adenocarcinoma of the uterine cervix has abnormal expression of sex steroid receptors, CA 125, and gastric mucin. Int J Gynecol Pathol 18:215–219, 1999.

Young RH, Scully RE. Mucinous tumors of the ovary associated with mucinous adenocarcinomas of the cervix: a clinicopathologic analysis of 16 cases. Int J Gynecol Pathol 7:99–111, 1988.

Young RH, Scully RE. Uterine carcinomas simulating microglandular hyperplasia: a report of six cases. Am J Surg Pathol 16:1092–1097, 1992.

Young RH, Scully RE. Villoglandular papillary adenocarcinoma of the uterine cervix: a clinicopathological analysis of 13 cases. Cancer 63:1773–1779, 1989.

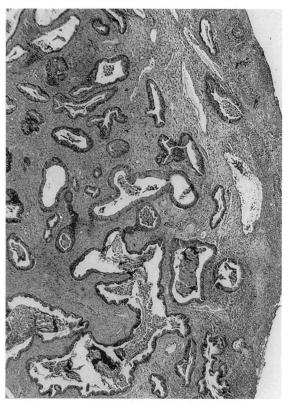

Figure 6–10. Invasive endocervical mucinous adenocarcinoma. The disorderly pattern and the marked irregularity of the gland profile indicate invasion. The tumor cells have intracellular mucin not clearly seen at this power (same tumor as in Fig. 6–11).

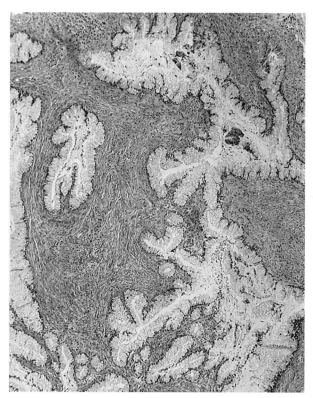

Figure 6–12. Adenoma malignum (i.e., minimal deviation adenocarcinoma of the endocervical type). Notice the complex and crowded gland arrangement and the marked irregularity of the size and shape of the glands.

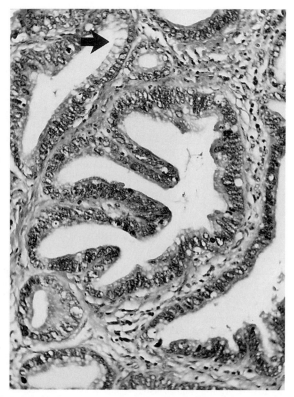

Figure 6–11. Invasive endocervical adenocarcinoma. Notice the intracellular mucin in some of the tumor cells (*arrow*).

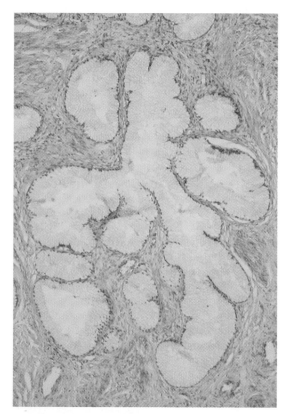

Figure 6–13. Adenoma malignum. A gland with a bizarre shape is lined by benign-appearing tumor cells.

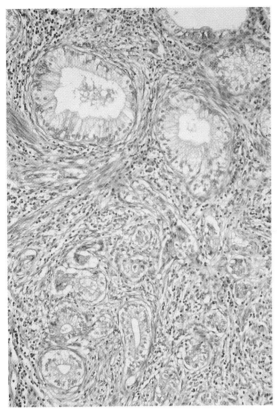

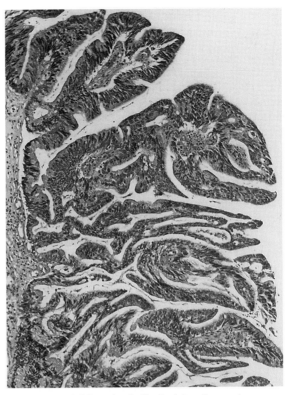

Figure 6–15. Well-differentiated villoglandular adenocarcinoma.

Figure 6–14. Adenoma malignum. Obviously malignant glands within a reactive stroma (*bottom*) formed a minor component of the tumor.

Figure 6–16. Well-differentiated villoglandular adenocarcinoma has only mild atypia.

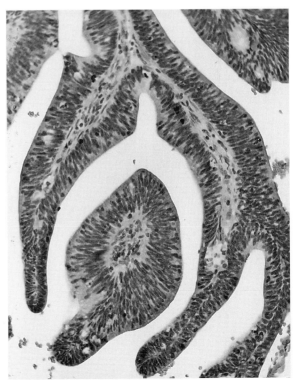

Intestinal-Type Mucinous Adenocarcinoma

■ Most of these rare adenocarcinomas contain intestinal-type cells, including goblet cells, Paneth cells, and argentaffin cells. Some may have the appearance of a colloid carcinoma. Intestinal-type mucins have also been demonstrated in these tumors. Some tumors have a superficial villous adenoma-like component (see Chapter 4).

References

Azzopardi JG, Hou LT. Intestinal metaplasia with argentaffin cells in cervical adenocarcinoma. J Pathol 90:686–690, 1985.

Fox H, Wells M, Harris M, et al. Enteric tumours of the lower female genital tract: a report of three cases. Histopathology 12:167–176, 1988.

Lewis TLT. Colloid (mucus secreting) carcinoma of the cervix. J Obstet Gynaecol Br Commonw 78:1128–1132, 1971.

Lee KR, Trainer TD. Adenocarcinoma of the uterine cervix of intestinal type containing numerous Paneth cells. Arch Pathol Lab Med 114: 731–733, 1990.

Savargaonkar PR, Hale RJ, Pope R, et al. Enteric differentiation in cervical adenocarcinomas and its prognostic significance. Histopathology 23:275–277, 1993.

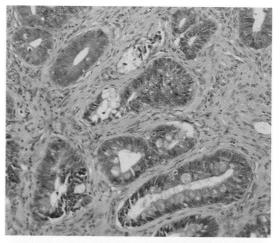

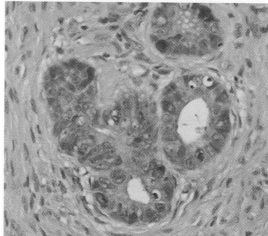

Figure 6–17. Intestinal-type endocervical mucinous adenocarcinoma. Notice the goblet cells (*top*) and argentaffin cells with red cytoplasmic granules (*bottom*).

Signet-Ring Cell Adenocarcinoma

- These tumors are rare in pure or almost pure form. Signet-ring cells occur more commonly as a focal finding in poorly differentiated adenocarcinomas of endocervical and intestinal type and in adenosquamous carcinomas (page 125).
- The differential diagnosis includes metastatic signet-ring cell carcinoma to the cervix (most commonly from gastric and breast primaries) and rare squamous cell carcinomas with signet-ring–like cells that are mucin negative.

References

Kupryjanczyk J, Kujawa M. Signet-ring cells in squamous cell carcinoma of the cervix and in non-neoplastic ectocervical epithelium. Int J Gynecol Cancer 2:152–156, 1992.

Moll UM, Chumas JC, Mann WJ, Patsner B. Primary signet ring cell carcinoma of the uterine cervix. NY State J Med 90:559–560, 1990.

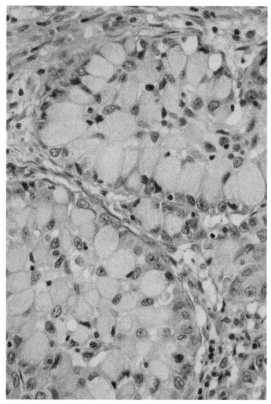

Figure 6–18. Signet-ring cell adenocarcinoma.

Endometrioid Adenocarcinoma

- These tumors, which account for 8% to 30% of cervical adenocarcinomas, have a clinical presentation and gross appearance similar to that of other cervical adenocarcinomas. In several studies, they have had a better prognosis than endocervical mucinous adenocarcinomas.
- The microscopic appearance is similar to endometrioid adenocarcinomas of the uterine corpus, except for a lower frequency of squamous differentiation.

Differential Diagnosis

- Mucin-poor adenocarcinomas of the endocervical type. These tumors contain cells with at least focal intracellular mucin, and mucin stains may be helpful.
- Cervical involvement by endometrial endometrioid carcinoma. Features that facilitate this differential include the site of a dominant mass determined by clinical and hysteroscopic examination, the distribution of tumor in fractional curettage specimens, the nature of any associated lesions (endometrial hyperplasia versus endocervical adenocarcinoma in situ), and the immunoprofile (i.e., CEA positive and vimentin negative favors endocervical origin; CEA negative and vimentin positive favors endometrial origin).

Variant: Endometrioid Minimal-Deviation Adenocarcinoma

- The patients, who are usually of reproductive age, may present with an abnormal Pap smear or abnormal bleeding, but in other cases, the tumor is an incidental finding in a hysterectomy or cone biopsy specimen.
- Endometrioid minimal-deviation adenocarcinomas consist of a deceptively benign-appearing proliferation of endometrioid glands and cysts with little or no stromal reaction. One to several layers of cells, often with cilia or apical snouts, line the glands. There is usually mild to moderate nuclear atypia; mitotic figures may be scarce or easily identified.
- Features of the tumor that help differentiate it from tuboendometrioid metaplasia include marked gland crowding, marked irregularity in gland size and shape, and in some cases, deep invasion, a focal stromal response, focal moderate atypia, and mitotic activity.

■ These tumors have a favorable prognosis; only one tumor has involved lymph nodes, and only one has been fatal.

References

Costa MJ, McIlnay KR, Trelford J. Cervical carcinoma with glandular differentiation: histological evaluation predicts disease recurrence in clinical stage I or II patients. Hum Pathol 26:829–837, 1995.

Dabbs DJ, Sturtz K, Zaino RJ. The immunohistochemical discrimination of endometrioid adenocarcinomas. Hum Pathol 27:172–177, 1996.

Kaminski PF, Norris HJ. Minimal deviation carcinoma (adenoma malignum) of the cervix. Int J Gynecol Pathol 2:141–153, 1983.

Rahilly MA, Williams ARW, Al-Nafussi A. Minimal deviation endometrioid adenocarcinoma of cervix: a clinicopathological and immunohistochemical study of two cases. Histopathology 20:351–354, 1992.

Saigo PE, Cain JM, Kim WS, et al. Prognostic factors in adenocarcinoma of the uterine cervix. Cancer 57:1584–1593, 1986.

Young RH, Scully RE. Minimal-deviation endometrioid adenocarcinoma of the uterine cervix: a report of five cases of a distinctive neoplasm that may be misinterpreted as benign. Am J Surg Pathol 17:660–665, 1993.

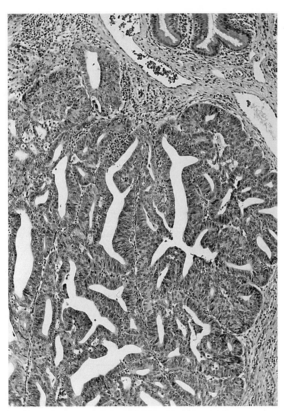

Figure 6–19. Endocervical endometrioid adenocarcinoma. Normal endocervical glands are on the upper right.

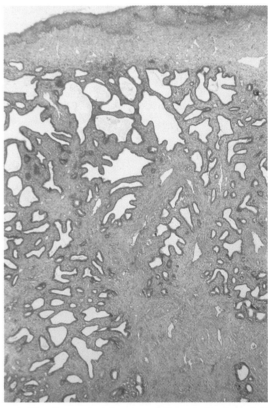

Figure 6–20. Minimal deviation–type endocervical endometrioid adenocarcinoma. Although the glands exhibited minimal atypia on higher-power examination, their pattern and depth as illustrated in this figure indicate invasion.

Clear Cell Adenocarcinoma

■ Clear cell adenocarcinomas were referred to as "mesonephric" or "mesonephroid" carcinomas in the older literature. Although rare cervical carcinomas of mesonephric origin occur (see page 124), clear cell carcinomas are now accepted as müllerian in origin.

■ Two thirds of cases in young patients reported over the past two decades have had in utero exposure to diethylstilbestrol (DES). The tumors are also encountered in the absence of DES exposure in females of all ages, with a peak frequency in postmenopausal women. These tumors accounted for 5% of cases of cervical adenocarcinomas before the DES era.

■ The tumors may be exocervical or endocervical; all of the DES-associated tumors have involved the exocervix, sometimes extending into the endocervix. The gross appearance is indistinguishable from other cervical adenocarcinomas.

- The basic microscopic patterns (see Chapter 14) are tubulocystic (i.e., tubules and cysts of various sizes lined by hobnail, flat, or clear cells), solid (i.e., nests and sheets of cells containing abundant, clear, glycogen-rich cytoplasm), and papillary (i.e., numerous papillae often with hyalinized cores, covered by clear and hobnail cells). The nuclear features are usually grade 2 or 3, and mitotic figures are usually numerous.
- Intraluminal, but not intracellular, mucin is usually present. In some tumors, intracellular mucin may result in tumor cells with a signet-ring–like appearance. Stromal hyalinization is often prominent.
- The differential diagnosis includes microglandular hyperplasia and Arias-Stella reaction (discussed in Chapter 4), cervical yolk sac tumors (usually in children, reticular pattern, Schiller-Duval bodies, a primitive nuclear appearance, and immunoreactivity for alpha-fetoprotein), and primary cervical alveolar soft part sarcomas (organoid pattern, cells with eosinophilic cytoplasm, periodic acid–Schiff (PAS)–positive intracytoplasmic crystals) (see Chapter 9).

References

Hart WR, Norris HJ. Mesonephric adenocarcinomas of the cervix. Cancer 29:106–113, 1972.

Fawcett KJ, Dockerty MB, Hunt AB. Mesonephric carcinomas and adenocarcinomas of the cervix in children. J Pediatr 69:104–110, 1966.

Kaminski PF, Maier RC. Clear cell adenocarcinoma of the cervix unrelated to diethylstilbestrol exposure. Obstet Gynecol 62:720–727, 1983.

Zaino RJ, Robbboy SJ, Bentley R, Kurman RJ. Diseases of the vagina. In Kurman RS (ed): Blaustein's Pathology of the Female Genital Tract, 4th ed. New York: Springer-Verlag, 1994:162–168.

Serous Adenocarcinoma

- Serous adenocarcinomas, which are much less common than serous carcinomas of endometrial origin, occur over a wide age range (26 to 70 years). A bimodal age distribution was found in one study, with one peak at less than 40 years and the second peak at more than 65 years.
- The presenting symptoms, in order of frequency, include abnormal vaginal bleeding, abnormal Pap smear, and watery vaginal discharge. Thirty percent of the cases are stage II or III.
- The gross appearance is indistinguishable from other cervical adenocarcinomas. The microscopic appearance is identical to that of papillary serous endometrial carcinoma (see Chapter 8). Another histologic subtype of adenocarcinoma is admixed in 40% of cases, most commonly low-grade villoglandular adenocarcinoma.
- Forty percent of patients had died of tumor or were alive with tumor on follow-up. An age older than 65 years, a stage greater than I, a diameter greater than 2 cm, tumor invasion of more than 10 mm, the presence of lymph node metastases, and an elevation of serum CA-125 were associated with a poor prognosis in the only reported series. Tumor grade and composition (pure or mixed) did not correlate with patient outcome.

References

Costa MJ, McIlnay KR, Trelford J. Cervical carcinoma with glandular differentiation: histological evaluation predicts disease recurrence in clinical stage I or II patients. Hum Pathol 26:829–837, 1995.

Zhou C, Gilks CB, Hayes M, Clement PB. Papillary serous carcinoma of the uterine cervix: a clinicopathologic study of 17 cases. Am J Surg Pathol 22:113–120, 1998.

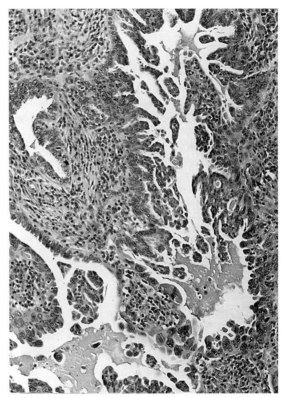

Figure 6–21. Endocervical serous adenocarcinoma. Notice the fine papillae and cellular buds. On high-power examination, the cells exhibited marked nuclear atypicality.

Mesonephric Adenocarcinoma

- Adenocarcinomas of mesonephric origin are a rare sub-type of cervical adenocarcinoma. Most "mesonephric" carcinomas reported in the older literature are examples of clear cell adenocarcinoma. All of the reported cases of mesonephric adenocarcinoma have been associated with mesonephric hyperplasia, which was usually florid.
- The age range is 34 to 73 years (mean, 50 years). Most patients present with abnormal vaginal bleeding. All of the reported tumors have been stage IB. Microscopic pelvic lymph node metastases, however, were found in two cases.
- The tumors are frequently bulky and deeply invasive without specific gross features. Involvement of the lower uterine segment may be more common than with other cervical adenocarcinomas.
- The microscopic appearance varies widely, even within a single tumor. Some tumors focally have patterns that are nonspecific or resemble endometrioid or serous adenocarcinoma. Distinctive patterns include "mesonephroid" (i.e., back-to-back small tubules with an eosinophilic luminal secretion), "retiform" (i.e., branching slit-like spaces with intraluminal fibrous papillae), sievelike, and sex cord–like. An admixed spindle cell sarcomatoid component is seen in rare cases.

- The disease has a malignant clinical course in about 50% of the cases. Some of the malignant tumors have had an indolent behavior with a tendency for late and, in some cases, multiple recurrences.

Differential Diagnosis

- Distinguish the mesonephroid pattern of carcinoma from diffuse mesonephric hyperplasia, which lacks a back-to-back pattern, malignant nuclear features, and other patterns of mesonephric carcinomas noted above, and from clear cell carcinoma, which has cystic, papillary and solid patterns, as well as clear cells and hobnail cells.
- Mesonephric tumors with an endometrioid appearance and those with spindle cells should be distinguished from endometrioid adenocarcinomas and endometrioid carcinosarcomas, respectively, which lack associated mesonephric hyperplasia and distinctive mesonephroid and retiform patterns.

Reference

Clement PB, Young RH, Keh P, et al. Mesonephric neoplasms of the uterine cervix: a report of eight cases, including four with a malignant spindle cell component. Am J Surg Pathol 19:1158–1171, 1995.

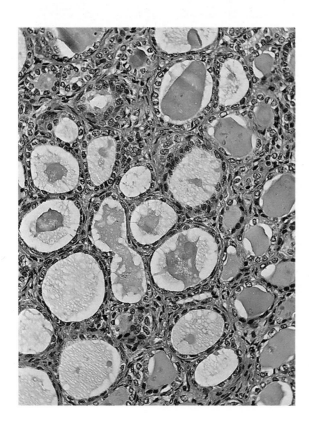

Figure 6–22. Mesonephric adenocarcinoma. Closely packed small to medium-sized tubules contain eosinophilic luminal secretion.

Adenosquamous Carcinoma

- Adenosquamous carcinomas are composed of a malignant glandular component and a malignant squamous component and account for one third of all cervical carcinomas with a glandular component. The prognosis has varied from better to worse than pure adenocarcinomas, depending on the study.
- The glandular component is almost always an endocervical-type adenocarcinoma; rarely, it is of the endometrioid or of signet-ring cell type. The squamous component is usually moderately to severely atypical. Benign-appearing squamous morules are rare.
- Sheets of clear cells with glycogenated cytoplasm in some tumors were interpreted as squamous in nature in one study (i.e., clear cell adenosquamous carcinoma). These tumors were all associated with HPV-18 and a high frequency (73%) of recurrence.
- The differential diagnosis includes squamous cell carcinomas with cytoplasmic mucin (see Chapter 5).

Variant: Glassy Cell Carcinoma

- Glassy cell carcinomas (GCCs) were considered a highly aggressive, undifferentiated form of adenosquamous carcinoma by Glucksmann and Cherry and in many subsequent studies. In the study by Glucksman and Cherry, GCCs accounted for 20% of adenosquamous carcinomas and for 1.6% of all cervical carcinomas.
- Costa and associates consider glassy cell features to be part of a spectrum of differentiation in adenosquamous carcinomas rather than a distinct histologic subtype with specific clinical significance.
- GCCs occur in a somewhat younger age group than adenocarcinomas in general; 83% of patients were younger than 35 years in one study. An association with pregnancy has been found in some series. The presenting clinical features and the gross appearance are similar to cervical adenocarcinomas in general.
- The characteristic microscopic features include nests and sheets of large cells with abundant eosinophilic or amphophilic, ground-glass or finely granular cytoplasm; prominent cell borders; large nuclei with macronucleoli; and a high mitotic rate. There is often a stromal inflammatory infiltrate composed predominantly of eosinophils and plasma cells. Rare foci of squamous or glandular differentiation and intracellular mucin are present in some cases.
- These tumors should be distinguished from large cell nonkeratinizing squamous cell carcinoma, which lacks ground-glass cytoplasm and macronucleoli and has more than a minor degree of squamous differentiation, and from lymphoepithelioma-like carcinoma, which contains tumor cells without the characteristic cytologic features of glassy cell carcinoma and that are singly disposed within a massive lymphoid infiltrate.

References

Costa MJ, Kenny MB, Hewan-Lowe K, Judd R. Glassy cell features in adenosquamous carcinoma of the uterine cervix: histologic, ultrastructural, immunohistochemical, and clinical findings. Am J Clin Pathol 96:520–528, 1991.

Costa MJ, McIlnay KR, Trelford J. Cervical carcinoma with glandular differentiation: histological evaluation predicts disease recurrence in clinical state I or II patients. Hum Pathol 26:829–837, 1995.

Fujiwara H, Mitchell MF, Arseneau J, et al. Clear cell adenosquamous carcinoma of the cervix: an aggressive tumor associated with human papillomavirus-18. Cancer 76:1591–600, 1995.

Gallup DG, Harper RH, Stock RJ. Poor prognosis in patients with adenosquamous cell carcinoma of the cervix. Obstet Gynecol 65:416–422, 1985.

Glucksmann A, Cherry CP. Incidence, histology, and response to radiation of mixed carcinomas (adenoacanthomas) of the uterus. Cancer 9:971–979, 1956.

Harrison TA, Sevin B, Koechli O, et al. Adenosquamous carcinoma of the cervix: prognosis in early stage disease treated by radical hysterectomy. Gynecol Oncol 50:310–315, 1993.

Maier RC, Norris HJ. Glassy cell carcinoma of the cervix. Obstet Gynecol 60:219–224, 1982.

Shingleton HM, Bell MC, Fremgen A, et al. Is there really a difference in survival of women with squamous cell carcinoma, adenocarcinoma, and adenosquamous carcinoma? Cancer 76:1948–1955, 1995.

Talerman A, Alenghat E, Okagaki T. Glassy cell carcinoma of the uterine cervix. APMIS 23:119–125, 1991.

Yazigi R, Sandstad J, Munoz AK, et al. Adenosquamous carcinoma of the cervix: prognosis in stage IB. Obstet Gynecol 75:1012–1015, 1990.

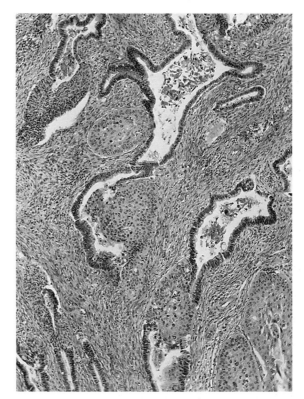

Figure 6–23. Adenosquamous carcinoma.

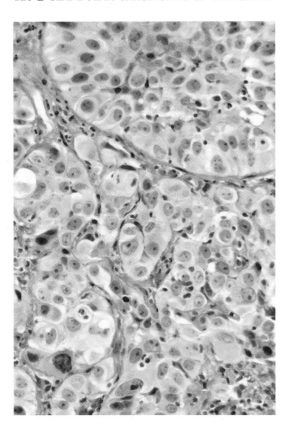

Figure 6–24. Glassy cell carcinoma. The tumor cells contain abundant eosinophilic "ground-glass" cytoplasm and large nuclei with macronucleoli.

Adenoid Basal Carcinoma

- About 50 cases of adenoid basal carcinoma (ABC) have been reported. The patients are typically postmenopausal, black, and asymptomatic. The presenting feature is usually an abnormal Pap smear. The cervix is usually normal on pelvic and gross pathologic examination.
- The characteristic microscopic appearance is that of widely separated or occasionally closed, packed, small, round, oval, or lobulated nests composed of uniform, mitotically inactive basaloid cells with peripheral palisading and no stromal response.
- Occasional gland lumens within the centers of the nests are lined by mucinous epithelium, cells with clear cytoplasm, basaloid cells, or flattened cells. Squamous or transitional cell differentiation is present within the nests in some cases.
- The neoplastic cells are typically immunoreactive for cytokeratin and HPV (typically HPV-16).

- Associated high-grade CIN is common. ABC may merge with a microinvasive or typical squamous cell carcinoma, and rare tumors have abutted a malignant müllerian mixed tumor. In such cases, the proportion of the tumor that is not ABC should be indicated in the pathology report.
- Typical ABCs have not been associated with metastases or tumor-related deaths. Brainard and Hart therefore prefer the appellation "adenoid basal epithelioma" for these tumors and for otherwise similar, superficial, microscopic lesions that have been referred to as adenoid basal hyperplasia.

References

Brainard JA, Hart WR. Adenoid basal epitheliomas of the uterine cervix: a reevaluation of distinctive cervical basaloid lesions currently classified as adenoid basal carcinoma and adenoid basal hyperplasia. Am J Surg Pathol 22:965–975, 1998.

Clement PB, Zubovits JT, Young RH, Scully RE. Malignant müllerian mixed tumors of the uterine cervix: a clincopathological study of 9 cases. Int J Gynecol Pathol 17:211–222, 1998.

Ferry JA. Adenoid basal carcinoma of the uterine cervix: evolution of a distinctive clinicopathological entity [Editorial]. Int J Gynecol Pathol 16:299–300, 1997.

Ferry JA, Scully RE. "Adenoid cystic" carcinoma and adenoid basal carcinoma of the uterine cervix: a study of 28 cases. Am J Surg Pathol 12:134–144, 1988.

Grayson W, Taylor LF, Cooper K. Adenoid basal carcinoma of the uterine cervix: detection of integrated human papillomavirus in a rare tumor of putative "reserve cell" origin. Int J Gynecol Pathol 16:307–312, 1997.

Grayson W, Taylor LF, Cooper K. Adenoid cystic and adenoid basal carcinoma of the uterine cervix. Comparative morphologic, mucin, and immunohistochemical profile of two rare neoplasms of putative "reserve" cell origin. Am J Surg Pathol 23:448–458, 1999.

Jones MW, Kounelis S, Papadaki H, et al. The origin and molecular characterization of adenoid basal carcinoma of the uterine cervix. Int J Gynecol Pathol 16:301–306, 1997.

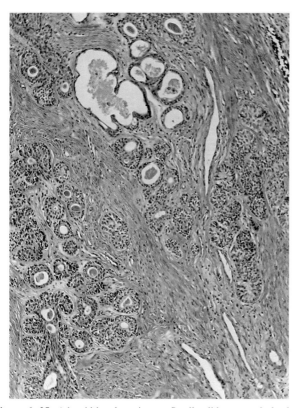

Figure 6–25. Adenoid basal carcinoma. Small solid nests and glands, a few of them cystically dilated, have an infiltrative pattern but lack a stromal response.

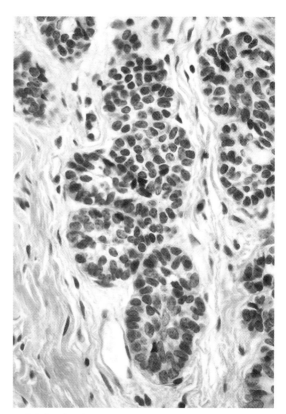

Figure 6–26. Adenoid basal carcinoma. Basaloid nests are composed of cells with bland nuclear features.

Adenoid Cystic Carcinoma

- Adenoid cystic carcinomas (ACCs) are similar, but not identical, to salivary gland cystic carcinomas on microscopic examination. The affected women are usually postmenopausal and black and present with abnormal uterine bleeding and an endophytic or exophytic cervical mass.
- The typical microscopic features include a cribriform pattern (the spaces of which may contain hyaline or mucinous material), nests, sheets, trabeculae, and cords. There is usually at least focal palisading of cells at the periphery of the tumor nests. The neoplastic cells are larger and have more pleomorphic, more mitotic nuclei than those of ABCs.
- Necrosis, which may be extensive, is common. There is usually a stromal response, which may be myxoid, fibroblastic, or hyaline.
- Uncommon findings include solid foci of undifferentiated carcinoma (i.e., "solid" variant of ACC) in 20%

of tumors, a minor component of small nests and cords of basaloid cells (similar to those of ABC) in 20% of tumors, and small foci of squamous differentiation.

■ Myoepithelial cells are absent by light microscopy, but ultrastructural examination in some cases has shown evidence of myoepithelial differentiation. In one such case, there was also ultrastructural evidence of neuroendocrine differentiation.

■ ACCs are aggressive tumors, including a propensity for hematogenous spread, and are associated with a poor prognosis. Two thirds of patients in the largest study were dead of tumor or were alive with tumor when last seen.

References

Albores-Saavedra J, Manivel C, Mora A, et al. The solid variant of adenoid cystic carcinoma of the cervix. Int J Gynecol Pathol 11:2–10, 1992.

Domínguez-Malagón HR, Flores-Flores G, Meneses Garcia A, Ro JY. Adenoid cystic carcinoma of the uterine cervix: a tumor with myoepithelial and neuroendocrine differentiation. Int J Surg Pathol 4:77–82, 1996.

Ferry JA, Scully RE. "Adenoid cystic" carcinoma and adenoid basal carcinoma of the uterine cervix: a study of 28 cases. Am J Surg Pathol 12:134–144, 1988.

Grayson W, Taylor LF, Cooper K. Adenoid cystic and adenoid basal carcinoma of the uterine cervix. Comparative morphologic, mucin, and immunohistochemical profile of two rare neoplasms of putative "reserve" cell origin. Am J Surg Pathol 23:448–458, 1999.

Mazur MT, Battifora HA. Adenoid cystic carcinoma of the uterine cervix: ultrastructure, immunofluorescence, and criteria for diagnosis. Am J Clin Pathol 77:494–500, 1982.

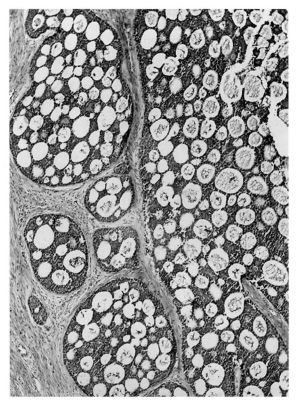

Figure 6–27. Adenoid cystic carcinoma with a cribriform pattern.

SMALL AND LARGE CELL NEUROENDOCRINE CARCINOMAS

Small Cell (Neuroendocrine) Carcinoma

Clinical Features

■ Small cell (neuroendocrine) carcinomas (SCCs) may arise from argyrophilic cells demonstrated within the ectocervical or endocervical epithelium in normal women and those with SCCs. Other tumors, particularly those with an admixed squamous or adenocarcinomatous component, may originate from subcolumnar reserve cells.

■ SCCs, which account for about 2% of cervical carcinomas, occur over a wide age range (21 to 87 years); the median and mean ages in most series are in the fifth decade.

■ The usual presenting manifestations are vaginal bleeding and a cervical mass identified on pelvic examination; some patients have an abnormal Pap smear. In rare cases, there is clinical or biochemical evidence of hormone production, including corticotropin (Cushing's syndrome), vasopressin (syndrome of inappropriate antidiuretic hormone), insulin (hypoglycemia), or serotonin (carcinoid syndrome).

■ About 75% of patients are clinical stage I or II, but as many as 60% of patients are surgical stage III or IV.

Pathologic Features

■ SCCs are grossly indistinguishable from squamous cell carcinomas. Some tumors are large, ulcerating masses that may encompass and destroy the cervix and extend into the surrounding organs.

■ SCCs are typically densely cellular and exhibit a variety of patterns, frequently admixed, including solid sheets, ill-defined or sharply defined nests, trabeculae, and single cells. Small rosette-like or acinar structures, sometimes containing PAS-positive material, may be present and, when numerous, impart a pseudoglandular pattern.

■ Characteristic small oval to spindle cells have scanty cytoplasm and hyperchromatic, molded nuclei with finely dispersed chromatin and indistinct nucleoli. Nuclear detail is often obscured by intense hyperchromasia, smudged chromatin, and crush artifact. The mitotic rate is usually higher than 20 mitotic figures (MF) per 10 high-power-fields (HPF)

■ Intermediate-type cells, which are admixed with small cells in some cases, have larger, round to oval nuclei that are more uniform and have coarser chromatin than the small cells and may have a prominent nucleolus.

■ Nuclear fragmentation (i.e., hematoxylin bodies) and single cell or confluent necrosis are common features. Lymphovascular invasion is usually prominent.

■ Foci of typical squamous cell carcinoma or adenocarcinoma (either of which may be in situ, invasive, or both) are found in up to 50% of the tumors. These invasive components may be discrete or intimately admixed with the neoplastic small cells.

Findings With Special Techniques

■ Neuroendocrine differentiation determined with one or more techniques is found in most cases. There is wide variation in the frequencuy of tumor cell arygyrophilia among series; the staining may be very focal and require prolonged search. Argentaffin cells have been demonstrated only in rare cases.

■ There is variable immunoreactivity for a wide variety of antigens, including low-molecular-weight cytokeratins (often focal punctate staining), epithelial membrane antigen, CEA, neuron-specific enolase, chromogranin, Leu-7, synaptophysin, and a variety of polypeptide and amine hormones (e.g., corticotropin, calcitonin, gastrin, serotonin, substance P, vasoactive intestinal peptide, pancreatic polypeptide, somatostatin). HPV (usually HPV-18) is present in most cases.

■ Dense-core granules have been found in most tumors on ultrastructural examination.

Differential Diagnosis

■ Small cell squamous carcinoma is discussed in Chapter 5.
■ Large cell neuroendocrine carcinomas (page 130).
■ Other small cell cancers, including lymphoepithelioma-like carcinoma, adenoid basal carcinoma, lymphoma and leukemia, and endometrial stromal sarcoma, are discussed elsewhere in this volume. Although their histologic distinction from SCCs may be difficult, particularly on a small biopsy specimen, routine light microscopic findings are usually diagnostic, and the histochemical and immunohistochemical findings facilitate the diagnosis in problem cases.

Behavior and Prognosis Factors

■ SCCs are highly aggressive neoplasms, with a propensity to metastasize early and widely. Involvement of regional and distant lymph nodes, lung, bone, brain, and liver is common.

■ Only about 25% of patients are alive and free of tumor on follow-up. The disease-free interval is usually less than 2 years. A more favorable prognosis (72% survival in one study) has been found for patients with pathologic stage I or II tumors.

References

Abeler VA, Holm R, Nesland JM, Kjorstad KE. Small cell carcinoma of the cervix: a clinicopathological study of 26 cases. Cancer 73:672–677, 1994.

Fetissof F, Serres G, Arbeille B, et al. Argyrophilic cells and ectocervical epithelium. Int J Gynecol Pathol 10:177–190, 1991.

Groben P, Reddick R, Askin F. The pathologic spectrum of small cell carcinoma of the cervix. Int J Gynecol Pathol 4:42–57, 1985.

Gersell DJ, Mazoujian G, Mutch DG, Rudloff MA. Small-cell undifferentiated carcinoma of the cervix: a clinicopathologic, ultrastructural, and immunocytochemical study of 15 cases. Am. J Surg Pathol 12:684–698, 1988.

Silva EG, Gershenson D, Sneige N, et al. Small cell carcinoma of the uterine cervix: "pathology and prognostic factors." Surg Pathol 2:105–115, 1989.

Stoler MH, Mills SE, Gersell DJ, Walker AN. Small-cell neuroendocrine carcinoma of the cervix: a human papillomavirus type 18–associated cancer. Am J Surg Pathol 15:28–32, 1991.

Van Nagell JR Jr, Powell DE, Gallion HH, et al. Small cell carcinoma of the uterine cervix. Cancer 62:1586–1593, 1988.

Walker AN, Mills SE, Taylor PT. Cervical neuroendocrine carcinoma: a clinical and light microscopic study of 14 cases. Int J Gynecol Pathol 7:64–74, 1988.

Wolber RA, Clement PB. In situ DNA hybridization of cervical small cell carcinoma and adenocarcinoma using biotin-labeled human papillomavirus probes. Mod Pathol 4:96–100, 1991.

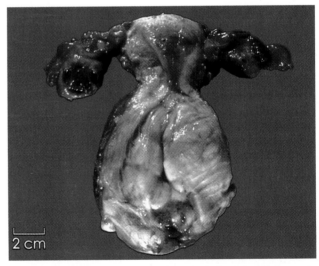

Figure 6–28. Small cell carcinoma has massively expanded the cervix and thickened its wall.

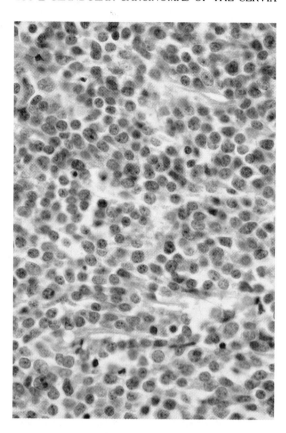

Figure 6–29. Small cell carcinoma.

Large Cell Neuroendocrine Carcinoma

- Large cell neuroendocrine carcinomas (LCNCs) occur over a wide age range (21 to 76 years; mean, 34 years in the largest series). The patients typically present with an abnormal Pap smear or vaginal bleeding and a cervical mass. Some patients have extrauterine spread at presentation.
- Insular, trabecular, glandular, and solid growth patterns, often with geographic areas of necrosis, are composed of medium to large cells with moderate to abundant cytoplasm that contains eosinophilic granules in 75% of the tumors.
- The tumor cells have high-grade nuclear features, often with prominent nucleoli, and a high mitotic rate (>10 MFs/10 HPFs and often >20 MFs/10 HPFs).
- Adenocarcinoma in situ is found adjacent to the tumor in more than one half the cases, and an associated invasive adenocarcinoma of nonneuroendocrine type was present in 25% of tumors in one study.
- Argyrophilia and immunoreactivity for chromogranin are present in almost all tumors. Serotonin and polypeptide hormones (somatostatin, glucagon) have been present in occasional tumors.

- The behavior of LCNCs is similar to that of small cell carcinomas. Seventy percent of patients with more than 1 year of follow-up died of tumor 6 to 24 months after hysterectomy in one study.

Differential Diagnosis

- LCNCs have larger cells than SCCs, with more abundant cytoplasm that frequently contains eosinophilic granules. Chromogranin immunoreactivity is usually more common and more diffuse in LCNCs than in SCCs.
- Carcinoid tumors and atypical carcinoid tumors are rarer in the cervix than LCNCs, and their clinical and pathologic features have not been well characterized. Criteria for their separation from LCNCs are the same as those for neuroendocrine tumors of the lung:
  - Typical carcinoid tumors have only rare mitotic figures, absent or mild nuclear atypia, and no necrosis.
  - Atypical carcinoid tumors have 5 to 10 MFs/10 HPFs, have mild to moderate nuclear atypia, and frequently have necrosis, although the latter tends to be less extensive than in LCNCs.

References

Albores-Saavedra J, Larraza O, et al. Carcinoid of the uterine cervix: additional observations on a new tumor entity. Cancer 38:2328–2342, 1976.

Albores-Saavedra J, Rodriguez-Martinez HA, Larraza-Hernandez O. Carcinoid tumors of the cervix. Pathol Annu 14:273–291, 1979.

Albores-Saavedra J, Gersell D, Gilks CB, et al. Terminology of endocrine tumors of the uterine cervix: results of a workshop sponsored by the College of American Pathologists and the National Cancer Institute. Arch Pathol Lab Med 121:34–39, 1997.

Gilks CB, Young RH, Gersell D, Clement PB. Large cell neuroendocrine carcinoma of the uterine cervix: a clinicopathologic study of 12 cases. Am J Surg Pathol 21:905–914, 1997.

Silva EG, Kott MM, Ordonez NG. Endocrine carcinoma intermediate cell type of the uterine cervix. Cancer 54:1705–1713, 1984.

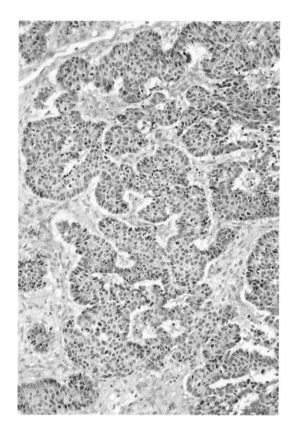

Figure 6–30. Large cell neuroendocrine carcinoma. Notice the trabecular pattern. The tumor cells were intensely immunoreactive for chromogranin.

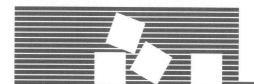

CHAPTER 7

Tumor-like and Inflammatory Lesions of the Uterine Corpus

EPITHELIAL METAPLASIAS

- Epithelial metaplasia may be overdiagnosed as endometrial adenocarcinoma on histologic examination. Conversely, it is important not to underdiagnose an unusual subtype of endometrial adenocarcinoma, e.g., oxyphilic or ciliated adenocarcinoma, as the corresponding metaplasia (oxyphilic or ciliated metaplasia).
- The extent of the change varies from one microscopic focus to most of the endometrium; endometrial polyps may be affected. Glandular and surface epithelium may be involved. Two or more types of metaplasia commonly coexist.
- Because endometrial metaplasias are often related to unopposed estrogen stimulation, underlying hyperplasia with architectural or cytologic atypia of the metaplastic glands is often present, or an endometrial hyperplasia or adenocarcinoma may be present elsewhere in the uterus. Metaplasia-associated adenocarcinomas usually occur in young patients and are well differentiated.

Squamous Metaplasia

- Squamous metaplasia is usually idiopathic, but potential predisposing factors in some cases include unopposed estrogen or progestin stimulation or inflammation (e.g., chronic endometritis, pyometra, an intrauterine device).
- Typically, intraglandular nests (morules) are composed of immature, round to spindled squamous cells, with indistinct cell borders and bland nuclear features. Maturation of the squamous cells with copious eosinophilic cytoplasm, intercellular bridges, keratin, and central necrosis occurs in some cases.
- Less commonly, the squamous metaplasia is a "flat" surface phenomenon with glycogenated epithelium, a finding that should be carefully distinguished from well-differentiated squamous cell carcinoma (see Chapter 8).
- The term *adenoacanthosis* has been used to refer to a complex endometrial hyperplasia with prominent squamous metaplasia. In such cases, confluent masses of squamous epithelium may be seen.

Mucinous Metaplasia

- Endometrial glands are lined by or the surface endometrial epithelium is replaced by columnar cells with mucin-rich cytoplasm, resembling endocervical epithelium. Rarely, the cells are of the goblet type, including the presence of intestinal-type mucin.
- Rare cases are accompanied by mucometra or mucinous lesions elsewhere in the female genital tract.
- The metaplastic mucinous glands may show architectural or cytologic atypia (i.e., atypical mucinous metaplasia). The differential diagnosis of atypical mucinous metaplasia with mucinous adenocarcinoma, which may be low grade and underdiagnosed as metaplasia, is discussed in Chapter 8.

Ciliated Metaplasia

- Endometrial glandular or surface epithelium consist predominantly of ciliated cells. The cells usually have eosinophilic or occasionally clear cytoplasm and are disposed in a single layer, but occasionally the cells stratify and form cribriform patterns.
- The glands with ciliated metaplasia may show architectural or cytologic atypia (i.e., atypical hyperplasia with ciliated cells). The differential diagnosis in these cases is with ciliated adenocarcinoma (see Chapter 8).

Eosinophilic and Oncocytic Metaplasia

- Endometrial glands are lined by or the surface epithelium is replaced by nonciliated cells with abundant eosinophilic cytoplasm that occasionally is granular (i.e., oncocytic metaplasia). The nuclei are uniform, round, and central, and mitotic figures are rare. Numerous mitochondria have been identified in some cases of oncocytic metaplasia.
- The lack of atypical features distinguish this alternation from endometrial hyperplasia with atypia, in which the cytoplasm is also typically eosinophilic, and from oxyphilic endometrioid adenocarcinomas (see Chapter 8).

132

Papillary Syncytial Metaplasia

- Papillary syncytial metaplasia (PSM), also called papillary syncytial change, involves the endometrial surface epithelium and, less commonly, the superficial endometrial glands. Cells, usually with eosinophilic cytoplasm, indistinct cell borders, and bland nuclear features are arrange in cellular aggregates, as well as in buds and papillae lacking stromal cores. A neutrophilic infiltrate is common.
- PSM probably represents a regenerative phenomenon after ovulatory or anovulatory menstrual bleeding, and it may be accompanied by signs of recent bleeding such as intraepithelial nuclear debris and aggregates of closely packed, degenerating endometrial stromal cells.
- Changes resembling PSM may occur as a surface change in some endometrioid endometrial adenocarcinomas (see Chapter 8).
- Features distinguishing PSM from carcinoma include its microscopic size, its usual confinement to the endometrial surface, and its generally bland nuclear features.

Hobnail Cell and Clear Cell Metaplasia

- Hobnail cell and clear cell metaplasia are rare, isolated findings with no apparent cause in a nonpregnant patient. Hobnail cells more often represent a reactive change, such as after a curettage (page 144) or within an infarcted polyp (page 146). Similar metaplastic changes in pregnancy are designated the Arias-Stella reaction or clear cell change of pregnancy (discussed later).
- Features that distinguish these conditions from clear cell carcinoma include the noninvasive, microscopic nature of the glands and an absence of mitotic activity.

References

Crum CP, Richart RM, Fenoglio CM. Adenoacanthosis of the endometrium: a clinicopathologic study in premenopausal women. Am J Surg Pathol 5:15–20, 1981.

Blaustein A. Morular metaplasia misdiagnosed as adenoacanthoma in young women with polycystic ovarian disease. Am J Surg Pathol 6: 223–228, 1982.

Demopoulos RI, Greco MA. Mucinous metaplasia of the endometrium: ultrastructural and histochemical characteristics. Int J Gynecol Pathol 1:383–390, 1983.

Hendrickson MR, Kempson RL. Endometrial epithelial metaplasias: proliferations frequently misdiagnosed as adenocarcinoma: report of 89 cases and proposed classification. Am J Surg Pathol 4:525–542, 1980.

Kaku T, Silverberg SG, Tsukamoto N, et al. Association of endometrial epithelial metaplasias with endometrial carcinoma and hyperplasia in Japanese and American women. Int J Gynecol Pathol 12:297–300, 1993.

Miranda MC, Mazur MT. Endometrial squamous metaplasia: an unusual response to progestin therapy of hyperplasia. Arch Pathol Lab Med 119:458–460, 1995.

Silver SA, Cheung ANY, Tavassoli FA. Oncocytic metaplasia and carcinoma of the endometrium: an immunohistochemical and ultrastructural study. Int J Gynecol Pathol 18:12–19, 1999.

Wells M, Tiltman A. Intestinal metaplasia of the endometrium. Histopathology 15:431–433, 1989.

Zaman SS, Mazur MT. Endometrial papillary syncytial change: a nonspecific alteration associated with active breakdown. Am J Clin Pathol 99:741–745, 1993.

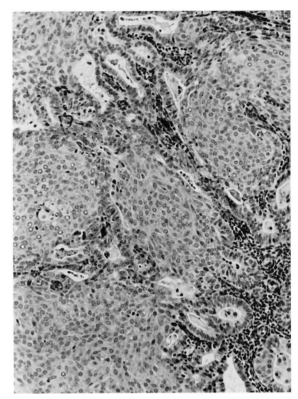

Figure 7–1. Squamous metaplasia. Extensive squamous (morular) metaplasia accompanies endometrial hyperplasia (i.e., adenoacanthosis). Many of the gland lumens are filled by the metaplastic squamous epithelium.

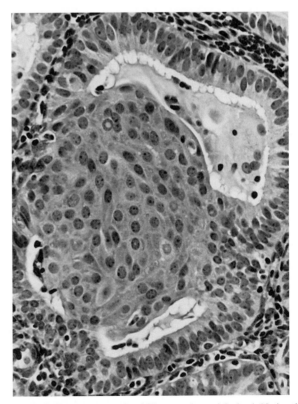

Figure 7–2. Squamous morule within an endometrial gland. Notice the bland appearance of the nuclei.

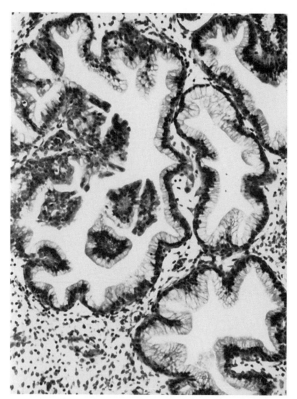

Figure 7–3. Mucinous metaplasia. Benign-appearing endocervical-type cells line endometrial glands and intraglandular stromal papillae.

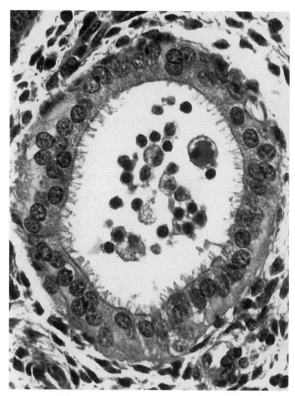

Figure 7–5. Ciliated metaplasia.

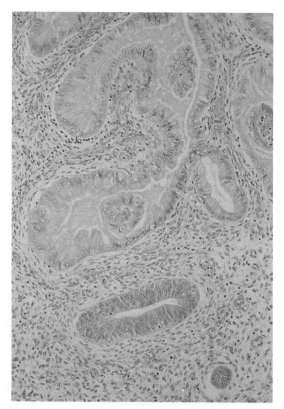

Figure 7–4. Atypical mucinous metaplasia. The large, irregular glands (*top*) are lined by pseudostratified mucinous cells with nuclear atypia.

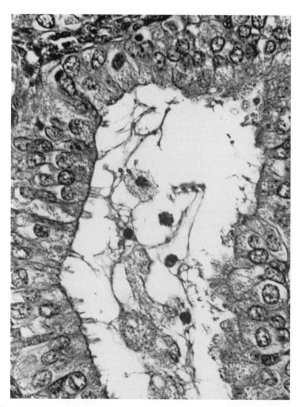

Figure 7–6. Atypical endometrial hyperplasia with ciliated metaplasia.

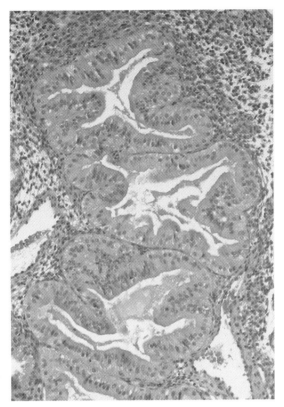

Figure 7–7. Eosinophilic metaplasia.

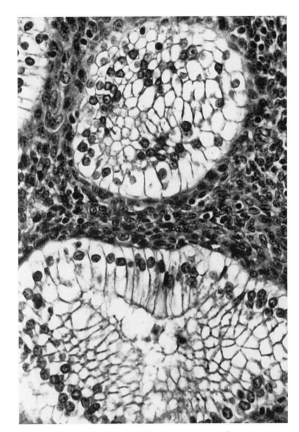

Figure 7–9. Clear cell metaplasia in nonpregnant patient.

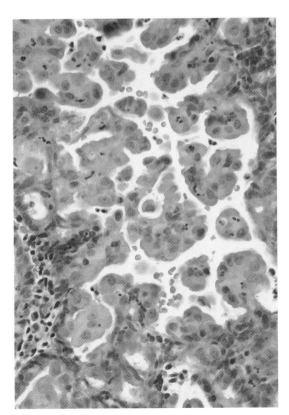

Figure 7–8. Papillary syncytial metaplasia.

PREGNANCY-RELATED AND HORMONAL CHANGES

- Misinterpreting pregnancy-related and hormonal changes as neoplastic or preneoplastic is more likely to occur if the pathologist is unaware that the patient is pregnant or if there is no trophoblastic tissue within the specimen.
- Similar findings occasionally occur in patients receiving progestins or rarely occur in patients with no apparent cause.

Arias-Stella Reaction

- The Arias-Stella reaction (ASR) is a characteristic histologic change within endometrial glands associated with an intrauterine or extrauterine pregnancy or trophoblastic disease. The ASR can also occur occasionally in premenopasual and postmenopausal women on hormonal medication.
- The ASR is typically located in the spongiosa, with involvement of a few to many glands. Regular papillary tufts are lined by cells with scanty cytoplasm and enlarged, pleomorphic, hyperchromatic nuclei, sometimes with a hobnail appearance. The nuclei are smudgy or optically clear; mitoses are absent or rare in our experience. In occasional cases, the nuclear atypia is striking.
- Features distinguishing the ASR from adenocarcinoma (especially clear cell carcinoma) include the typical association with clinical or other histologic evidence of pregnancy, its focal microscopic nature, an absence of invasion, and the usual mitotic inactivity.

Clear Cell Change

- The endometrial alteration called "clear cell change" is related to pregnancy and may accompany the ASR or occur in its absence.
- Glandular epithelial cells contain abundant, clear, glycogen-rich cytoplasm. The clear cells may stratify as regular papillary tufts or as solid nests or sheets with luminal obliteration. Nuclei similar to those of the ASR may or may not be present.
- Features distinguishing clear cell change from adenocarcinoma are the same as those for the ASR (described earlier).

Optically Clear Nuclei

- Optically clear nuclei, a characteristic alteration of nuclei within endometrial glandular epithelium, have been found in 7% of first-trimester abortion specimens and less commonly later in pregnancy or at term. The finding is often associated with the ASR.
- The appearance is similar to that of herpetic inclusions, but ultrastructural examination shows a network of fine filamentous material rather than herpesvirus DNA. The presence of biotin within the clear nuclei can result in a false-positive immunohistochemical reaction for herpetic antigens.

Decidual Reaction

- A decidual reaction is almost invariably confined to pregnant women and those being treated with progestins. However, rare examples of a florid decidual reaction have occurred in premenopausal or postmenopausal women with no apparent cause.
- Unusual microscopic features that are occasionally associated with diagnostic problems include the following:
  - Nuclear pleomorphism and hyperchromasia of decidual cells may mimic a sarcoma.
  - Unusual degrees of cytoplasmic vacuolation may mimic a signet-ring carcinoma (a similar finding may occur in predecidual cells in nonpregnant women); in contrast to metastatic signet-ring adenocarcinoma, however, the vacuoles contain acid, rather than neutral mucin.
  - The tissue in some cases of idiopathic decidual reaction in postmenopausal women may be polypoid and necrotic, with nuclear atypia and signet-ring–like cells.

Heterotopic Tissues

- Heterotopic tissues are usually an incidental microscopic finding in women of reproductive age. There may be an association with infertility in some cases.
- The tissues are most commonly cartilage, bone, glia, and fat, and they are usually within the endometrium and less commonly in the cervix or myometrium.
- Implantation of fetal parts during therapeutic or spontaneous abortion is the presumed pathogenetic mechanism in most cases. Other possible sources include metaplasia (as in nodules of endometrial smooth muscle), true heterotopia, or a dystrophic origin. Fragments of adipose tissue in a curettage specimen may be related to uterine perforation or derived from a submucosal lipoleiomyoma or lipoma.

Tumor-like Changes Associated with Menses

- Several tumor-like changes are associated with menses:
  - A pseudohyperplastic or pseudocarcinomatous appearance caused by menses-related fragmentation and crowding of endometrial glands and surface epithelium, features that may be accentuated by the curettage procedure
  - Compact, densely cellular nests of degenerating endometrial stromal cells with scanty cytoplasm and small, sometimes spindled hyperchromatic nuclei, changes that can be mistaken for a small cell carcinoma or sarcoma
  - Menstrual endometrium within uterine blood vessels
- Features distinguishing these changes from hyperplasia and carcinoma include the fragmented nature of the epithelium, the frequent presence of residual secretory changes within the epithelium, and the usual absence of nuclear atypicality and mitotic activity.

References

Arias-Stella J. Atypical endometrial changes associated with the presence of chorionic tissue. Arch Pathol Lab Med 58:112–128, 1954.

Arias-Stella J Jr, Arias-Velasquez A, Arias-Stella J. Normal and abnormal mitoses in the atypical endometrial change associated with chorionic tissue effect. Am J Surg Pathol 18:694–701, 1994.

Banks ER, Mills SE, Frierson HF Jr. Uterine intravascular menstrual endometrium simulating malignancy. Am J Surg Pathol 15:407–412, 1991.

Clement PB, Young RH, Scully RE. Nontrophoblastic pathology of the female genital tract and peritoneum associated with pregnancy. Semin Diagn Pathol 6:372–406, 1989.

Clement PB, Scully RE. Idiopathic postmenopausal decidual reaction of the endometrium: a clinicopathologic analysis of four cases. Int J Gynecol Pathol 7:152–161, 1988.

Doss BJ, Logani S, Jacques SM, et al. The Arias-Stella reaction and its variants: histopathologic and immunohistochemical features [Abstract]. Mod Pathol 11:102A, 1998.

Huettner PC, Gersell DJ. Arias-Stella reaction in nonpregnant women: a clinicopathologic study of nine cases. Int J Gynecol Pathol 13:241–247, 1994.

Jacques SM, Qureshii F, Ramirez NC, Lawrence WD, Unusual endometrial stromal cell changes mimicking metastatic carcinoma. Pathol Res Pract 192:33–36, 1996.

Mazur MT, Hendrickson MR, Kempson RL. Optically clear nuclei: an alteration of endometrial epithelium in the presence of trophoblast. Am J Surg Pathol 7:415–423, 1983.

Nogales FF, Pavcovich M, Medina MT, Palomino M. Fatty change in the endometrium. Histopathology 20:362–363, 1992.

Roca AN, Guajardo M, Estrada WJ. Glial polyp of the cervix and endometrium: report of a case and review of the literature. Am J Clin Pathol 73:718–720, 1980.

Schammel DP, Mittal KR, Kaplan K, et al. Endometrial adenocarcinoma associated with intrauterine pregnancy: a report of five cases and a review of the literature. Int J Gynecol Pathol 17:327–335, 1998.

Scully RE. Smooth-muscle differentiation in genital tract disorders. Arch Pathol Lab Med 105:505–507, 1981.

Tyagi SP, Saxena K, Rizvi R, Langley FA. Foetal remnants in the uterus and their relation to other uterine heterotopia. Histopathology 3:339–345, 1979.

Yokoyama S, Kshima K, Inoue S, et al. Biotin-containing intranuclear inclusions in endometrial glands during gestation and puerperium. Am J Clin Pathol 99:13–17, 1993.

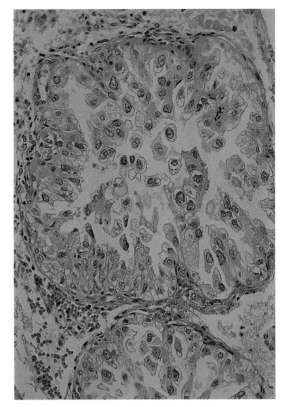

Figure 7–10. Arias-Stella reaction in a pregnant woman.

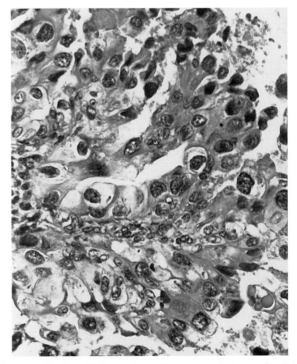

Figure 7–11. Arias-Stella reaction with an unusual degree of cellular stratification and nuclear atypia.

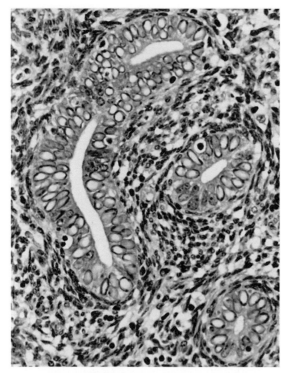

Figure 7–12. Optically clear nuclei, a finding characteristic of pregnancy.

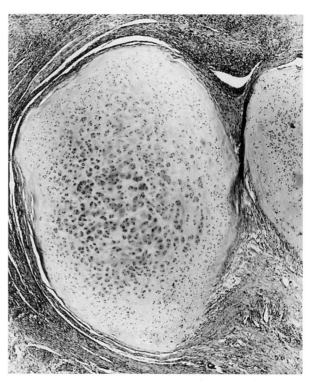

Figure 7–14. Nodules of hyaline cartilage within the superficial myometrium.

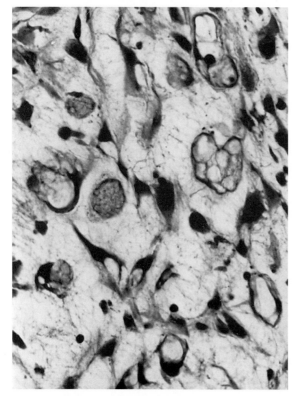

Figure 7–13. Endometrial decidual reaction with signet-ring–like cells in a patient taking progestins. The decidual cells have atypical, hyperchromatic nuclei that are displaced by cytoplasmic vacuoles that contain acid mucin.

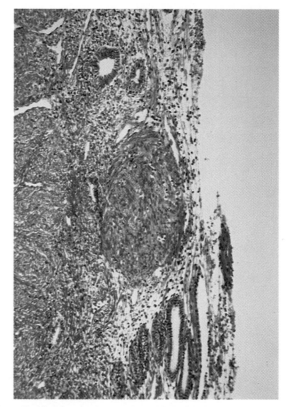

Figure 7–15. Metaplastic smooth muscle in the endometrium.

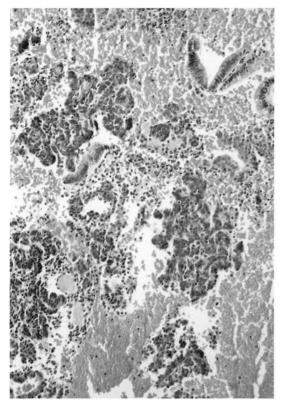

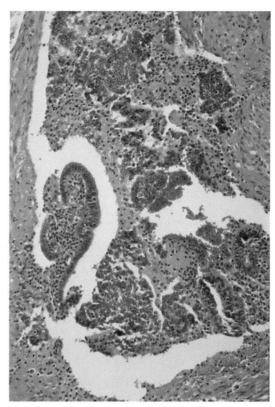

Figure 7–16. Normal postovulatory menstrual endometrium. The degenerating stromal cells were initially misdiagnosed as representing an undifferentiated small cell carcinoma.

Figure 7–17. Menstrual endometrium within a myometrial vein.

INFLAMMATORY AND REPARATIVE LESSIONS

Chronic Endometritis

- The histologic findings in most cases of endometritis associated with pelvic inflammatory disease (PID) are nonspecific; culture or other special techniques are usually necessary to identify the infectious agents.
- The term "chronic" endometritis is used here and elsewhere to refer to the presence of plasma cells within the endometrium (i.e., plasma cell endometritis). However, in virtually all such cases, including PID-related endometritis, acute and other chronic inflammatory cells are present.
- The sine qua non for a histologic diagnosis of chronic endometritis is the presence of plasma cells within the endometrial stroma, most commonly beneath the surface epithelium, around glands, at the periphery of lymphoid follicles, or around distended sinusoids; the basalis and the superficial myometrium may be infiltrated in severe cases.
- A diagnosis of chronic endometritis rarely rests exclusively on the presence of plasma cells. Lymphoid follicles with or without germinal centers are a frequent finding, and their numbers usually correlate with the number of plasma cells.
- Other common inflammatory cells include neutrophils within the surface epithelium and gland lumens (sometimes with microabscess formation), subepithelial lymphocytic infiltrates, hemosiderin-laden stromal histiocytes, and occasional eosinophils.
- Superficial stromal edema, increased stromal density, periglandular palisading of the stromal cells, fibroblastic or predecidual-like alteration of the stromal cells, stromal necrosis, and intrasinusoidal fibrin thrombi may also be seen.
- The normal cyclic response of the glands and stroma to the hormonal milieu of the menstrual cycle is variably diminished often resulting in an inactive appearance or marked variation between glands or between glands and stroma. Histologic dating of the endometrium is not reliable in the presence of endometritis.
- Other epithelial findings may include squamous metaplasia, including morule formation, and regenerative changes such as cellular stratification, increased

amounts of eosinophilic cytoplasm, prominent nucleoli, cleared chromatin, and mitotic figures.

■ The typical findings in chlamydial endometritis are nonspecific, but the diagnosis should be suspected in cases with dense and diffuse infiltrates of plasma cells and lymphocytes, stromal lymphoid follicles with transformed lymphocytes, stromal necrosis, and reparative atypia. Chlamydial inclusions may be identified in some cases, but their localization typically requires immunohistochemical staining.

References

Cadena D, Cavanzo FJ, Leone CL, Taylor HB. Chronic endometritis: a comparative clinicopathologic study. Obstet Gynecol 41:733–738, 1973.

Greenwood SM, Moran JJ. Chronic endometritis: morphologic and clinical observations. Obstet Gynecol 58:176–184, 1981.

Kiviat NB, Wolner-Hanssen P, Eschenbach DA, et al. Endometrial histopathology in patients with culture-proven upper genital tract infection and laparoscopically diagnosed acute salpingitis. Am J Surg Pathol 14:167–175, 1990.

Rotterdam H. Chronic endometritis: a clinicopathologic study. Pathol Annu 13:209–231, 1978.

Winkler B. Gallo L, Reumann W, et al. Chlamydial endometritis: a histological and immunohistochemical analysis. Am J Surg Pathol 8: 771–778, 1984.

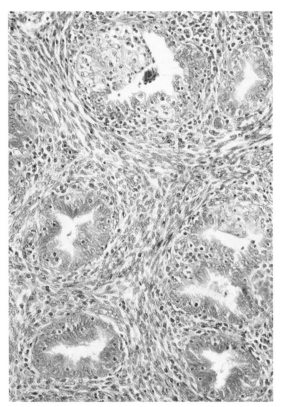

Figure 7–19. Chronic endometritis. The endometrial stromal cells are spindle shaped, and there is focal squamous metaplasia of the glands.

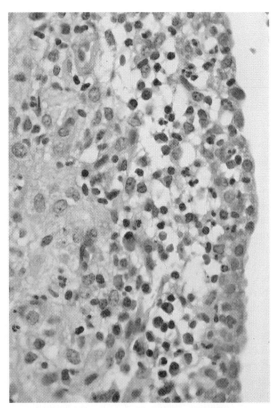

Figure 7–18. Chronic endometritis. Numerous plasma cells occur within the subepithelial stroma. Occasional neutrophils involve the surface epithelium.

Focal Necrotizing Endometritis

- This recently described lesion is typically encountered in premenopausal women who present with abnormal vaginal bleeding.
- The lesion is characterized by a focal inflammatory infiltrate of lymphocytes and neutrophils centered around occasional glands; plasma cells are not present. The infiltrate typically extends into the gland lumen with disruption or partial or subtotal necrosis of the glandular epithelium, the appearance resembling a crypt abscess.
- The clinical significance, if any, of this lesion is not yet known.

Reference

Bennett AE, Rathore S, Rhatigan RM. Focal necrotizing endometritis: A clinicopathologic study of 15 cases. Int J Gynecol Pathol 18:220–225, 1999.

Lymphoma-like Lesions

- Lymphoma-like lesions typically occur in women of reproductive age who present with abnormal bleeding, although in some patients the lesion is an incidental microscopic finding. All of the reported cases were discovered in curettage specimens, often in a background of typical chronic endometritis.
- The microscopic findings are generally similar to those of lymphoma-like lesions of the uterine cervix (see Chapter 4); differences include an absence of a band-like distribution and more numerous, focal, ill-defined aggregates of large lymphoid cells with an appearance resembling reactive germinal centers; a peripheral mantle of mature lymphocytes, however, is usually absent.
- Features distinguishing lymphoma-like lesions from uterine lymphoma include an absence of a grossly evident mass, reactive germinal centers within the lymphoid aggregates, a mixed inflammatory infiltrate at the periphery of the aggregates and sometimes within it, and the presence of typical chronic endometritis elsewhere in the specimen.

Reference

Young RH, Harris NL, Scully RE. Lymphoma-like lesions of the lower female genital tract: a report of 16 cases. Int J Gynecol Pathol 4:289–299, 1985.

Massive Lymphoid Infiltration in Leiomyomas (see Chapter 9)

Granulomatous Endometritis, Including Effects of Thermal Ablation

- Granulomatous endometritis usually results from tuberculous, fungal, or parasitic infection, foreign material, or sarcoidosis. In such cases, discrete granulomas are typically found, sometimes accompanied by granulomatous myometritis.
- Necrotic granulomas, in which palisaded histiocytes surround necrotic zones, have been described after diathermy or laser ablation of the endometrium. In other cases, the granulomas are associated with refractile, brown, hematoidin-like pigment or uniform black pigment.

References

Davis JR, Maynard KK, Brainard CP, et al. Effects of thermal endometrial ablation. Am J Clin Pathol 109:96–100, 1998.

Silvernagel SW, Harshbarger KE, Shevlin DW. Postoperative granulomas of the endometrium: histological features after endometrial ablation. Ann Diagn Pathol 1:82–90, 1997.

Xanthogranulomatous or Histiocytic Endometritis

- Xanthogranulomatous or histiocytic endometritis typically occurs in postmenopausal women who present with vaginal bleeding or discharge. In some cases, there is a history of radiation treatment for endometrial adenocarcinoma or squamous cell carcinoma of the cervix.
- Pelvic examination reveals cervical stenosis, pyometra, or both. Necrotic, friable, yellow-brown tissue may be found within a curettage specimen, or similar tissue lines the endometrial cavity in a hysterectomy specimen.
- Microscopically, the lesion is characterized by sheets of histiocytes in the endometrium (and in some cases, myometrium) with abundant, eosinophilic, granular or foamy cytoplasm in the absence of Michaelis-Gutmann bodies. The cytoplasm of the histiocytes is typically rich in lipid and, in some cases, ceroid pigment.
- A common admixture of other inflammatory cells includes neutrophils, lymphocytes, plasma cells, hemosiderin-laden histiocytes, and foreign-body giant cells. Other findings in some cases include cholesterol crystals, focal calcification, necrosis, and radiation-induced changes. Bacteria have been cultured in rare cases.
- The pathogenesis probably is related to cervical obstruction resulting in pyometra, hematometra, endometrial necrosis, or combinations thereof. Radiation-induced tumor necrosis and bacterial infection may be additional factors in some cases.
- The differential diagnosis includes malacoplakia and endometrial stromal foam cells occurring in some cases of endometrial hyperplasia and carcinoma (see Chapter 8).

References

Ladefoged C, Lorentzen M. Xanthogranulomatous inflammation of the female genital tract. Histopathology 13:541–551, 1988.

Russack V, Lammers RJ. Xanthogranulomatous endometritis: report of six cases and a proposed mechanism for development. Arch Pathol Lab Med 114:929–932, 1990.

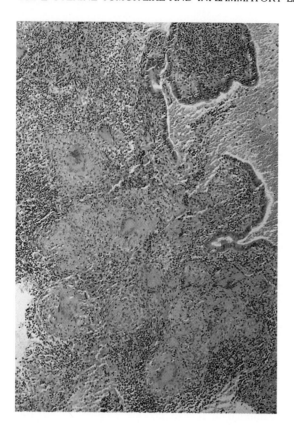

Figure 7–20. Granulomatous (tuberculous) endometritis.

Figure 7–21. Xanthogranulomatous endometritis.

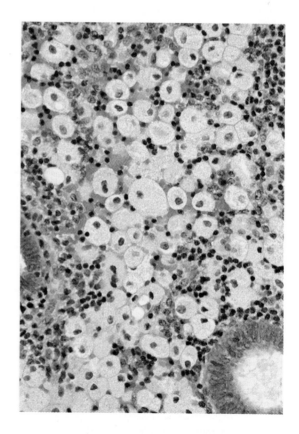

Malacoplakia

- Uterine malacoplakia typically occurs in postmenopausal women who present with abnormal vaginal bleeding or spotting. Other parts of the female genital tract (e.g., cervix, broad ligament) or inguinal region have been involved in some cases.
- The endometrium may be grossly thickened, nodular or polypoid, soft, yellow to brown, and focally hemorrhagic.
- The typical microscopic features include sheets of histiocytes with copious granular cytoplasm (i.e., von Hansemann cells), Michaelis-Gutmann bodies, and intracellular bacilli. Other inflammatory cells are typically present.

Reference

Kawai K, Fukuda K, Tsuchiyama H. Malacoplakia of the endometrium: an unusual case studied by electron microscopy and a review of the literature. Acta Pathol Jpn 38:531–540, 1988.

Eosinophilic Infiltrates

- Eosinophils in the uterine corpus are typically a response to a local operation. The eospinophils are usually an incidental microscopic finding in the endometrium and myometrium in a hysterectomy specimen days to weeks after a curettage.

Reference

Miko TL, Lampe LG, Thomazy VA, et al. Eosinophilic endomyometritis associated with diagnostic curettage. Int J Gynecol Pathol 7:162–172, 1988.

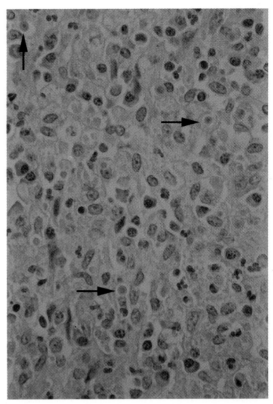

Figure 7–22. Endometrial malacoplakia. Notice the Michaelis-Gutmann bodies (*arrows*).

Mast Cell Infiltrates

- Small to moderate numbers of endometrial and myometrial mast cells are considered a normal finding.
- Mast cells may occur in striking numbers associated with intrauterine devices (IUDs), within the stroma of endometrial polyps, in areas of hyperplastic glands, and within leiomyomas. Their presence appears to have no clinical significance.

References

Crow J, Wilkins M, Howe S, et al. Mast cells in the female genital tract. Int J Gynecol Pathol 10:230–237, 1991.
Orii A, Mori A, Zhai Y-L, et al. Mast cells in smooth muscle tumors of the uterus. Int J Gynecol Pathol 17:336–342, 1998

Inflammatory Pseudotumor

- Three uterine examples of inflammatory pseudotumor with uneventful follow-up have been reported for symptomatic or asymptomatic patients 6 to 30 years of age.
- Gross examination revealed a solitary, well-circumscribed, leiomyoma-like myometrial mass up to 12.5 cm in diameter. The lesions were composed of an admixture of uniform, mitotically inactive, spindled myofibroblasts and a mixed inflammatory infiltrate rich in plasma cells.

References

Gilks CB, Taylor GP, Clement PB. Inflammatory pseudotumor of the uterus. Int J Gynecol Pathol 6:275–286, 1987.

Kargi HA, Ozer E, Gokden N. Inflammatory pseudotumor of the uterus: a case report. Tumori 81:454–456, 1995.

Postoperative Spindle Cell Nodule

■ One endometrial example of a spindle cell nodule was described in a hysterectomy specimen 2.5 weeks after a dilatation and curretage procedure in a 75-year-old woman.

■ A 1.0-cm nodule in the endometrium and superficial myometrium was composed of a densely cellular proliferation of mitotically active spindle cells, small blood vessels, and a sprinkling of inflammatory cells.

Reference

Clement PB. Postoperative spindle-cell nodule of the endometrium. Arch Pathol Lab Med 112:566–568, 1988.

Viral Lesions

■ Two cases of endometrial condyloma acuminatum have been reported as "diffuse viral papillomatosis" or "condylomatous atypia." Viral lesions must be distinguished from the equally rare verrucous carcinomas and other well-differentiated squamous carcinomas that may occur in this site (see Chapter 8). Features favoring condyloma include premenopausal age, associated cervical condyloma, prominent koilocytosis, prominent papillomatosis with central fibrovascular cores, and no myoinvasion.

■ Herpetic endometritis is a rare finding that may be associated with herpetic cervicitis or diagnosed at autopsy in patients with disseminated infection. The typical microscopic features include extensive necrosis and acute inflammation, multinucleated giant cells, and ground-glass nuclei with intranuclear inclusions. The stromal, epithelial, or endothelial cells are immunoreactive for herpes simplex virus in some cases. The differential diagnosis includes glands lined by optically clear nuclei, a pregnancy-related change (page 136).

■ Cytomegalovirus infection of the endometrium is relatively common in pregnant women and their infants and may be a significant cause of fetal mortality and morbidity. However, cytomegalovirus endometritis is only rarely encountered as a microscopic finding. The diagnosis rests on finding the characteristic intranuclear inclusion bodies in occasional cells lining otherwise typical endometrial glands. The surrounding endometrial stroma may contain prominent numbers of lymphocytes, lymphoid follicles with germinal centers, and plasma cells.

References

Duncan DA, Varner RE, Mazur MT. Uterine herpes virus infection with multifocal necrotizing endometritis. Hum Pathol 20:1021–1024, 1989.
Roberts PF, Brown JC. Condylomatous atypia of the endometrial cavity: case report. Br J Obstet Gynaecol 92:535–538, 1985.
Venkataseshan VS, Woo TH. Diffuse viral papillomatosis (condyloma) of the uterine cavity. Int J Gynecol Pathol 4:370–377, 1985.
Wenckebach GFC, Curry B. Cytomegalovirus infection of the female genital tract: histologic findings in three cases and review of the literature. Arch Pathol Lab Med 100:609–612, 1976.

Postcurettage Reparative Changes

■ Postcurettage epithelial atypia, which may be striking, is typically confined to the surface epithelium and superficial glands. The reactive cells may have enlarged and hyperchromatic nuclei with prominent nucleoli; some of the cells may have a hobnail appearance.

■ Papillary syncytial metaplasia (page 133) may sometimes represent a postcurettage reparative change.

■ The diagnosis is facilitated by awareness of a recent curettage, the superficial location of the changes, and an absence of significant architectural changes in the underlying glands.

Changes Related to an Intrauterine Device

■ IUD-related changes vary with the type of device and duration of use, and they include chronic (plasma cell) endometritis (with or without an associated salpingitis or tubo-ovarian abscess), squamous metaplasia, reparative hobnail cell metaplasia, and interglandular or gland-stromal dyssynchrony. Progestational changes (e.g., atrophic glands, decidua) may be seen in patients with progestin-releasing IUDs.

■ Actinomycosis infection (colonies of gram-positive bacteria [sulfur granules], neutrophilic infiltrate) is a recognized complication of IUDs. The differential diagnosis includes pseudoactinomycotic radiate granules.

■ Pseudoactinomycotic radiate granules (pseudosulfur granules) are a tissue response to the IUD. They are composed of neutral glycoproteins, lipid, and calcium, and lack the central branching filaments and diphtheroid forms of a true actinomycotic granule.

References

Bhagavan BS, Ruffier J, Shinn B. Pseudoactinomycotic radiate granules in the lower female genital tract: relationship to the Splendore-Hoeppli phenomenon. Hum Pathol 13:898–904, 1982.
Czernobilsky B, Rotenstreich L, Mass N, Lancet M. Effect of intrauterine device on histology of endometrium. Obstet Gynecol 45:64–66, 1975.
Lane ME, Dacalos E, Sobrero AJ, Ober WB. Squamous metaplasia in the endometrium in women with an intrauterine contraceptive device: follow-up study. Am J Obstet Gynecol 119:693–697, 1974.
Miller-Holzner E, Ruth NR, Abfalter E, et al. IUD-associated pelvic actinomycosis: a report of five cases. Int J Gynecol Pathol 14:70–74, 1995.
Schmidt WA. IUDs, inflammation, and infection: assessment after two decades of IUD use. Hum Pathol 10:878–881, 1982.
Silverberg SG, Haukkamaa M, Arko H, et al. Endometrial morphology during long-term use of levonorgestrel-releasing intrauterine devices. Int J Gynecol Pathol 5:235–241, 1986.

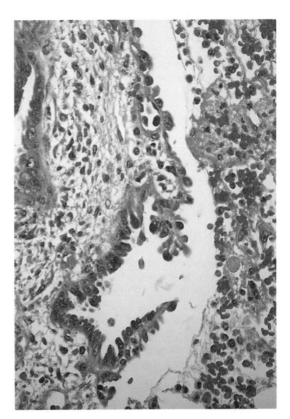

Figure 7–23. Postcurettage regenerative atypia of endometrial surface epithelium. Some cells are the hobnail type.

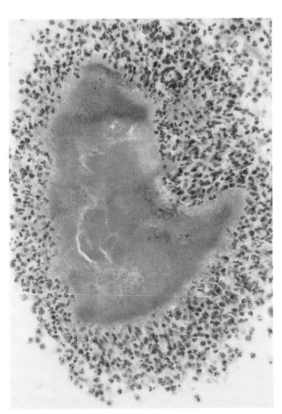

Figure 7–24. Endometrial actinomyocosis ("sulfur granule").

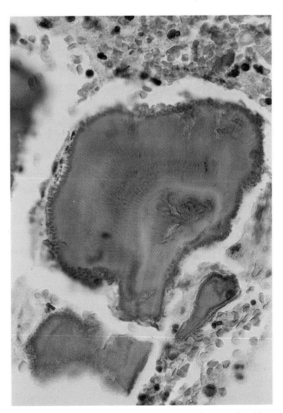

Figure 7–25. Pseudoactinomycotic radiate granule (pseudosulfur granule) related to an intrauterine device. Unlike a true sulfur granule, its features include the characteristic laminations (i.e., "tidewater" marks) and lack of a filamentous interior.

Ligneous Endometritis

- At least one, possibly two cases of ligneous endometritis have been reported; neither were associated with conjunctival disease at the time of reporting. Fallopian tubes were involved in one case.
- The histology is similar to that of ligneous cervicitis (see Chapter 4).

Reference

Scurry J, Planner R, Fortune DW, et al. Ligneous (pseudomembranous) inflammation of the female genital tract: a report of two cases. J Reprod Med 38:407–412, 1993.

Radiation-Induced Changes

- Radiation-induced changes, which may also occur in adenomyosis, are similar to those occurring in the cervix (see Chapter 4). Radiation changes tended to be more severe in normal endometrial glands than in carcinomatous glands in one study.
- Distinction from preneoplastic or neoplastic changes is facilitated by awareness of the history and appreciation of the typical histologic findings, including an absence of glandular crowding and mitotic activity.

References

Kraus FT. Irradiation changes in the uterus. In Norris HJ, Hertig AT (eds): The Uterus. Internal Academy of Pathology Monographs in Pathology. Baltimore: Williams & Wilkins, 1973:457–488.
Silverberg SG, DeGiorgi LS. Histopathologic analysis of preoperative radiation therapy in endometrial carcinoma. Am J Obstet Gynecol 119:698–704, 1974.

ENDOMETRIAL POLYPS

- Endometrial polyps were identified in 24% of consecutive endometrial biopsy specimens in one study. A recent association with chronic tamoxifen therapy has been found; in these cases, the polyps may be unusually large or multiple. One study (Pettersson and colleagues) considered endometrial polyps a risk factor for endometrial carcinoma.
- Polyps may mimic benign or malignant polypoid neoplasms on clinical or gross examination, but they typically have a smooth surface compared with the more irregular surface of most endometrial carcinomas, may contain cysts separated by fibrous tissue, and lack the fleshy, sometimes necrotic sectioned surface and myometrial invasion that are common in malignant tumors.

- Variable glandular morphology, including inactive and cystic glands, functional (normal proliferative or secretory appearance) glands, metaplastic glands, and hyperplastic or even adenocarcinomatous glands may be seen microscopically.
- The glandular morphology within the polyp may reflect the appearance of endometrial glands adjacent to or a distance from the polyp.
- Rarely, small serous carcinomas (see Chapter 8) are confined to a polyp, sometimes confined to a single layer of cells on its surface, and consequently may be overlooked. In tamoxifen-treated women, small endometrioid carcinomas may arise within and be confined to a polyp.
- The stroma of endometrial polyps is typically fibrotic with thick-walled blood vessels at the base of polyp, but it occasionally may resemble normal endometrial stroma or be hypercellular. Uncommon stromal findings include foci of smooth muscle, multinucleated stromal giant cells, and decidua; the latter finding usually reflects exogenous progestin use.
- Vascular thrombosis and hemorrhagic necrosis within the polyp are common. Reactive atypia of the glands or stroma of the polyp may be seen in such cases.
- The distinction from benign and low-grade müllerian mixed tumors (müllerian adenofibroma and adenosarcoma) is discussed in Chapter 9.

References

Berezowsky J, Chalvardjian A, Murray D. Iatrogenic endometrial megapolyps in women with breast carcinoma. Obstet Gynecol 84:727–730, 1994.
Corley D, Rowe J, Curtis MT, et al. Postmenopausal bleeding from unusual endometrial polyps in women on chronic tamoxifen therapy. Obstet Gynecol 79:111–116, 1992.
Creagh TM, Krausz T, Flanagan AM. Atypical stromal cells in a hyperplastic polyp. Histopathology 27:386–387,1995.
De Muylder, Neven P, De Somer M, et al. Endometrial lesions in patients undergoing tamoxifen therapy. Int J Gynecol Obstet 36:127–130, 1991.
Pettersson B, Adami H, Lindgren A, Hesselius I. Endometrial polyps and hyperplasia as risk factors for endometrial carcinoma. Acta Obstet Gynecol Scand 64:653–659, 1985.
Ramondetta LM, Sherwood JB, Dunton CJ, Palazzo JP. Endometrial cancer in polyps associated with tamoxifen use. Am J Obstet Gynecol 180:340–341, 1999.
Schlaen I, Bergeron C, Ferenczy A, et al. Endometrial polyps: a study of 204 cases. Surg Pathol 1:375–382, 1988.
Schlesinger C, Kamoi S, Ascher SM, et al. Endometrial polyps: a comparison of patients receiving tamoxifen with two control groups. Int J Gynecol Pathol 17:302–311, 1998.
Silva EG, Jenkins R. Serous carcinoma in endometrial polyps. Mod Pathol 3:120–128, 1990.
Van Bogaert L-J. Clinicopathologic findings in endometrial polyps. Obstet Gynecol 71:771–773, 1988.

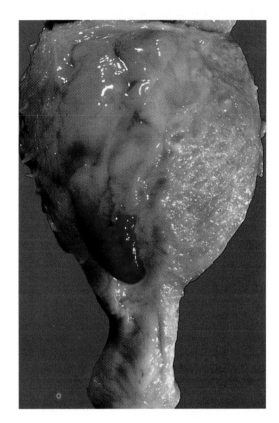

Figure 7–26. Endometrial polyp with a hemorrhagic tip. Notice the adenomyosis involving the right wall of the uterus.

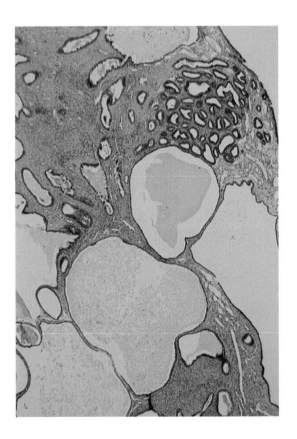

Figure 7–27. Endometrial polyp. Most of the polyp shows the typical features of an endometrial polyp with atropic cystic glands within a fibrotic stroma, but a focus of hyperplastic glands is in the upper right portion.

ADENOMYOSIS

- Adenomyosis is a common disorder that may cause tumor-like enlargement of the uterus on clinical examination. There is a wide variation in the diagnostic frequency between institutions and pathologists because of a lack of uniform diagnostic criteria.

- Gross examination may reveal a focally or diffusely thickened, trabeculated myometrium, occasionally with small cysts that may be blood filled. A discrete, leiomyoma-like, mural mass composed of adenomyosis and surrounding neoplastic, benign smooth muscle is designated *adenomyoma* (see Chapter 9)

- Adenomyosis is usually arbitrarily defined as the presence of endometrial tissue within the myometrium at least one 100× microscopic field below the endomyometrial junction.

- Adenomyotic foci almost always contain endometrial glands and stroma, and they are typically surrounded by hyperplastic myometrium. Hyperplastic or carcinomatous changes may involve adenomyotic glands.

- Adenomyosis with sparse glands (typically in postmenopausal women) may be confused with low-grade endometrial stromal sarcoma, the differential diagnosis of which is discussed in Chapter 9.

- Adenomyosis with atrophic stroma (typically in postmenopausal women), in which glands deep within the myometrium are surrounded directly by hyperplastic smooth muscle, may be confused with invasive adenocarcinoma. The atrophic appearance of the adenomyotic glands, the lack of mitotic activity, the presence of typical adenomyosis elsewhere, and the lack of an endometrial neoplasm facilitate the diagnosis.

- Intravascular endometrium (stroma only or glands and stroma) has been documented in 18% of women with adenomyosis, which was usually extensive (Sahin and coworkers). This finding appears to have no clinical significance.

References

Goldblum J, Clement PB, Hart WR. Adenomyosis with sparse glands: a potential mimic of low-grade endometrial stromal sarcoma. Am J Clin Pathol 103:218–223, 1995.

Sahin AA, Silva EG, Landon G, et al. Endometrial tissue in myometrial vessels not associated with menstruation. Int J Gynecol Pathol 8:139–146, 1989.

Seidman JD, Kjerulff KH. Pathologic findings from the Maryland Women's Health Study: practice patterns in the diagnosis of adenomyosis. Int J Gynecol Pathol 15:217–221, 1996.

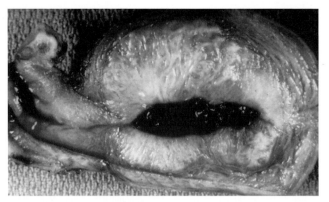

Figure 7–28. Adenomyosis. Notice the diffusely thickened, trabeculated myometrium (also see Fig. 7–26).

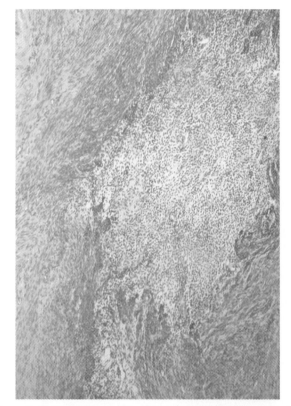

Figure 7–29. Adenomyosis with sparse glands. Notice the characteristic concentric zonal organization in which a pale-staining area of loosely aggregated stromal cells is surrounded by a more cellular rim of stromal and smooth muscle cells.

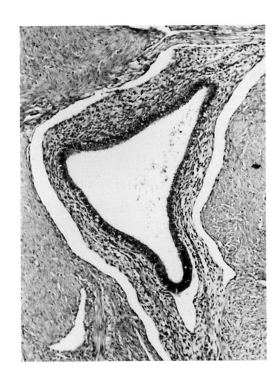

Figure 7–30. Intravascular adenomyosis.

IDIOPATHIC MYOMETRIAL HYPERTROPHY

■ Idiopathic myometrial hypertrophy (IMH) is a rarely diagnosed lesion arbitrarily defined as a uterine weight of more than 120 g in the absence of any other lesion. It was documented in 5.7% of consecutive hysterectomies in one series.

■ There is usually only moderate uterine enlargement; the heaviest uterus in the aforementioned series was 230 g. The uterus is typically symetrically enlarged with a diffusely thickened myometrium (potentially mimicking adenomyosis) on gross examination. The micronodularity of diffuse leiomyomatosis (see Chapter 9) is absent.

■ The myometrium is microscopically normal, although the smooth muscle fibers are hypertrophied, as evidenced by a decrease in the number of muscle fibers per unit area.

■ The finding is of uncertain clinical significance, although 75% of patients in the Lewis series complained of excessive menstrual bleeding.

Reference

Lewis PL, Lee ABH, Easler RE. Myometrial hypertrophy: a clinical pathologic study and review of the literature. Am J Obstet Gynecol 84:1032–1041, 1962.

CONGENITAL MYOMETRIAL CYSTS

■ Affected patients are usually of reproductive age and present with symptoms related to uterine enlargement.

■ Gross examination typically reveals a unilocular cyst surrounded by myometrium and filled with clear to amber fluid.

■ The cysts are usually of the müllerian type, located in the midline of the anterior or posterior uterine wall, and a lining typically composed of a single layer of columnar cells that may be ciliated (tubal), endometrioid, or endocervical in type.

■ Rare cysts of mesonephric origin are situated in the lateral walls of the corpus (usually below the insertion of the round ligaments) or cervix, with a lining of mucin-free, typically nonciliated columnar or cuboidal epithelium.

■ The differential diagnosis is with other myometrial cysts, including adenomyotic cysts (with surrounding endometrial stroma), cystic adenomyoma (with myomatous muscle surrounding the epithelium), echinococcal cysts, and cysts caused by hydrosalpinx of the intrauterine portion of the fallopian tube.

References

Buerger PT, Petzing HE. Congenital cysts of the corpus uteri. Am J Obstet Gynecol 67:143–151, 1954.

Chongchitnant N, Otken LB Jr. Intrauterine hydrosalpinx. Hum Pathol 15:592–594, 1984.

Sherrick JC, Vega JG. Congenital intramural cysts of the uterus. Obstet Gyencol 19:486–493, 1962.

Welcker ML, Kaneb GO, Goodale RH. Primary echinococcal cyst of the uterus. N Engl J Med 223:574–575, 1940.

EXTRAMEDULLARY HEMATOPOESIS

◼ Extramedullary hematopoeisis is rare in the endometrium and even more so in the myometrium and cervix.

◼ It is associated with hematologic disease in some cases; in others, it appears to represent an isolated finding without clinical significance.

References

Creagh TM, Bain BJ, Evans DJ, et al. Endometrial extramedullary haemopoeisis. J Pathol 176:99–104, 1995.

Pandey U, Aluwihare N, Light A, Hamilton M. Extramedullary haematopoiesis in the cervix. Letter. Histopathology 34:556–557, 1999.

Sirgi KE, Swanson PE, Gersell DJ. Extramedullary hematopoeisis in the endometrium: report of four cases and review of the literature. Am J Clin Pathol 101:643–646, 1994.

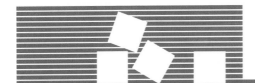

CHAPTER 8

Endometrial Hyperplasia and Carcinoma

ENDOMETRIAL HYPERPLASIA

Classification

- Formulated by the World Health Organization and International Society of Gynecological Pathologists (WHO/ISGP):

1. Simple hyperplasia
   a. Without atypia
   b. With atypia
2. Complex hyperplasia
   a. Without atypia
   b. With atypia

- We also use the classification proposed by Welch and Scully:

1. Cystic hyperplasia
2. Atypical hyperplasia
   - The degree of the architectural atypia, if present, is indicated as mild, moderate, or severe.
   - The degree of the cytological atypia, if present, is indicated as mild, moderate or severe.
   - The extent of the process (focal, multifocal, or diffuse) is also indicated.

Clinical Features

- An unknown proportion of endometrial carcinomas is preceded by precancerous hyperplasia. Knowledge of the natural history of these precancerous changes is confined to women with endometrial sampling before the appearance of the endometrial adenocarcinoma (<10% of women with endometrial adenocarcinoma).
- Endometrial hyperplasia is frequently associated with hyperestrinism (i.e., exogenous estrogen use, polycystic ovarian disease, obesity). Hyperplasia-associated adenocarcinomas are usually prognostically favorable (i.e., a grade 1 endometrial carcinoma with no or superficial myometrial invasion).

Pathologic Features

- In the WHO/ISGP classification, *simple hyperplasia* indicates lesions formerly designated as cystic hyperplasia and those with mild and moderate degrees of architectural complexity. *Complex hyperplasia* refers to lesions with marked glandular complexity.
- Atypia refers to cellular atypia characterized by nuclear changes, including enlargement, rounding, variation in size and shape, and hyperchromatism, nucleolar prominence, and loss of polarity. The nuclear changes are usually accompanied by increased amounts of eosinophilic cytoplasm.
- Findings that may occasionally occur in any type of hyperplasia include
  - Intraglandular papillae with connective tissue cores
  - Cellular stratification, including cellular buds, intraglandular bridges, or luminal obliteration; a cribriform pattern is uncommon and favors the diagnosis of adenocarcinoma
  - Superimposed metaplastic changes (see Chapter 7)
  - Superimposed secretory changes characterized by subnuclear and sometimes supranuclear glycogen-rich vacuoles in the glandular epithelium; these changes typically occur in young women who have a corpus luteum and a normal secretory endometrium adjacent to the carcinoma
  - Focal menstrual-type breakdown (e.g., compact stroma, nuclear debris, regenerating surface epithelium)
  - Dilatation and thrombosis of endometrial sinusoids and focal infarct-like necrosis
  - Stromal foam cells (more common in adenocarcinoma, page 155)
  - Synchronous adenocarcinoma (discussed later)
- Genest and colleagues described localized endometrial proliferations as an incidental finding in gestational endometria:
  - The finding is confined to a few glands or a small aggregate of glands, and is characterized by glandular

expansion with smooth external contours, epithelial stratification (4 to 15 layers), a cribriform pattern, mitotic activity, bland to mildly atypical nuclear features, and intraglandular calcification.

- The natural history of the change is not known with certainty. Follow-up of the cases in the study by Genest and colleagues suggested a benign behavior. Schammel and coworkers, however, found similar proliferations accompanying endometrial adenocarcinomas in pregnancy, suggesting that this lesion may represent a pregnancy-related atypical hyperplasia.

Behavior

■ Progression to carcinoma is associated with cytological atypia. Kurman and associates found progression to carcinoma in fewer than 3% of cases of hyperplasia without atypia (simple and complex), compared with 22% to 24% of patients with atypia (simple and complex).

■ Because no follow-up studies of hyperplasias associated with superimposed metaplastic or secretory changes have been published, the frequency of progression to carcinoma of these uncommon forms of hyperplasia is unknown.

Differential Diagnosis

■ Artifactual changes resulting from the fragmentation and crowding of glands induced by the curettage procedure. These include artifactual crowding, telescoping of the glands (i.e., glands within glands), and strips of crowded surface epithelium that may have a pseudo-papillary pattern, a finding that is often associated with an atrophic endometrium.

■ Epithelial metaplasias, pregnancy-related and other hormonal changes, and postmenstrual and postcurettage reparative changes (see Chapter 7).

■ Atypical polypoid adenomyoma (see Chapter 9).

■ Cystic atrophy (possible confusion with simple hyperplasia with cystic glands). Cystic atophy is a regressive change in elderly women, characterized by a fibrotic stroma and cystic glands lined by simple, flattened epithelium devoid of mitotic activity.

■ "Persistent" or "disordered" proliferative endometrium. An otherwise typical proliferative endometrium contains occasional cystic glands and minimal focal glandular crowding and budding (the gland to stroma ratio is about 1:1). The appearance merges with that of mild simple hyperplasia. Huang and associates found this lesion regressed in almost 80% of cases and the remainder progressed to hyperplasia; no cases progressed to carcinoma.

■ Grade 1 endometrioid adenocarcinoma. This differential diagnosis, which can be difficult and subjective, is based on the evaluation of architectural and nuclear changes that usually parallel each other, but occasionally the diagnosis is based on only architectural or only nuclear features.

- Architectural patterns indicating adenocarcinoma include a confluent, haphazard glandular pattern in which individual glands merge, resulting in interconnecting gland lumens; a cribriform pattern in more than a rare gland; and an extensive or confluent papillary pattern (coarse or fine papillae or branching villi with stromal cores).

- Many carcinomas retain some interglandular stroma, at least focally, a finding that in our experience often leads to underdiagnosis of carcinoma.

- Nuclear changes favoring adenocarcinoma include grade 2 or 3 nuclear pleomorphism and prominent nucleoli.

- Nonspecific findings that favor a diagnosis of adenocarcinoma over that of complex atypical hyperplasia include glands surrounded by granulation tissue–type stroma or a desmoplastic stroma, necrosis, numerous neutrophils, numerous mitotic figures, and atypical mitotic figures.

- "At least complex atypical hyperplasia; grade 1 adenocarcinoma cannot be excluded" is a reasonable diagnosis to render in borderline lesions for which distinction between the two processes is problematic.

References

Genest DR, Brodsky G, Lage JA. Localized endometrial proliferations associated with pregnancy: clinical and histopathologic features in 11 cases. Hum Pathol 26:1233–1240, 1995.

Hendrickson MR, Ross JC, Kempson RL. Toward the development of morphologic criteria for well-differentiated adenocarcinoma of the endometrium. Am J Surg Pathol. 7:819–838, 1983.

Huang SJ, Amparo EG, Fu YS. Endometrial hyperplasia: Histologic classification and behavior. Surg Pathol 1:215–229, 1988.

Kendall BS, Ronnett BM, Isacson C, et al. Reproducibility of the diagnosis of endometrial hyperplasia, atypical hyperplasia, and well-differentiated carcinoma. Am J Surg Pathol 22:1012–1019, 1998.

Kurman RJ, Kaminski PF, Norris HJ. The behavior of endometrial hyperplasia: a long-term study of "untreated" hyperplasia in 170 patients. Cancer 56:403–412, 1985.

Kurman RJ, Norris HJ. Evaluation of criteria for distinguishing atypical endometrial hyperplasia from well-differentiated carcinoma. Cancer 49:2547–2559, 1982.

Longacre TA, Chung MH, Jensen DN, Hendrickson MR. Proposed criteria for the diagnosis of well-differentiated endometrial carcinoma: a diagnostic test for myoinvasion. Am J Surg Pathol 19:371–406, 1995.

Norris HJ, Tavassoli FA, Kurman RJ. Endometrial hyperplasia and carcinoma: diagnostic considerations. Am J Surg Pathol 7:839–847, 1983.

Silverberg SG. Hyperplasia and carcinoma of the endometrium. Semin Diagn Pathol 5:135–153, 1988.

Welch WR, Scully RE. Precancerous lesions of the endometrium. Hum Pathol 8:503–512, 1977.

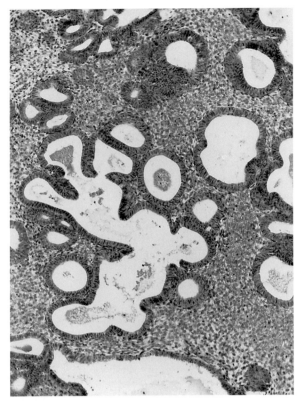

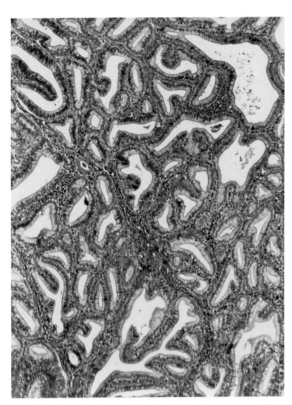

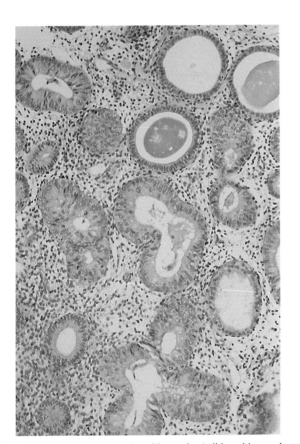

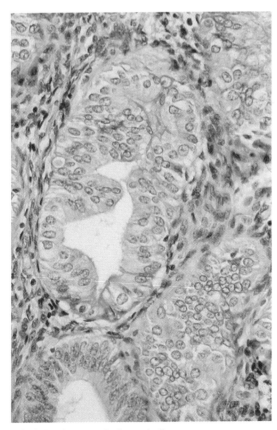

Figure 8–1. Simple hyperplasia (mild architectural atypicality). No cytological atypia is present.

Figure 8–3. Complex hyperplasia (moderate to severe architectural atypicality).

Figure 8–2. Simple hyperplasia with atypia (mild architectural and moderate cytologic atypicality).

Figure 8–4. Moderate cytologic atypicality.

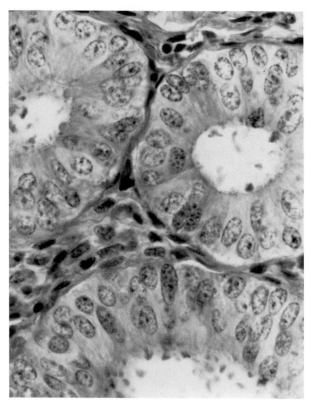

Figure 8–5. Severe cytologic atypicality. Notice the rounding of nuclei, clumped chromatin, and moderate amounts of eosinophilic cytoplasm.

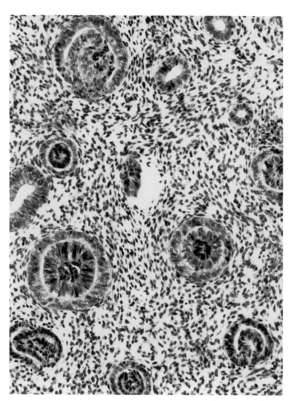

Figure 8–7. Telescoping of glands, an appearance that should not be confused with simple hyperplasia.

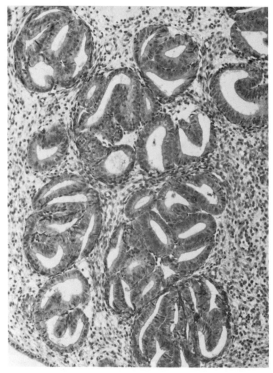

Figure 8–6. Artifactual crowding of glands.

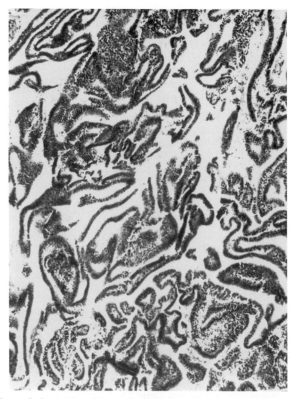

Figure 8–8. Artifactual crowding of strips of surface epithelium in a curettage specimen. This appearance is usually associated with an atrophic endometrium.

ENDOMETRIAL CARCINOMA

Classification

■ The current classification of endometrial carcinomas used by the ISGP and the WHO is based primarily on the cell type of the tumor. The classification that follows is based on the ISGP/WHO classification, with any additions marked with an asterisk (*).

ENDOMETRIOID
  TYPICAL
  VARIANTS
    Villoglandular*
    With squamous differentiation
    Secretory
    Ciliated
    Oxyphilic*
    Sertoliform*
    With trophoblastic differentiation*
    With giant cell component*
    (With argyrophil cells)*
SEROUS PAPILLARY ADENOCARCINOMA
CLEAR CELL ADENOCARCINOMA
MUCINOUS ADENOCARCINOMA
SQUAMOUS CELL CARCINOMA
TRANSITIONAL CELL CARCINOMA*
HEPATOID CARCINOMA*
LYMPHOEPITHELIOMA-LIKE CARCINOMA*
UNDIFFERENTIATED CARCINOMA
  LARGE CELL*
  SMALL CELL*
MIXED CARCINOMA

Gross Features

■ The various subtypes are indistinguishable on gross examination and vary from sessile, polypoid masses that may fill the endometrial cavity to irregular thickened plaques that may be localized or diffuse. The surface of the tumor is typically irregular or shaggy. Some tumors are confined to the lower uterine segment.

■ The neoplastic tissue is typically pale tan to white, fleshy, and firm or gritty. Foci of hemorrhage, necrosis, or both are often visible, especially in poorly differentiated tumors.

■ Myometrial invasion by similar tissue is grossly evident in some cases. In others, myometrial invasion is detectable only microscopically, especially if the invasive tumor is confined to lymphatic spaces.

Grading

■ The 1988 FIGO/ISGP grading (with suggested modifications by Zaino and colleagues in 1995) for endometrioid adenocarcinomas is by pattern and nuclear features. A similar grading system can be applied to mucinous adenocarcinomas.

  • Tumors that are less than 5% solid are grade 1; 5% to 50% solid are grade 2; and more than 50% solid are grade 3. The assessment of the solid growth is based only on the glandular component and not any squamous component that may be present.

  • The presence of grade 3 nuclear features (e.g., marked nuclear pleomorphism, coarse chromatin, prominent nucleoli) in most neoplastic cells in architecturally grade 1 or 2 tumors increases their grade by 1. Takeshima and coworkers found that architectural grade 1 or 2 tumors with more than 25% of grade 3 nuclei had a similar behavior to those with more than 50% grade 3 nuclei.

■ The WHO/ISGP grading for serous and clear cell adenocarcinomas and squamous carcinomas uses nuclear grade only.

Endometrioid Carcinomas

■ Endometrioid carcinomas, which account for 80% of endometrial carcinomas, typically occur in postmenopausal women, but a minority occur in younger women, including pregnant women, and tumors rarely occur in adolescents. The typical symptom is abnormal menstrual bleeding, usually postmenopausal bleeding. The uterus may be enlarged.

■ Some endometrioid carcinomas are related to unopposed estrogenic stimulation of the endometrium, which may be related to chronic anovulation, obesity, estrogen-secreting ovarian tumors, exogenous estrogens, or chronic tamoxifen therapy. Such tumors are typically preceded by hyperplasia and are usually well differentiated.

■ Endometrioid carcinomas are composed of tubular glands lined by stratified or pseudostratified columnar cells. Mucin is usually absent or confined to luminal tips of the cells, but minor foci of mucinous differentiation (i.e., cells with intracellular mucin) are present in almost one half the tumors. When luminal mucin is prominent, the term "mucin-rich" endometrioid carcinoma is appropriate.

■ Rare variants include tumors in which the cells have abundant oxyphilic cytoplasm (i.e., oxyphilic or oncocytic endometrioid carcinomas); clear, glycogen-rich cytoplasm; or foamy, lipid-rich cytoplasm.

■ Epithelial changes are found on the surface of the tumors in as many as 50% of cases, including squamous metaplasia or changes resembling papillary syncytial metaplasia or microglandular hyperplasia. The degree of nuclear atypia in these surface areas is usually less than that of the underlying tumor.

■ Stromal foamy histiocytes occur in about 15% of tumors, which are usually well differentiated. Rare findings include psammoma bodies or benign heterologous elements (e.g., fat, osteoid).

■ Associated endometrial hyperplasia, which occurs in 20% to 40% of endometrioid adenocarcinomas, should be identified (discussed later).

■ The carcinoma may extend into or rarely arise within areas of adenomyosis. When the tumor in the myometrium is confined to adenomyotic foci, the prognosis is not adversely affected.

■ Some tumors have a distinctive pattern of myoinvasion in which individual, deceptively benign glands are

Table 8–1
FIGO STAGING OF ENDOMETRIAL CARCINOMA

Stage	Characteristics
Ia	Tumor limited to endometrium
Ib	Invasion to less than one half of myometrium
Ic	Invasion to more than one half of myometrium
IIa	Endocervical glandular involvement only
IIb	Cervical stromal invasion
IIIa	Tumor invades serosa and/or adnexa and/or positive peritoneal cytology
IIIb	Vaginal metastases
IVa	Tumor invasion of bladder and/or bowel mucosa
IVb	Distant metastases including intraabdominal tumor and/or inguinal lymph nodes

widely spaced in the myometrium (minimal-deviation endometrioid adenocarcinoma; "diffusely infiltrating" pattern). This pattern lacks special prognostic significance.

■ These tumors should be distinguished from endometrioid carcinomas of the uterine cervix by colposcopic and hysteroscopic findings and by the nature of any benign glands and stroma contiguous with tumor.

• Vimentin positivity and carcinoembryonic antigen (CEA) negativity favor an endometrial over an endocervical endometrioid carcinoma.

Prognostic Factors

■ Prognostic factors to include in the pathology report, in addition to the histologic type or subtype, for endometrioid and other types of endometrial carcinoma include the grade, depth of myometrial invasion, and the presence or absence of involvement of the following: lymphovascular spaces, the cervix, the adnexa, and other submitted tissues, such as lymph nodes. Some studies have found aneuploidy to be an independent adverse prognostic factor.

■ The foregoing information allows assessment of the clinical stage (Table 8–1).

■ Coexistent endometrial hyperplasia is a favorable prognostic factor. The difference in prognosis between hyperplasia-related and atrophy-related endometrioid carcinomas is related to the higher grade of the latter tumors.

References

Beckner ME, Mori T, Silverberg SG, Endometrial carcinoma: nontumor factors in prognosis. Int J Gynecol Pathol 4:131–145, 1985.

Dabbs DJ, Sturtz K, Zaino RJ. The immunohistochemical discrimination of endometrioid adenocarcinomas. Hum Pathol 17:172–177, 1996.

Jacques SM, Lawrence WD. Endometrial adenocarcinoma with variable-level myometrial involvement limited to adenomyosis: a clinicopathologic study of 23 cases. Gynecol Oncol 37:401–407, 1990.

Jacques SM, Qureshi F, Lawrence WD. Surface epithelial changes in endometrial adenocarcinoma: diagnostic pitfalls in curettage specimens. Int J Gynecol Pathol 14:191–197, 1995.

Jacques SM, Qureshi F, Ramirez NC, et al. Tumors of the uterine isthmus: clinicopathologic features and immunohistochemical characterization of p53 expression and hormone receptors. Int J Gynecol Pathol 16:38–44, 1997.

Lee KR, Scully RE. Complex endometrial hyperplasia and carcinoma in adolescents and young women 15 to 20 years of age: a report of 10 cases. Int J Gynecol Pathol 8:201–213, 1989.

Longacre TA, Hendrickson MR. Diffusely infiltrative endometrial adenocarcinoma: an adenoma malignum pattern of myoinvasion Am J Surg Pathol 23:69–78, 1999.

Nogales FF, Gomez-Morales M, Raymundo C, Aguilar D. Benign heterologous tissue components associated with endometrial carcinoma. Int J Gynecol Pathol 1:286–291, 1982.

Parkash V, Carcangiu ML. Endometrioid endometrial adenocarcinoma with psammoma bodies. Am J Surg Pathol 21:399–406, 1997.

Pitman MB, Young RH, Clement PB, et al. Endometrioid carcinoma of the ovary and endometrium, oxyphilic cell type: a report of nine cases. Int J Gynecol Pathol 13:290–301, 1994.

Schammel DP, Mittal KR, Kalpan K, et al. Endometrial adenocarcioma associated with intrauterine pregnancy: a report of five cases and a review of the literature. Int J Gynecol Pathol 17:327–335, 1998.

Silver SA, Cheung ANY, Tavassoli FA. Oncocytic metaplasia and carcinoma of the endometrium: an immunohistochemical and ultrastructural study. Int J Gynecol Pathol 18:12–19, 1999.

Silver SA, Sherman ME. Morphologic and immunophenotypic characterization of foam cells in endometrial lesions. Int J Gynecol Pathol 17:140–145, 1998.

Sivridis E, Fox H, Buckley CH. Endometrial carcinoma: two or three entities? Int J Gynecol Cancer 8:183–188, 1998.

Takeshima N, Hirai Y, Hasumi K. Prognostic validity of neoplastic cells with notable nuclear atypia in endometrial cancer. Obstet Gynecol 92:119–123, 1998.

Yorishima M, Hiura M, Moriwaki S, et al. Clear cell carcinoma of the endometrium with lipid-producing activity: histologic and ultrastructural study suggesting a unique neoplasm. Int J Gynecol Pathol 8:286–295, 1989.

Zaino RJ, Davis ATL, Ohlsson-Wilhelm, Brunneto VL. DNA content is an independent prognostic indicator in endometrial adenocarcinoma: a Gynecology Group Study. Int J Gynecol Pathol 17:312–319, 1998.

Zaino RJ, Kurman RJ, Diana KL, Morrow CP. The utility of the revised International Federation of Gynecology and Obstetrics histologic grading of endometrial adenocarcinoma using a defined nuclear grading system: a Gyncology Oncology Group study. Cancer 75:81–86, 1995.

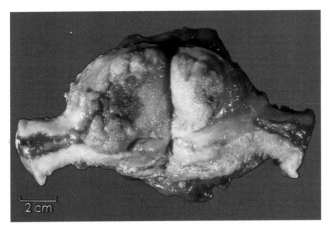

Figure 8–9. Gross appearance of an endometrioid-type endometrial carcinoma. A polypoid mass fills the endometrial cavity and invades the myometrium.

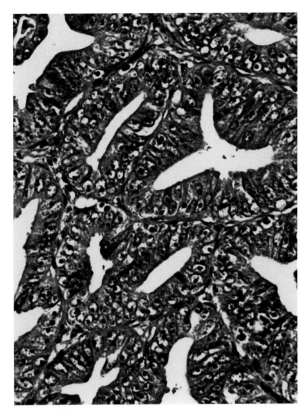

Figure 8–11. Grade 1 endometrial endometrioid adenocarcinoma. Notice the prominent nucleoli.

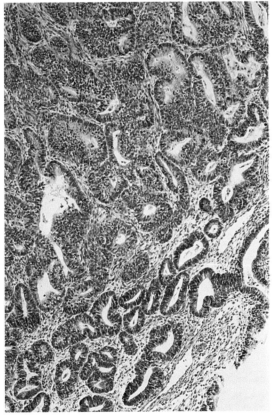

Figure 8–10. Grade 1 endometrial endometrioid adenocarcinoma.

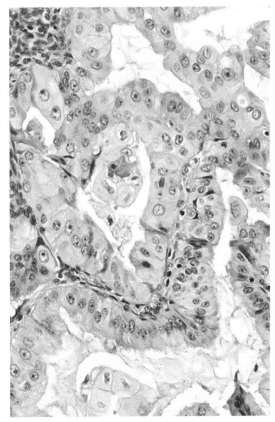

Figure 8–12. Oxyphilic endometrioid adenocarcinoma.

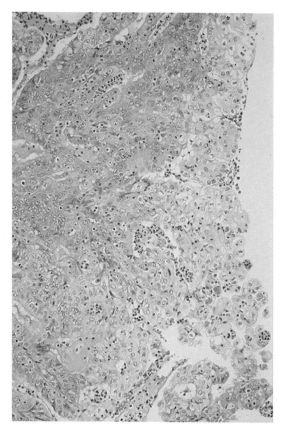

Figure 8–13. Papillary syncytial-like change on the surface of an endometrioid adenocarcinoma. Notice the obvious nuclear atypicality in the carcinoma (*extreme left*) compared with the milder atypia in the surface cells (*extreme right*).

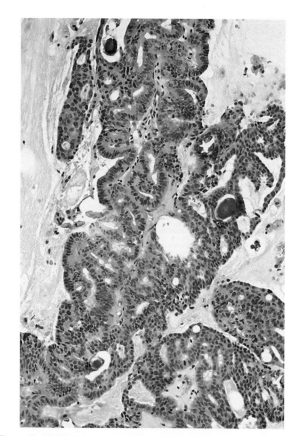

Figure 8–15. Endometrioid adenocarcinoma with psammoma bodies.

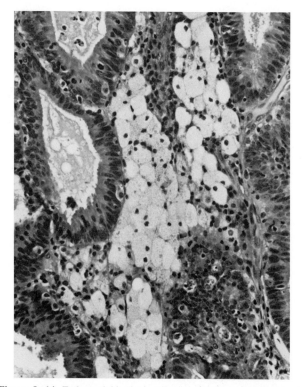

Figure 8–14. Endometrioid adenocarcinoma with foamy histiocytes in the stroma.

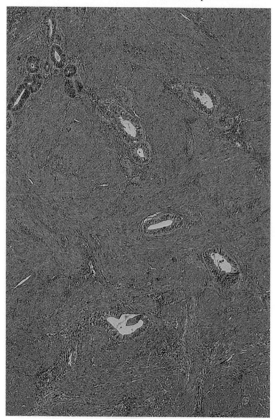

Figure 8–16. Endometrioid adenocarcinoma of the adenoma malignum type. Well-differentiated glands are widely spread in the myometrium with no periglandular stromal response.

Villoglandular Endometrioid Carcinoma

■ Villoglandular endometrioid carcinomas (VGECs) account for 2.5% to 22% of endometrioid carcinomas. About 40% of the tumors are pure, whereas the rest are mixed with typical endometrioid carcinoma or occasionally with a more aggressive histologic type, such as serous papillary carcinoma.

■ The tumors are typically grade 1 or 2 and contain villus-like papillae with thin fibrovascular cores, admixed with a variable proportion of endometrioid glands.

■ The behavior is similar to that of typical endometrioid carcinoma of similar grade in most studies. Ambros and colleagues, however, found that myoinvasive VGECs had a higher frequency of vascular invasion and nodal involvement and worse outcome than myoinvasive endometrioid carcinoma of usual type. The two types, however, had a similar behavior when confined to the endometrium.

■ The differential diagnosis is with papillary serous carcinomas (page 166).

References

Ambros RA, Ballouk F, Malfetano JH, Ross JS. Significance of papillary (villoglandular) differentiation in endometrioid carcinoma of the uterus, Am J Surg Pathol 18:569–575, 1994.

Chen JL, Trost DC, Wilkinson EJ. Endometrial papillary adenocarcinomas: two clinicopathological types. Int J Gynecol Pathol 4:279–288, 1985.

Hendrickson MR, Ross J, Eifel P, et al. Uterine papillary serous carcinoma: a highly malignant form of endometrial adenocarcinoma. Am J Surg Pathol 6:93–108, 1982.

O'Hanlan KA, Levine PA, Harbatkin D, et al. Virulence of papillary endometrial carcinoma. Gynecol Oncol 37:112–119, 1990.

Zaino RJ, Kurman RJ, Brunetto VL, et al. Villoglandular adenocarcinoma of the endometrium: a clinicopathologic study of 61 cases. A Gynecologic Oncology Group Study. Am J Surg Pathol 22:1379–1385, 1998.

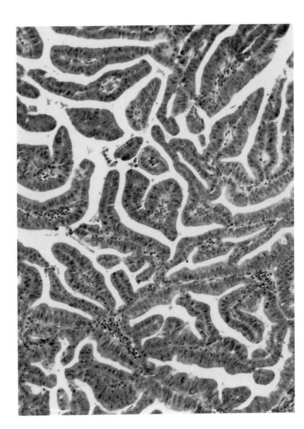

Figure 8–17. Villoglandular endometrioid adenocarcinoma.

Endometrioid Carcinomas with Squamous Differentiation

- These tumors, which account for about 25% of endometrioid carcinomas, contain focal to extensive squamous elements ranging from intraluminal morules of immature squamous cells with bland nuclear features to obvious squamous cell carcinoma.
- Rare features include squamous cells with a spindle shape (with an appearance resembling sarcomatoid carcinoma) or those with clear glycogen-rich cytoplasm. A rare variant is characterized by a similarity to glassy cell carcinoma of the uterine cervix (see Chapter 6).
- In most recent series, the behavior depends on the grade of glandular component and is similar to that of typical endometrioid carciomas when matched for grade and depth of myometrial invasion.
- Peritoneal granulomas, present in rare cases and attributable to exfoliation and transtubal spread of keratin, are not associated with a worse prognosis (see Chapter 20).

References

Abeler VM, Kjorstad KE. Endometrial adenocarcinoma with squamous cell differentiation. Cancer 69:488–495, 1992.

Christopherson WM, Alberhasky RC, Connelly PJ. Glassy cell carcinoma of the endometrium. Hum Pathol 13:418–421, 1982.

Hachisuga T, Sugimori H, Kaku T, et al. Glassy cell carcinoma of the endometrium. Gynecol Oncol 36:134–138, 1990.

Zaino RJ, Kurman RJ. Squamous differentiation in carcinoma of the endometrium: a critical appraisal of adenoacanthoma and adenosquamous carcinoma. Semin Diagn Pathol 5:154–171, 1988.

Zaino RJ, Kurman R, Herbold D, et al. The significance of squamous differentiation in endometrial carcinoma: data from a Gynecologic Oncology Group study. Cancer 68:2293–2302, 1991.

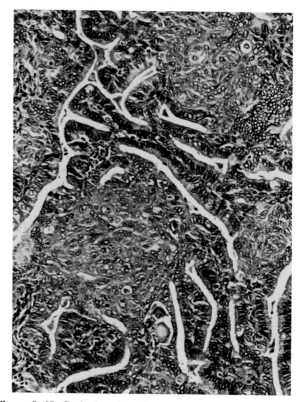

Figure 8–18. Grade 1 endometrioid adenocarcinoma with squamous differentiation (i.e., adenoacanthoma), which consists of well-circumscribed morules of immature squamous cells with bland nuclear features.

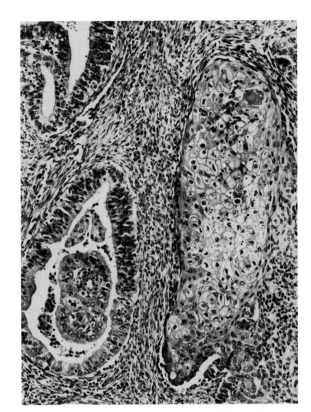

Figure 8–19. Endometrioid adenocarcinoma with squamous differentiation (i.e., adenosquamous carcinoma). Glandular and squamous elements are invading the myometrium and are surrounded by a reactive stroma. The squamous component has malignant cytologic features.

Secretory Carcinoma

■ Rare endometrioid carcinomas, which are usually well differentiated, contain cells with subnuclear or supranuclear glycogen vacuoles. The appearance is attributable to an endogenous or exogenous progestational stimulus in a few cases, but in most cases, there is no obvious cause.

■ The behavior is similar to that of other endometrioid carcinomas of similar grade.

■ The differential diagnosis is with clear cell carcinoma (page 169).

References

Christopherson WM, Alberhasky RC, Connelly PJ. Carcinoma of the endometrium: I. A clinicopathologic study of clear-cell carcinoma and secretory carcinoma. Cancer 49:1511–1523, 1982.

Silverberg SG, Makowski EL, Roche WD. Endometrial carcinoma in women under 40 years of age: comparison of cases in oral contraceptive users and non-users: Cancer 39:592–598, 1977.

Tobon H, Watkins GJ. Secretory adenocarcinoma of the endometrium. Int J Gynecol Pathol 4:328–335, 1985.

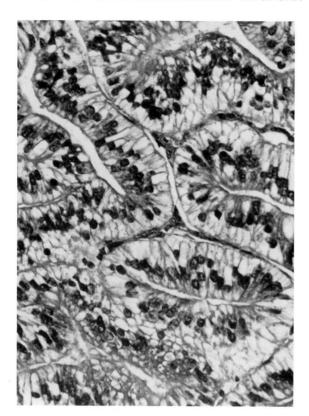

Figure 8–20. Secretory-type endometrioid adenocarcinoma.

Ciliated Carcinoma

■ Most of these rare carcinomas resemble typical well-differentiated endometrioid adenocarcinomas, except that the glands are lined predominantly by ciliated cells.
■ Distinctive features of an unusual type of ciliated carcinoma reported by Hendrickson and Kempson include sheets of cells punctured by small extracellular lumina (imparting a cribriform appearance) lined by cells with grade 1 nuclear features and cilia that project into the extracellular and intracellular lumina.

■ The behavior is similar to that of typical endometrioid carcinoma.

References

Haibach H, Oxenhandler RW, Luger AM. Ciliated adenocarcinoma of the endometrium. Acta Obstet Gynecol Scand 64:457–462, 1985.
Hendrickson MR, Kempson RI. Ciliated carcinoma—a variant of endometrial adenocarcinoma: a report of 10 cases. Int J Gynecol Pathol 2: 1–12, 1983.

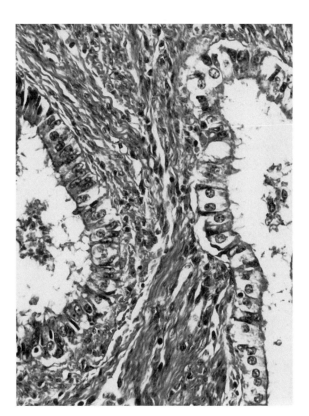

Figure 8–21. Ciliated endometrioid adenocarcinoma.

Sertoliform Endometrioid Carcinomas

- These are rare endometrioid carcinomas with a focal to predominant pattern resembling that of ovarian Sertoli cell tumors. The sertoliform component is composed of small, hollow tubules lined by columnar cells with apical, occasionally clear cytoplasm and short, slender cords.
- The cells in the sertoliform component are immunoreactive for cytokeratin, epithelial membrane antigen, and vimentin but not for actin or desmin.
- Based on a small number of cases, the behavior of these tumors does not differ from endometrioid carcinomas of the usual type.
- They must be distinguished from endometrial stromal sarcomas with sex cord–like elements and uterine tumors resembling ovarian sex cord tumors (see Chapter 9) by the presence of typical endometrioid carcinoma, squamous elements, and nonimmunoreactivity of the sertoliform component for smooth muscle antigens.

Reference

Eichhorn JH, Young RH, Clement PB. Sertoliform endometrial adenocarcinoma: a study of four cases. Int J Gynecol Pathol 15:119–126, 1996.

Endometrioid Carcinomas With Trophoblastic Differentiation

- These carcinomas are rare, otherwise typical endometrioid adenocarcinomas with focal trophoblastic differentiation, ranging from isolated syncytiotrophoblastic cells to typical choriocarcinoma. The trophoblastic elements are immunoreactive for human chorionic gonadotropin (hCG).
- The tumors are typically associated with elevated serum levels of hCG that decline after hysterectomy. The clinical course is usually rapid, with most patients dead of disease or alive with tumor at the time of last follow-up.

References

Bradley CS, Benjamin I, Wheeler JE, Rubin SC. Endometrial adenocarcinoma with trophoblastic differentiation. Gynecol Oncol 69:74–77, 1998.

Kalir T, Seijo L, Deligdisch L, Cohen C. Endometrial adenocarcinoma with choriocarcinomatous differentiation in an elderly virginal woman. Int J Gynecol Pathol 14:266–269, 1995.

Endometrioid Carcinomas With Giant Cell Carcinoma

■ These carcinomas are rare, otherwise typical endometrioid adenocarcinomas with a malignant giant cell component. The tumors were stage III of IV in three of the six reported cases.

■ Poorly cohesive sheets and nests of bizarre, multinucleated giant cells are admixed with mononucleate tumor cells; sarcomatoid carcinoma may also be present. There is a marked inflammatory infiltrate in one half the cases; the inflammatory cells may be found within the giant cells.

■ The malignant giant cells are immunoreactive for cytokeratin and epithelial membrane antigen.

■ Four of the six patients were dead of tumor or alive with tumor at the last follow-up.

Reference

Jones MA, Young RH, Scully RE. Endometrial adenocarcinoma with a component of giant cell carcinoma. Int J Gynecol Pathol 10:260–270, 1991.

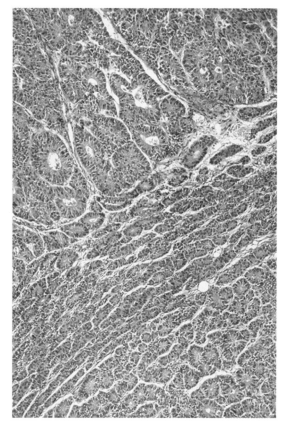

Figure 8–22. Endometrioid adenocarcinoma with a focal sertoliform pattern. Typical endometrioid carcinoma is visible at the top.

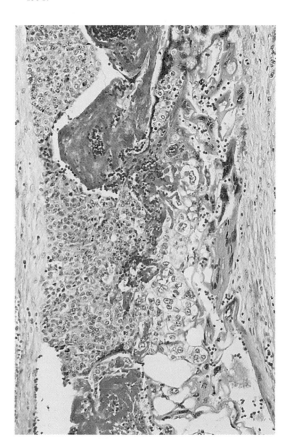

Figure 8–23. Endometrioid adenocarcinoma (not illustrated) with choriocarcinomatous differentiation.

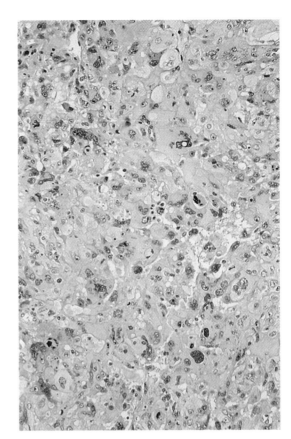

Figure 8–24. Endometrioid carcinoma (not illustrated) with foci of giant cell carcinoma.

Endometrioid Carcinomas With Argyrophil Cells

- Twenty-two percent to 70% of otherwise typical endometrioid adenocarcinomas contain argyrophil cells. In some of these tumors, the argyrophilia is apical and is related to apical mucin granules. In other cells, diffuse cytoplasmic argyrophilia in columnar or squamous cells results from glycogen granules.
- Argyrophilia in 10% to 12% of endometrioid carcinomas results from enterochromaffin cells (ECs) that appear as round, ovoid, or flask-shaped cells individually disposed within the glandular epithelium; occasional cells contain long cytoplasmic processes.
- ECs are typically immunoreactive for chromogranin, serotonin, and occasionally one or more polypeptide hormones, including calcitonin, somatostatin, and corticotropin. Ultrastructural examination of ECs reveals granules 80 nm in diameter.
- No patients with endometrioid carcinomas containing ECs have had endocrine manifestations. Because the behavior of argyrophilic endometrioid carcinomas is similar to that of typical endometrioid carcinomas in most studies, the designation "argyrophil cell carcinoma" is unnecessary for clinical usage.

References

Aguirre P, Scully RE, Wolfe HJ, DeLellis RA. Endometrial carcinoma with argyrophil cells: a histochemical and immunohistochemical analysis. Hum Pathol 15:210–217, 1984.

Bannatyne P, Russell P, Wills EJ. Argyrophilia and endometrial carcinoma. Int J Gynecol Pathol 2:235–254, 1983.

Inoue M, DeLellis RA, Scully RE. Immunohistochemical demonstration of chromogranin in endometrial carcinomas with argyrophil cells. Hum Pathol 17:841–847, 1986.

Inoue M, Ueda G, Yamasaki M, et al. Immunohistochemical demonstration of peptide hormones in endometrial carcinoma. Cancer 54:2127–2131, 1984.

Sivridis E, Buckley CH, Fox H. Argyrophil cells in normal, hyperplastic, and neoplastic endometrium. J Clin Pathol 37:378–381, 1984.

Ueda G, Nishino T, Saito J, et al. Detection of chromogranin in argyrophil cells of endometrial carcinoma. Gynecol Oncol 27:159–165, 1987.

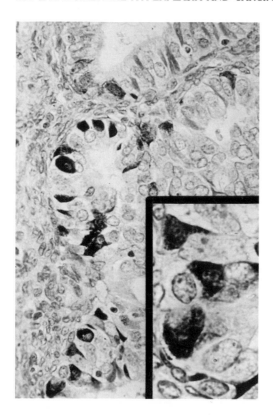

Figure 8–25. Endometrioid carcinoma with argyrophilic cells. The argyrophilic cells are individually disposed and have the appearance of enterochromaffin cells. *Inset,* Some cells are flask shaped.

Serous Papillary Adenocarcinoma

Clinical Features

■ Serous papillary adenocarcinomas (SPAs), which account for 1% to 10% of endometrial carcinomas, occur in women with an average age that is 10 years older than that of patients with endometrioid carcinoma. The usual symptom is postmenopausal bleeding, but there is occasionally a serous or serosanguinous vaginal discharge. In some studies, most women have had malignant cells in their cervicovaginal smears at the time of presentation.

■ Endometrial SPA is occasionally an incidental finding in a woman with a clinically evident serous carcinoma involving the fallopian tubes, ovaries, peritoneum, or combinations thereof. In such cases, clonality studies may be required to determine if the tumors represent multifocal primaries or a unicentric tumor with widespread metastases.

■ Estrogen use is less common than in patients with endometrioid carcinoma. Some patients have a history of pelvic irradiation.

■ The surgical stage is III or IV in as many as 75% of patients, with frequent involvement of pelvic and paraaortic lymph nodes, the ovaries, and the peritoneum, including upper abdominal peritoneum.

Pathologic Features

■ There are no distinctive gross features. The uterus may be small and atrophic in the presence of extensive myometrial and myometrial lymphatic involvement.

■ Usually, there is a complex papillary pattern of papillae with fibrovascular stalks covered by stratified epithelial cells and cellular buds. Other patterns, which occasionally may predominate, include irregular, slitlike glandular spaces and solid sheets of cells. Psammoma bodies occur in 10% to 60% of cases.

■ The nuclear features are almost always high grade (grade 3), often with marked nuclear pleomorphism, hyperchromasia, macronucleoli, and frequent mitotic figures. Hobnail-type cells and giant cells with bizarre nuclear features are present in some cases.

■ Although SPAs are occasionally confined to the endometrium or an endometrial polyp, most tumors invade the myometrium and myometrial lymphatics; lymphatic invasion of the cervix or adnexa may also occur.

- Fifty percent of tumors are admixed with other types of endometrial carcinoma, including endometrioid (typical and villoglandular forms) and clear cell carcinoma. The proportion of the tumor that is papillary serous should be specified in the pathology report.
- "Endometrial intraepithelial carcinoma" (EIC) (noninvasive serous carcinoma or uterine surface carcinoma) is focally present in the endometrium adjacent to SPAs in most cases. The endometrial surface and glandular epithelium is replaced by high-grade malignant cells that frequently form papillary tufts. Rarely, EIC with or without foci of microinvasion or lymphatic invasion occurs in the absence of an overt SPA.
- The endometrium not involved by SPA or EIC is usually atrophic.
- SPAs and EIC exhibit a high frequency of aneuploidy, oncogene expression (C-myc, C-erB-2) amplification, and p53 overexpression, and a low frequency of estrogen and progesterone receptors.

Behavior and Prognostic Factors

- SPAs are the most aggressive of the major subtypes of endometrial carcinoma: survival rates for surgical stage I tumors vary from 33% to 50%. Tumors confined to the endometrium (stage Ia), however, have had a survival rate of more than 80% in two studies. Thorough sampling of the myometrium is important to ensure accurate staging in these cases.
- Lymphovascular space invasion is associated with an increased risk of extrauterine disease in some studies but has had no impact on survival in other studies. The risk of lymph node metastases has not depended on the presence or absence or depth of myometrial invasion in some studies.
- Prognostic significance of mixed carcinomas with a component of SPA:
  - If SPA accounts for more than 25% of a mixed carcinoma, the behavior was that of pure SPA in two studies. In a third study, if SPA accounted for 10% to 25% of the tumor, the behavior was that of the lower-grade tumor, but the number of cases was small.
  - A preliminary Gynecologic Oncology Group (GOG) study found that mixed SPA-endometrioid carcinomas had a better outcome (65% at 5 years) than pure SPAs (42% at 5 years). The prognostic significance of small foci of serous carcinoma in a mixed carcinoma remains to be determined.
- DNA studies indicate that peritoneal serous tumor associated with minimally invasive SPA or EIC is metastatic from the endometrial tumor.

Differential Diagnosis

- Villoglandular endometrioid carcinoma (page 159). These tumors lack the complex papillarity, marked cel-

lular stratification, and usually the high-grade nuclear features of serous carcinomas.

- Papillary clear cell carcinoma (page 169). Features favoring this diagnosis include papillae with hyalinized cores, a tubulocystic pattern, a prominent component of clear cells or hobnail cells, or combinations thereof. Psammoma bodies may occur in clear cell carcinomas but are more common in SPAs. The distinction between papillary clear cell carcinoma and SPA with foci of clear cells may be arbitrary in some cases.

References

Ambros RA, Sherman ME, Zahn CM, et al. Endometrial intraepithelial carcinoma: a distinctive lesion specifically associated with tumors displaying serous differentiation. Hum Pathol 26:1260–1267, 1995.

Carcangiu ML, Chambers JT. Uterine papillary serous carcinoma: a study on 108 cases with emphasis on the prognostic significance of associated endometrioid carcinoma, absence of invasion, and concomitant ovarian carcinoma. Gynecol Oncol 47:298–305, 1992.

Carcangiu ML, Tan LK, Chambers JT. Stage IA uterine serous carcinoma: a study of 13 cases. Am J Surg Pathol 21:1507–1514, 1997.

Goff BA, Kato D, Schmidt RA, et al. Uterine papillary serous carcinoma: patterns of metastatic spread. Gynecol Oncol 54:264–268, 1994.

Grice J, Ek M, Greer B, et al. Uterine papillary serous carcinoma: evaluation of long-term survival in surgically staged patients. Gynecol Oncol 69:69–73, 1998.

Hendrickson MR, Longacre TA, Kempson RL. Uterine papillary serous carcinoma revisited. Gynecol Oncol 54:261–263, 1994.

Isacson C, Kurman RJ, Ellenson LH. p53 mutation analyses support the use of broad histopathologic criteria for the diagnosis of uterine serous carcinoma. [Abstract]. Mod Pathol 12:118A, 1999.

Kato DT, Ferry JA, Goodman A, et al. Uterine papillary serous carcinoma (UPSC): a clinicopathologic study of 30 cases. Gynecol Oncol 59:384–389, 1995.

King SA, Adas AA, LiVolsi VA, et al. Expression and mutation analysis of the p53 gene in uterine papillary serous carcinoma. Cancer 75:2700–2705, 1995.

Lee KR, Belinson JL. Recurrence in noninvasive endometrial carcinoma: relationship to uterine papillary serous carcinoma. Am J Surg Pathol 15:965–973, 1991.

Prat J, Oliva E, Lerma E, et al. Uterine papillary serous adenocarcinoma: a 10-case study of p53 and c-erbB-2 expression and DNA content. Cancer 74:1778–1783, 1994.

Sasano H, Comerford J, Wilkinson DS, et al. Serous papillary adenocarcinoma of the endometrium: analysis of proto-oncogene amplification, flow cytometry, estrogen and progesterone receptors, and immunohistochemistry. Cancer 65:1545–1551, 1990.

Sherman ME, Bitterman P, Rosenshein NB, et al. Uterine serous carcinoma: a morphologically diverse neoplasm with unifying clinicopathologic features. Am J Surg Pathol 16:600–610, 1992.

Silva EG, Jenkins R. Serous carcinoma in endometrial polyps. Mod Pathol 3:120–128, 1990.

Spiegel GW. Endometrial carcinoma in situ in postmenopausal women. Am J Surg Pathol 19:417–432, 1995.

Warren CD, Horak S, Isacson C, et al. Extrauterine serous tumors in minimally invasive USC are metastatic [Abstract]. Mod Pathol 11:116A, 1998.

Williams KE, Waters ED, Woolas RP, et al. Mixed serous-endometrioid carcinoma of the uterus: pathologic and cytopathologic analysis of a high-risk endometrial carcinoma. Int J Gynecol Cancer 4:7–18, 1994.

Zheng W, Khurana R, Farahmand S, et al. p53 immunostaining as a significant adjunct test for uterine surface carcinoma: precursor of uterine papillary serous carcinoma. Am J Surg Pathol 22:1463–1473, 1998.

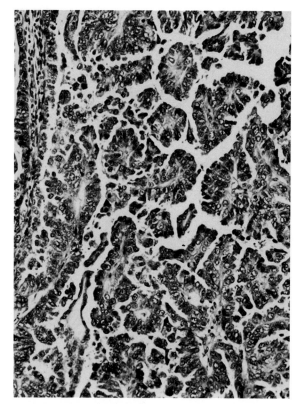

Figure 8–26. Serous papillary adenocarcinoma.

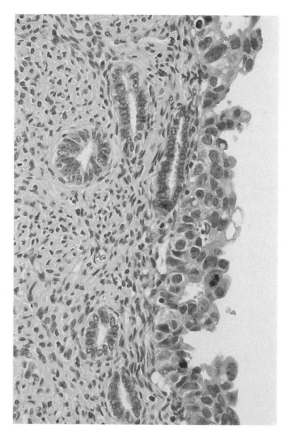

Figure 8–28. Serous carcinoma lining the endometrial surface (endometrial intraepithelial carcinoma or noninvasive serous carcinoma). This focus was found in otherwise atrophic endometrium adjacent to a typical serous papillary carcinoma.

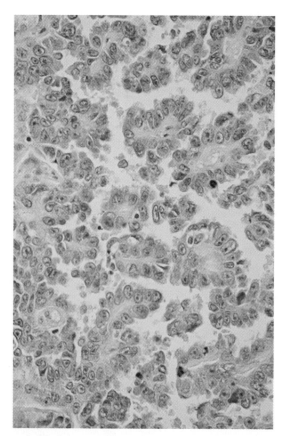

Figure 8–27. Serous papillary adenocarcinoma. Notice the cellular buds and high-grade nuclear features.

Clear Cell Adenocarcinoma

Clinical Features

- Clear cell adenocarcinomas (CCAs), which account for 1% to 6.6% of endometrial carcinomas, occur in women with a mean age of about 65 years. The presenting features are similar to those of women with endometrioid endometrial carcinoma. Thirty percent of cases are surgicopathologic stage II or higher.
- A history of pelvic irradiation was present in 16% of cases in one study. There has been no association with in utero exposure to diethylstilbestrol, but an association with the use of tamoxifen or synthetic progestins was found in one study.

Pathologic Features

- There are no characteristics gross features. CCAs are occasionally confined to an endometrial polyp.
- CCAs are characterized by tubulocystic, papillary, or solid patterns (alone or in combination) and one or more of four cell types: polygonal cells with abundant, clear, glycogen-rich cytoplasm and generally eccentric nuclei, hobnail cells, polygonal cells with oxyphilic cytoplasm, and flattened cells. The nuclei features are typically grade 2 or 3.
- Intraluminal mucin is typical. Eosinophilic hyaline mucin droplets in intracytoplasmic vacuoles (signet-ring–like or targetoid cells) are present focally in up to one-half of the cases.
- Stromal hyalinization and deposition of basement membrane material, especially within the cores of the papillae, may be prominent. Psammoma bodies are present in about 10% of the cases, usually in association with a papillary pattern. A stromal lymphoplasmacytic infiltrate is common.
- Myometrial invasion occurs in about 80% of cases. Lymphovascular space invasion is present in about 25% of cases.

Differential Diagnosis

- Serous papillary carcinoma (page 166).
- Secretory carcinomas (page 161). Features indicating a secretory carcinoma include a purely or predominantly glandular pattern, columnar cells with subnuclear vacuoles, and low-grade nuclear features.
- Rare, glycogen-rich endometrioid carcinomas. The distinctive patterns and the hobnail cells of CCCs are absent.

Behavior and Prognostic Features

- The 5-year survival rates (5YSR) have ranged from 34% to 75% (all stages). The stage is the most important prognostic parameter. The 5YSR of pathologic stage I tumors has ranged from 59% to 72%, a survival similar to that for grade III endometrioid carcinoma and significantly better than that for serous carcinomas. A preliminary GOG study, however, found only a 41% 5YS for stage I and occult stage II CCCs.
- Myometrial and lymphovascular space invasions have been adverse prognostic features in some studies. An admixture with endometrioid carcinoma was not prognostically significant in one study.
- The recurrent tumor was extrapelvic (including upper abdomen, liver, and lungs) in two thirds of cases with relapse in one study.

References

Abeler VM, Kjorstad KE. Clear cell carcinoma of the endometrium: a histopathological and clinical study of 97 cases. Gynecol Oncol 40:207–217, 1991.

Abeler VM, Vergote IB, Kjorstad KE, Trope CG. Clear cell carcinoma of the endometrium: prognosis and metastatic pattern. Cancer 78:1740–1707, 1996.

Carcangiu ML, Chambers JT. Early pathologic stage clear cell carcinoma and uterine papillary serous carcinoma of the endometrium: comparison of clinicopathologic features and survival. Int J Gynecol Pathol 14:30–38, 1995.

Chew S-H, Zaino RJ, Lax SP, et al. Carcinoma of the endometrium with clear cells: two distinct subtypes with differing prognosis [Abstract]. Mod Pathol 12:114A, 1999.

Christopherson WM, Alberhasky RC, Connelly PJ. Carcinoma of the endometrium: I. A clinicopathologic study of clear-cell carcinoma and secretory carcinoma. Cancer 49:1511–1523, 1982.

Dallenbach-Hellweg G, Hahn U. Mucinous and clear cell adenocarcinomas of the endometrium in patients receiving antiestrogens (tamoxifen) and gestagens. Int J Gynecol Pathol 14:7–15, 1995.

Kanbour-Shakir A, Tobon H. Primary clear cell carcinoma of the endometrium: a clinicopathologic study of 20 cases. Int J Gynecol Pathol 10:67–78, 1991.

Kurman RJ, Scully RE. Clear cell carcinoma of the endometrium: an analysis of 21 cases. Cancer 37:872–882, 1976.

Malpica A, Tornos C, Burke TW, Silva EG. Low-stage clear-cell carcinoma of the endometrium. Am J Surg Pathol 19:769–774, 1995.

Zaino RJ. Pathologic indicators of prognosis in endometrial adenocarcinoma. Selected aspects emphasizing the GOG experience. Pathol Annu 30(1):1–28, 1995.

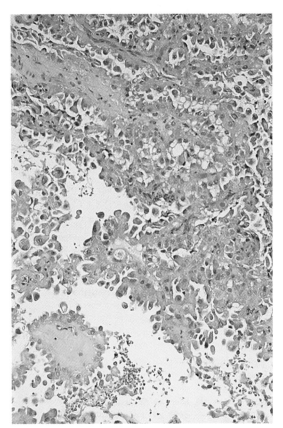

Figure 8–29. High-grade papillary clear cell adenocarcinoma of the endometrium. Notice the hyalinized stromal papilla (*bottom left*), clear cells, and hobnail cells.

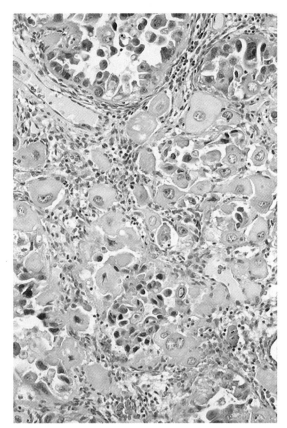

Figure 8–31. Oxyphilic clear cell carcinoma. Some typical hobnail cells are also present.

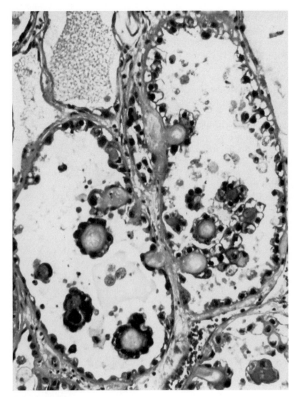

Figure 8–30. Clear cell carcinoma with tubulocystic pattern. Intracystic papillae have hyalinized cores.

Mucinous Adenocarcinoma

Clinical Features

- Mucinous tumors account for about 10% of pathologic stage I endometrial carcinomas. The tumors are almost invariably stage I.
- The age range in one study was 47 to 89 years (mean, 60.2 years). One study found an association with the use of tamoxifen or synthetic progestins.

Pathologic Features

- The cardinal feature is a predominant (>50%) component of endocervical-type tumor cells with mucin-rich cytoplasm. Mucinous metaplasia of nonneoplastic endometrium is present in some cases.
- The tumors are almost always well or moderately differentiated, with complex glandular, cribriform, villoglandular, and villous patterns or, rarely, with foci resembling microglandular hyperplasia. Cystically dilated, mucin-filled glands and neutrophils within the luminal mucin or within intracellular mucin-filled spaces are common.
- Focal epithelial stratification and loss of nuclear polarity are typical. Foci of moderate nuclear atypia are often admixed with areas of only mild atypia or even small foci of benign-appearing mucinous epithelium. Focal marked atypia is present in only a minority of cases. Mitotic figures are uncommon. Myometrial invasion occurs in about 50% of tumors.
- The neoplastic cells are typically immunoreactive for CEA and vimentin.
- A rare intestinal variant is characterized by goblet cells. Some of these tumors may also contain Paneth cells, argyrophilic enterochromaffin-like cells, argentaffin cells, and cells immunoreactive for chromogranin, serotonin, synaptophysin, neuron-specific enolase (NSE), gastrin, and somatostatin.

Behavior

- The posthysterectomy relapse rate is not significantly different from that of endometrioid carcinoma with minor mucinous differentiation or typical endometrioid carcinoma.

Differential Diagnosis

- Endometrioid carcinomas with minor foci of mucinous differentiation (page 155).

- Typical and atypical mucinous metaplasia. Distinguishing a complex mucinous metaplasia from a mucinous carcinoma may be difficult, especially in a biopsy or curettage specimen. Features favoring a carcinoma include abundant tissue, architectural complexity, epithelial stratification, loss of nuclear polarity, and moderate nuclear atypia, although the latter feature may be only focal.
- Endocervical mucinous adenocarcinoma. Colposcopy, hysteroscopy, and examination of both specimens from a fractional curettage with close attention to the nature of any nonneoplastic glands and stroma contiguous to the carcinoma establish the diagnosis in most cases. A CEA-positive, vimentin-positive immunoprofile favors an endometrial origin, whereas a CEA-positive vimentin-negative profile favors an endocervival origin.
- Microglandular hyperplasia (versus mucinous carcinomas with microglandular patterns). Features favoring or establishing a diagnosis of carcinoma include postmenopausal age, more than moderate degrees of nuclear atypia, merging of microglandular patterns with typical mucinous carcinoma, and immunoreactivity for CEA.

References

Czernobilsky B, Katz Z, Lancet M, Gaton E. Endocervical-type epithelium in endometrial carcinoma: a report of 10 cases with emphasis on histochemical methods for differential diagnosis. Am J Surg Pathol 4: 481–489, 1980.

Dallenbach-Hellweg G, Hahn U. Mucinous and clear cell adenocarcinomas of the endometrium in patients receiving antiestrogens (tamoxifen) and gestagens. Int J Gynecol Pathol 14:7–15, 1995.

Mannion CM, Branton PA, Tavassoli FA. Microglandular variant of endometrial carcinoma: light microscopic and immunohistochemical evaluation [Abstract]. Mod Pathol 11:109A, 1998.

Melham MF, Tobon H. Mucinous adenocarcinoma of the endometrium: a clinico-pathological review of 18 cases. Int J Gynecol Pathol 6: 347–355, 1987.

Ross JC, Eifel PJ, Cox RS, et al. Primary mucinous adenocarcinoma of the endometrium: a clinicopathologic and histochemical study. Am J Surg Pathol 7:715–729, 1983.

Young RH, Scully RE. Uterine carcinomas simulating microglandular hyperplasia: a report of six cases. Am J Surg Pathol 16:1092–1097, 1992.

Zheng W, Yang GCH, Godwin TA, et al. Mucinous adenocarcinoma of the endometrium with intestinal differentiation: a case report. Hum Pathol 26:1385–1388, 1995.

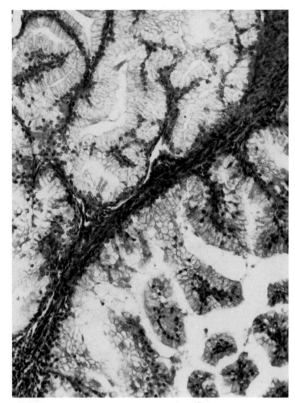

Figure 8–32. Well-differentiated mucinous adenocarcinoma. Notice the villoglandular pattern. The tumor is invading the myometrium.

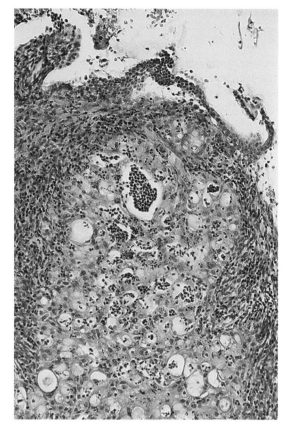

Figure 8–34. Mucinous adenocarcinoma of the endometrium with a focal microglandular pattern.

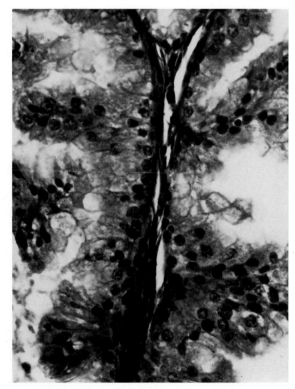

Figure 8–33. Well-differentiated mucinous adenocarcinoma (higher-power view of the tumor seen in Figure 8–32). Notice the cellular stratification and nuclear atypia.

Squamous Cell Carcinoma

Clinical Features

- Squamous cell carcinomas (SCCs), which account for about 0.5% of endometrial carcinomas, occur in patients 47 to 85 years old (mean, 67 years). The tumors are stage III or IV in one third of cases.
- Predisposing factors in some cases include cervical stenosis, pyometra, uterine prolapse, extensive endometrial squamous metaplasia, and a history of pelvic irradiation.
- The survival is 80% with stage I tumors, 20% with stage II tumors, and 0% with stage IV tumors.

Pathologic Features

- SCCs may resemble endometrioid carcinomas on gross examination, although occasionally they appear white and may have a condylomatous appearance.
- Criteria for diagnosis include an absence of a coexisting adenocarcinoma, a lack of contiguity between the tumor and the cervical squamous epithelium, and an absence of a concurrent or preexisting invasive cervical squamous cell carcinoma. If an in situ cervical squamous carcinoma exists, there must be no connection between it and the endometrial carcinoma.
- Most SCCs are obviously malignant on histologic examination, but rare, typical verrucous carcinomas of the endometrium have been reported. Some nonverrucous SCCs are extremely well differentiated. In such cases, a curettage may yield only fragments of almost-normal-appearing, glycogenated squamous epithelium devoid of cellular atypia.

References

Goodman A, Zukerberg LR, Rice LW, et al. Squamous cell carcinoma of the endometrium: a report of eight cases and a review of the literature. Gynecol Oncol 61:54–60, 1996.

Dalyrymple JC, Russell P. Squamous endometrial neoplasia—are Fluhmann's postulates still relevant? Int J Gynecol Cancer 5:421–425, 1995.

Hussain SF. Verrucous carcinoma of the endometrium. APMIS 96:1075–1078, 1988.

Ryder DE. Verrucous carcinoma of the endometrium—a unique neoplasm with a long survival. Obstet Gynecol 59:78S–80S, 1982.

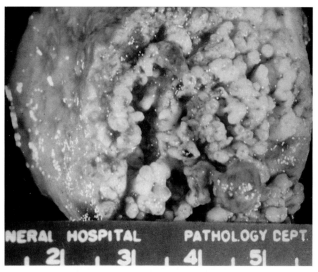

Figure 8–35. Squamous cell carcinoma of the endometrium.

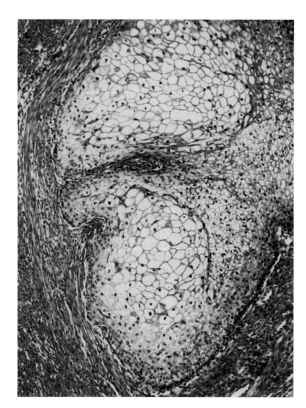

Figure 8–36. Highly differentiated endometrial squamous cell carcinoma invading the myometrium. The tumor cells have glycogenated cytoplasm and an essentially benign appearance.

Transitional Cell Carcinoma

- Ten endometrial transitional cell carcinomas (TCCs) have been reported in patients between the ages of 41 and 83 (mean, 63.9 years), who usually presented with abnormal uterine bleeding.
- The tumors were polypoid, resembled grade 2 to 3 papillary TCCs of the urinary tract, and infiltrated the myometrium to various degrees. The TCCs were almost always admixed with other types of endometrial carcinoma, including endometrioid, squamous, serous, sarcomatoid, or poorly differentiated. The proportion of the tumor that was TCC varied from 5% to 95%.
- The immunoreactivity of the tumors (mostly cytokeratin 7 positive and cytokeratin 20 negative, less commonly cytokeratin 7 and 20 negative) suggest a müllerian rather than a urothelial phenotype. Two of eight tumors were human papillomavirus type 16 positive.
- In three cases, the tumors were stage III because of spread to the ovary or paraovarian area. Foci of TCC were present in the mucosa of both fallopian tubes in one of the cases.
- Of seven patients with follow-up, five were alive with no evidence of tumor at intervals of 0.3 to 8.2 years; one was alive with recurrence at 1 year; and one died of other causes at 12.9 years.

References

Chen KTK. Extraovarian transitional cell carcinoma of female genital tract [Letter]. Am J Clin Pathol 94:670–671, 1990.

Lininger RA, Ashfag R, Albores-Saavedra J, Tavassoli FA. Transitional cell carcinoma of the endometrium and endometrial carcinoma with transitional cell differentiation. Cancer 79:1933–1943, 1997.

Lininger RA, Wistuba I, Gazdar A, et al. Human papillomavirus type 16 is detected in transitional cell carcinomas and squamotransitional cell carcinomas of the cervix and endometrium. Cancer 83:521–527, 1998.

Spiegel GW, Austin RM, Gelven PL. Transitional cell carcinoma of the endometrium. Gynecol Oncol 60:325–330, 1996.

Hepatoid Carcinoma

- The two patients described with hepatoid carcinoma were in their seventh decade and presented with vaginal bleeding and an elevated serum alpha-fetoprotein (AFP) level. The tumors were fatal for both patients.
- Both tumors were microscopically similar to hepatocellular carcinoma, including AFP immunoreactivity. One tumor contained an admixed component of typical endometrioid carcinoma.

References

Hoshida Y, Nagakawa T, Mano S, et al. Hepatoid adenocarcinoma of the endometrium associated with alpha-fetoprotein production. Int J Gynecol Pathol 15:266–269, 1996.

Yamamoto R, Ishikura H, Azuma M, et al. Alpha-fetoprotein production by a hepatoid adenocarcinoma of the uterus. J Clin Pathol 49:420–422, 1996.

Lymphoepithelioma-like Carcinoma

- Two endometrial lymphoepithelioma-like carcinomas have been described in postmenopausal women. One

patient with stage IVb disease was treated with chemotherapy and was alive with no evidence of tumor 9 months later. The other patient with stage IIIc disease received irradiation and chemotherapy and died of disease 1 year after diagnosis.
- Both tumors resembled lymphoepithelioma-like carcinomas in other sites. There was no evidence of Epstein-Barr virus in either tumor.

Reference

Vargas MP, Merino MJ. Lymphoepitheliomalike carcinoma: an unusual variant of endometrial cancer. A report of two cases. Int J Gynecol Pathol 17:272–276, 1998.

Undifferentiated Carcinoma

- The term undifferentiated carcinoma (UC) is applied to endometrial carcinomas that are too poorly differentiated to be categorized as one of the other subtypes.
- UCs accounted for 1.6% of endometrial carcinomas in a study by Abeler and coworkers. About 50% of the tumors were of the large cell type, and the remainder were of the intermediate or small cell type. The patients were 45 to 86 years old (mean, 63.9 years).

Large Cell Undifferentiated Carcinoma

- One third of the large cell undifferentiated carcinomas in the Abeler study were surgical stage III or IV. Seventy-eight percent of the tumors invaded the outer half of the myometrium, and 62% invaded lymphatics or blood vessels.
- All of the tumors were immunoreactive for cytokeratin and less frequently vimentin (64%), CEA (18%), and NSE (36%).
- The 5- and 10-year survival rates were 54% and 39%, respectively.

Small Cell Undifferentiated Carcinoma

- Endometrial small cell undifferentiated carcinomas (SCUCs), which are much less common that those of cervical origin, occur in patients 30 to 78 years old (mean, 60 years).
- About two thirds of the patients are stage II to IV (i.e., spread to cervix, adnexa, pelvic lymph nodes, vagina, or peritoneum). A similar proportion of patients were dead of disease or alive with disease on follow-up.
- Microscopic examination reveals sheets, cords, nests, and rosettes of small or intermediate-sized cells with scanty cytoplasm, hyperchromatic nuclei, and a high mitotic rate. Single cell and zonal necrosis and myometrial and vascular invasion are present in most cases.
- An admixed endometrial endometrioid carcinoma with or without squamous differentiation is present in about 50% of the cases. Rare malignant müllerian mixed tumors have contained a component of SCUC.
- Neuroendocrine differentiation has been found with special techniques in most tumors, including immunoreactivity for one or more neuroendocrine markers (i.e.,

NSE, chromogranin, Leu-7, synaptophysin, bombesin, insulin, calcitonin, or glucagon) and dense core granules on ultrastructural examination.

Differential Diagnosis

- Endometrioid carcinomas with argyrophil cells (page 165).
  - Secondary endometrial involvement by small cell carcinomas of the cervix. An obvious mass found on clinical examination and the distribution of tumor in a fractional curettage specimen facilitate the diagnosis in most cases. A synchronous cervical adenocarcinoma or squamous cell carcinoma or an endometrial adenocarcinoma may provide additional evidence for an origin of the small cell carcinoma within the cervix or endometrium, respectively.
- Malignant lymphomas and leukemias. Routine light microscopic findings are usually diagnostic, and the histo-chemical, immunohistochemical, and ultrastructural findings facilitate the diagnosis in problem cases.
- Primitive neuroectodermal tumors (see Chapter 10). These tumors are characterized by true rosettes and Homer-Wright and perivascular pseudorosettes; glial, ependymal, and medulloepithelial differentiation; and immunoreactivity for glial fibrillary acidic protein.

References

Abeler VM, Kjorstad KE, Nesland JM. Undifferentiated carcinoma of the endometrium: a histopathologic and clinical study of 31 cases. Cancer 68:98–105, 1991.

Huntsman DG, Clement PB, Gilks CG, Scully RE. Small cell carcinoma of the endometrium: a clinicopathologic analysis of sixteen cases. Am J Surg Pathol 18:376–390, 1994.

van Hoeven KH, Hudock JA, Woodruff JM, Sutherland MJ. Small cell neuroendocrine carcinoma of the endometrium. Int J Gynecol Pathol 14:21–29, 1995.

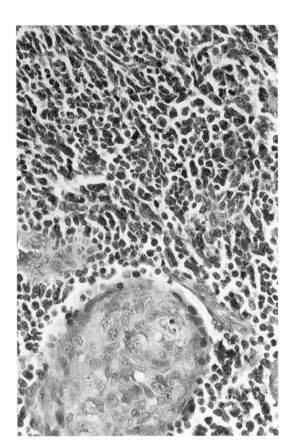

Figure 8–37. Undifferentiated small cell carcinoma of the endometrium. A focus of squamous cell carcinoma is also seen; the small cell carcinoma was admixed with an endometrioid adenocarcinoma with squamous differentiation.

Mixed Carcinomas

- Mixed carcinomas consist of two or more subtypes in which each component accounts for at least 10% of the tumor. The proportion of each subtype should be specified in the pathology report, because this information may have prognostic and therapeutic importance.
- In our experience, the most common admixtures are endometrioid-serous, serous-clear cell, endometrioid-mucinous, and transitional-squamous types.

CHAPTER 9

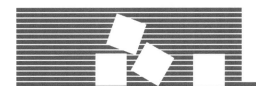

Mesenchymal and Mixed Epithelial-Mesenchymal Tumors of the Uterine Corpus and Cervix

SMOOTH MUSCLE TUMORS

Leiomyomas

Usual-Type Leiomyoma

Clinical Features

- Leiomyomas are the most common uterine tumor, occurring in up to 75% of hysterectomy specimens, but the tumors are symptomatic in only about one third of cases. The tumors are most common in the fourth and fifth decades. Postmenopausal regression occurs in some cases.
- The clinical manifestations are related to their number, size, and location and typically include pelvic pain, abnormal vaginal bleeding, and uterine enlargement. Pedunculated submucosal tumors may appear at the external os. Large tumors may produce pressure symptoms on adjacent pelvic organs (e.g., bowel, bladder) or complicate pregnancy or delivery.

Typical Gross Features

- Leiomyomas are multiple in 65% to 80% of cases. They are typically confined to the corpus; fewer than 2% of uteri harbor cervical leiomyomas. The tumors are typically round, well-circumscribed, nonencapsulated myometrial masses (that can be enucleated) with white, whorled, bulging, solid sectioned surfaces. Infarction (see below) may impart a brown color. Leiomyomas may be intramural, submucosal, or subserosal.
- Submucosal tumors are contiguous with or close to the endometrium, which may be compressed. They may be nonpolypoid or polypoid; the latter may be sessile or pedunculated. Pedunculated tumors occasionally prolapse through the cervical os. Ulcerative necrosis is found in some submucosal tumors (page 178).

- Subserosal leiomyomas are contiguous with or close to the serosa. They are occasionally pedunculated; torsion of the pedicle of subserosal or submucosal tumors may lead to hemorrhagic infarction. Rarely, hemoperitoneum may occur after rupture of distended veins on the surface of the leiomyoma. Loss of attachment to the uterus in some cases can result in a "parasitic leiomyoma" (page 191).

Typical Microscopic Features

- Elongated spindle cells with scanty eosinophilic cytoplasm and central, pale, fusiform nuclei form intersecting fascicles. Rarely, nuclear palisading is a prominent feature (i.e., schwannoma-like leiomyoma).
- The smooth muscle cells are separated by variable amounts of collagen, which typically increases with age. Leiomyomas may be richly vascular with numerous vessels, including large muscular arteries, arterioles, and veins.
- There is a sharp border with the surrounding myometrium in most cases, but occasionally there is limited focal extension of the tumor into the contiguous myometrium. The latter is a much more common finding in highly cellular leiomyomas (page 181).

Degenerative Changes

- These features can alter the gross appearance of the leiomyoma to the extent that it can resemble that of leiomyosarcoma; when a leiomyosarcoma is present in a myomatous uterus, it is almost always the largest mass. Sections should be taken from any leiomyoma exhibiting other than the usual gross appearance and from the largest tumor if multiple tumors are present.
- Focal necrosis may be found in some tumors and may be of two types.

- Infarct-type necrosis (referred to by Bell and colleagues as "hyaline" necrosis) is characterized by a zone of granulation or fibrous tissue separating the necrotic areas from the viable areas, a mummified appearance of the necrotic smooth muscle cells and blood vessels, and areas of hemorrhage. It should be distinguished from tumor cell necrosis, which commonly occurs in leiomyosarcomas (page 183).
- Ulcerative necrosis typically involves the ulcerated surface of submucosal leiomyomas and is characterized by numerous inflammatory cells surrounding necrotic foci that contain necrotic debris more often than ghost outlines of dead cells.

■ Hyaline change is common and appears as homogenization of the collagen within the leiomyoma. The hyalinization occasionally replaces large portions of the neoplasm, obscuring its smooth muscle nature.

■ Hydropic degeneration (i.e., accumulation of edema fluid), which often accompanies hyaline degeneration, may progress to cystification. Perinodular hydropic degeneration in which nodules of nonhydropic tumor are surrounded by hydropic connective tissue may mimic intravenous leiomyomatosis (page 188) grossly and microscopically. The nodules, however, are not within vascular spaces as in intravenous leiomyomatosis.

■ Myxoid degeneration, sometimes seen during pregnancy, may result in a grossly gelatinous appearance. Stellate tumor cells are separated by an accumulation of abundant weakly basophilic, alcianophilic material. A well-circumscribed border distinguishes a myxoid leiomyoma from myxoid leiomyosarcoma (page 183), a distinction not usually possible in a curettage specimen.

■ Dystrophic calcification may be extensive, particular in postmenopausal women, and be visible radiologically.

Hormonal and Pregnancy-Related Changes

■ "Red degeneration," which typically occurs in pregnant women or less commonly in those on oral contraceptives, results in a beefy red appearance. Red degeneration probably results from various degrees of infarction and hemorrhage with subsequent hemolysis.

■ Although some studies have found no significant difference in gonadotropin-releasing hormone–treated leiomyomas compared with those from control patients, changes have been described in other studies:
- Irregular borders, focal hypercellularity, focal hyalinization, hyaline necrosis, massive lymphoid infiltrates, and vascular changes (e.g., decreased vessel number, decreased vessel caliber, mural smooth muscle proliferation, myxoid change, fibrinoid degeneration)
- Decreased cellular proliferation index (by proliferating cell nuclear antigen test) and a decrease in estrogen and progesterone receptors

■ Hemorrhagic cellular ("apoplectic") leiomyomas are typically associated with oral contraceptive use or pregnancy.
- Acute abdominal signs may occur from rupture of the tumor into the peritoneal cavity. Hemorrhage is usually seen grossly within one or more leiomyomas.
- Microscopic examination reveals densely cellular proliferations of bland, occasionally mitotically active smooth muscle cells surrounding stellate zones of recent hemorrhage. Vascular alterations in the leiomyomas and the surrounding myometrium may include intimal myxoid change and fibrosis, medial hypertrophy, fibrinoid necrosis, and thrombosis.

Heterologous Elements

■ Heterologous elements within otherwise typical leiomyomas have included fat (i.e., lipoleiomyomas), bone, cartilage, skeletal muscle cells, and tubules lined by mesothelial cells; all except the first are rare.

■ Prominent inflammatory cell infiltrates within otherwise typical leiomyomas have consisted of histiocytes, mast cells, eosinophils, neutrophils (i.e., pyomyomas, a result of bacterial infection within a leiomyoma), and mixed, often dense infiltrates of variably sized lymphocytes and plasma cells.

■ In leiomyomas with dense lymphoid infiltrates, the polymorhism of the lymphoid infiltrate, the presence of occasional germinal centers, and confinement of the infiltrate to the leiomyoma facilitate distinction from lymphoma.

References

Clement PB, Young RH, Scully RE. Diffuse, perinodular, and other patterns of hydropic degeneration within and adjacent to uterine leiomyomas: problems in differential diagnosis. Am J Surg Pathol 16:26–32, 1992.

Colgan TJ, Pendergast S, LeBlanc M. The histopathology of uterine leiomyomas following treatment with gonadotropin releasing hormone analogues. Hum Pathol 24:1073–1077, 1993.

Demopoulos RI, Jones KY, Mittal KR, Vamvakas EC. Histology of leiomyomata in patients treated with leuprolide acetate. Int J Gynecol Pathol 16:131–137, 1997.

Ferry JA, Harris NL, Scully RE. Uterine leiomyomas with lymphoid infiltration simulating lymphoma: a report of seven cases. Int J Gynecol Pathol 8:263–270, 1989.

Fornelli A, Pasquinelli G, Eusebi V. Leiomyoma of the uterus showing skeletal muscle differentiation: a case report. Hum Pathol 30:356–358, 1999.

Hart WR. Problematic uterine smooth muscle neoplasms [Letter]. Am J Surg Pathol 21:252, 1997.

Kalir T, Goldstein M, Dottino P, et al. Morphometric and electron-microscopic analyses on the effects of gonadotropin-releasing hormone agonists on uterine leiomyomas. Arch Pathol Lab Med 122:442–446, 1998.

Mazur MT, Kraus FT. Histogenesis of morphologic variations in tumors of the uterine wall. Am J Surg Pathol 4:59–74, 1980.

Myles JL, Hart WR. Apoplectic leiomyomas of the uterus: a clinicopathologic study of five distinctive hemorrhagic leiomyomas associated with oral contraceptive usage. Am J Surg Pathol 9:798–805, 1985.

Norris HJ, Hilliard GD, Irey NS. Hemorrhagic cellular leiomyomas ("apoplectic leiomyoma") of the uterus associated with pregnancy and oral contraceptives. Int J Gynecol Pathol 7:212–224, 1988.

Scully RE. Pathology of leiomyomas. Semin Reprod Endocrinol 10:325–331, 1992.

Sreenan JJ, Prayson RA, Biscotti CV, et al. Histopathologic findings in 107 uterine leiomyomas treated with leuprolide acetate compared with 126 controls. Am J Surg Pathol 20:427–432, 1996.

Tiltman AJ. Leiomyomas of the uterine cervix: a study of frequency. Int J Gynecol Pathol 17:231–234, 1998.

Vu K, Greenspan DL, Wu T-C, et al. Cellular proliferation, estrogen receptor, progesterone receptor, and bcl-2 expression in GnRH agonist-treated uterine leiomyomas. Hum Pathol 29:359–363, 1998.

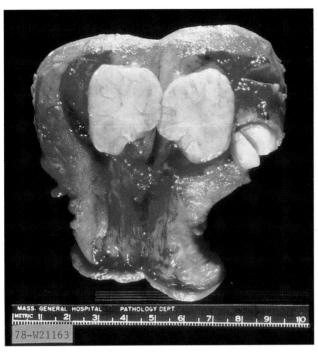

Figure 9–1. Uterus with two leiomyomas; both have been bisected. The larger tumor is submucosal, and the smaller one is mural.

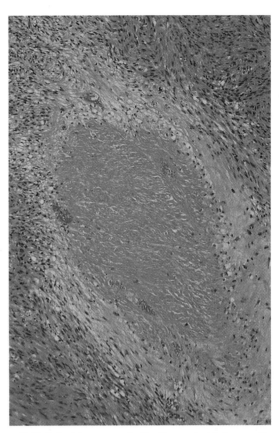

Figure 9–3. Infarct-type necrosis (hyaline necrosis) in an otherwise typical leiomyoma. Notice the hyalinized fibrous tissue separating the zone of necrosis from the viable tumor.

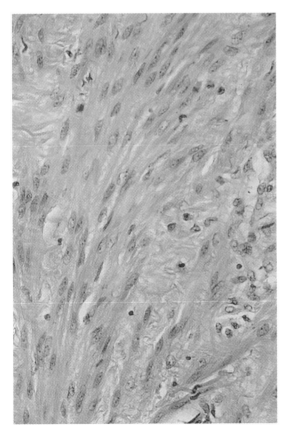

Figure 9–2. Typical leiomyoma.

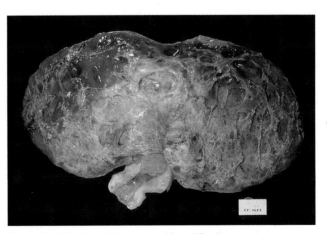

Figure 9–4. Hydropic leiomyoma with cystification.

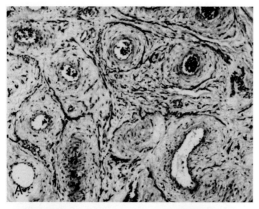

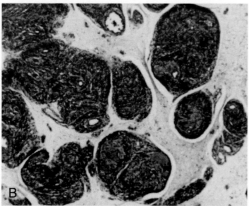

Figure 9–5. Hydropic leiomyoma. *A,* Most of the smooth muscle cells are replaced by hydropic fibrous tissue, with only cords of residual smooth muscle cells and thick-walled blood vessels remaining. *B,* Perinodular hydropic degeneration. Nodules of cellular nonhydropic smooth muscle are separated by hydropic fibrous tissue, and there is some retraction artifact around the nodules.

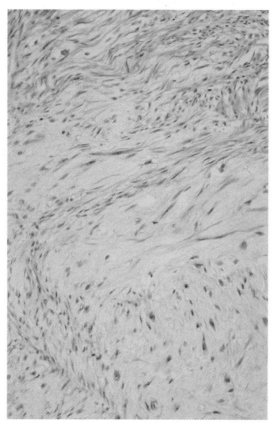

Figure 9–6. Myxoid change in an otherwise typical leiomyoma.

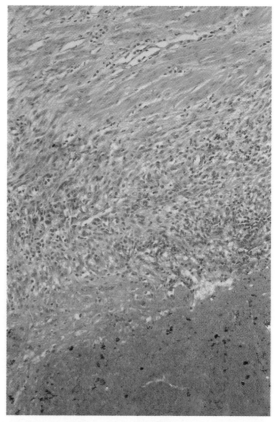

Figure 9–7. Apoplectic leiomyoma. Notice the hypercellular zone of smooth muscle around an area of hemorrhage.

Cellular Leiomyoma and Highly Cellular Leiomyoma

- Cellular leiomyomas (CLs) and highly cellular leiomyomas (HCLs) grossly may resemble typical leiomyomas but sometimes have a more fleshy, soft, tan-brown sectioned surface, with hemorrhage, necrosis, or both in some cases.
- CLs are defined as leiomyomas that are "significantly" more cellular than the normal myometrium but that are otherwise typical (i.e., devoid of nuclear atypia, a mitotic rate of 4 or fewer mitotic figures [MF] per 10 high-power-fields [HPF], and no tumor cell necrosis).
- HCLs are characterized by a cellularity similar to that of endometrial stromal tumors and may be misdiag-

nosed as an endometrial stromal nodule when well-circumscribed or a low-grade endometrial stromal sarcoma when poorly circumscribed.
- HCLs are distinguished from an endometrial stromal tumor by a fascicular growth pattern, blood vessels with thick muscular walls, fusiform nuclei, cleftlike spaces, focal merging with the adjacent myometrium, and desmin immunoreactivity.

References

Oliva E, Young RH, Clement PB, et al. Cellular benign mesenchymal tumors of the uterus: a comparative morphologic and immunohistochemical analysis of 33 highly cellular leiomyomas and seven endometrial stromal nodules, two frequently confused tumors. Am J Surg Pathol 19:757–768, 1995.

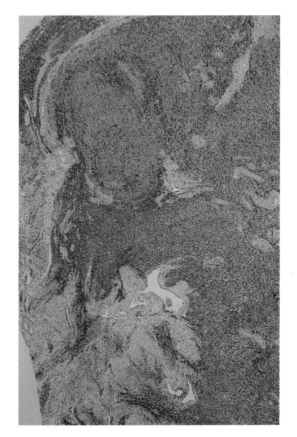

Figure 9–8. Highly cellular leiomyoma. The tumor has irregular borders and thick-walled blood vessels.

Leiomyoma with Bizarre Nuclei

- The gross appearance of leiomyomas with bizarre nuclei (i.e., symplastic leiomyomas) usually resembles that of typical leiomyomas, but yellow to tan areas, softening, cysts, or myxoid change are seen in a minority of cases.
- The cardinal microscopic feature is the presence of large cells with eosinophilic cytoplasm and bizarrely shaped, multilobated or multinucleated, hyperchromatic, often "smudged" nuclei but an absence of other worrisome histological features.
- The foci of cells with bizarre nuclei may be unifocal but are more commonly multifocal or diffusely distributed on a background of an otherwise typical leiomyoma.
- Mitotic activity is low compared with that of leiomyosarcomas. Downes and Hart found 0 to 7 MF per 10 HPF (mean, 1.6) using the highest count method and 0 to 2.8 MF per 10 HPF (mean, 0.8) using the average count method. Degenerating or karyorrhectic nuclei may be mistaken for typical or atypical mitotic figures.
- They can be distinguished from leiomyosarcomas by an absence of tumor cell necrosis and a usual paucity of mitotic figures. The combination of aneuploidy and high MIB-1 activity strongly favors a diagnosis of leiomyosarcoma.

References

Downes KA, Hart WR. Uterine bizarre ("symplastic") leiomyomas: morphology and behavior. Am J Surg Pathol 21:1261–1270, 1997.

Downes KA, Hart WR. Bizarre uterine leiomyomas: Ki-67 activity and DNA ploidy [Abstract]. Mod Pathol 12:116A, 1999.

Mitotically Active Leiomyoma

- Mitotically active leiomyomas (MALs) are otherwise typical or cellular leiomyomas with more than 4 but less than 20 MF per 10 HPF; most have mitotic counts between 5 and 9 MF per 10 HPF. Otherwise similar tumors with 20 or more MF per 10 HPF are referred to by Bell and colleagues as "leiomyomas with increased mitotic index but experience limited."
- The cellularity is variable, and nuclear atypia is absent or mild. Infarct-type necrosis may be present.
- MALs are frequently submucosal and often associated with the secretory phase of the menstrual cycle, pregnancy, or the use of exogenous hormones.
- Distinguish from leiomyosarcoma by the absence of both diffuse moderate to marked atypia and tumor cell necrosis. The differential also includes leiomyomas with focal mitotic activity around foci of ulcerative necrosis (page 178) and areas of hemorrhage (apoplectic leiomyomas, page 178).

References

Bell SW, Kempson RL, Hendrickson MR. Problematic uterine smooth muscle neoplasms: a clinicopathologic study of 213 cases. Am J Surg Pathol 18:535–558, 1994.

O'Connor DM, Norris HJ. Mitotically active leiomyomas of the uterus. Hum Pathol 21:223–227, 1990.

Perrone T, Dehner LP. Prognostically favorable "mitotically active" smooth-muscle tumors of the uterus: a clinicopathologic study of 10 cases. Am J Surg Pathol 12:1–8, 1988.

Prayson RA, Hart WR. Mitotically active leiomyomas of the uterus. Am J Clin Pathol 97:14–20, 1992.

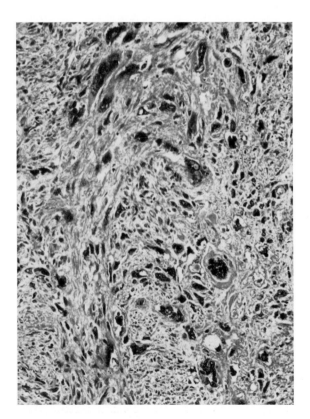

Figure 9–9. Leiomyoma with bizarre nuclei.

Leiomyosarcoma

Clinical Features

- Leiomyosarcomas (LMSs) account for about 45% of uterine sarcomas or for more than 80% of uterine sarcomas if, as they should be, malignant müllerian mixed tumors are excluded from the category of uterine sarcomas.
- Affected patients are in the third to ninth decade of life. Most are older than 40 years of age. The clinical presentation is usually abnormal vaginal bleeding, pain, and an enlarged uterus on pelvic examination. Extrauterine extension is found at presentation in one sixth to one half of the cases.

Gross Features

- LMSs are typically solitary but are frequently associated with leiomyomas in the uterus. In such cases, the LMS is almost always the largest mass. An origin from a leiomyoma can be demonstrated in rare cases.
- LMSs have a mean diameter of 10 cm. Two thirds are intramural, one fifth submucosal, and one tenth subserosal; fewer than 5% arise in the cervix.
- The borders of the tumors are typically less well circumscribed than leiomyomas and LMSs usually cannot be readily shelled out from the adjacent myometrium. The sectioned surface is typically bulging, soft, fleshy, and focally necrotic and hemorrhagic, without the whorled appearance characteristic of a leiomyoma.
- Myxoid LMSs are characterized by a gelatinous appearance and often a deceptively well-circumscribed border. Some tumors may extend into the broad ligament.

Typical Microscopic Features

- The typical features are hypercellularity of at least a moderate degree, diffuse moderate to marked nuclear atypia, a high mitotic rate (usually 10 MF or more per 10 HPF), and tumor cell necrosis.[1] According to Bell and associates, *any two of the latter three features* are sufficient to diagnose LMS.
- Tumor cell necrosis is characterized by an abrupt transition from viable cells to necrotic cells, ghost outlines of pleomorphic and hyperchromatic nuclei of the necrotic cells, and perivascular viable tumor cells.
- Other common LMS features include atypical mitotic figures, an infiltrative border, and in a few cases, vascular invasion.
- Immunoreactivity for smooth muscle markers (e.g., actin, smooth muscle actin, desmin) may facilitate the diagnosis, but these procedures are rarely necessary.

Uncommon Variants

- Epithelioid LMS (page 186).
- Myxoid LMSs are paucicellular tumors with neoplastic cells widely separated by a myxoid stroma.

- The neoplastic cells may be uniformly distributed, arranged in cords, or surround spaces filled with myxoid material.
- The oval to spindle to stellate tumor cells have scanty cytoplasm, usually only mild to moderate nuclear atypia, and a low mitotic rate (<2 MF per 10 HPF).
- Nonmyxoid areas, if present, may exhibit obvious smooth muscle differentiation and more overtly malignant features.
- Leiomyosarcoma with a prominent component of osteoclastic-type giant cells may resemble benign or malignant giant cell tumor of bone or a giant cell variant of malignant fibrous histiocytoma.
- Xanthomatous LMSs are characterized by a prominent component of large xanthomatous cells with abundant cytoplasm containing lipid vacuoles and multiple or multilobulated nuclei that are sometimes disposed in a wreathlike arrangement.

Behavior and Prognosis

- Survival rates in most series are 15% to 30%. The median survival has ranged from 13 to 43 months. Tumor-related deaths are usually related to distant metastases, frequently accompanied by local recurrence.
- A size of less than 5 cm is a favorable prognostic feature. Tumor size larger than 8 cm, vascular invasion, and infiltrating (versus pushing) margins were adverse prognostic factors in one study.
- Myxoid LMSs have a less predictable behavior, resulting in death in several to many years or long-term survival, even after discovery of a recurrence.

Differential Diagnosis

- Leiomyoma variants (discussed earlier) that exhibit some of the features of LMS, including cellular leiomyomas, mitotically active leiomyomas, and leiomyomas with bizarre nuclei, as well as leiomyomas with necrosis other than tumor cell necrosis. Myxoid leiomyomas are distinguished from myxoid LMS by a well-circumscribed border with the myometrium, a distinction that may not be possible in a curettage specimen.
- Benign smooth muscle tumors with unusual growth patterns (page 188).
- Smooth muscle tumors with atypical features but not diagnostic for LMS as categorized by Bell and colleagues include:
  - "Atypical leiomyoma with low risk of recurrence" (1 of 46 tumors was clinically malignant): diffuse, moderate to severe atypia; no tumor cell necrosis; and fewer than 10 MF per 10 HPF.
  - "Atypical leiomyoma but experience limited" (5 of 5 tumors were clinically benign): focal, moderate to severe atypia; fewer than 20 MF per 10 HPF; and no coagulative tumor cell necrosis.
  - "Smooth muscle tumor of low malignant potential" (1 of 4 tumors was clinically malignant): tumor cell necrosis; fewer than 10 MF per 10 HPF, and no or mild atypia.
- "Smooth muscle tumors of uncertain malignant poten-

---

[1]Bell and associates use the term *coagulative tumor cell necrosis,* but we prefer *tumor cell necrosis,* as suggested by Hart.

tial" are nonleiomyosarcomatous smooth muscle tumors with atypical features that do not belong in any of the previous categories.

References

Bell SW, Kempson RL, Hendrickson MR. Problematic uterine smooth muscle neoplasms: a clinicopathologic study of 213 cases. Am J Surg Pathol 18:535–558, 1994.

Burch DM, Tavassoli FA. Myxoid leiomyosarcoma of the uterus [Abstract]. Mod Pathol 11:101A, 1998.

Chen KTK. Leiomyosarcoma with osteoclast-like giant cells. Am J Surg Pathol 19:487–488, 1995.

Devaney K, Tavassoli FA Immunohistochemistry as a diagnostic aid in the interpretation of unusual mesenchymal tumors of the uterus. Mod Pathol 4:225–231, 1991.

Evans HL. Smooth muscle neoplasms of the uterus other than ordinary leiomyoma: a study of 46 cases, with emphasis on diagnostic criteria and prognostic factors. Cancer 62:2239–2247, 1988.

Hart WR. Problematic uterine smooth muscle neoplasms [Letter]. Am J Surg Pathol 21:252, 1997.

Jones MW, Norris HJ. Clinicopathologic study of 28 uterine leiomyosarcomas with metastasis. Int J Gynecol Pathol 14:243–249, 1995.

King ME, Dickersin GR, Scully RE Myxoid leiomyosarcoma of the uterus: a report of six cases. Am J Surg Pathol 6:589–598, 1982.

Major FI, Blessing JA, Silverberg SG, et al. Prognostic factors in early-stage uterine sarcoma: a Gynecologic Oncology Group Study. Cancer 71:1702–1709, 1993.

Marshall RJ, Braye SG, Jones DB. Leiomyosarcoma of the uterus with giant cells resembling osteoclasts. Int J Gynecol Pathol 5:260–268, 1986.

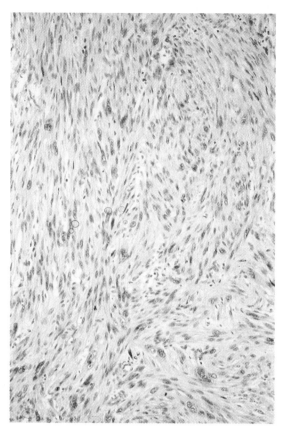

Figure 9–11. Leiomyosarcoma with diffuse, moderate to severe atypia. Mitotic figures were numerous but are not clearly visible at this magnification.

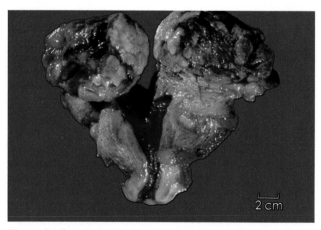

Figure 9–10. Leiomyosarcoma. The tumor is poorly circumscribed, with a fleshy sectioned surface that is focally necrotic and hemorrhagic.

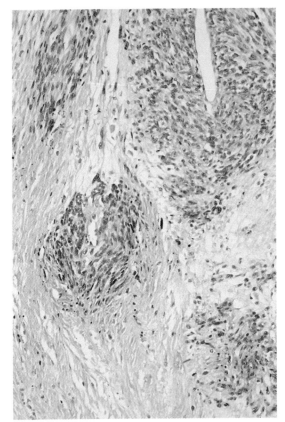

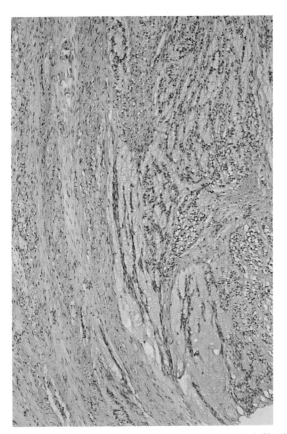

Figure 9–12. Leiomyosarcoma with tumor cell necrosis. Perivascular tumor directly abuts areas of necrosis with no interposed connective tissue. Necrotic debris exists within the areas of necrosis.

Figure 9–14. Myxoid leiomyosarcoma. The tumor has an infiltrative border with the myometrium.

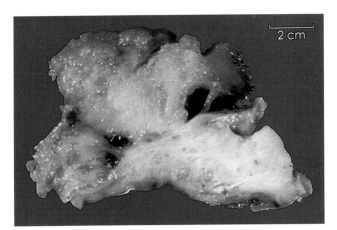

Figure 9–13. Myxoid leiomyosarcoma. The tumor has a gelatinous sectioned surface.

Epithelioid Smooth Muscle Tumors
General Features

- The designation "epithelioid smooth muscle tumor" refers to rare smooth muscle tumors composed predominantly or entirely of polygonal cells. The term *leiomyoblastoma* has also been used, but this designation incorrectly implies a tumor composed of primitive cells.
- The designation *epithelioid* should not be applied to smooth muscle tumors in which edema, hyalinization, or other changes cause cordlike or other epithelial-like appearances in the absence of the typical cellular features.
- The clinical presentation is similar to that of patients with typical leiomyomas.

Pathologic Features

- The tumors may grossly resemble typical leiomyomas, but some benign tumors and some epithelioid LMSs have worrisome gross features, including a fleshy appearance, a poorly circumscribed margin, and hemorrhage or necrosis. Occasional tumors arise in the cervix.
- The tumor cells are typically arranged in sheets, nests, or long cords that are sometimes disposed in a focal plexiform pattern. Tumors that are entirely plexiform and smaller than 1 cm in diameter (usually microscopic in size), so-called *plexiform tumorlets,* are frequently multiple and are more common in the myometrium but occasionally involve or are confined to the endometrium.
- The tumor cells are predominantly or exclusively round or polygonal with eosinophilic to clear cytoplasm (i.e., clear cell leiomyoma). Spindle-shaped smooth muscle cells are present in 50% of the tumors. In such cases, the epithelioid cells may be scattered throughout a leiomyoma or leiomyosarcoma composed predominantly of spindle cells.
- The nucleus is typically central and round with variable degrees of pleomorphism that tend to parallel malignant potential. Rare benign tumors, however, may have cells with bizarre nuclei similar to those in the usual leiomyoma with bizarre nuclei (page 182).
- Mitotic figures are rare (0 to 1 MF per 10 HPF) in benign tumors. In contrast, most epithelioid LMSs have at least 3 or 4 MF per 10 HPF but occasionally as few as 2 MF per 10 HPF.
- Stromal hyalinization is variable. In some tumors, particularly in plexiform tumors, the extent of stromal hyalinization may be striking.
- The tumors tend to be less well circumscribed than spindle cell smooth muscle tumors. Vascular invasion occurs with occasional benign tumors and with epithelioid LMSs.
- Epithelioid smooth muscle tumors are more frequently positive for cytokeratins and are less frequently positive for muscle markers, vimentin, and CD34 than typical smooth muscle tumors.

Behavior and Criteria for Epithelioid Leiomyosarcoma

- The proportion of tumors that are clinically malignant is higher than with spindle-cell smooth muscle tumors, ranging from 10% to 40% in the three largest series (predominantly consultation cases). In one study of metastasizing uterine LMSs (all histologic types included), 36% were the epithelioid type.
- No single microscopic feature is predictive of metastatic potential. Epithelioid LMSs typically have significant nuclear atypia (grade 2 or 3 nuclear features) and some mitotic activity (usually at least 3 or 4 MF per 10 HPF). Most also have tumor cell necrosis. Until more cases are reported, Prayson and colleagues tentatively regard tumors with grade 2 nuclear features but without increased mitotic activity or tumor cell necrosis as "epithelioid smooth muscle tumor, probably benign."
- Epithelioid LMSs may have a more protracted clinical course than typical LMSs. Patients may die of tumor, often after multiple recurrences, 5, 10, or more years after hysterectomy.

Differential Diagnosis

- Poorly differentiated or undifferentiated carcinomas or melanomas. Evidence of a mucosal origin (except metastatic carcinomas or melanomas), focal glandular or papillary differentiation, mucin production, and in melanomas, immunoreactivity for S-100 and HMB-45 facilitate the diagnosis. Epithelioid smooth muscle tumors may be immunoreactive for cytokeratin and lack immunoreactivity for smooth muscle markers.
- Placental site trophoblastic tumors (PSTTs). PSTTs may be associated with an elevated serum level of human chorionic gonadotropin (hCG) and typically exhibit a permeative growth pattern within the myometrium and replacement of blood vessel walls. They are immunoreactive for placental lactogen and hCG.
- Uterine tumors resembling ovarian sex cord tumors (page 206).

References

Jones MW, Norris HJ. Clinicopathologic study of 28 uterine leiomyosarcomas with metastasis. Int J Gynecol Pathol 14:243–249, 1995.

Kaminski PF, Tavassoli FA. Plexiform tumorlet: a clinical and pathologic study of 15 cases with ultrastructural observations. Int J Gynecol Pathol 3:124–134, 1984.

Kurman RJ, Norris HJ Mesenchymal tumors of the uterus. VI. Epithelioid smooth muscle tumors including leiomyoblastoma and clear-cell leiomyoma: a clinical and pathological analysis of 26 cases. Cancer 37:1853–1865, 1976.

Oliva E, Nielsen PG, Clement PB. et al. Epithelioid smooth muscle tumors of the uterus: a clinicopathologic analysis of 80 cases. Mod Pathol 10:107A, 1997.

Prayson RA, Goldblum JR, Hart WR. Epithelioid smooth-muscle tumors of the uterus: a clinicopathologic study of 18 patients. Am J Surg Pathol 21:383–391, 1997.

Rizeq MN, Van de Rijn M, Hendrickson MR, Rouse RV. A comparative immunohistochemical study of uterine smooth muscle neoplasms with emphasis on the epithelioid variant. Hum Pathol 25:671–677, 1994.

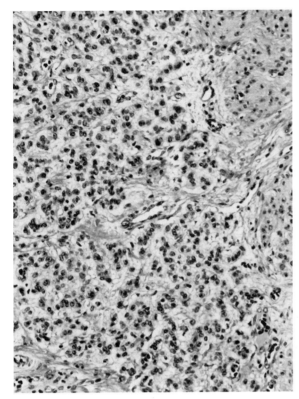

Figure 9–15. Plexiform tumorlets within the myometrium.

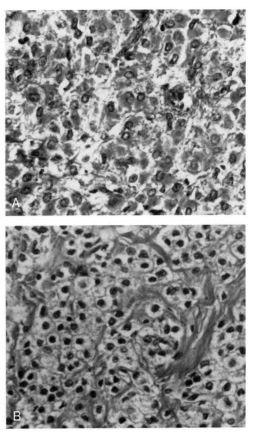

Figure 9–16. Epithelioid leiomyoma. *A,* Epithelioid leiomyoma of the usual type with eosinophilic cells. *B,* Epithelioid leiomyoma with clear cells.

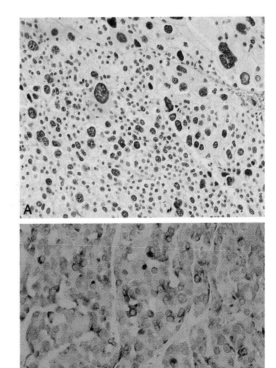

Figure 9–17. Epithelioid leiomyosarcoma. *A,* There is marked nuclear atypicality. Mitotic figures were numerous but are not seen at this magnification. *B,* Another epithelioid leiomyosarcoma, showing immunoreactivity for desmin.

Smooth Muscle Tumors With Unusual Growth Patterns

Diffuse Uterine Leiomyomatosis

- Diffuse uterine leiomyomatosis is a rare, benign disorder characterized by symmetric uterine enlargement caused by countless, confluent, leiomyomatous myometrial nodules.
- The nodules, including many not appreciable grossly, are composed of cytologically benign, typically cellular, mitotically inactive smooth muscle.
- The differential diagnosis includes uterine involvement by lymphangioleiomyomatosis (LAL). Some patients with uterine LAL have other stigmata of tuberous sclerosis. In uterine LAL, the myometrium is involved by microscopic, ill-defined nodules of smooth muscle surrounding lymphatics and protruding into their lumens. The smooth muscle cells are immunoreactive for HMB-45.

References

Clement PB, Young RH. Diffuse leiomyomatosis of the uterus: a report of four cases. Int J Gynecol Pathol 6: 322–330, 1987.

Gyure KA, Hart WR, Kennedy AW. Lymphangiomyomatosis of the uterus associated with tuberous sclerosis and malignant neoplasia of the female genital tract: a report of two cases. Int J Gynecol Pathol 14:344–351, 1995.

Longacre TA, Hendrickson MR, Kapp DS, Teng NNH. Lymphangioleiomyomatosis of the uterus simulating high-stage endometrial stromal sarcoma. Gynecol Oncol 63:404–410, 1996.

Mulvany NJ, Östör AG, Ross I. Diffuse leiomyomatosis of the uterus: Histopathology 27:175–179, 1995.

Dissecting Leiomyomas, Including Cotylenoid Dissecting Leiomyoma

- Rare leiomyomas, including hydropic leiomyomas and intravenous leiomyomatosis (see below), may have a dissecting growth pattern. Grossly, dissecting leiomyomas are often lobulated with irregular, indistinct margins. On microscopic examination, columns of neoplastic smooth muscle dissect into the surrounding myometrium or, occasionally, into the broad ligament.
- One specific type of dissecting leiomyoma is the cotylenoid dissecting leiomyoma (CDL) (i.e., Sternberg tumor). CDLs occur in women of reproductive age who present with a pelvic mass, an enlarged uterus, menstrual irregularities, or combinations thereof. Follow-up in three cases revealed a benign clinical course.
- The most distinctive feature of CDL is its appearance at laparotomy and on gross examination: congested exophytic placental-like masses extend from the uterus into the broad ligament and pelvic cavity. In one case, the tumors were bilateral.
- Microscopic examination of CDLs reveals a sinuous dissecting pattern at the periphery of the tumors, micronodules of smooth muscle with a swirling (rather than fascicular) growth pattern, marked vascularity, and extensive hydropic and hyaline degeneration.

References

Brand AH, Scurry JP, Planner RS, Grant PT. Grapelike leiomyoma of the uterus. Am J Obstet Gynecol 173:956–961, 1995.

Fukunaga M, Ushigome S. Dissecting leiomyoma of the uterus with extrauterine extension. Histopathology 32:160–164, 1998.

Roth LM, Reed RJ. Dissecting leiomyomas of the uterus other than cotylenoid dissecting leiomyoma a report of 8 cases. Am J Surg Pathol 23:1032–1039, 1999.

Roth LM, Reed RJ, Sternberg WH. Cotylenoid dissecting leiomyoma of the uterus: the Sternberg tumor. Am J Surg Pathol 20:1455–1461, 1996.

Leiomyoma With Vascular Invasion

- Leiomyoma with vascular invasion refers to rare, otherwise typical leiomyomas or leiomyoma variants with microscopic intravascular growth confined to the tumor.
- The finding is probably clinically inconsequential in most cases, although no large series of these tumors has been reported. Occasionally, the tumors are associated with benign smooth muscle nodules in the lungs (i.e., benign metastasizing leiomyoma, discussed later).
- Some cases may represent an early stage of intravenous leiomyomatosis (see below).

Reference

Canzonieri V, D'Amore ESG, Bartoloni G, et al. Leiomyomatosis with vascular invasion. Virchows Arch A 425:541–545, 1994.

Intravenous Leiomyomatosis

General Features

- Intravenous leiomyomatosis (IVL) is an uncommon uterine tumor characterized by the presence of intravenous proliferations of benign-appearing smooth muscle in the absence of or outside the confines of a leiomyoma. The clinical presentation is usually similar to that of typical uterine leiomyomas.
- Extrauterine extension into the veins of the broad ligament or, less often, ovarian and vaginal veins, occurs in 30% of cases. The extrauterine extension may be noticed intraoperatively or on gross examination of the hysterectomy specimen.
- Extension of intravascular tumor into the inferior vena cava and the right side of the heart occurs in rare cases. These patients may present initially or many years after hysterectomy with cardiac manifestations.
- Rare cases are associated with solitary metastases (e.g., lungs, pelvic lymph nodes), so-called benign metastasizing leiomyoma (discussed later).

Pathologic Features

- Gross examination reveals multinodular, rubbery, gray-white myometrial masses, at least some of which take the form of wormlike plugs of tumor within myometrial and occasionally parametrial vessels. The intravascular involvement, however, is frequently not grossly appreciated by the initial examiner.

- On microscopic examination, endothelium-coated plugs of cytologically benign smooth muscle occupy the lumens of myometrial veins outside one or more leiomyomas. Extravascular leiomyomas are usually present and are often less well circumscribed, occasionally dissecting, and more hydropic than usual leiomyomas.
- The intravascular tumor usually resembles a typical or hydropic leiomyoma but occasionally resembles a leiomyoma variant, including cellular leiomyoma, leiomyoma with bizarre nuclei, lipoleiomyoma, myxoid leiomyoma, or epithelioid leiomyoma.
- Common features of the intravascular tumor that should suggest the diagnosis of IVL include a clefted or lobulated contour, hyalinization, numerous thick-walled vessels, or combinations thereof.

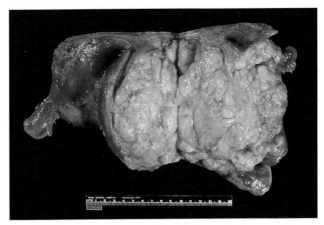

Figure 9–18. Intravenous leiomyomatosis. Intravascular wormlike projections of yellow tumor project from the sectioned surface.

Differential Diagnosis

- Typical leiomyomas may be partly surrounded by compressed slitlike spaces that may represent retraction artifact or compressed vascular spaces. In these cases, the tumor does not have the intraluminal location or typical appearance of IVL.
- Endometrial stromal sarcomas (ESSs) (page 191). ESSs, like IVL, are characterized by prominent intravascular growth, but unlike IVL, typically involve the endometrium, have permeative myoinvasion, constituent endometrial stromal-type cells, and have a network of small arterioles. Features that aid in the distinction of cellular IVL from ESS are the same as those that distinguish highly cellular leiomyomas from endometrial stromal tumors (page 181).
- Leiomyoma with vascular invasion (page 188).
- Leiomyomas with perinodular hydropic change (page 178).

Behavior

- Recurrences may appear months to years after hysterectomy because of continued growth of residual intravenous tumor within the pelvic veins. The tumor may reach the inferior vena cava and the right side of the heart.
- Rare cases of IVL are associated with lymph node or pulmonary involvement (i.e., benign metastasizing leiomyoma).
- The recurrence rate ranges from a high of 30% (based on a literature review) to less than 5% (based on a series of cases from one institution (Mulvaney and coworkers).

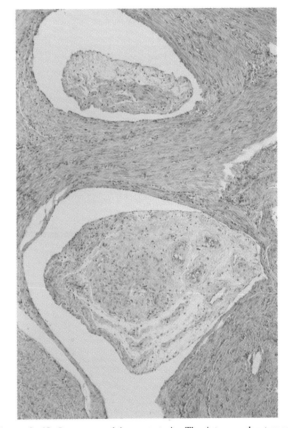

Figure 9–19. Intravenous leiomyomatosis. The intravascular tumor is focally hydropic.

References

Clement PB. Intravenous leiomyomatosis. Pathol Annu 23(2):153–183, 1988.

Clement PB, Young RH, Scully RE. Intravenous leiomyomatosis of the uterus: a clinicopathological analysis of 16 cases with unusual histologic features. Am J Surg Pathol 12:932–945, 1988.

Mulvany NJ, Slavin JL, Östör AG, Fortune DW. Intravenous leiomyomatosis of the uterus: a clinicopathologic study of 22 cases. Int J Gynecol Pathol 13:1–9, 1994.

Norris HJ, Parmley T. Mesenchymal tumors of the uterus. V. Intravenous leiomyomatosis: a clinical and pathological study of 14 cases. Cancer 36:2164–2178, 1975.

Benign Metastasizing Leiomyoma

■ Benign metastasizing leiomyoma (BML) is a rare disorder characterized by the presence of single or multiple pulmonary nodules composed of benign-appearing, mitotically inactive smooth muscle in women with typical uterine leiomyomas or rarely leiomyomas with vascular invasion or IVL. Involvement of extrapulmonary sites (e.g., retroperitoneal and mediastinal lymph nodes, bone, soft tissue) has been reported in rare cases.

■ The pulmonary nodules range up to 10 cm in diameter (but are usually smaller) and are circumscribed, solid, or solid and cystic. Microscopic examination reveals benign smooth muscle, often with entrapment of bronchioalveolar epithelium. The smooth muscle cells are frequently immunoreactive for progesterone and estrogen receptors.

■ The diagnosis of BML is only appropriate in cases in which the uterine leiomyomas have been thoroughly sampled to exclude leiomyosarcoma. The possibility of an extrauterine leiomyosarcoma should also be investigated.

■ The differential diagnosis includes pulmonary lymphangioleiomyomatosis (page 188).

References

Abell MR, Littler ER. Benign metastasizing uterine leiomyoma. Cancer 36:2206–2213, 1975.

Cramer SF, Meyer JS, Kraner JF, et al. Metastasizing leiomyoma of the uterus. Cancer 45:932–937, 1980.

Jautzke G, Müller-Ruchholtz E, Thalmann U. Immunohistological detection of estrogen and progesterone receptors in multiple and well differentiated leiomyomatous lung tumors in women with uterine leiomyomas (so-called benign, metastasizing leiomyomas): a report of 5 cases. Pathol Res Pract 192:215–223, 1996.

Wolff M, Silva F, Kaye G. Pulmonary metastases (with admixed epithelial elements) from smooth muscle neoplasms. Am J Surg Pathol 3: 325–342, 1979.

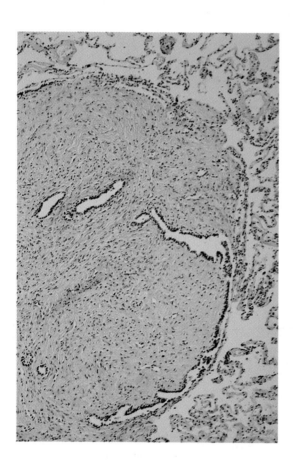

Figure 9–20. Benign, metastasizing leiomyoma in the lung. Notice the entrapped bronchoalveolar epithelium.

Peritoneal Leiomyomas

- Peritoneal ("parasitic") leiomyoma refers to otherwise unremarkable, usually solitary or occasionally a few, leiomyomas or leiomyoma variants attached to the pelvic peritoneum in women who usually have uterine leiomyomas.
- The presumed origin is from subserosal pedunculated uterine leiomyomas that become attached to and vascularized by the pelvic peritoneum, eventually losing their attachment to the uterus.

Diffuse Peritoneal Leiomyomatosis (see Chapter 19).

ENDOMETRIAL STROMAL AND RELATED TUMORS

- Most endometrial stromal tumors are composed of neoplastic cells that resemble the endometrial stromal cells of a proliferative endometrium. Such tumors are subdivided into well-circumscribed tumors (stromal nodules) and infiltrative tumors (low-grade endometrial stromal sarcomas [LGESS]).
- Pure high-grade endometrial sarcomas, which are rare, usually lack overt stromal differentiation and have been referred to as "poorly differentiated endometrial sarcoma" or "high-grade undifferentiated uterine sarcoma." These tumors are of uncertain histogenesis but are most conveniently discussed in this section, as are similar tumors that arise in the endocervix (i.e., endocervical stromal sarcomas).
- Rare tumors that have prominent endometrial stromal and smooth muscle differentiation are also included in this section.

Endometrial Stromal Nodule

- Endometrial stromal nodules (ESNs) have a nonspecific presentation resembling that of uterine leiomyomas.
- Gross examination reveals a well-circumscribed, nonencapsulated, usually solitary, round to oval tumor with a soft, fleshy, tan to yellow sectioned surface. ESNs are almost always located in the myometrium or myometrium and endometrium. The median diameter in one series was 4.0 cm (range, 0.8 to 15 cm).
- Although the tumors are usually well circumscribed on microscopic examination, occasional finger-like projections of up to several millimeters long are considered diagnostically allowable. Myometrial and vascular invasion is absent. ESNs are otherwise histologically identical to low-grade endometrial stromal sarcomas (discussed later).
- The differential diagnosis is primarily with highly cellular leiomyomas (page 181) and LGESSs. Distinction from the latter is based on evaluation of the border with the surrounding myometrium, a feature that is not usually evaluable in a curettage specimen. Circumscribed tumors with focal endometrial stromal differentiation but with a predominance of epithelial patterns

are placed in the category of "uterine tumor resembling ovarian sex cord tumor" (page 206).

- ESNs are benign tumors adequately treated by hysterectomy. If an ESN is a diagnostic consideration in a curettage specimen in a woman who desires to retain her uterus and diagnostic imaging can confirm that the lesion is well circumscribed, local excision may be technically feasible.

References

Oliva E, Young RH, Clement PB, et al. Cellular benign mesenchymal tumors of the uterus: a comparative morphologic and immunohistochemical analysis of 33 highly cellular leiomyomas and seven endometrial stromal nodules, two frequently confused tumors. Am J Surg Pathol 19:757–768, 1995.

Tavassoli FA, Norris HJ. Mesenchymal tumours of the uterus. VII. A clinicopathological study of 60 endometrial stromal nodules. Histopathology 5:1–10, 1981.

Low-Grade Endometrial Stromal Sarcoma

Clinical Features

- LGESSs account for 10% to 15% of uterine cancers with a mesenchymal component. Middle-aged women are usually affected. Seventy-five percent of patients are younger than 50 years of age, including rare cases in adolescents and children.
- The presenting features are usually abnormal vaginal bleeding and less commonly pelvic or abdominal pain; some patients are asymptomatic. Pelvic examination usually reveals an enlarged uterus and, in some cases, tumor protruding through the external os.
- Extrauterine pelvic extension at presentation is found in up to one third of patients. Rarely, the patient presents with tumor at a metastatic site, such as the ovary.
- Rare cases are associated with prolonged estrogenic stimulation, tamoxifen treatment, or prior pelvic irradiation.

Pathologic Features

- Gross examination reveals single or multiple, predominantly intramural masses with frequent protrusion into the endometrial cavity. There is often nodular or diffuse permeation of the myometrium, including wormlike plugs of tumor in myometrial or parametrial veins. The sectioned surface of the tumor is typically soft, fleshy, bulging, and tan to yellow.
- On microscopic examination, the endometrium is typically involved, and the tumor permeates the myometrium as irregular tongues. Myometrial and extrauterine veins and lymphatics are frequently invaded.
- The tumors are cellular, with uniform, oval to spindle-shaped, endometrial stromal-type cells. The neoplastic cells are often focally disposed in a whorled pattern around numerous arterioles. Significant degrees of nuclear pleomorphism and tumor giant cells are absent. There are usually fewer than 3 MF per 10 HPF, but

higher mitotic rates do not exclude the diagnosis of ESN or LGESS.

- Other findings include cells with foamy cytoplasm, which may be tumor cells, foamy histiocytes, or both; hyalinized, occasionally calcified, plaques or perivascular hyalinization; foci of sex cord–like elements consisting of cells, sometimes with an epithelioid appearance and variable amounts of eosinophilic cytoplasm, arranged in small nests, cords, trabeculae, and solid or hollow tubules; benign or malignant endometrioid glands; extensive fibrotic or myxoid areas; and foci of rhabdoid-like cells.

- The neoplastic cells are typically immunoreactive for vimentin, muscle-specific actin, and smooth muscle actin. In some studies, the tumors cells stain for desmin. The tumor cells are often immunoreactive for estrogen, progesterone, or both types of receptors.

- Sex cord–like elements are frequently immunoreactive for vimentin, muscle-specific actin, desmin, and in some cases, cytokeratin. One recent study also found variable immunoreactivity for inhibin, CD99, or both, suggesting true sex-cord differentiation in at least some cases.

Differential Diagnosis

- Highly cellular leiomyoma (page 181) and highly cellular variant of intravenous leiomyomatosis (page 188).
- Adenosarcoma (page 199). In contrast to the occasional low-grade ESSs with glands, the glands of adenosarcomas are usually present more diffusely throughout the tumor, are typically surrounded by cellular condensations of the sarcomatous stroma, and may contain intraglandular polypoid stromal projections. Adenosarcomas only rarely permeate the myometrium and its vessels in the distinctive manner of stromal sarcomas.
- Adenomyosis with sparse glands (see Chapter 7). Features favoring this diagnosis include a postmenopausal age, no grossly evident mass, a concentric zonal organization (i.e., central, pale-staining area of loosely aggregated stromal cells surrounded by a more cellular rim of more darkly staining stromal and smooth muscle cells), atrophic-appearing stromal cells, the presence of typical adenomyosis elsewhere in the uterus, and an absence of sclerosis, foam cells, sex cord–like areas, prominent vascular invasion, and extrauterine extension.
- Uterine tumors resembling ovarian sex cord tumors (page 206). These tumors, in contrast to endometrial stromal sarcoma with focal sex cord–like elements, have pure or predominant sex cord–like patterns.

Behavior and Prognostic Features

- Low-grade ESSs are tumors with a low malignant potential; pelvic or abdominal recurrences develop in one third to one half of patients. The tumors are typically indolent, with a tendency for late recurrence, sometimes many years after hysterectomy.
- Chang and associates found that stage I tumors had a recurrence rate of 36% and survival rate of 92%, whereas stage III and IV tumors had a recurrence rate

of 76% and a survival of 66%. Tumor size, mitotic rate, and nuclear atypia were not predictive of recurrence in patients with stage I tumors.

References

Baker RJ, Hildebrandt RH, Rouse RV, et al. Inhibin and CD99 (MIC2) expression in uterine stromal neoplasms with sex-cord–like elements. Hum Pathol 30:671–679, 1999.

Chang KL, Crabtree GS, Lim-Tan SK, et al. Primary uterine endometrial stromal neoplasms: a clinicopathologic study of 117 cases. Am J Surg Pathol 14:415–438, 1990.

Clement PB, Scully RE. Endometrial stromal sarcomas of the uterus with extensive endometrioid glandular differentiation: a report of three cases that caused problems in differential diagnosis. Int J Gynecol Pathol 11:163–173, 1992.

Evans HL. Endometrial stromal sarcoma and poorly differentiated endometrial sarcoma. Cancer 50:2170–2182, 1982.

Fekete PS, Vellios F. The clinical and histologic spectrum of endometrial stromal neoplasms: a report of 41 cases. Int J Gynecol Pathol 3:198–212, 1984.

Hart WR, Yoonessi M. Endometrial stromatosis of the uterus. Obstet Gynecol 49:393–403, 1977.

Kempson RL, Hendrickson MR. Pure mesenchymal neoplasms of the uterine corpus: selected problems. Semin Diagn Pathol 5:172–198, 1988.

Lillemoe TJ, Perrone T, Norris HJ, Dehner LP. Myogenous phenotype of epithelial-like areas in endometrial stromal sarcomas. Arch Pathol Lab Med 115:215–219, 1991.

McCluggage WG, Date A, Bharucha H, Toner PG. Endometrial stromal sarcoma with sex cord–like areas and focal rhabdoid differentiation. Histopathology 29:369–374, 1996.

Norris HJ, Taylor HB. Mesenchymal tumors of the uterus. I. A clinical and pathologic study of 53 endometrial stromal tumors. Cancer 19:755–766, 1966.

Oliva E, Young RH, Clement PB, Scully RE. Myxoid and fibrous endometrial stromal tumors of the uterus: a report of ten cases. Int J Gynecol Pathol 18:310–319, 1999.

Tanimoto A, Sasaguri T, Arima N, et al. Endometrial stromal sarcoma of the uterus with rhabdoid features. Pathol Int 46:231–237, 1996.

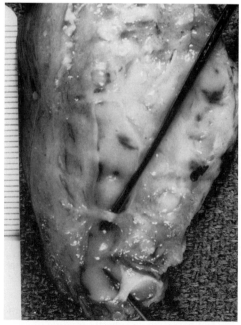

Figure 9–21. Low-grade endometrial stromal sarcoma. Fleshy tumor has extensively replaced the myometrium and extends into a blood vessel at the tip of the probe.

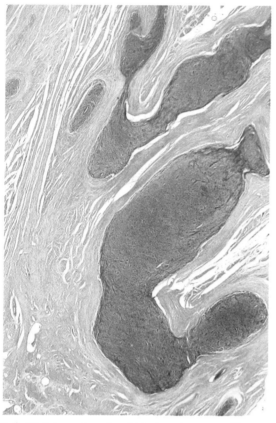

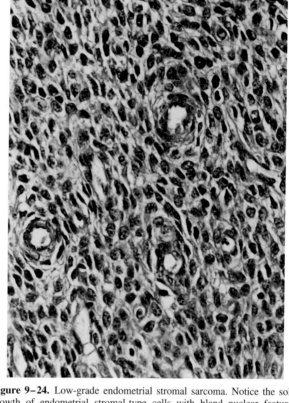

Figure 9–24. Low-grade endometrial stromal sarcoma. Notice the solid growth of endometrial stromal-type cells with bland nuclear features. Several small arterioles are present.

Figure 9–22. Low-grade endometrial stromal sarcoma. The tumor is infiltrating the myometrium and the myometrial vessels.

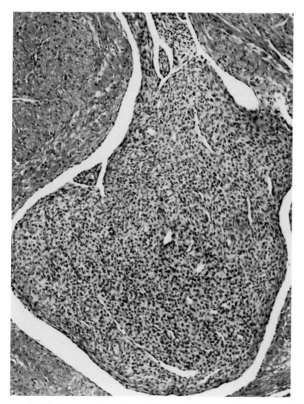

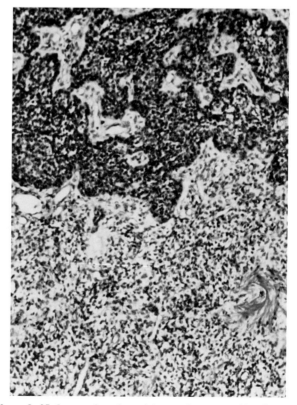

Figure 9–23. Low-grade endometrial stromal sarcoma. The tumor fills the lumen of a myometrial vein.

Figure 9–25. Low-grade endometrial stromal sarcoma with a focal sex cord–like pattern.

High-Grade Endometrial Sarcoma

- High-grade endometrial sarcomas tend to occur in postmenopausal women who present with bleeding and an enlarged uterus.
- Gross examination usually reveals polypoid or plaque-like, fleshy, gray-white to gray-yellow endometrial masses, often with prominent hemorrhage and necrosis. Myometrial invasion is common, but the intravascular wormlike plugs characteristic of LGESS are usually not seen.
- On microscopic examination, the tumors are typically composed of spindle to polygonal cells with marked degrees of nuclear pleomorphism, including multinucleated giant cells, and a high mitotic rate (usually more than 10 MF per 10 HPF, often more than 20 MF per 10 HPF). There is usually destructive myometrial invasion, in contrast to the permeative invasion of LGESSs; microscopic vascular invasion is common.
- These sarcomas can be distinguished from LGESS by a lack of typical growth patterns and vascularity, and presence of greater cytologic atypia; from malignant müllerian mixed tumors by an absence of a carcinomatous component; from leiomyosarcoma by the absence of smooth muscle differentiation; and from rhabdomyosarcoma by an absence of rhabdomyoblasts. Desmin stains may be helpful.
- The tumors are typically aggressive and usually associated with death from abdominopelvic recurrence and lymphatic and hematogenous metastases within 3 years after hysterectomy in most cases. Tumors limited to the endometrium may have a more favorable prognosis. Higher survival rates have been reported in some series in which the tumors were considered high grade based solely on a high mitotic rate, but at least some of these tumors would be considered LGESSs by current criteria.

References

Evans HL. Endometrial stromal sarcoma and poorly differentiated endometrial sarcoma. Cancer 50:2170–2182, 1982.

Kempson RL, Hendrickson MR. Pure mesenchymal neoplasms of the uterine corpus: selected problems. Semin Diagn Pathol 5:172–198, 1988.

Norris HJ, Taylor HB. Mesenchymal tumors of the uterus. I. A clinical and pathologic study of 53 endometrial stromal tumors. Cancer 19:755–766, 1966.

Yoonessi M, Hart WR. Endometrial stromal sarcomas. Cancer 40:898–906, 1977.

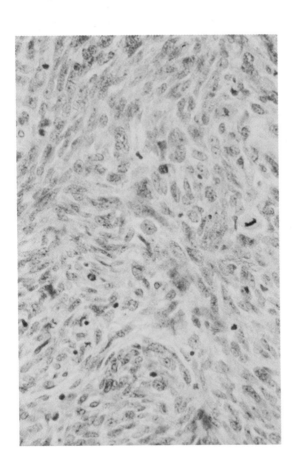

Figure 9–26. High-grade endometrial sarcoma.

Endocervical Stromal Sarcoma

■ Endocervical stromal sarcomas are rare tumors that are usually polypoid or diffusely infiltrative.

■ On microscopic examination, spindle to stellate cells with scanty cytoplasm are arranged in sheetlike, fascicular, or storiform patterns. The tumor cells exhibit various degrees of nuclear pleomorphism and hyperchromasia. Mitotic activity has exceeded 10 MF per 10 HPF in all of the reported cases.

■ Death from recurrent or metastatic tumor has occurred within 2 years of treatment in about 50% of the reported patients.

References

Abdul-Karim FW, Bazi TM, Sorensen K, Nasr MF. Sarcoma of the uterine cervix: clinicopathologic findings in three cases. Gynecol Oncol 26:103–111, 1987.
Abell MR, Ramirez JA. Sarcomas and carcinosarcomas of the uterine cervix. Cancer 31:1176–1192, 1973.

Tumors With Endometrial Stromal and Smooth Muscle Differentiation

■ Only one series of 15 of these rare tumors has been fully reported. The preliminary results of another series of 38 cases has been also published. More than 30% of each component was a criterion for inclusion in both studies.

■ The patients were 20 to 68 years old (mean, 46 years); the presenting features did not differ from those of typical endometrial stromal tumors.

■ The 15 tumors in one series had diameters of 3 to 27 cm (mean, 9.6 cm); only one tumor had grossly infiltrating margins, although six had infiltrating margins microscopically. In some tumors, firm, white, whorled areas alternated with soft, tan-yellow areas. In the abstracted study 22 of 38 tumors were stromal–smooth muscle nodules, and 16 of 38 were low-grade sarcomas.

■ The endometrial stromal component resembles that of pure endometrial stromal tumors. The smooth muscle component is composed of spindle cells in disorganized, short and long fascicles or nodules with prominent central hyalinization (sometimes with a radiating "starburst" pattern of collagen). The nodular pattern may simulate epithelial differentiation.

■ Desmin staining facilitates distinction of the smooth muscle component, which is desmin reactive, from the stromal component, which is usually desmin negative.

■ In the study of 15 cases follow-up for more than 1 year was available for seven patients. The tumors of six patients had benign clinical courses, whereas one tumor with an infiltrating border recurred at 48 months as a pure endometrial stromal sarcoma.

■ In the abstracted series, all the patients with nodules had an uneventful course whereas three of the patients with sarcomas had extrauterine spread at presentation, recurrences, or both.

■ We report these tumors as endometrial stromal nodules or ESSs with smooth muscle differentiation (depending on the margins), with the designation of mixed endometrial stromal–smooth muscle tumor given in parentheses.

References

Devaney K, Tavassoli FA. Immunohistochemistry as a diagnostic aid in the interpretation of unusual mesenchymal tumors of the uterus. Mod Pathol 4:225–231, 1991.
Oliva E, Clement PB, Young RH, Scully RE. Mixed endometrial stromal and smooth muscle tumors of the uterus: a clinicopathologic study of 15 cases. Am J Surg Pathol 22:997–1005, 1998.
Schammel DP, Silver SA, Tavassoli FA. Combined endometrial stromal/ smooth muscle neoplasms of the uterus: a clinicopathological study of 38 cases [Abstract]. Mod Pathol 12:124A, 1999.

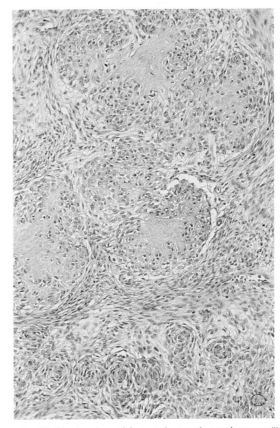

Figure 9–27. Mixed endometrial stromal–smooth muscle tumor ("stromomyoma")). The smooth muscle component takes the form of nodules with central hyalinization. The endometrial stromal component is seen on the extreme bottom.

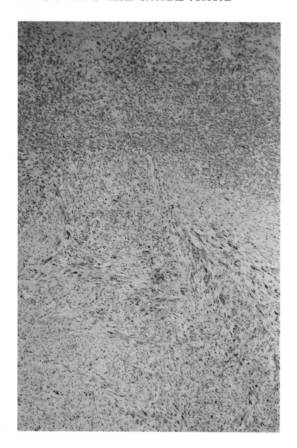

Figure 9–28. Mixed endometrial stromal–smooth muscle tumor, desmin stain. The endometrial stromal component (*top*), which is desmin negative, abuts an area exhibiting smooth muscle differentiation (*bottom*), which is immunoreactive for desmin.

TUMORS WITH MIXED EPITHELIAL AND MESENCHYMAL ELEMENTS

Malignant Müllerian Mixed Tumor

Clinical Features

■ Malignant müllerian mixed tumors (MMMTs) occur almost exclusively in postmenopausal women; rare cases, however, have been reported in females younger than 40 years of age, including children. The risk factors (e.g., excess weight, exogenous estrogen use, nulliparity) are similar to those of women with endometrial adenocarcinoma. A history of pelvic irradiation exists in some cases.

■ The patients present with abnormal vaginal bleeding and an enlarged uterus in most cases; pelvic or abdominal pain is common. The serum CA-125 level is elevated in most cases. Extrauterine spread (stages III and IV) is identified in as many as one third of cases.

Gross Appearance

■ Large, soft broad-based, polypoid tumors typically fill the endometrial cavity and, in some cases, protrude through the external os. Grossly evident myometrial invasion is common. Rare tumors arise in the cervix.

■ The tumor usually has a fleshy cut surface, often with areas of hemorrhage, necrosis, and cystic degeneration.

Microscopic Appearance

■ MMMTs are characterized by an intimate admixture of carcinomatous and sarcomatous components, although one component may focally predominate. The sarcomatous elements of MMMTs are homologous or heterologous.

■ The carcinomatous and sarcomatous components in most MMMTs are high grade, but in some tumors, both components are low grade; we refer to such tumors as low-grade MMMTs. These tumors may have a better prognosis than typical MMMTs.

- The carcinomatous component is usually high-grade endometrioid or serous and less often clear cell, mucinous, nonspecific adenocarcinoma, squamous carcinoma, or undifferentiated carcinoma (including small cell carcinoma), alone or in combination. MMMTs arising in the cervix frequently have nonglandular carcinomatous elements that are exclusively or predominantly squamous or basaloid or resemble adenoid cystic carcinoma.
- Homologous sarcoma is usually a nonspecific spindle-cell sarcoma or may resemble high-grade ESS, leiomyosarcoma, malignant fibrous histiocytoma, undifferentiated sarcoma, or any combination thereof.
- Heterologous sarcomas may contain or consist of rhabdomyoblasts; mature-appearing cartilage or chondrosarcoma; osteoid, bone, or osteosarcoma; and liposarcoma. The heterologous foci typically merge with and appear to be derived from undifferentiated homologous sarcoma, but they occasionally appear intimately associated with the epithelial component, with little nonspecific sarcomatous component.
- Intracellular and extracellular eosinophilic hyaline droplets are common, especially in the sarcomatous elements.
- Rare types of differentiation include neuroectodermal tissue, yolk sac tumor, and malignant rhabdoid tumor.
- Myometrial invasion beyond the inner third occurs in 80% of cases; 40% of cases have deep myometrial invasion. Myometrial lymphatic and vascular invasion is detected in most cases.
- Atypical endometrial hyperplasia or pure endometrial carcinoma (endometrioid or serous) is present in the endometrium uninvolved by MMMT in as many as one half of cases.
- The metastatic and recurrent tumor may be exclusively carcinomatous, sarcomatous, or carcinosarcomatous.

Immunohistochemical Findings

- Carcinomatous elements are typically immunoreactive for epithelial markers (cytokeratin, epithelial membrane antigen [EMA]) and, like typical endometrial adenocarcinomas, vimentin.
- The sarcomatous elements are typically immunoreactive for vimentin and frequently for actin. Weak and focal positivity for epithelial markers may be seen in the sarcomatous areas. Myoglobin appears to be the most specific but least sensitive marker for rhabdomyoblasts.

Differential Diagnosis

- Endometrioid carcinoma with spindled epithelial cells (i.e., sarcomatoid carcinoma). Features favoring sarcoma (and thus MMMT) include sharp demarcation from the obvious epithelial component, a dense pattern of reticulin fibers, the presence of heterologous elements, and strong and diffuse vimentin, actin, or desmin immunoreactivity.
- High-grade endometrial sarcomas (page 194) and pure heterologous sarcomas (page 208). These tumors lack the integral carcinomatous component of MMMTs.

- Endometrial adenocarcinomas with heterologous elements. These tumors are rare, otherwise typical adenocarcinomas with minor foci of benign heterologous elements (e.g., cartilage, fat) but lacking a sarcomatous component.

Behavior and Prognostic Factors

- The 5-year survival rates range from 5 to 40% (all stages) and from 40 to 60% (stages I and II). The median survival time in most studies is less than 2 years.
- The most important pathologic prognostic factors are stage, size of tumor, and depth of invasion. Tumors confined to the endometrium (or an endometrial polyp) or with only superficial myometrial invasion are associated with a better prognosis. Low survival is associated with deep myometrial invasion because of the high frequency of lymphatic and hematogenous involvement.
- Adverse prognostic indicators in some studies include vascular or lymphatic invasion or a component of serous or clear cell carcinoma.
- Patients usually die of tumor growth within the pelvis and abdomen, although most such patients also have hematogenous spread, most commonly to the lungs, liver, bone, and brain.

References

Clement PB, Zubovits JT, Young RH, Scully RE. Malignant mullerian mixed tumors of the uterine cervix: a clinicopathological study of 9 cases. Int J Gynecol Pathol 17:211–222, 1998.

Costa MJ, Khan R, Judd R. Carcinosarcoma (malignant mixed müllerian [mesodermal] tumor) of the uterus and ovary: correlation of clinical, pathologic, and immunohistochemical features in 29 cases. Arch Pathol Lab Med 115:583–590, 1991.

Bitterman P, Chun B, Kurman RJ. The significance of epithelial differentiation in mixed mesodermal tumors of the uterus: a clinicopathologic and immunohistochemical study. Am J Surg Pathol 14:317–328, 1990.

Fukunuga M, Nomura K, Endo Y, et al. Carcinosarcoma of the uterus with extensive neuroectodermal differentiation. Histopathology 29:565–560, 1996.

Gagne E, Tetu B, Blondeau L, et al. Morphologic prognostic factors of malignant mixed müllerian tumor of the uterus: a clinicopathologic study of 58 cases. Mod Pathol 2:433–438, 1989.

George E, Manivel JC, Dehner LP, Wick WR. Malignant mixed müllerian tumors: an immunohistochemical study of 47 cases, with histogenetic considerations and clinical correlation. Hum Pathol 22:215–223, 1991.

Iwasa Y, Haga H, Konishi I, et al. Prognostic factors in uterine carcinosarcoma: a clinicopathologic study of 25 patients. Cancer 82:512–519, 1998.

Meis JM, Lawrence WD. The immunohistochemical profile of malignant mixed müllerian tumor: overlap with endometrial adenocarcinoma. Am J Clin Pathol 94:1–7, 1990.

Nordal RR, Kristensen GB, Stenwig AE, et al. An evaluation of prognostic factors in uterine carcinosarcoma. Gynecol Oncol 67:316–321, 1997.

Silverberg SG, Major FJ, Blessings JA, et al: Carcinosarcoma (malignant mixed mesodermal tumor) of the uterus: a Gynecologic Oncology Group pathologic study of 203 cases. Int J Gynecol Pathol 9:1–19, 1990.

Zelmanowicz A, Hildesheim A, Sherman ME, et al. Evidence for a common etiology for endometrial carcinomas and malignant mixed müllerian tumors. Gynecol Oncol 69:253–257, 1998.

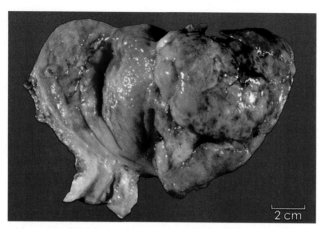

Figure 9–29. Malignant müllerian mixed tumor. A fleshy, polypoid tumor fills the endometrial cavity.

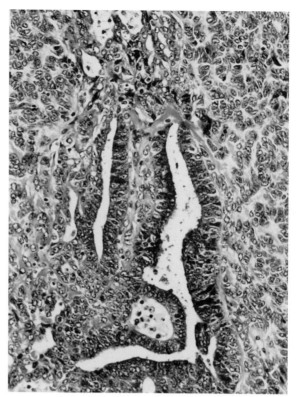

Figure 9–31. Low-grade malignant müllerian mixed tumor. The tumor is composed of a grade 1 endometrioid adenocarcinoma admixed with a low-grade sarcomatous component resembling a low-grade endometrial stromal sarcoma that focally exhibits a cordlike pattern.

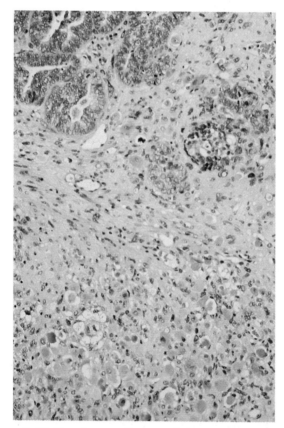

Figure 9–30. Heterologous malignant müllerian mixed tumor. The tumor consists of a high-grade endometrioid adenocarcinoma (*top*) and a sarcomatous component (*bottom*) that contains numerous rhabdomyoblasts that were immunoreactive for myoglobin.

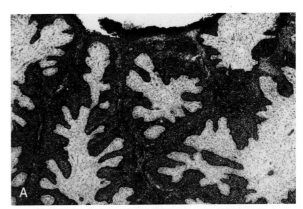

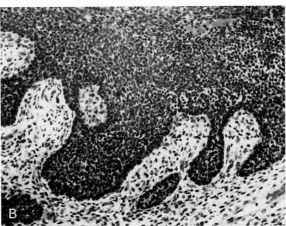

Figure 9–32. Malignant müllerian mixed tumor of the uterine cervix. *A,* The tumor consists of a basaloid carcinoma that forms interconnecting trabeculae. *B,* The basaloid carcinoma abuts a sarcomatous component resembling a low-grade endometrial stromal sarcoma.

Müllerian Adenosarcoma

Clinical Features

- Adenosarcomas typically occur in postmenopausal women, but 30% occur in premenopausal women. The usual presentation is abnormal vaginal bleeding, often accompanied by pelvic pain and an enlarged uterus. Tumor protrudes through the external os in one half of cases.
- The presenting feature in some cases is recurrent endometrial or endocervical "polyps," which on retrospective microscopic review are found to be adenosarcoma.
- Some tumors are associated with hyperestrinism (including tamoxifen therapy) or prior pelvic irradiation.
- Adenosarcomas are almost always stage I at presentation. Rare cases with extraovarian adenosarcoma (e.g., ovary, cul-de-sac) at presentation may represent a multicentric origin rather than a metastatic tumor.

Gross Appearance

- The tumors are typically polypoid, sometimes villous, broad-based masses. Ninety percent are endometrial, and 10% are endocervical. In rare cases, the corpus and endocervix are involved by separate primary tumors, or the tumor is confined to the myometrium.
- The sectioned surface is frequently spongy, with cystic spaces filled with a watery or mucoid fluid surrounded by white to tan tissue. Myometrial invasion is grossly evident only rarely.

Microscopic Appearance

- Low-power examination reveals a biphasic tumor in which glands, which are often cystically dilated, are scattered throughout a mesenchymal component. Thin papillae or broad polypoid fronds may project into the glands or form the surface of the tumor.

- The glands are lined by a variety of benign or atypical müllerian epithelia, most commonly of proliferative-endometrial type with mitotic figures. Endocervical (mucinous), tubal (ciliated), secretory-endometrial (with subnuclear vacuoles), hobnail, or indifferent epithelia may also be seen. Metaplastic squamous epithelium, typically nonkeratinizing, may line or fill the gland lumens.
- Focal architectural or cytologic atypia of the glandular epithelium is identified in one third of cases, and small foci of adenocarcinoma have been rarely encountered in otherwise typical adenosarcomas. In such cases, the endometrium elsewhere in the uterus may be atypically hyperplastic or carcinomatous.
- The mesenchymal component usually consists of a low-grade sarcoma, usually resembling an endometrial stromal sarcoma, fibrosarcoma, or combinations thereof. Minor or, uncommonly, extensive foci of smooth muscle differentiation have been encountered in some cases.
- The sarcoma is typically more cellular around the glands, and in these areas, 4 or more MF per 10 HPF are present in more than 80% of the tumors. In other areas, the sarcoma may be sparsely cellular or replaced by myxoid or hyalinized fibrous tissue that may have a deceptively benign appearance.
- Heterologous elements are found in about 20% of tumors, varying from small foci of fat, cartilage, or rhabdomyoblasts to extensive embryonal rhabdomyosarcoma occupying most or all of the stroma.
- Myometrial invasion is found in about one sixth of tumors; it is superficial (inner one half of myometrium) in 80%. The invasive border of the tumor is usually well circumscribed, but occasional tumors invade in irregular tongues. Rare tumors invade myometrial vessels.
- Overgrowth of more than 25% of the tumor by a pure homologous or heterologous sarcoma occurs in about 10% of cases. The pure sarcoma is typically of higher grade and more mitotic than the sarcoma of the associated adenosarcoma. These tumors invade the myometrium more commonly and more deeply than typical adenosarcomas.
- Foci of sex cord–like elements occur within the sarcomatous component in rare tumors. These sex cord–like elements consist of benign-appearing cells of epithelial type arranged in solid nests, trabeculae, and solid or hollow tubules. The cells often contain abundant eosinophilic or foamy, lipid-rich cytoplasm.

Differential Diagnosis

- Adenofibromas. Features favoring adenofibroma include diffusely paucicellular stroma with no periglandular stromal cuffs, no stromal atypia, and no or rare mitotic figures (<2 MF per 10 HPF). Adenofibromas account for only 5% of tumors in the adenofibroma-adenosarcoma spectrum and should be diagnosed only after the tumor has been extensively sampled to exclude foci with 2 or more MF per 10 HPF, marked cellularity, or stromal cell atypia, any of which warrant a diagnosis of adenosarcoma rather than adenofibroma.
- Benign endometrial or endocervical polyp. Features favoring a benign polyp include inactive glands and a diffusely paucicellular, fibrotic stroma with no periglandular stromal hypercellularity; no stromal mitoses and no intraluminal stromal papillae. Some polyps have a cellular stroma and stromal mitotic figures but no other features that indicate adenosarcoma.
- Atypical polypoid adenomyoma (APA) (page 204). Features favoring APA include a predominant component of cellular smooth muscle and a glandular component that is less cystic, generally more atypical, and with more prominent squamous morules than in adenosarcomas.
- MMMTs. Most or all of the glandular component is frankly carcinomatous.
- ESSs. ESSs lack the integral glandular component of the adenosarcoma, although their periphery may contain occasional entrapped glands or, in a minority of cases, there may be focal prominent endometrioid glandular differentiation. ESSs, unlike most adenosarcomas, typically have highly infiltrative borders with extensive myometrial and vascular penetration.

Behavior

- Adenosarcomas are tumors with low malignant potential, a behavior manifested primarily by vaginal or abdominopelvic recurrence in about 25% of the cases, often at posthysterectomy intervals of 5 years or more. Hematogenous spread occurs in fewer than 5% of cases. The risk of recurrence is greater with myoinvasive tumors (46%) than in nonmyoinvasive tumors (12.7%).
- The histology of the recurrent tumor is pure sarcoma in 70% of the cases, adenosarcoma in almost 30%, and a carcinosarcoma in rare cases. Recurrent tumor rarely may contain heterologous elements or foci of carcinoma not present in the primary tumors. Blood-borne metastases have been purely sarcomatous.
- Sarcomatous overgrowth is associated with recurrence, hematogenous metastases, and death from tumor in 70%, 40%, and 60% of patients, respectively. Adenosarcomas with sarcomatous overgrowth therefore have a malignant potential similar to that of other high-grade uterine sarcomas such as MMMT and leiomyosarcoma.

References

Clement PB. Müllerian adenosarcomas of the uterus with sarcomatous overgrowth: a clinicopathological analysis of 10 cases. Am J Surg Pathol 13:28–38, 1989.

Clement PB, Scully RE. Müllerian adenosarcomas of the uterus with sex cord–like elements: a clinicopathological analysis of eight cases. Am J Clin Pathol 91:664–672, 1989.

Clement PB, Scully RE. Müllerian adenosarcoma of the uterus: a clinicopathological analysis of 100 cases with a review of the literature. Hum Pathol 21:363–381, 1990.

Clement PB. Oliva E, Young RH. Müllerian adenosarcoma of the uterus associated with tamoxifen therapy: a report of six cases and a review of tamoxifen-associated endometrial lesions. Int J Gynecol Pathol 25:222–229, 1996.

Hattab EM, Allam-Nandyala P, Rhatigan RM. The stromal component of large endometrial polyps. Int J Gynecol Pathol 18:332–337, 1999.

Kaku T, Silverberg SG, Major FJ, et al. Adenosarcoma of the uterus: a Gynecologic Oncology Group clinicopathologic study of 31 cases. Int J Gynecol Pathol 11:75–88, 1992.

Zaloudek CJ, Norris HJ. Adenofibroma and adenosarcoma of the uterus: a clinicopathologic study of 35 cases. Cancer 48:354–366, 1981.

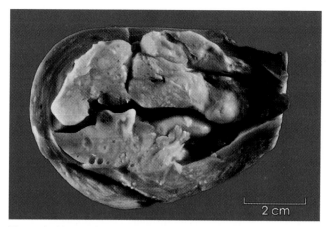

Figure 9–33. Müllerian adenosarcoma. A polypoid mass fills the endometrial cavity. Cysts are visible on the sectioned surface of the tumor.

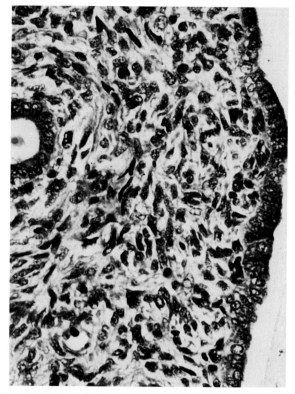

Figure 9–35. Müllerian adenosarcoma. The sarcomatous stromal component resembles low-grade endometrial stromal sarcoma.

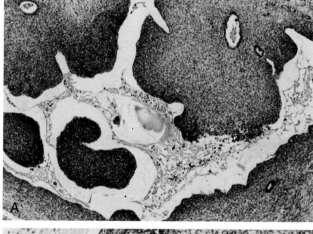

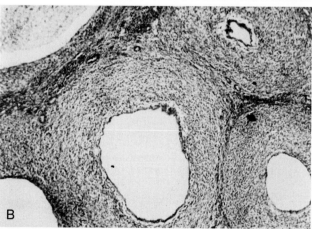

Figure 9–34. Müllerian adenosarcoma. Notice the variably sized glands and cysts admixed with a cellular stromal component, which forms intracystic polypoid projections (A) and periglandular stromal cuffs (A and B).

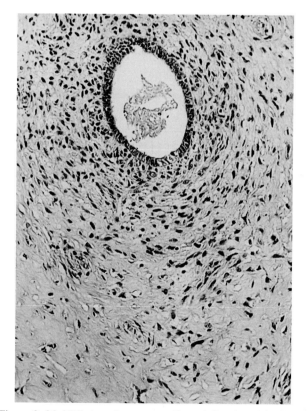

Figure 9–36. Müllerian adenosarcoma. Stromal fibrosis and hyalinization impart a deceptively benign appearance; periglandular stromal condensation, however, is still apparent. The stromal component was more overtly sarcomatous in other areas of the tumor.

Müllerian Adenofibroma

- Müllerian adenofibromas, which are much less common than adenosarcomas, have a clinical presentation and gross appearance that is similar to that of adenosarcoma.
- The glandular or villoglandular epithelial component is similar to that of adenosarcoma.
- The benign stromal component has variable cellularity, with a composition of cells resembling fibroblasts or endometrial stromal cells that exhibit absent or minimal nuclear pleomorphism and are mitotically inactive (see differential diagnosis with adenosarcoma earlier).
- Heterologous stromal elements are absent, except for fat in a single case (i.e., lipoadenofibroma).
- The tumors are usually noninvasive, but rare examples have invaded the endocervical wall, myometrium, or myometrial vessels.
- The postoperative course is usually uneventful, although the tumors may recur after local excision.

References

Clement PB, Scully RE. Müllerian adenofibroma of the uterus with invasion of myometrium and pelvic veins. Int J Gynecol Pathol 9: 363–371, 1990.

Miller KN, McClure SP. Papillary adenofibroma of the uterus: report of a case involved by adenocarcinoma and review of the literature. Am J Clin Pathol 97:806–809, 1992.

Vellios F, Ng ABP, Reagan JW. Papillary adenofibroma of the uterus: a benign mesodermal mixed tumor of mullerian origin. Am J Clin Pathol 60:543–551, 1973.

Zaloudek CJ, Norris HJ. Adenofibroma and adenosarcoma of the uterus: a clinicopathologic study of 35 cases. Cancer 48:354–366, 1981.

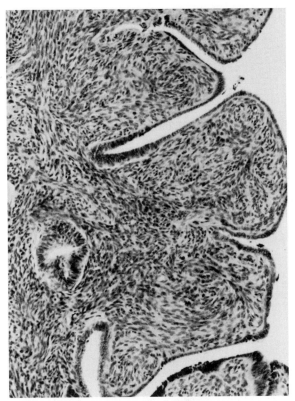

Figure 9–37. Müllerian adenofibroma. Benign endometrioid epithelium lines surface stromal papillae and a few glands. The stroma is composed of benign fibroblasts that were devoid of mitotic activity.

Müllerian Carcinofibroma and Carcinomesenchymoma

- These rare uterine tumors have a malignant epithelial component and a benign mesenchymal component. Tumors with a mesenchymal element of abundant fibromatous tissue have been designated *carcinofibroma,* although in such cases the fibrous component may be reactive. *Carcinofibroma* has also been applied (inappropriately in our opinion) to otherwise typical tumors in the adenofibroma-adenosarcoma spectrum with foci of in situ or invasive adenocarcinoma.
- Another example of a tumor in this category (i.e., carcinomesenchymoma) was composed of adenocarcinoma admixed with benign smooth muscle, cartilage, and adipose tissue.

References

Chen KTK, Vergon JM. Carcinomesenchymoma of the uterus. Am J Clin Pathol 75:746–748, 1981.

Peters WM, Wells M, Bryce FC. Müllerian clear cell carcinofibroma of the uterine corpus. Histopathology 8:1069–1078, 1984.

Thompson M, Husemeyer R. Carcinofibroma—a variant of the mixed müllerian tumor. Br J Obstet Gynaecol 88:1151–1155, 1981.

Adenomyomas

Adenomyoma of Endocervical Type (see Chapter 4)

Typical Endometrioid-Type Adenomyoma

- In one series, the patients were 26 to 64 years old (median, 49 years). The usual presentation was abnormal vaginal bleeding; some tumors were an incidental finding on clinical or pathologic examination.

- Most tumors are submucosal, grossly resembling a typical endometrial polyp; some tumors are mural or subserosal. Submucosal and subserosal tumors may be pedunculated. In the series mentioned earlier, the tumor diameters were 0.3 to 17 cm (median, 3.8 cm). The sectioned surfaces are predominantly solid but may contain small, sometimes blood-filled, cysts.
- The tumors are composed of benign, widely spaced endometrial glands with periglandular endometrial stroma embedded within smooth muscle. Occasional tumors may also contain a minor component of glands lined by tubal or endocervical-type epithelium.
- The tumors are distinguished from APA (discussed

later) by an absence of architectural and, more importantly, cytologic atypia. Typical adenomyomas also usually lack the conspicuous squamous metaplasia and the cellularity of the smooth muscle component typical of APAs. In contrast to adenomyosis, typical adenomyomas are usually sharply circumscribed masses that have a prominent component of smooth muscle of myomatous type.

References

Cullen TS. Adenomyoma of the Uterus. Philadelphia: WB Saunders, 1908.

Gilks CB, Clement PB, Young RH, Scully RE. Uterine adenomyomas of endometrioid type other than atypical polypoid adenomyoma (in preparation).

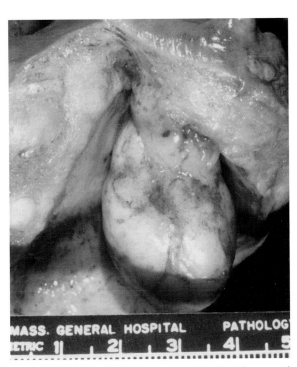

Figure 9–38. Typical polypoid adenomyoma. A polypoid mass projects into the endometrial cavity.

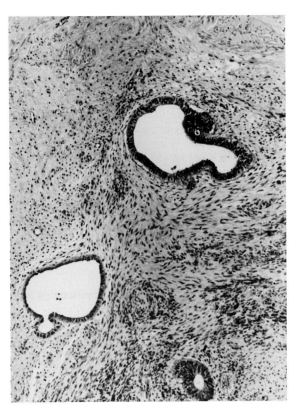

Figure 9–39. Typical polypoid adenomyoma. The tumor is composed of benign endometrial glands, endometrial stroma, and smooth muscle.

Atypical Polypoid Adenomyoma

Clinical and Gross Findings

- Most APAs are encountered in reproductive age women (average age, 39 years), but occasional tumors have occurred after the menopause. Rare cases are associated with long-term estrogen therapy.
- The patients typically present with abnormal vaginal bleeding. Pelvic examination is usually negative, although a polypoid mass may project through the external os in some cases.
- APAs frequently involve the lower uterine segment, but they may arise in the endocervix or corpus. The tumors are usually solitary, well circumscribed, pedunculated or sessile, and typically less than 2 cm in maximum dimension. The sectioned surfaces are yellow-tan to gray to white, solid, and firm to rubbery.

Microscopic Findings

- Endometrioid glands with various degrees of architectural and cytologic atypia and mitotic activity are admixed with a myofibromatous stroma.
- Squamous morules occur in 90% of cases. The morules may obliterate glandular lumens and occasionally contain areas of central necrosis. Keratin from the morules may rarely implant on the peritoneum, resulting in keratin granulomas (see Chapter 20).
- Rare features include a cribriform glandular pattern, severe cytologic epithelial atypia, or both. Forty-five percent of APAs in one study (Longacre and coworkers) had foci that architecturally resembled well-differentiated adenocarcinomas and were designated "APAs of low malignant potential" (APAs-LMP). Rare APAs are contiguous to, and appear to be the origin of, a well-differentiated myoinvasive endometrioid adenocarcinoma.
- The stromal component consists of interlacing bundles of cellular smooth muscle or myofibroblasts. The stromal cells appear benign but exhibit mild to moderate atypia in a minority of cases. A few mitotic figures are usually present.
- APAs are usually noninvasive, with a well-circumscribed border in hysterectomy specimens, although some tumors involve the superficial myometrium. In one study (Longacre and coworkers), none of the typical APAs invaded the myometrium, whereas 2 of 12 APAs-LMP superficially invaded the myometrium.
- The uninvolved endometrium is typically estrogenic (i.e., normal proliferative, endometrial hyperplasia) but rarely is normal secretory.

Differential Diagnosis

- Endometrial adenocarcinoma. Features favoring this diagnosis over APA in a curettage specimen include a postmenopausal age and the presence of glands with overtly malignant features (e.g., marked nuclear pleomorphism, prominent nucleoli) with or without invasion of normal myometrium. Both APAs and endometrial adenocarcinomas, however, may have a similar myofibromatous stroma.
- MMMT or adenosarcoma (if cellular stroma of APA is mistaken for sarcoma). Differential features that distinguish these tumors from APA include the usual absence of a prominent smooth muscle stromal component (MMMT and adenosarcoma), periglandular stromal condensation and intraglandular stromal papillae (adenosarcoma), a glandular component that is often predominantly cystic and less atypical than that of the APA (adenosarcoma), and overtly malignant epithelial and stromal components (MMMT).
- Typical polypoid adenomyomas. The features that distinguish these adenomyomas from APA include the usual absence of architectural and cytologic atypia of the glands and a paucicellular smooth muscle component.

Behavior

- Longacre and colleagues found intrauterine persistence or recurrence in as many as 45% of patients if treated conservatively (e.g., dilatation and curettage, polypectomy). The conservatively treated AMPs-LMP had a higher local persistence or recurrence rate than the APAs of usual type (60% versus 33%).
- Conservatively treated APAs rarely have progressed to adenocarcinoma.

References

Clement PB, Young RH. Atypical polypoid adenomyoma of the uterus associated with Turner's syndrome: a report of three cases, including a review of "estrogen-associated" endometrial neoplasms and neoplasms associated with Turner's syndrome. Int J Gynecol Pathol 6: 104–113, 1987.

Longacre TA, Chung MH, Rouse RV, Hendrickson MR. Atypical polypoid adenomyofibromas (atypical polypoid adenomyomas) of the uterus: a clinicopathologic study of 55 cases. Am J Surg Pathol 20:1–20, 1996.

Mazur MT. Atypical polypoid adenomyomas of the endometrium. Am J Surg Pathol 5:473–482, 1981.

Soslow RA, Chung MH, Rouse RV, et al. Atypical polypoid adenomyofibroma (APA) versus well-differentiated endometrial carcinoma with prominent stromal matrix: an immunohistochemical study. Int J Gynecol Pathol 15:209–216, 1996.

Sugiyama T, Ohta S, Nishida T, et al. Two cases of endometrial adenocarcinoma arising from atypical polypoid adenomyoma. Gynecol Oncol 71:141–144, 1998.

Young RH, Treger T, Scully RE. Atypical polypoid adenomyoma of the uterus: a report of 27 cases. Am J Clin Pathol 86:139–145, 1986.

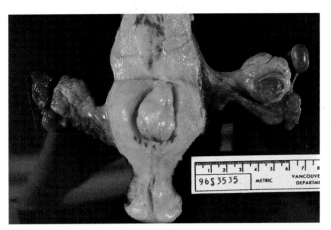

Figure 9–40. Atypical polypoid adenomyoma. A polypoid mass projects into the endometrial cavity.

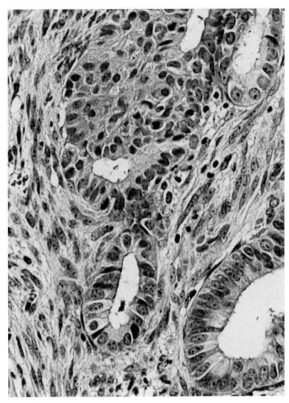

Figure 9–42. Atypical polypoid adenomyoma. Atypical endometrial glands, one with a squamous morule, are separated by a cellular fibromuscular stroma.

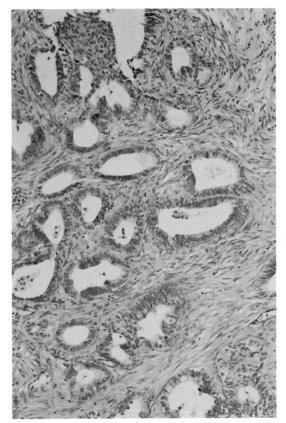

Figure 9–41. Atypical polypoid adenomyoma. Crowded atypical endometrial glands lie within a cellular smooth muscle stroma. Notice the squamous morule in upper left corner.

Uterine Tumors Resembling Ovarian Sex Cord Tumors

Clinical Features

- The typical presenting clinical manifestations of these uncommon tumors, which occur in the reproductive and postmenopausal age groups, are abnormal vaginal bleeding and uterine enlargement or a pelvic mass. Some patients may be asymptomatic.
- Uterine tumors resembling ovarian sex cord tumors (UTROSCTs) are almost invariably confined to the uterus at presentation.

Pathologic Features

- UTROSCTs are generally solid, round, well-circumscribed myometrial masses (mean diameter, 5.7 cm). Occasional tumors are submucosal or subserosal and may be polypoid. Rare tumors are predominantly cystic. The sectioned surfaces are yellow, grey, or tan; soft; and fleshy, without the whorled pattern of a leiomyoma.
- UTROSCTs are characterized microscopically by a variety of epithelial and stromal patterns that create a resemblance to those of ovarian sex cord tumors, especially granulosa cell and Sertoli cell tumors, including the retiform-type tumors. These patterns include anastomosing cords one to two cells in width or broader trabeculae, small nests, and sertoliform tubular structures; occasionally, Call-Exner–like bodies may be present.
- The neoplastic cells in the sex cord–like areas range from small and round with scanty cytoplasm to larger cells with abundant eosinophilic, clear, or foamy cytoplasm that is often lipid rich.
- The nuclei are generally small and regular, with indis-

tinct nucleoli. Nuclear grooves are rare or absent, and mitotic figures are typically scarce.
- The sex cord–like elements are separated by a scanty to abundant stroma that varies from moderately cellular to hypocellular and hyalinized. Occasionally, the stroma has the features of benign-appearing smooth muscle.
- The borders of the tumor may be well circumscribed or infiltrative. Vascular invasion occurs in rare cases.
- The tumor cells are immunoreactive for mesenchymal (e.g., vimentin, desmin) and epithelial markers (e.g., cytokeratin, EMA) and for estrogen and progesterone receptors in most cases. One study found immunoreactivity for one or more markers of sex cord differentiation (e.g., inhibin, O13, A103) in all the tumors studied, providing evidence for the presence of true sex cord elements in these tumors.

Behavior

- UTROSCTs are considered to be tumors with low malignant potential. Recurrences develop in approximately 15% of cases at intervals of 2 to 12 years after hysterectomy.
- Features predictive of recurrence include serosal rupture, vessel invasion, stromal predominance, and cytologic atypia.

References

Baker RJ, Hildebrandt RH, Rouse RV, et al. Inhibin and CD99 (MIC2) in uterine stromal neoplasms with sex-cord-like elements. Hum Pathol 30:671–679, 1999.

Clement PB, Scully RE. Uterine tumors resembling ovarian sex-cord tumors: a clinicopathologic analysis of fourteen cases. Am J Clin Pathol 66:512–525, 1976.

Krishnamurthy S, Jungbluth AA, Busam KJ, Rosai J. Uterine tumors resembling ovarian sex-cord tumors have an immunophenotype consistent with true sex-cord differentiation. Am J Surg Pathol 22:1078–1082, 1998.

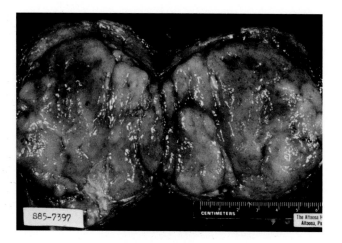

Figure 9–43. Uterine tumor resembling ovarian sex cord tumor. The well-circumscribed tumor is surrounded by myometrium and has a fleshy, lobulated cut surface, which was tan.

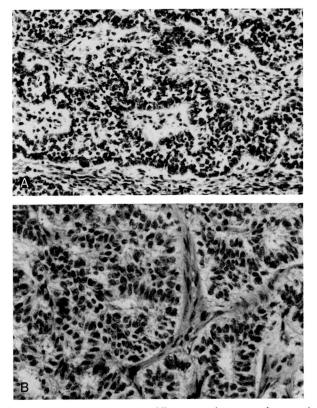

Figure 9–44. Uterine tumor resembling an ovarian sex cord tumor. *A,* One tumor is composed of cellular trabeculae arranged in a plexiform pattern simulating a granulosa cell tumor. *B,* Another tumor is composed of solid and hollow sertoliform tubules lined by cells with abundant vacuolated cytoplasm, which was rich in lipid.

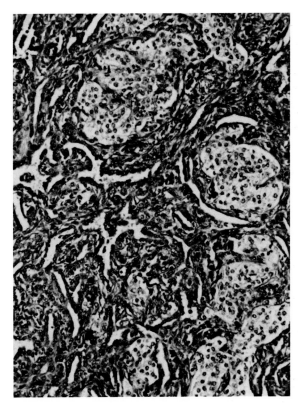

Figure 9–45. Uterine tumor resembling an ovarian sex cord tumor. Tumor cells with scant cytoplasm line ramifying slitlike spaces, imparting a retiform pattern. Admixed are solid nests of cells with abundant foamy cytoplasm.

RARE SARCOMAS

Homologous Sarcomas

Vascular Tumors

- About 15 uterine angiosarcomas have been reported in females 17 to 76 years of age, but most patients are perimenopausal or postmenopausal. The patients typically present with uterine bleeding and anemia.
- Grossly, the tumors usually are large with deep myometrial invasion.
- The tumors are morphologically similar to angiosarcomas in other sites. Two of the tumors were epithelioid angiosarcomas that arose in a uterine leiomyoma; one of them was associated with ovarian and tubal angiomatosis.
- Immunoreactivity for endothelial markers (CD31, factor VIII, CD43) and lack of reactivity for smooth muscle actin, keratin, and estrogen receptor facilitate the diagnosis.

- Most of the tumors had a clinically malignant course, with death from tumor within a year of presentation.

Reference

Schammel DP, Tavassoli FA. Uterine angiosarconas: a morphologic and immunohistochemical study of four cases. Am J Surg Pathol 22:246–250, 1998.

Malignant Fibrous Histiocytoma

- About 12 uterine malignant fibrous histiocytomas (MFHs) or variants thereof (including fibroxanthosarcoma and malignant giant cell tumor) have been reported in patients 43 to 75 years of age.
- Patients typically present with abnormal vaginal bleeding and a large pelvic mass. Several patients had hematogenous metastases at presentation.
- Gross examination reveals large, fleshy polypoid masses with prominent hemorrhage and necrosis involving the endometrium and myometrium.

- The microscopic appearance is similar to MFH in other sites, with various combinations of pleomorphic epithelioid and spindled mononuclear cells, benign-appearing multinucleated cells resembling osteoclasts or Touton giant cells, malignant giant cells with multiple bizarre nuclei, and foamy histiocytes.
- Nine of 12 patients died of tumor or were alive with tumor at follow-up.

References

Isaksen CV, Lindboe CF, Hagen B. Malignant fibrous histiocytoma of the uterus. Acta Obstet Gynecol Scand 74:224–226, 1995.

Kawai K, Senba M, Tagawa H, et. al. Osteoclast-type giant cell tumor of the endometrium: an immunohistochemical study. Zentralbl Allgemeine Pathol Pathologische Anat 135:743–749, 1989.

Magni E, Lauritzen AF, Wilken-Jensen C, Horn T. Malignant giant cell tumour of the uterus. APMIS Suppl 23:113–118, 1991.

Selvaggi L, Di Vagno G, Maiorano E, et. al. Giant malignant fibrous histiocytoma of the uterus. Arch Gynecol Obstet 259:197–200, 1997.

Neurogenic Sarcomas (see Chapter 10)

Heterologous Sarcomas

Embryonal Rhabdomyosarcoma

- Most uterine embryonal rhabdomyosarcomas (i.e., sarcoma botryoides) are of cervical origin. Some cases have been confined to the corpus or have involved the corpus and cervix.
- The tumors typically occur in young women (mean age, 18 years) but may be encountered in females of any age. The patients typically present with vaginal bleeding, tissue protruding from the introitus, or both.
- On gross examination, the tumors are usually 3 to 4 cm in the maximal dimension, smooth, and polypoid, with a myxoid sectioned surface. Occasional tumors have an overtly botryoid appearance.
- The tumors microscopically resemble their vaginal counterparts (see Chapter 3); nodules of hyaline cartilage, however, are more common, occurring in about 50% of the tumors. Invasion of the cervical wall or myometrium may occur but is uncommon.
- The prognosis is favorable in most cases, with an 80% survival rate for patients with cervical tumors (88% for stage I tumors). The main adverse pathologic prognostic factor is deep invasion. Rare tumors with foci resembling alveolar rhabdomyosarcoma may be more aggressive.

Differential Diagnosis

- Pleomorphic rhabdomyosarcoma. These tumors usually occur in an older age group and are usually more diffusely cellular, with numerous bizarre cells, more plentiful rhabdomyoblasts, and no cambium layer.
- Benign endocervical (see Chapter 4) or endometrial polyps (see Chapter 10). Polyps are rare in the first two decades of life and lack a cambium layer, mitotic figures, and rhabdomyoblasts.
- Rhabdomyomas (see Chapter 3). These benign tumors lack a cambium layer, mitoses, and stromal invasion.

Rare cases of rhabdomyosarcoma mixed with rhabdomyoma have been reported.

- Poorly differentiated endometrial and endocervical stromal sarcomas (page 194). These tumors usually occur in older women and lack rhabdomyoblasts.
- Müllerian adenosarcomas (page 199). These tumors contain an integral glandular component in contrast to absent or rare entrapped glands in embryonal rhabdomyosarcomas.
- Fibroepithelial polyps with stromal atypia (see Chapter 3). These lesions lack a cambium layer, small malignant cells with mitotic activity, and rhabdomyoblasts.

References

Brand E, Berek JS, Nieberg RK, Hacker NF. Rhabdomyosarcoma of the uterine cervix: sarcoma botryoides. Cancer 60:1552–1560, 1987.

Copeland LJ, Gershenson DM, Saul PB, et. al. Sarcoma botryoides of the female genital tract. Obstet Gynecol 66:262–266,1985.

Daya D, Scully RE. Sarcoma botryoides of the uterine cervix in young women: a clinicopathological analysis of 13 cases. Gynecol Oncol 29:290–304, 1988.

Emerich J, Senkus E, Konefka T. Alveolar rhabdomyosarcoma of the uterine cervix. Gynecol Oncol 63:398–403, 1996.

Jacques SM, Lawrence WD, Malviya VK. Uterine mixed embryonal rhabdomyosarcoma and fetal rhabdomyoma. Gynecol Oncol 48:272–276, 1993.

Zeisler H, Mayerhofer K, Joura EA, et. al. Embryonal rhabdomyosarcoma of the uterine cervix: case report and review of the literature. Gynecol Oncol 69:78–83, 1998.

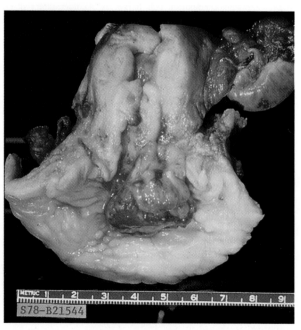

Figure 9–46. Embryonal rhabdomyosarcoma of the uterine cervix. The tumor forms a polypoid mass.

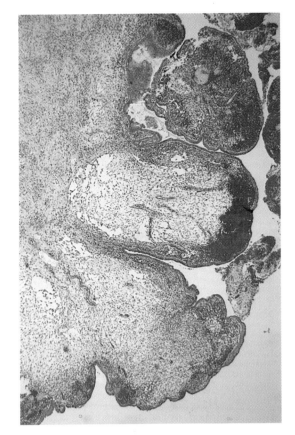

Figure 9–47. Embryonal rhabdomyosarcoma of the uterine cervix (i.e., sarcoma botryoides). Notice the subepithelial cambium layer that is demarcated from the underlying edematous stroma.

Rare Heterologous Sarcomas

- Rare cases of pleomorphic rhabdomyosarcoma, chondrosarcoma, osteosarcoma, and liposarcoma have been reported, typically in elderly women who present with abnormal vaginal bleeding and an enlarged uterus.
- Large polypoid masses usually fill the endometrial cavity, often prolapsing through the external os, and frequently invade the myometrium. Some tumors are confined to the myometrium or cervix.
- The sectioned surface of the tumors and their microscopic appearance are similar to those of their extrauterine counterparts.
- These sarcomas are distinguished from MMMTs with heterologous elements by the absence of a glandular component. The distinction of pleomorphic from embryonal rhabdomyosarcoma was discussed previously.
- Most cases are associated with a malignant clinical course with local recurrence and hematogenous dissemination.

References

Bapat K, Brustein S. Uterine sarcoma with liposarcomatous differentiation: report of a case and review of the literature. Int J Gynecol Obstet 28:71–75, 1989.

De Young B, Bitterman P, Lack EE. Primary osteosarcoma of the uterus: report of a case with immunohistochemical study. Mod Pathol 5:212–215, 1992.

Kofinas AD, Suarez J, Calame RJ, Chipeco Z. Chondrosarcoma of the uterus. Gynecol Oncol 19:231–237. 1984.

Ordi J, Stamatakos MD, Tavassoli FA. Pure pleomophic rhabdomyosarcoma of the uterus. Int J Gynecol Pathol 16:369–377, 1997.

Sarcomas of Uncertain Histogenesis

Alveolar Soft Part Sarcomas

- Nineteen uterine alveolar soft part sarcomas (ASPSs) have been reported, approximately two thirds of which have involved the cervix, the lower uterine segment, or both. The remainder have arisen in the corpus.
- The patients have ranged in age from 8 to 50 years of

age (mean 30 years) and usually presented with abnormal vaginal bleeding, a cervical mass that was sometimes polypoid, or both.

- Gross examination usually reveals a well-circumscribed, solid mass that is yellow, tan, gray, or white and 0.4 to 7 cm in diameter. The tumors are usually within the superficial cervical stroma, endometrium, or myometrium.
- The tumors microscopically resemble ASPS in other sites. Metastasis to a pelvic lymph node was found at the time of hysterectomy in only one patient.
- Follow-up in 17 cases was uneventful, although in one half of the cases the follow-up period was 12 months or less.

References

Nielsen GP, Oliva E, Young RH, et. al. Alveolar soft-part sarcoma of the female genital tract. Int J Gynecol Pathol 14:283–292, 1995.

Radig K, Buhtz P, Roessner A. Alveolar soft part sarcoma of the uterine corpus: report of two cases and review of the literature. Pathol Res Pract 194:59–63. 1998.

Malignant Rhabdoid Tumors

- Five examples of malignant rhabdoid tumor have been described in women 39 to 56 years of age, two with intraabdominal metastases at presentation. Four patients with published follow-up data died of tumor-related causes.
- There was endometrial, myometrial, or both types of involvement in each case. The tumors microscopically resembled rhabdoid tumors in other sites. One tumor abutted a grade 1 endometrial endometrioid adenocarcinoma ("collision tumor").
- The differential diagnosis includes the rare endometrial stromal sarcoma with rhabdoid differentiation (page 192).

References

Gaertner EM, Farley JH, Taylor RR, Silver SA. Collision of uterine rhabdoid tumor and endometrioid adenocarcinoma: a case report and review of the literature. Int J Gynecol Pathol 18:396–401, 1999.

Hseuh S, Chang T-C. Malignant rhabdoid tumor of the uterine corpus. Gynecol Oncol 61:142–146, 1996.

RARE BENIGN MESENCHYMAL TUMORS

- This category includes pure lipomas, rhabdomyomas (see Chapter 3), vascular tumors (hemangiomas and lymphagiomas of both typical and cavernous type, hemangiomyomas), and a "fibro-osteochondroma."
- Rare examples of myometrial myxomas have been associated with the complex of myxomas (usually of the heart, skin, and breast) and primary pigmented nodular adrenocortical disease (i.e., Carney's complex). The differential in these cases is with myxoid leiomyoma (page 178).

References

Carney JA, Young WF Jr. Primary pigmented nodular adrenocortical disease and its associations. Endocrinologist 2:6–21, 1992

Chestnut DH, Szpak CA, Fortier KJ, Hammond CB. Uterine hemangioma associated with infertility. South Med J 81:926–928, 1988

Dharkar DD, Kraft JR. Gangadharam D. Uterine lipomas. Arch Pathol Lab Med 105:43–45, 1981.

Fukuoka M, Fujii S, Konishi I, et al. Fibro-osteochondroma of the uterus. Obstet Gynecol 70:517–521, 1987

Gantchev S. Vascular abnormalities of the uterus, concerning a case of diffuse cavernous angiomatosis of the uterus. Gen Diagn Pathol 143:71–74, 1997.

Jameson CF. Angiomyoma of the uterus in a patient with tuberous sclerosis. Histopathology 16:202–203, 1990

CHAPTER 10

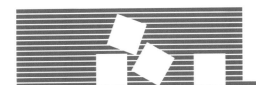

Trophoblastic Lesions, Miscellaneous Primary Uterine Neoplasms, and Metastatic Neoplasms to the Uterus

TROPHOBLASTIC LESIONS

- Gestational trophoblastic lesions can be subdivided into those with villi and those without villi (Table 10–1). The World Health Organization classification of these lesions is given in Table 10–2. The International Federation of Gynecology (FIGO) and tumor, node, and metastasis (TNM) staging for gestational trophoblastic disease is given in Table 10–3.

Hydatidiform Moles

- Hydatidiform moles (HMs) may be partial (PM) or complete (CM) and occur in the reproductive age group (mean age, 28 years; range, 14 to 53). HMs occur in 1 of 4500 deliveries in the United States but are much more common in other parts of the world, particularly the Far East.
- Risk factors include personal or family history of gestational trophoblastic disease (GTD), two or more previous spontaneous abortions, infertility, smoking, and increased maternal age.
- Most CMs are diploid (i.e., only paternal genomic DNA), and most PMs are triploid (one maternal and two paternal haploid sets of DNA, i.e., diandric), although exceptions occur. Most but not all diandric triploid gestations have the features of PMs. Thus studies using flow cytometry, image cytometry, or cytogenetics to determine the DNA content of a mole can aid in their histologic classification.

Complete Hydatidiform Mole

Clinical Features

- CMs have been traditionally considered the most common form of molar pregnancy, but PMs have been underdiagnosed in the past. Two recent studies found that the frequency of PMs is similar to (Fukunaga and Ushigome) or as much as 3 times more common (Jeffers and colleagues) than that of CMs.
- Patients most frequently present with vaginal bleeding or passage of molar vesicles, no fetal heart sounds, and a uterus that is large for gestational age; in one third of cases, however, the uterus is small for dates. Occasionally, CMs are found unexpectedly in elective abortion specimens. The mean gestational age at abortion or evacuation was about 12 weeks in one study.
- About 10% of patients have manifestations related to high human chorionic gonadotropin (hCG) levels (e.g., hyperreactio luteinalis [page 275], preeclampsia in early gestation, hyperemesis gravidarum, hyperthyroidism). Rarely, metastases (e.g., lung, vagina) are a presenting feature.
- Pathologic diagnosis of early CMs (<12 weeks' gestational age) has become more common because of early termination of pregnancy based on abnormal sonographic findings. In one study, 80% of CMs were early compared with only 17% of CMs diagnosed 25 years earlier.

Pathologic Features

- Grossly evident hydropic villi (i.e., villous vesicles) are characteristic of CMs. Because hydrops increases with gestational age, this finding may not be grossly evident in an early CM or if there has been extensive villous disruption by the curette, resulting in collapse of the vesicles.
- The cardinal histologic features of the well-developed CM are diffuse villous hydrops of variable degree and diffuse trophoblastic hyperplasia.

Table 10–1
TYPES OF GESTATIONAL TROPHOBLASTIC DISEASE

With villi
  Hydatidiform mole
    Complete mole
    Partial mole
  Invasive mole
  Persistent mole
  Chorangiocarcinoma
Without villi
  Placental site nodules and plaques
  Placental site trophoblastic tumor
  Epithelioid trophoblastic tumor
  Choriocarcinoma

Table 10–3
TNM AND FIGO STAGING OF GESTATIONAL
TROPHOBLASTIC DISEASE

TNM	FIGO*	Characteristics
Tx		Primary tumor cannot be assessed
T0		No evidence of primary tumor
T1	I	Tumor confined to the uterus
T2	II	Tumor extends by metastases or direct extension to other genital structures: vagina, ovaries, broad ligament, or fallopian tubes
M1a	III	Metastases to the lungs
M1b	IV	Other distant metastases, with or without lung involvement

TNM, tumor, nodes, and metastasis staging: FIGO, International Federation of Gynecology and Obstetrics.
* FIGO stages are subdivided into A (no risk factors), B (one risk factor), and C (two risk factors). The risk factors are serum level of human chorionic gonadotropin of more than 100,000 IU/mL and duration of disease longer than 6 months from the termination of an antecedent pregnancy.

■ In contrast to PMs (discussed later), intact hydropic villi are spherical, exhibit a spectrum of sizes, and may have polypoid or clublike projections. Cisterns (cavities) are present within the larger villi and increase in number with the age of the mole; they may be absent in early CMs.

■ The hyperplastic villous trophoblast tends to be circumferential, ensheathing the entire villus, and involves most of the villi in mature CMs. The degree and extent of trophoblastic hyperplasia, however, can vary, and in some cases is no greater (or less) than that of a normal first-trimester placenta.

■ The cytotrophoblast (CT) may exhibit marked nuclear pleomorphism. The cells of the syncytiotrophoblast (ST), which usually contain cytoplasmic vacuoles, form lacy protrusions from the villous surface. Extravillous or intermediate trophoblast in the intervillous space and the implantation site is also hyperplastic, often showing marked nuclear atypia and hyperchromasia.

■ The molar villi usually appear avascular with routine staining, but immunostaining for CD34 indicates vessels in numbers similar to those of normal villi of 8 to 12 weeks' gestational age.

■ Karyorrhectic debris within the villous stroma is characteristic of CMs; similar debris within vessels occurs in CMs and PMs.

■ Fetal tissues, including intravascular fetal blood cells, are uncommon in CMs but do not exclude the diagnosis. Their presence suggests the possibility of a PM or twin gestation.

■ Early CMs (<12 weeks' gestational age) are more difficult to diagnose because only one third have gross

Table 10–2
WORLD HEALTH ORGANIZATION CLASSIFICATION OF
GESTATIONAL TROPHOBLASTIC LESIONS

Hydatidiform mole
  Complete
  Partial
Invasive hydatidiform mole
Choriocarcinoma
Placental site trophoblastic tumor
Trophoblastic lesions, miscellaneous
  Exaggerated placental site
  Placental site nodule or plaque
Unclassified trophoblastic lesion

vesicles. Microscopic features include variably edematous villi with clubbing and occasional cisterns, focal to circumferential trophoblastic hyperplasia, atypia of intermediate trophoblast, villous karyorrhexis, persistent villous vessels with nucleated erythrocytes in some, and no fetal parts.

Differential Diagnosis

■ A CM should be distinguished from a PM and a hydropic abortus. The differential features are indicated in Table 10–4. Fox indicates that the most reliable features distinguishing an early CM from a PM are the presence in the former of villi with polypoid projections and stromal karyorrhexis.

Behavior

■ Most CMs are cured by uterine evacuation or, if preservation of fertility is not desired, hysterectomy. The serum hCG levels are measured weekly until normal and then monthly for 6 months.

■ Persistent mole
  • Persistence occurs in 8% to 20% of unselected CMs, including early CMs. Hallmarks are failure of hCG levels to normalize after initial evacuation and residual molar villi in a repeat curettage.
  • The risk increases with maternal age older than 40 years, previous molar pregnancy, pre-evacuation hCG levels higher than 100,000 mIU/mL, uterine size large for dates, and the presence of hyperreactio luteinalis (page 275), preeclampsia, hyperthyroidism, or trophoblastic emboli.
  • The management is chemotherapy, hysterectomy, or both, depending on the stage, the hCG levels, and the patient's wishes to retain reproductive function. About 15% of patients with CMs require chemotherapy.

■ Invasive mole (chorioadenoma destruens)
  • Invasion, which occurs with 5% to 10% of CMs, is suggested by failure of hCG levels to decline after evacuation combined with an absence of molar villi on a repeat curettage.

Table 10–4
FEATURES OF COMPLETE HYDATIDIFORM MOLE, PARTIAL HYDATIDIFORM MOLE, AND HYDROPIC ABORTUS*

Feature	Complete Mole	Partial Mole	Hydropic Abortus
Mean of highest hCG level†	184,056 IU/mL	66,259 IU/mL	7942 IU/mL
Mean gestational age at abortion or evacuation†	12.1 wk	15.4 wk	10.7 wk
Amount of placental tissue compared with norm for gestational age	Voluminous (5- to 10-fold increase)‡	Moderately increased (2-fold)	Scanty tissue, far less than normal
Mean maximal villous diameter§	0.71 cm	0.53 cm	0.28 cm
Villous population	Spectrum of sizes	Two populations	Spectrum of sizes
Polypoid/clublike projections from main villi	Common	Rare	Rare
Scalloped villous contours with round trophoblastic inclusions	Rare	Common	Rare
Villous trophoblast	Diffusely hyperplastic	Focally hyperplastic	Attenuated; focal polar trophoblast in some cases
Trophoblastic atypia	Prominent	Rare	None
Cisterns	In many villi	In some villi	In few villi
Karyorrhexis in villous vessels	Common, intense	Absent or inconspicuous	Absent or inconspicuous
Ectatic anastomosing villous vessels	Rare	About 20% (usually second trimester PMs)	Rare
Fetal tissue	Usually none	Present in most cases and abnormal	Usually none
DNA content	Diploid/tetraploid#	Triploid**	Diploid
Chromosome number by cytogenetic analysis	46††	69‡‡	46 ± a few
Postevacuation normalization of hCG without chemotherapy†	78.3 days	62.8 days	46.7 days

hCG, human chorionic gonadotropin; PM, partial mole.
* Adapted from Lage JL, Young RH. Pathology of trophoblastic disease In Clement PB, Young RH (eds): Contemporary Issues in Surgical Pathology, vol 19. Tumors and Tumorlike Lesions of the Uterine Cervix. New York: Churchill Livingstone, 1993.
† Data from Paradinas FJ, Browne P, Fisher RA, et al. A clinical, histopathological and flow cytometric study of 149 complete moles, 146 partial moles and 107 hydropic abortions. Histopathology 28:101–109, 1996.
‡ Excludes first trimester complete moles.
§ Data from Lage JM, Mark SD, Roberts DJ, et al. A flow cytometric study of 137 fresh hydropic placentas: correlation between types of hydatidiform moles and DNA ploidy. Obstet Gynecol 79:403–410, 1992.
# A minority are haploid, triploid, or polyploid.
** A minority are haploid, diploid, tetraploid, aneuploid, or polyploid.
†† Usually 46,XX; 15% to 25% are 46,XY.
‡‡ 69,XXX; 69,XXY; or 69,XYY.

- The diagnosis requires the presence of myometrial and vascular invasion by the molar villi (findings that usually require a hysterectomy, an uncommon procedure in this clinical setting) or the presence of metastases (e.g., lungs, vagina, vulva, broad ligament) containing molar villi.
- The management is the same as for persistent mole.
■ Postmolar choriocarcinoma occurs in about 5% of cases (see Choriocarcinoma, page 218.)
■ Nodules of intermediate trophoblast (Silva and colleagues)
  - These patients present with vaginal bleeding or a mildly elevated serum hCG. Two cases were associated with choriocarcinoma. Successful treatment includes curettage, hysterectomy, chemotherapy, or combinations thereof.
  - This lesion may be similar or identical to the epithelioid trophoblastic tumor (page 227).
■ Recurrent GTD (i.e., new episode of GTD after complete postchemotherapy remission) is indicated by a repeat elevation of the hCG level after three consecutive weekly normal hCG values.
  - One hundred percent cure rates are achieved for these patients who have nonmetastatic disease or good-prognosis metastatic disease (i.e., lung or vaginal metastases, hCG levels <40,000 mIU/mL, short duration of disease).
- Cure rates of 83% have been achieved even in patients with bad-prognosis metastatic disease (i.e., brain, liver, kidney metastases; hCG levels >40,000 mIU/mL; gestational tumor after a term gestation).

Partial Hydatidiform Mole

Clinical Features

■ Women with PMs usually present with late first-trimester bleeding (range, 9th to 34th weeks) and a uterus that is small or normal for dates. Less common presentations include no fetal heart beat or preeclampsia. One study found that early PMs (< 12 weeks) accounted for 90% of PMs in the 1990s, compared with 62% in the 1980s.
■ The pre-evacuation hCG levels are in the low to normal range for gestational age, although rarely they are as high as in CMs. The most common pre-evacuation diagnosis is a missed or incomplete abortion; most PMs escape clinical detection.

Pathologic Features

- On gross examination, villous vesicles in PMs tend to be smaller and less numerous than those of a CM and are admixed with a population of normal-sized villi.
- The two cardinal findings on microscopic examination are two populations of villi, with one composed of enlarged hydropic villi and the other composed of normal to fibrotic villi that are normal in size or small for gestational age, and focal trophoblastic hyperplasia.
- The larger villi have irregularly scalloped contours, resulting in trophoblastic invaginations and round gland-like trophoblastic inclusions within the villous stroma.
- Cisterns within the hydropic villi are fewer than in a CM, and their presence is not required for a diagnosis of PM. Large cavitated villi (>4 mm in greatest dimension), however, were found to be the single most useful criterion in one study of possible PMs for distinguishing between triploid cases (those most likely to be true PMs) and nontriploid cases.
- The stroma contains well-formed blood vessels that usually contain fetal erythrocytes. Thin-walled, ectatic, anastomosing vascular channels occur within the villi in about 20% of second-trimester PMs, and their presence suggests the diagnosis.
- Villous trophoblastic hyperplasia is usually more focal and mild than in CMs, although it occasionally can be exuberent and circumferential. ST tends to predominate, often as small papillary projections or knuckles extending from the villous surfaces.
- Fetal tissues are present in most cases. The nature of such tissues depends on the gestational age and whether fetal death has occurred. Rarely, liveborn but nonviable malformed infants are delivered at term.

Differential Diagnosis

- CM and hydropic abortus (see Table 10–4).
- CM associated with a normal twin pregnancy. In this circumstance, the vesicular villi have the features of a CM rather than a PM, and ploidy can indicate that, although all the villi are diploid, some are biparental, and others are androgenetic.
- Triploid conceptus with a maternal extra haploid set of DNA. These conceptuses lack the gross and microscopic features of PM, except for an excess of trophoblastic knuckles in some cases.

Behavior

- The management of PMs is similar to that of CMs.
- Sequelae including persistence, invasion, metastasis, and postmolar choriocarcinoma are much less common than after CMs. Only about 5% of patients with a PM have persistent or metastatic disease.

References

Fox H. Differential diagnosis of hydatidiform moles. Gen Diagn Pathol 143:117–125, 1997.

Fukunaga M, Ushigome S. Early partial hydatidiform mole: prevalence, histopathology, DNA ploidy, and persistence rate [Abstract]. Mod Pathol 12:117A, 1999.

Fukunaga M, Ushigome, S. Incidence of hydatidiform mole: a 10-year (1989–1998) prospective clinicopathological and flow cytometric study [Abstract]. Mod Pathol 12:117A, 1999.

Jeffers MD, O'Dwyer P, Curran B, et al. Partial hydatidiform mole: a common but underdiagnosed condition. Int J Gynecol Pathol 12:315–323, 1993.

Lage JM, Bagg A. Hydatidiform moles: DNA flow cytometry, image analysis and selected topics in molecular biology. Histopathology 28:379–382, 1996.

Lage JM, Mark SD, Roberts DJ, et al. A flow cytometric study of 137 fresh hydropic placentas: correlation between types of hydatidiform moles and DNA ploidy. Obstet Gynecol 79:403–410, 1992.

Lage JL, Young RH. Pathology of trophoblastic disease. In Clement PB, Young RH (eds): Contemporary Issues in Surgical Pathology, vol 19: Tumors and Tumorlike Lesions of the Uterine Corpus and Cervix. New York: Churchill Livingstone, 1993.

Montes M, Roberts D, Berkowitz RS, Genest DR. Prevalence and significance of implantation site trophoblastic atypia in hydatidiform moles and spontaneous abortions. Am J Clin Pathol 105:411–416, 1996.

Mosher R, Genest DR. Early complete hydatidiform mole: prevalence, histopathology, and persistence [Abstract]. Mod Pathol 11:109A, 1998.

Paradinas FJ. The histological diagnosis of hydatidiform moles. Curr Diagn Pathol 1:24–31, 1994.

Paradinas FJ, Browne P, Fisher RA, et al. A clinical, histopathologial and flow cytometric study of 149 complete moles, 146 partial moles and 107 hydropic abortions. Histopathology 28:101–109, 1996.

Qiao S, Nagasaka T, Nakashima N. Numerous vessels detected by CD34 in the villous stroma of complete hydatidiform moles. Int J Gynecol Pathol 16:233–238, 1997.

Redline RW, Hassold T, Zaragoza MV. Prevalence of the partial molar phenotype in triploidy of maternal and paternal origin. Hum Pathol 28:505–511, 1998.

Sheikh SS, Lage JM. Diagnosis of early complete hydatidiform mole: a study of 35 cases [Abstract]. Mod Pathol 11:114A, 1998.

Silva EG, Tornos C, Lage J, et al. Multiple nodules of intermediate trophoblast following hydatidiform moles. Int J Gynecol Pathol 12:324–332, 1993.

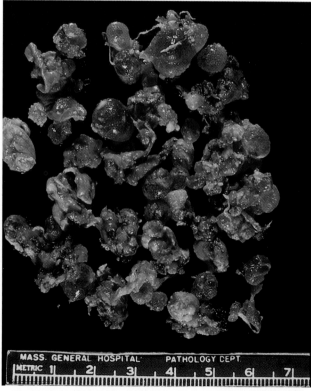

Figure 10–1. Complete hydatidiform mole in a curettage specimen.

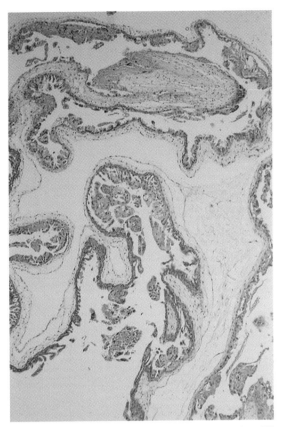

Figure 10–2. Complete hydatidiform mole, showing molar villi with cisterns and circumferential trophoblastic hyperplasia.

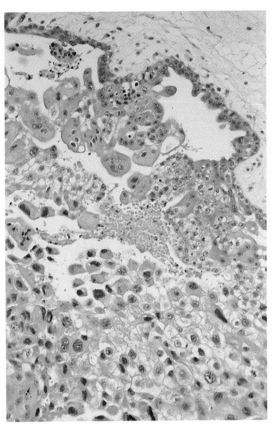

Figure 10–3. Complete hydatidiform mole with marked trophoblastic hyperplasia of villous and extravillous trophoblast. The latter in particular shows marked nuclear atypia (*bottom*).

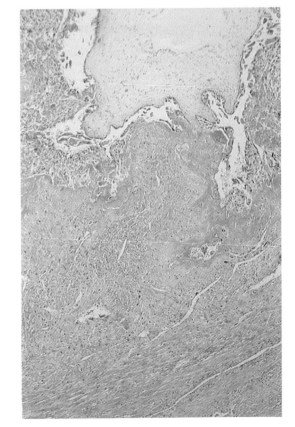

Figure 10–4. Invasive hydatidiform mole. A molar villus with hyperplastic trophoblast is in the myometrium.

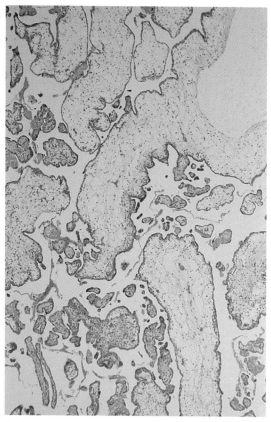

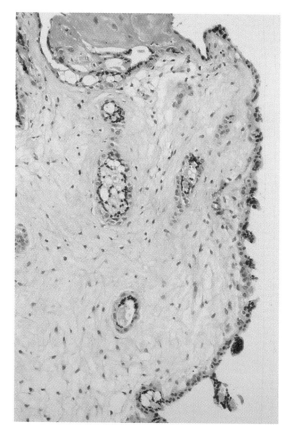

Figure 10–5. Partial hydatidiform mole. Notice the two populations of villi (i.e., large hydropic villi with scalloped outlines and small fibrotic villi) and focally hyperplastic trophoblast, including trophoblastic knuckles. The villus in the upper right contains a cistern.

Figure 10–6. Partial hydatidiform mole. Notice the trophoblastic knuckles (*bottom right*) and trophoblastic inclusions.

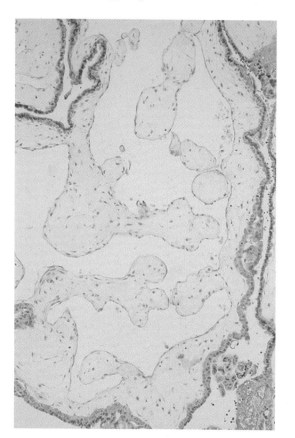

Figure 10–7. Partial hydatidiform mole. Notice the ectatic, anastomosing villous vessels.

Hydropic Abortus

- The evacuated tissue in a hydropic abortus (HA) is typically scanty, with complete examination of the chorionic tissue (which should be performed in any suspected case) requiring only one or two blocks.
- Hydropic villi on gross or microscopic examination can equal in size those of a CM, but such villi are rare, and the mean villous size is much smaller than that of CMs and PMs (see Table 10–4). Cisterns are rare and less than 3 mm in diameter or absent. Some villi may be avascular and fibrotic or contain vessels with fetal erythrocytes.
- In contrast to CMs and PMs, the trophoblast of an HA is usually diffusely attenuated or, if present, is predominantly polar and less atypical than that of CMs and PMs.
- Villous trophoblastic hyperplasia, however, is common in abortions with an abnormal karyotype, especially triploidy abortuses. Between 4% and 14% of HAs are triploid as a result of an extra maternal set of chromosomes. Hyperplasia similar to that of CMs is frequent in cases of trisomy 7, 15, 21, and 22. Hyperplasia is more common in abortions older than 8.5 weeks' gestational age, those that lack uniformly hydropic villi, and those without fetal tissue.
- The differential diagnosis is usually with a PM (see Table 10–4). There is considerable interobserver variation in making this distinction, and in occasional cases, a definite histologic distinction between the two lesions may not be possible, necessitating hormonal surveillance. Diploidy essentially excludes a PM; triploidy, however, may indicate PM or a triploid HA, as discussed previously.

References

Fox H. Differential diagnosis of hydatidiform moles. Gen Diagn Pathol 143:117–125, 1997.

Lage JL, Young RH. Pathology of trophoblastic disease. In Clement PB, Young RH (eds): Contemporary Issues in Surgical Pathology, vol 19: Tumors and Tumorlike Lesions of the Uterine Corpus and Cervix. New York: Churchill Livingstone, 1993.

Paradinas FJ. The histological diagnosis of hydatidiform moles. Curr Diagn Pathol 1:24–31, 1994.

Redline RW, Hassold T, Zaragoza M. Determinants of villous trophoblastic hyperplasia in spontaneous abortions. Mod Pathol 11:762–768, 1998.

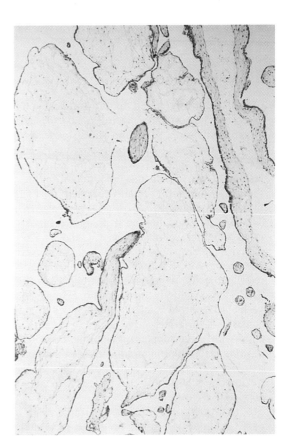

Figure 10–8. Hydropic abortus. Notice the diffusely attenuated trophoblast. A villus (*upper right*) contains a cistern.

Choriocarcinoma

Clinical Features

- Choriocarcinomas (CCAs) in the United States complicate about 1 of 25,000 pregnancies; they are about twice as common among blacks and other races compared with whites. The incidence of CCA is 20 to 40 times higher in Asia, Africa, and Latin America.
- Hertig and Mansell found that 50% of CCAs were preceded by a CM (CCA followed 1 of 40 molar gestations), 25% by an abortion (1 of 15,386), 22.5% by a normal pregnancy (1 of 160,000), and 2.5% by an ectopic pregnancy (1 of 5333). Later studies have found a lower risk of CCA after CMs.
- Rarely, CCA is found in a term placenta; such tumors are often small. If missed on pathologic examination of the placenta, these tumors may account for some CCAs after a "normal" pregnancy.
- The most common presentation is vaginal bleeding and an elevated serum hCG level; the levels may be very high if metastases exist. Some patients may be asymptomatic because the CCA is confined to the myometrium.
- Many patients have manifestations related to hematogenous spread, most commonly to the lungs, brain, liver, kidney, intestinal tract, and skin. In rare cases, CCA is initially diagnosed in the infant; in a few such cases, no tumor is found in the mother.

Pathologic Features

- CCA is typically a red to brown, fleshy tumor with extensive hemorrhage, necrosis, and destructive myometrial invasion. The superficial part of the tumor may be polypoid. Rare primary tumors arise in the cervix. Some patients with metastatic CCA have no residual gross or microscopic tumor in the hysterectomy specimen, presumably because of regression of the primary tumor.
- The sine qua non for the histologic diagnosis of CCA is an admixture of malignant CT and ST. A plexiform pattern is commonly formed by large sheets of CT alternating with ST (which may line spaces containing red blood cells) or intermediate trophoblast (IT).
- The ST has densely eosinophilic cytoplasm and large vesicular multiple nuclei with clumped chromatin. CT consists of discrete, mononucleate, oval to polygonal cells with clear to pale cytoplasm, convoluted nuclei, macronucleoli, and numerous mitoses that may be atypical. The IT resembles that in placental site trophoblastic tumors (PSTT) (discussed later), including marked atypia.
- The term *atypical CCA* has been applied to rare cases of CCA in which some or all of the tumor consists predominantly of CT or IT with scanty ST. This pattern may be found in the primary or metastatic tumor, and in some cases, it occurs after chemotherapy. Some or all of these tumors may be identical to epithelioid trophoblastic tumor (page 227).
- CCAs usually invade the myometrium and myometrial vessels. Extensively infarcted and hemorrhagic CCAs may require numerous sections to demonstrate viable tumor, which is often confined to a thin peripheral zone surrounding necrotic areas.

Differential Diagnosis

- Trophoblastic tissue obtained in curretage specimens other than CCA. Elston and Bagshawe classified such tissues as villous trophoblast, simple trophoblast, and trophoblast suspicious for CCA; IT should also be added to this list.
  - Villous trophoblast. The interpretation rests on evaluation of the associated villi (i.e., normal, HA, PM, or CM). Evacuation of a spontaneous abortion may leave residual avillous trophoblast that may be sampled in a later procedure. Knowledge of the history in such cases and examination of the prior specimen containing normal villi is important to avoid a misdiagnosis of CCA.
  - Simple trophoblast. Small amounts of undifferentiated trophoblast exist in the absence of villi. Such trophoblast includes the often malignant-appearing and invasive trophoblast of the normal blastocyst. The diagnosis of simple trophoblast requires sampling the entire specimen and that the trophoblast be scanty and exhibit only minimal differentiation toward CT or ST. Vascular invasion does not exclude the diagnosis.
  - IT. IT can be derived from a normal or exaggerated implantation site, a placental site nodule or plaque, or a PSTT. The differential diagnosis of CCA with PSTT is discussed on page 224.
  - Trophoblast suspicious for CCA. Moderate to large amounts of trophoblast exist with differentiation into ST and CT or IT. No villous tissue is present, and there is endomyometrial invasion. Women with suspicious or simple trophoblast in a currettage specimen who have had a previous normal pregnancy almost always develop malignant or metastatic trophoblastic disease, in contrast to only 50% of patients with similar findings who have had a previous molar gestation.
- Nongestational CCA, including CCAs of germ cell origin (see Chapter 15) metastatic to the uterus and endometrial adenocarcinomas with trophoblastic differentiation (see Chapter 8).
- Chorangiocarcinoma (page 220).
- Other malignant epithelial and mesenchymal tumors. These tumors are most likely to be simulated by atypical CCAs. The diagnosis is facilitated by a history of a recent pregnancy or mole, thorough sampling to demonstrate ST, and the serologic and immunohistochemical detection of hCG. Other markers of ST that may be useful in this differential include inhibin and human placental lactogen (hPL).

Behavior

- The survival rate after chemotherapy for patients with choriocarcinoma is about 80% of all patients and about 70% in those with metastases.

- Adverse prognostic factors include pretreatment hCG levels higher than 100,000 mIU/mL, liver or brain metastases, lack of immediate chemotherapy because of a delayed diagnosis, and in postterm CCAs, an interval of more than 4 months since the antecedent pregnancy.
- Death is usually caused by hemorrhagic events within the metastases or pulmonary insufficiency from tumor burden or the effects of treatment.

References

Brewer JI, Mazur MT. Gestational choriocarcinoma: its origin in the placenta during seemingly normal pregnancy. Am J Surg Pathol 5: 267–277, 1981.

Elston CW, Bagshawe KD. The diagnosis of trophoblastic tumours from uterine curettings. J Clin Pathol 25:111–118, 1972.

Hertig AT, Mansell H. Tumors of the female sex organs. Part 1. Hydatidiform mole and choriocarcinoma. In Atlas of Tumor Pathology, sect 9, fasc 33. Washington, DC: Armed Forces Institute of Pathology, 1956;7.

Lage JL, Young RH. Pathology of trophoblastic disease. In Clement PB, Young RH (eds): Contemporary Issues in Surgical Pathology, vol 19. Tumors and Tumorlike Lesions of the Uterine Corpus and Cervix. New York: Churchill Livingstone, 1993.

Mazur MT. Metastatic gestational choriocarcinoma: unusual pathologic variant following therapy. Cancer 63:1370–1377, 1989.

Paradinas FJ. The histological diagnosis of hydatidiform moles. Curr Diagn Pathol 1:24–31, 1994.

Pelkey TJ, Frierson HF Jr, Mills SE, Stoler MH. Detection of the alpha-subunit of inhibin in trophoblastic neoplasia. Hum Pathol 30:26–31, 1999.

Rodabaugh KJ, Bernstein MR, Goldstein DP, Berkowitz RS. Natural history of postterm choriocarcinoma. J Reprod Med 43:75–80. 1998.

Shih I-M, Kurman RJ. Immunohistochemical localization of inhibin-alpha in the placenta and gestational trophoblastic lesions. Int J Gynecol Pathol 18:144–150, 1999.

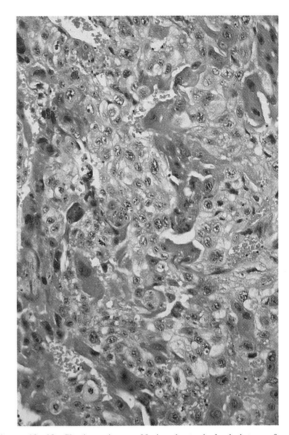

Figure 10–10. Choriocarcinoma. Notice the typical admixture of cytotrophoblast and syncytiotrophoblast and focal hemorrhage.

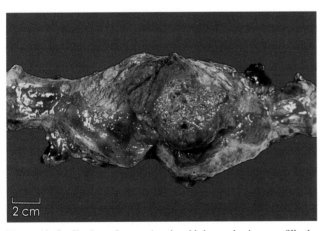

Figure 10–9. Choriocarcinoma. A polypoid, hemorrhagic mass fills the endometrial cavity.

Chorangiocarcinoma

- These are rare tumors composed of nonhydropic villi lined by malignant trophoblast associated with a villous vascular proliferation.
- There have been no malignant sequelae in the mothers or infants.

Reference

Trask C, Lage JM, Roberts DJ. A second case of "chorangiocarcinoma" presenting in asymptomatic twin pregnancy: choriocarcinoma in situ with associated villous vascular proliferation. Int J Gynecol Pathol 13:87–91, 1994.

Lesions of Intermediate Trophoblast

Normal Intermediate Trophoblast

- According to Shih and colleagues, there appear to be three subpopulations of IT with distinctive morphologic and immunohistochemical features (Table 10–5): villous IT (i.e., IT cells in the trophoblastic columns) and the two types of IT that originate from it, implantation site IT and chorion-type IT.
- The lesional cells of exaggerated placental site and its neoplastic counterpart, placental site trophoblastic tumor, are derived from implantation site IT, whereas placental site nodule and its neoplastic counterpart, epithelioid trophoblastic tumor, are derived from chorionic-type IT.
- In the absence of chorionic villi and fetal tissues, the identification of IT cells in a curettage specimen is useful in establishing the diagnosis of an intrauterine pregnancy and excluding an ectopic pregnancy. In such cases, it is important that IT cells are distinguished from decidual cells, which they can resemble.
  - In contrast to the nuclei of decidual cells, the nuclei of IT cells tend to be more variable in size and shape, are more hyperchromatic, and often have convoluted outlines because of clefts of variable length and orientation.
  - IT cells, in contrast to decidual cells, are immunoreactive for cytokeratin and the other antigens indicated in Table 10–5.

References

Daya D, Sabet L. The use of cytokeratin as a sensitive and reliable marker for trophoblastic tissue. Am J Clin Pathol 95:137–141, 1991.

Kurman RJ, Main CS, Chen H-C. Intermediate trophoblast: a distinctive form of trophoblast with specific morphological, biochemical and functional features. Placenta 5:349–370, 1984.

Kurman RJ, Young RH, Main CA, et al. Immunohistochemical localization of placental lactogen and chorionic gonadotropin in the normal placenta and trophoblastic tumors with emphasis on intermediate trophoblast and the placental-site trophoblastic tumor. Int J Gynecol Pathol 3:101–121, 1984.

O'Connor DM, Kurman RJ. Intermediate trophoblast in uterine curettings in the diagnosis of ectopic pregnancy. Obstet Gynecol 72:665–670, 1988.

Shih I-M Kurman RJ. Immunohistochemical localization of inhibin-alpha in the placenta and gestational trophoblastic lesions. Int J Gynecol Pathol 18:144–150, 1999.

Shih I-M, Seidman JD, Kurman RJ. Placental site nodule and characterization of distinctive types of intermediate trophoblast. Hum Pathol 30:687–694, 1999.

Wan SK, Lam PWY, Pau MY, Chan JKC. Multiclefted nuclei: a helpful feature for identification of intermediate trophoblastic cells in uterine curetting specimens. Am J Surg Pathol 16:1226–1232, 1992.

Yeh I-T, O'Connor DM, Kurman RJ. Intermediate trophoblast: further immunocytochemical characterization. Mod Pathol 3:282–287, 1990.

Exaggerated Placental Site

- Exaggerated placental site (EPS) refers to the occasionally extensive involvement of the myometrium at the placental site by IT. Synonymous terms used in the past have included *syncytial endometritis* and *exaggerated placental site reaction.*
- An EPS may be worrisome if the atypia that is seen in the giant cells at the placental base and the extent to which they can infiltrate the myometrium is not known to be a normal phenomenon.
- The differential diagnosis is with PSTT. Features favoring PSTT are a mass and confluent aggregates of mitotically active cells that destroy the myometrium rather than infiltrate between its muscle bundles. Nuclear atypia is not helpful, because it is striking in EPS. The Ki-67 proliferative index is much higher in PSTTs than in an EPS (14% ± 6.9% versus near zero).
- In the rare curettage specimens for which a definite distinction between a PSTT and an EPS cannot be made, follow-up should include a repeat curettage and serum hCG and hPL determinations, although the latter may be negative in the presence of a PSTT. Imaging studies of the uterus may reveal a mass in cases of PSTT.

Placental Site Nodules and Plaques

- Placental site nodules and plaques (PSNPs) are foci of chorionic-type IT that are usually an incidental finding in the reproductive era but occasionally are discovered in the early postmenopausal years. PSNPs are nonneoplastic lesions that have an uneventful follow-up (except for subsequent PSNPs in rare patients) and no malignant potential.
- The interval from the most recent known pregnancy may be up to 8 years (average of 3 years in one series). Some patients have a history of tubal ligation several years before presentation or a history of HM.
- PSNPs are usually found in an endometrial curettage specimen but occasionally in an endocervical or hysterectomy specimen. PSNPs were grossly visible in only 25% of cases in one series, had a maximal size of 2.5 cm, and have a predilection for the lower uterine segment, the endometrium immediately above this area, or the endocervix.
- Microscopic examination reveals single or multiple, typically well-circumscribed nodules or plaques, sometimes with lobulated margins, on the surface of the endometrium, within it, within the adjacent myometrium, or in the superficial endocervical stroma.
- PSNPs typically contain densely eosinophilic hyalinized material surrounding single cells or those in small, ir-

Table 10–5
MORPHOLOGIC FEATURES, GROWTH PATTERN, AND IMMUNOSTAINING OF DIFFERENT POPULATIONS OF INTERMEDIATE TROPHOBLASTIC CELLS

Type of Intermediate Trophoblast	Location	Cellular Morphology	Growth Pattern	Immunostaining*					
				hPL	Mel-CAM	OF-FN	PLAP	HNK-1†	Ki-67
Villous	Trophoblastic column	Polyhedral with clear to eosinophilic cytoplasm	Cohesive	−/+++‡	−/++++‡	−/++++‡	−	+++	>90%
Implantation site	Placental site (basal plate)	Pleomorphic with abundant eosinophilic cytoplasm	Infiltrative	+++	+++	+++	+	−	0%
Chorionic type	Chorion laeve of fetal membrane	Uniform and round with clear or eosinophilic cytoplasm	Cohesive	+	+	+	++	−	5%

hPL, human placental lactogen; OF-FN, oncofetal fibronectin; PLAP, placental alkaline phosphatase; Mel-CAM, melanoma cell adhesion molecule (also known as MUC18 and CD146).
*The percentage of positive cells was scored as follows: −, no staining; +, <25%; ++, 25%–75%; +++, >75%.
† Data from Shih IM, et al. Distribution of cells bearing the HNK-1 epitope in the human placenta. Placenta 18:67–74, 1997.
‡ The percentage of positive cells increased from the proximal to the distal end of the trophoblastic column.
Reproduced from Shih I-M, Seidman JD, Kurman RJ. Placental site nodule and characterization of distinctive types of intermediate trophoblast. Hum Pathol 30:687–694, 1999.

221

regular clusters, cords, or rounded nests. Focal necrosis, cystic degeneration, or calcification may occur.

■ Small, rounded pseudopods often project from the periphery of PSNPs and may be associated with brightly eosinophilic fibrin-like material that may resemble keratin; a misdiagnosis of an early invasive squamous cell carcinoma may result.

■ The lesional cells (IT) are often degenerative, with cytoplasm that varies from abundant and amphophilic to scanty and clear or vacuolated; rounded eosinophilic hyaline bodies may be seen. One or more irregular, often lobulated nuclei vary from hyperchromatic to pale and vesicular; mitotic figures are typically absent or rare.

■ PSNPs are occasionally associated with evidence of a remote pregnancy in the form of necrotic or hyalinized chorionic villi.

■ The IT cells are strongly and diffusely immunoreactive for cytokeratin, placental alkaline phosphatase, and epithelial membrane antigen and less frequently and more focally for hPL and hCG.

Differential Diagnosis

■ Placental site trophoblastic tumor (PSTT). Features favoring or indicating a diagnosis of PSNP rather than PSTT include small size, circumscription, extensive hyalinization, degenerative appearance of the cells, and lack or rarity of mitotic figures.

■ Hyalinized squamous cell carcinoma. The typical features of PSNPs and the absence of squamous differentiation help distinguish PSNPs from this rare carcinoma of the cervix.

■ Hyalinized decidua. The distinction between decidual cells and IT has been discussed (page 220).

■ EPS. PSNP differs from EPS by its distinctive shape, circumscription, extensive hyalinization, and lack of association with a current or recent pregnancy.

■ Epithelioid trophoblastic tumor (page 227).

■ Nodules of IT after HM (page 213).

References

Huettner PC, Gersell D. Placental site nodule: a clinicopathologic study of 38 cases. Int J Gynecol Pathol 13:191–198, 1994.

Shih I-M, Seidman JD, Kurman RJ. Placental site nodule and characterization of distinctive types of intermediate trophoblast. Hum Pathol 30:687–694, 1999.

Shih I-M, Kurman RJ. Immunohistochemical localization of inhibin-alpha in the placenta and gestational trophoblastic lesions. Int J Gynecol Pathol 18:144–150, 1999.

Shitabata PK, Rutgers JL. The placental site nodule: an immunohistochemical study. Hum Pathol 25:1295–1301, 1994.

Young RH, Kurman RJ, Scully RE. Proliferations and tumors of intermediate trophoblast of the placental site. Semin Diagn Pathol 5:223–237, 1988.

Young RH, Kurman RJ, Scully RE. Placental site nodules and plaques: A clinicopathologic analysis of 20 cases. Am J Surg Pathol 14:1001–1009, 1990.

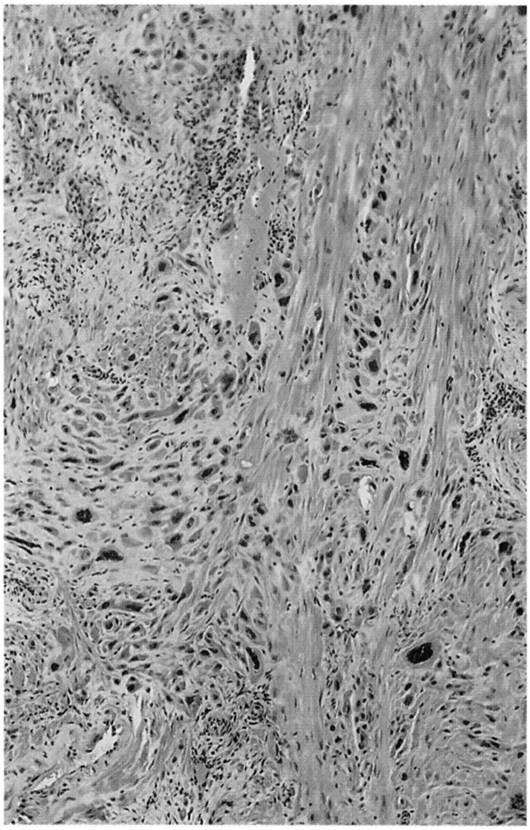

Figure 10–11. Exaggerated placental site.

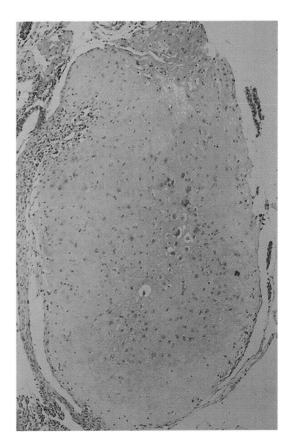

Figure 10–12. Placental site nodule. Notice the circumscribed border, intermediate trophoblastic cells with clear cytoplasm, and hyalinized stroma.

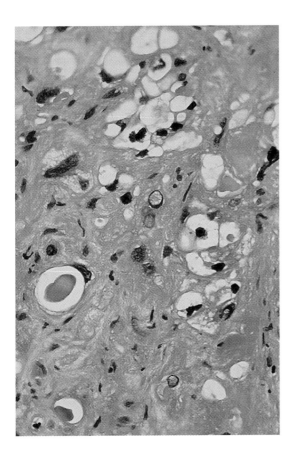

Figure 10–13. Placental site nodule. The intermediate trophoblast cells focally contain cytoplasmic vacuoles and eosinophilic hyaline bodies and have hyperchromatic nuclei that vary considerably in size and shape.

Placental Site Trophoblastic Tumor

Clinical Features

- PSTTs typically occur in women of reproductive age (mean, 28 years), but rare tumors have occurred as late as 5 years after the menopause. Amenorrhea, menorrhagia, or metrorrhagia and an enlarged uterus are common presenting manifestations.
- There is usually a history of an antecedent normal pregnancy. In about 5% of cases, there is a history of a spontaneous abortion or an HM, although a history of the latter is much less common than in cases of choriocarcinoma.
- The serum hCG levels are slightly elevated in about 45% and moderately elevated in about 30% of the cases and normal in the remainder. The clinical findings, alone or in combination, may lead to misdiagnoses of a normal pregnancy or a missed abortion.
- Uncommon or rare presentations or manifestations include
  - Spontaneous uterine perforation (although this is more often a complication of uterine curettage of a PSTT)
  - Virilization from ovarian stromal hyperthecosis caused by elevated hCG levels
  - Erythrocytosis or hyperprolactinemia, which disappears after removal of the tumor
  - The nephrotic syndrome caused by a distinctive glomerular lesion probably related to chronic intravascular coagulation

Gross Pathologic Features

- A mass is usually visible except in occasional cases in which most of the lesion has been removed by curettage. The mass may be largely polypoid, sometimes filling the endometrial cavity, or predominantly infiltrative of the myometrium, which may be perforated. Involvement of the cervix has occasionally resulted in a polypoid endocervical mass.
- PSTTs may be well circumscribed, but the border with the underlying myometrium is often ill defined, or there is diffuse uterine enlargement without a discrete mass. The sectioned surface is typically soft; tan, white, or yellow; and in some cases, focally or massively hemorrhagic. Rare findings have included cystification and spread to an ovary.

Microscopic Features

- PSTTs are composed of an ill-defined mass of polyhedral, rounded, or occasionally spindle-shaped cells of IT, most of which are mononucleate but some of which are binucleate or multinucleate. Rare multinucleated cells may resemble ST.
- The cytoplasm is typically abundant and amphophilic but may be eosinophilic or clear. The nuclei vary from small, round, and pale to large, convoluted, and hyperchromatic or smudgy. Nucleoli are usually visible and may be prominent. Intranuclear cytoplasmic pseudoinclusions may be seen.

- The mitotic count averages about 2 mitotic figures (MF) per 10 high-power-fields (HPF), although in rare tumors it exceeds 5 MF per 10 HPF; abnormal mitotic figures are not uncommon.
- PSTTs usually exhibit myoinvasion as cellular aggregates or single cells dissecting between muscle fibers. Rare PSTTs have a pushing border and the hyalinization characteristic of a placental site nodule. The tumor extends to the serosa in about one third of cases and occasionally extends to the endocervix.
- PSTTs frequently invade blood vessels, with tumor cells and fibrin replacing the vessel walls and lining the lumen. Fibrin-like material may be focally or diffusely distributed throughout the tumor.
- The endometrium adjacent to a PSTT may be the site of a decidual reaction, the Arias-Stella phenomenon, or both. Chorionic villi are present only rarely.
- PSTTs usually stain diffusely for cytokeratin, hPL, and inhibin; hCG is present only focally.

Differential Diagnosis

- EPS (page 220).
- CCA (page 218).
  - Differential features indicating or favoring CCA include a hemorrhagic mass, an admixture of CT and ST, and extensive immunoreactivity for hCG. CCAs usually lack the fibrinoid material and the distinctive pattern of vascular invasion of PSTTs. The Ki-67 proliferative index is much higher in choriocarcinomas than in PSTTs (Shih and Kurman).
  - Poorly differentiated PSTTs may not be readily distinguishable from atypical CCAs (page 218), and some CCAs have areas that resemble PSTTs. A definite diagnosis of pure PSTT probably should not be made until a hysterectomy specimen has been thoroughly examined.
- Sarcomas, particularly epithelioid leiomyosarcoma (see Chapter 9). The clinical setting, associated symptoms, and pattern of growth of the PSTT usually differ from those of a leiomyosarcoma. Immunoreactivity for hCG and hPL and negative staining for desmin favor PSTT.
- Uterine carcinomas (e.g., clear cell carcinoma, cervical squamous cell carcinomas with necrosis and hyalinization).
  - The clinical and laboratory features of PSTT (young patient age, amenorrhea, history of pregnancy, or HM, elevated hCG level in some cases) and its microscopic features (characteristic myoinvasion and vascular invasion, hPL or hCG immunoreactivity, progestational endometrial changes) differ from those of most uterine carcinomas.
  - The presence of more typical invasive squamous cell carcinoma or adjacent carcinoma in situ and keratinization also facilitate the differential diagnosis with hyalinizing squamous cell carcinoma.

Behavior

- In addition to rare patients with PSTT who have died as a result of uterine perforation, 15% to 20% of

PSTTs have had a malignant behavior with metastasis. The malignant PSTTs frequently spread to the lungs, liver, and central nervous system.

■ The malignant tumors have usually had more than 4 MF per 10 HPF, whereas clinically benign PSTTs with rare exceptions have had mitotic rates below this level. Rare malignant PSTTs have had only 2 MF per 10 HPF, indicating the necessity for long-term follow-up of all patients with PSTTs.

■ Some of the fatal tumors have had extensive necrosis and many cells with clear cytoplasm, in contrast to the usual absence of these findings in benign tumors.

■ PSTTs are typically resistant to chemotherapy compared with other types of gestational trophoblastic disease. Successful treatment of metastatic disease with chemotherapy, however, has been reported.

References

Brewer CA, Adelson MD, Elder RC. Erythrocytosis associated with a placental-site trophoblastic tumor. Obstet Gynecol 79:846–849, 1992.

Finkler NJ, Berkowitz RS, Driscoll SG, et al. Clinical experience with placental site trophoblastic tumors at the New England Trophoblastic Disease Center. Obstet Gynecol 71:854–857, 1988.

Fukunaga M, Ushigome S. Metastasizing placental site trophoblastic tumor: an immunohistochemical and flow cytometric study of two cases. Am J Surg Pathol 17:1003–1010, 1993.

Kurman RJ, Young RH, Main CA, et al. Immunohistochemical localization of placental lactogen and chorionic gonadotropin in the normal placenta and trophoblastic tumors with emphasis on intermediate trophoblast and the placental-site trophoblastic tumor. Int J Gynecol Pathol 3:101–121, 1984.

Nagamani M, Kaspar HG, Van Dinh T, et al. Hyperthecosis of the ovaries in a woman with a placental site trophoblastic tumor. Obstet Gynecol 76:931–935, 1990.

Pelkey TJ, Frierson HF Jr, Mills SE, Stoler MH. Detection of the alpha-subunit of inhibin in trophoblastic neoplasia. Hum Pathol 30:26–31, 1999.

Rhoton-Vlasak A, Wagner JM, Rutgers JL, et al. Placental site trophoblastic tumor: human placental lactogen and pregnancy-associated major basic protein as immunohistologic markers. Hum Pathol 29:280–288, 1998.

Shih I-M, Kurman RJ. Immunohistochemical localization of inhibin-alpha in the placenta and gestational trophoblastic lesions. Int J Gynecol Pathol 18:144–150, 1999.

Shih I-M, Kurman RJ. Ki-67 labelling index in the differential diagnosis of exaggerated placental site, placental site trophoblastic tumor, and choriocarcinoma: a double immunohistochemical staining technique using Ki-67 and Mel-CAM antibodies. Hum Pathol 28:27–33, 1998.

Swisher E, Drescher CW. Metastatic placental site trophoblastic tumor: long-term remission in a patient treated with EMA/CO chemotherapy. Gynecol Oncol 68:62–65, 1998.

Young, RH, Scully RE. Placental-site trophoblastic tumor: current status. Clin Obstet Gynecol 27:248–257, 1984.

Young RH, Scully RE, McCluskey RT. A distinctive glomerular lesion complicating placental site trophoblastic tumor: report of two cases. Hum Pathol 16:35–42, 1985.

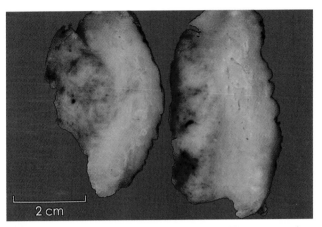

Figure 10–14. Placental site trophoblastic tumor. Two cross sections show a mass that is only focally hemorrhagic, and invades the myometrium.

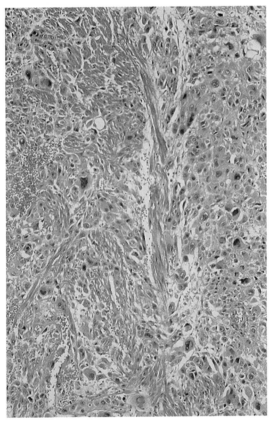

Figure 10–15. Placental site trophoblastic tumor. Sheets of tumor cells (i.e., neoplastic intermediate trophoblast) invade between bundles of myometrial smooth muscle.

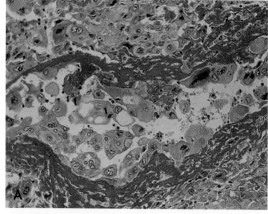

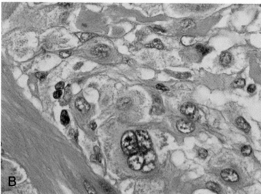

Figure 10–16. Placental site trophoblastic tumor. *A,* The tumor cells have invaded a myometrial vessel and replaced the normal endothelial cells. Notice the fibrin deposits in the vessel wall. *B,* High-power view of tumor cells shows the typical cytologic features. Notice the amphophilic cytoplasm and striking variation in nuclear size. The multinucleated cells differ in appearance from syncytiotrophoblast.

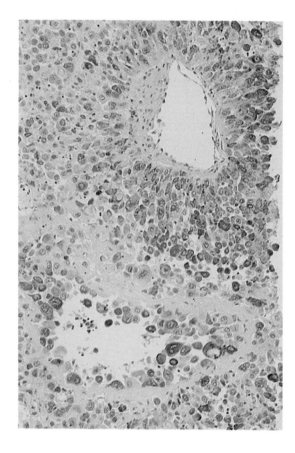

Figure 10–17. Placental site trophoblastic tumor. The tumor cells are immunoreactive for human placental lactogen.

Epithelioid Trophoblastic Tumor

- The term epithelioid trophoblastic tumor (ETT) has been applied by Shih and Kurman to a rare trophoblastic tumor distinct from CCA and PSTT that resembles a poorly differentiated carcinoma. ETTs are composed of chorion-type IT.
- The patients typically present with abnormal vaginal bleeding, a history of a recent or remote gestational event, and an elevated hCG level. Rare patients present with an extrauterine ETT without a history of a uterine lesion.
- Gross examination reveals a discrete, hemorrhagic, solid and cystic, deeply invasive tumor that may involve any part of the uterus, including the cervix.
- ETTs have nodular expansile borders surrounded by a lymphocytic infiltrate and are composed of uniform, rounded mononucleated IT cells in nests and cords associated with eosinophilic hyaline material and necrosis. The mean mitotic count was 2 MF per 10 HPF in the Shih study.
- The cells are diffusely immunoreactive for cytokeratin, EMA, and inhibin-alpha but are only focally reactive for hPL, hCG, PLAP, and Mel-CAM.
- Two of 12 uterine ETTs metastasized, and one of two cases that presented with extrauterine disease was fatal.

Differential Diagnosis

- PSTT. In contrast to ETTs, PSTTs have an infiltrative and sheetlike pattern, prominent vascular invasion, larger and more pleomorphic cells, and strong diffuse immunoreactivity for hPL and Mel-CAM.
- Squamous cell carcinoma of cervix. These tumors, in contrast to ETTs, may contain keratin and lack immunoreactivity for inhibin and cytokeratin 18.
- Epithelioid smooth muscle tumors. These tumors usually contain a component of typical smooth muscle cells and express muscle markers but lack immunoreactivity for inhibin-alpha, hCG, and hPL.

References

Parkash V, Tan LK, Carcangiu ML. Poorly differentiated trophoblastic tumor simulating squamous cell carcinoma [Abstract]. Mod Pathol 11: 111A, 1998.

Shih I-M, Kurman RJ. Epithelioid trophoblastic tumor: a neoplasm distinct from choriocarcinoma and placental site trophoblastic tumor simulating carcinoma. Am J Surg Pathol 22:1393–1403, 1998.

Tumor-like Abnormalities of Placentation

Placental Polyps

- Placental polyps refer to polypoid fragments of retained placental tissue obtained by postpartum curettage. Retention probably results from focal failure or delay in the involution of the placental bed. Microscopic examination reveals retained villi admixed with blood, fibrin, and uteroplacental vessels.

Placenta Accreta, Increta, and Percreta

- Abnormal adherence of the placenta to the myometrium can lead to failure of normal postpartum placental separation. Placental villi may adhere to but not invade the myometrium (i.e., placenta accreta), invade into the myometrium (i.e., placenta increta), or invade through the myometrium (i.e., placenta percreta). The latter can result in potentially fatal uterine perforation and hemoperitoneum.
- Predisposing factors include placenta previa, prior cesarean section, previous placental retention requiring manual removal, and prior curettage.
- Microscopic examination of the hysterectomy specimen or occasionally the placenta reveals villi in contact with or invading myometrial smooth muscle without intervening decidua.

References

deRoux SJ, Prendergast NC, Adsay NV. Spontaneous uterine rupture with fatal hemoperitoneum due to placenta accreta percreta: a case report and review of the literature. Int J Gynecol Pathol 18:82–86, 1999.

Fox H. Placenta accreta, 1945–69. Obstet Gynecol 27:475–486, 1972.

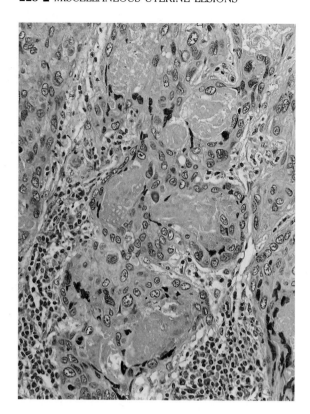

Figure 10–18. Epithelioid trophoblastic tumor. Tumor nests contain hyaline material that was eosinophilic, resembling keratin. A lymphocytic infiltrate is at the tumor margin. (From Shih I-M, Kurman RJ. Epithelioid trophoblastic tumor: a neoplasm distinct from choriocarcinoma and placental site trophoblastic tumor simulating carcinoma. Am J Surg Pathol 22:1393–1403, 1998.)

Figure 10–19. Placental polyp.

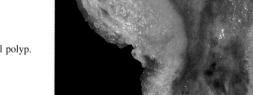

MISCELLANEOUS PRIMARY TUMORS

Adenomatoid Tumors

General Features

- Adenomatoid tumors are benign tumors of mesothelial origin that are often misinterpreted grossly and sometimes even microscopically as leiomyomas.
- The patients are usually of reproductive age, and the tumors are typically an incidental pathologic finding, but occasional larger examples have been symptomatic. The presenting feature in one case was signet-ring–like cells within an endometrial curettage specimen.

Pathologic Features

- On gross examination, the tumors are typically solitary, subserosal, myometrial masses, often located near a cornu and smaller than 4 cm in diameter, with a solid, grey-tan to grey-pink to yellow, trabeculated cut surface that is usually less well circumscribed than that of a leiomyoma.
- Unusual gross features include a diameter larger than 10 cm, diffuse replacement of the myometrium, multiple tumors, bilateral cornual tumors, transmural involvement with endometrial extension, predominantly or entirely cystic tumors (fluid-filled locules separated by thin septa), an exophytic serosal component, and an association with a similar tumor in the fallopian tube.
- Microscopic examination reveals distinctive patterns of mesothelial cells scattered irregularly on a background of myometrial smooth muscle; the border of the lesion is often ill defined.
- The patterns, in order of frequency, include
  - Adenoid pattern: anastomosing glandlike spaces lined by cuboidal cells that often contain cytoplasmic vacuoles
  - Angiomatoid pattern: larger spaces lined by flattened cells mimicking a vascular tumor
  - "Solid" pattern: polygonal cells with eosinophilic cytoplasm and occasional vacuoles growing in sheets, columns, or plexiform cords
  - Cystic pattern: large spaces lined by flattened cells separated by thin fibrous septa
  - Papillary pattern: a rare pattern characterized by papillae with stromal cores that resemble those in well-differentiated papillary mesotheliomas
- The lesional cells contain bland, round to oval, mitotically inactive nuclei with no or rare mitotic figures.
- The "stroma" of the tumor characteristically consists of hyperplastic myometrial smooth muscle. In many cases, the smooth muscle may predominate to the extent that the diagnosis of an adenomatoid tumor may be overlooked. Occasionally, there is also a fibrous stroma that varies from loose and edematous to hyalinized.
- In some cases, continuity with the uterine serosa is seen; it may be focally replaced by tumor or exhibit papillary mesothelial hyperplasia, mesothelial inclusions, endosalpingiosis, fibrous adhesions, or combinations thereof.
- Mucin stains reveal the usual presence of acid mucins (predominantly hyaluronic acid) within the vacuoles and lumina of the tumor. The neoplastic cells are typically immunoreactive for cytokeratin and vimentin.

Differential Diagnosis

- Leiomyoma. Gross features favoring adenomatoid tumor include a posterior, especially cornual, subserosal location; abnormalities of the overlying serosa; tan-gray to pink to yellow color (rather than white); and absence of a sharply circumscribed border. Microscopically, leiomyomas lack the characteristic patterns of adenomatoid tumors.
- Vascular tumors. Unlike adenomatoid tumors, these tumors immunoreact for endothelial markers but not cytokeratin.
- Metastatic adenocarcinoma, particularly of signet-ring cell type. These tumors, in contrast to adenomatoid tumors, contain neutral mucin and exhibit malignant nuclear features.
- Peritoneal inclusion cysts (versus cystic adenomatoid tumors). Peritoneal inclusion cysts (see Chapter 20) may be adherent to the uterine serosa, but in contrast to adenomatoid tumors, they do not involve the myometrium.

References

Carlier MT, Dardick I, Lagace AF, Sreeram V. Adenomatoid tumor of the uterus: presentation in endometrial curettings. In J Gynecol Pathol 5:69–74, 1986.

Chan JKC, Fong MH. Composite multicystic mesothelioma and adenomatoid tumour of the uterus: different morphological manifestations of the same process? Histopathology 29:375–377, 1996.

De Rosa G, Boscaino A, Terracciano LM, Giordano G. Giant adenomatoid tumors of the uterus. Int J Gynecol Pathol 11:156–160, 1992.

Goddard MR, Grant JW. Adenomatoid tumours: a mucin histochemical and immunohistochemical study. Histopathology 20:57–61, 1992.

Livingstone EG, Guis MS, Pearl ML, et al. Diffuse adenomatoid tumor of the uterus with a serosal papillary cystic component. Int J Gynecol Pathol 11:288–292, 1992.

Otis CN. Uterine adenomatoid tumors: immunohistochemical characteristics with emphasis on Ber-EP4 immunoreactivity and distinction from adenocarcinoma. Int J Gynecol Pathol 15:146–151, 1996.

Quigley JC, Hart WR. Adenomatoid tumors of the uterus. Am J Clin Pathol 76:627–635, 1981.

Srigley JR, Colgan TJ. Multifocal and diffuse adenomatoid tumor involving uterus and fallopian tube. Ultrastruct Pathol 12:351–355, 1988.

Tiltman AJ. Adenomatoid tumours of the uterus. Histopathology 4:437–443, 1980.

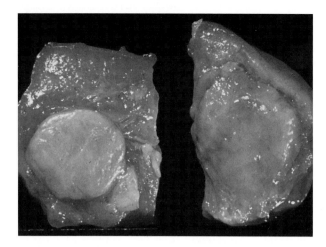

Figure 10–20. Adenomatoid tumor within the myometrium (*right*) is contrasted with a typical uterine leiomyoma (*left*). The adenomatoid tumor, which is subserosal, has a less well delineated border than the leiomyoma.

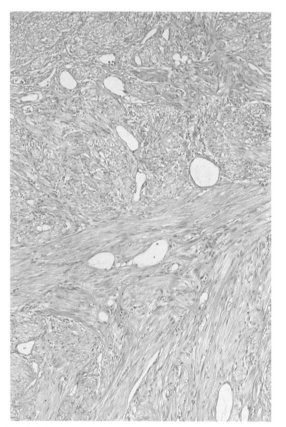

Figure 10–21. Adenomatoid tumor. Vessel-like spaces lined by flattened cells are widely separated by hyperplastic myometrial smooth muscle.

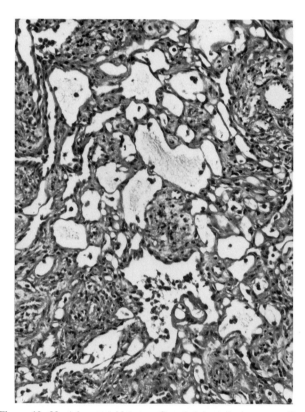

Figure 10–22. Adenomatoid tumor. Crowded, irregular spaces are lined by flattened and cuboidal cells.

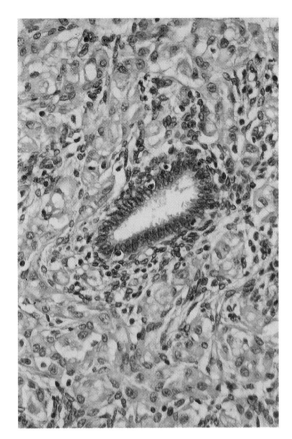

Figure 10–23. Adenomatoid tumor involving the endometrium. Notice the signet ring–like cells. The tumor initially was identified in a curettage specimen, and the prehysterectomy diagnostic considerations included signet ring adenocarcinoma and an epithelioid smooth muscle tumor.

Germ Cell Tumors

Yolk Sac Tumor

- About 12 cases of yolk sac tumors (YSTs) have been reported in the cervix or the cervix and vagina of infants or the endometrium or outer aspect of the uterus in women of reproductive age.
- The presentation is typically vaginal bleeding, pelvic pain, or combinations thereof; an elevated serum level of alpha-fetoprotein is usual.
- Two thirds of patients are cured by excision of the tumor (usually hysterectomy) and chemotherapy. The other patients, one of whom did not receive chemotherapy, died of tumor.
- Grossly, the tumors are typically soft, friable, grey-tan polypoid masses that are less than 6 cm in the maximum dimension. The cervical stroma or myometrium is usually invaded, sometimes deeply.
- The tumors are usually pure YSTs with typical patterns on microscopic examination. One juxtauterine YST had an endometrioid-like pattern and was associated with a teratoma.

References

Clement PB, Young RH, Scully RE. Extraovarian pelvic yolk sac tumors. Cancer 62:620–626, 1988.

Copeland LJ, Sneige N, Ordonez NG, et al. Endodermal sinus tumor of the vagina and cervix. Cancer 55:2558–2565, 1985.

Joseph MG, Fellows FG, Hearn SA. Primary endodermal sinus tumor of the endometrium. Cancer 65:297–302, 1990.

Ohta M, Sakakibara K, Mizuno K, et al. Successful treatment of primary endodermal sinus tumor of the endometrium. Gynecol Oncol 31:357–364, 1988.

Pileri S, Martinelli G, Serra L, Bazzocchi F. Endodermal sinus tumor arising in the endometrium. Obstet Gynecol 56:391–396, 1980.

Teratomas

- About 12 uterine lesions have been reported as "mature teratomas" in women of reproductive age who presented with abnormal vaginal bleeding and a polypoid, solid to cystic, endocervical or endometrial mass. The tumors were composed of an admixture of mature heterotopic tissues; one tumor consisted entirely of lung tissue.
- There is one report of a 10-cm pedunculated endometrial mass composed of endometrial adenocarcinoma

admixed with immature neuroepithelium, squamous and mucinous epithelium, cartilage, bone, and a tooth bud; glial implants were found on the peritoneal surfaces of the ovaries.

■ The differential diagnosis of mature teratomas includes heterotopic tissues of fetal origin. Some authorities believe that most or all mature uterine "teratomas" represent implants of fetal tissue.

■ The differential diagnosis of immature teratomas includes neuroectodermal tumors (page 232).

References

Ansah-Boateng Y, Wells M, Poole DR. Coexistent immature teratoma of the uterus and endometrial adenocarcinoma complicated by gliomatosis peritonei. Gynecol Oncol 21:106–110, 1985.

Bell MC, Schmidt-Grimminger D, Connor MG, Alvarez RD. A cervical teratoma with invasive squamous cell carcinoma in an HIV-infected patient: a case report. Gynecol Oncol 60:475–479, 1996.

Dallenbach-Hellweg G, Wittlinger H. Benign solid teratoma of the uterus. Beitr Pathol Bd 158:307–314, 1976.

Khoor A, Fleming MV, Purcell CA, et al. Mature teratoma of the uterine cervix with pulmonary differentiation. Arch Pathol Lab Med 119:848–850, 1995.

Martin E, Scholes J, Richart RM, Fenoglio CM. Benign cystic teratoma of the uterus. Am J Obstet Gynecol 135:429–431, 1979.

Mihailovici A, Radulescu D, Bendescu M, Paraschiv L. Teratoma of the uterine cervix. Morphol Embryol 135:191–193, 1976.

Hanai J, Tsuji M. Uterine teratoma with lymphoid hyperplasia. Acta Pathol Jpn 31:153–159, 1981.

Iwanaga S, Ishii H, Nagano H, et al. Mature cystic teratoma of the uterine cervix. Asia Oceania J Obstet Gynaecol 16:363–366, 1990.

Tyagi SP, Saxena K, Rizvi R, Langley FA. Foetal remnants in the uterus and their relation to other uterine heterotopia. Histopathology 3:339–345, 1979.

Neuroectodermal Tumors

Primitive Neuroectodermal Tumors

■ Ten uterine primitive neuroectodermal tumors (PNETs) have been described, mostly in postmenopausal women, although two women were young adults. The typical presentation was abnormal vaginal bleeding and an enlarged uterus, a pelvic mass, or a visible lesion on the cervix. One half of the patients had stage II to IV disease, including evidence of pelvic nodal or distant metastases in some cases.

■ One of the patients with stage I tumor and all but one of the patients with higher-stage disease died of tumor progression within 2 years of presentation.

■ Eight tumors arose in the corpus: one involved the corpus and cervix, and one was confined to the cervix. The cervical tumor was considered a primary endocervical extraosseous Ewing's sarcoma or PNET because of immunoreactivity for p30/32^{mic2} and characteristic ultrastructural findings.

■ Gross examination has usually revealed polypoid endometrial or endocervical masses with mural invasion in most of them and soft, fleshy, and gray to white sectioned surfaces.

■ The tumors contained a wide range of neural, glial, ependymal, and medulloepithelial differentiation on microcopic examination. One tumor exhibited cartilagi-

nous differentiation. Eight tumors were pure, whereas two were admixed with another neoplasm (an endometrial stromal sarcoma and a grade 1 endometrial adenocarcinoma).

■ Differential diagnosis
  • Other neuroectodermal tumors discussed in this section, mature and immature teratomas with neuroectodermal differentiation (discussed earlier), and malignant müllerian mixed tumors with neuroectodermal differentiation (page 197).
  • Fetal neuroectodermal remnants, in contrast to PNETs, are usually microscopic and multifocal, consist predominantly or entirely of mature glial tissue, and are occasionally associated with other heterotopic elements, such as cartilage, bone, and adipose tissue.

References

Cenacchi G, Pasquinelli G, Montanaro L, et al. Primary endocervical extraosseus Ewing's sarcoma/PNET. Int J Gynecol Pathol 17:83–88, 1998.

Daya D, Lukka H, Clement PB. Primitive neuroectodermal tumors of the uterus: a report of four cases. Hum Pathol 23:1120–1129, 1992.

Fragetta F, Magro G, Vasquez E. Primitive neuroectodermal tumour of the uterus with focal cartilaginous differentiation. Histopathology 30: 483–485, 1997.

Molyneux AJ, Deen S, Sundaresan V. Primitive neuroectodermal tumour of the uterus. Histopathology 21:584–585, 1992.

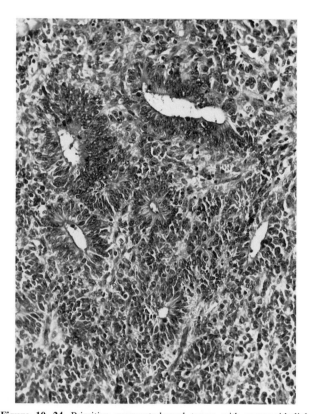

Figure 10–24. Primitive neuroectodermal tumor with neuroepithelial-type tubules.

Pigmented Neuroectodermal Tumor of Infancy

- Of the two uterine examples of pigmented neuroectodermal tumor of infancy (PNTI) (retinal anlage tumor, melanotic progonoma) that have been reported, one was a polypoid, invasive endocervical mass in a 57-year-old woman who was free of tumor 5 years after hysterectomy. The other tumor was a polypoid endometrial mass in a 69-year-old woman who died of tumor 2 months after presentation.
- Microscopic examination of the endocervical tumor revealed a cellular tumor composed of small, nonpigmented cells with scanty cytoplasm (neuroblasts) and melanin-laden cuboidal cells (melanocytes) with mildly pleomorphic nuclei in nests, cords, sheets, tubules, and pseudopapillae. The endometrial tumor consisted of a malignant müllerian mixed tumor with focal PNTI.

References

Schulz DM. A malignant, melanotic neoplasm of the uterus, resembling the "retinal anlage" tumors. Arch Pathol 28:524–532, 1957.

Sobel N, Carcangiu ML. Primary pigmented neuroectodermal tumor of the uterine cervix. Int J Surg Pathol 2:31–36, 1994.

Uterine Gliomas

- One of the two reported such tumors was in a 15-year-old girl who presented with vaginal bleeding. Examination of the hysterectomy specimen revealed a polypoid endometrial tumor that was myoinvasive and that microscopically was a low-grade fibrillary astrocytoma. The patient had an uneventful 6-year follow-up. The other case was not described in detail but was associated with metastatic nodules on the uterine serosa.
- Gliomas can be distinguished from uterine PNETs by their monotonous proliferation of pure glial tissue and an absence of the diverse differentiation that characterizes PNETs. They are also usually less cellular and less mitotically active.

References

Liao SY, Choi BH. Expression of glial fibrillary acidic protein by neoplastic cells of müllerian origin. Virchows Arch (Cell Pathol) 52: 185–193, 1986.

Young RH, Kleinman GM, Scully RE. Glioma of the uterus: report of a case with comments on histogenesis. Am J Surg Pathol 5:695–699, 1981.

Other Neuroectodermal Tumors

- Rare reported examples of neuroectodermal tumors include neurofibromatosis, benign paraganglioma of typical and melanotic types, malignant paraganglioma, ganglioneuroma, granular cell tumors, and benign and malignant schwannomas.
- Malignant schwannomas can be confused with leiomyosarcomas and endocervical stromal sarcomas and can occasionally have a biphasic pattern that can suggest a malignant müllerian mixed tumor. Rarely, the tumors are pigmented. Immunoreactivity for S-100 and vimentin and negativity for cytokeratin, HMB-45, and desmin facilitate the diagnosis.
- A "pigmented myomatous neurocristoma" formed a focally pigmented myometrial mass that was approximately 4 cm in diameter and composed of pigmented and nonpigmented melanocytes in a matrix of altered smooth muscle cells.

References

Beham A, Schmid C, Fletcher CDM, et al. Malignant paraganglioma of the uterus. Virchows Arch A 420:453–457, 1992.

Fingerland A. Ganglioneuroma of the cervix uteri. J Pathol Bacteriol 47: 631–634, 1938.

Gersell DJ, Fulling KH. Localized neurofibromatosis of the female genitourinary tract. Am J Surg Pathol 13:873–878, 1989.

Gordon MD, Weilert M. Ireland K. Plexiform neurofibromatosis involving the uterine cervix, endometrium, myometrium, and ovary. Obstet Gynecol 88:699–701, 1996.

Keel SB, Clement PB, Prat J, Young RH. Primary malignant schwannoma of the uterine cervix: a study of three cases. Int J Gynecol Pathol 17:223–230, 1998.

Martin PC, Pulitzer DR, Reed RJ. Pigmented myomatous neurocristoma of the uterus. Arch Pathol Lab Med 113:1291–1295, 1989.

Tavassoli FA. Melanotic paraganglioma of the uterus. Cancer 58:942–948, 1986.

Terzakis JA, Opher E, Melamed J, et al. Pigmented melanocytic schwannoma of the uterine cervix. Ultrastruct Pathol 14:357–366, 1990.

Young TW, Thrasher TV. Nonchromaffin paraganglioma of the uterus: a case report. Arch Pathol Lab Med 106:608–609, 1982.

Wilms' Tumor

- Four uterine cases have been reported in females 11 to 22 years of age. Bulky polypoid, pedunculated masses were attached to the endocervix, the lower segment, or the endometrium. One tumor was superficially invasive and infiltrated the pouch of Douglas and the left broad ligament.
- Microscopic examination revealed typical Wilms' tumors. Smooth and skeletal muscle were identified in three cases, one of which also contained hyaline cartilage.
- One patient had an intraabdominal recurrence at 7 months; the other patients had benign clinical courses.

Reference

Benatar B, Wright C, Freinkel AL, Cooper K. Primary extrarenal Wilms' tumor of the uterus presenting as a cervical polyp. Int J Gynecol Pathol 17:277–280, 1998.

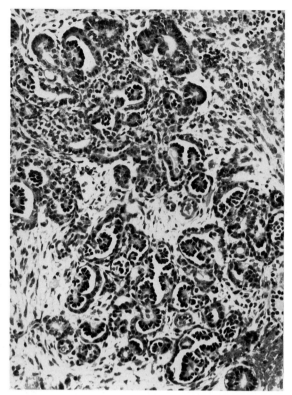

Figure 10–25. Uterine Wilms' tumor.

Malignant Melanoma

Clinical Features

■ About 45 primary or probably primary malignant melanomas have been reported in the cervix, a site of origin consistent with melanin-containing cells (presumably melanocytes) found in cervical epithelium in 3% of women.

■ The tumors have occurred over a wide age range (26 to 83 years), although most women have been between 50 and 70 years of age (mean, 56 years). The presenting symptoms are usually vaginal bleeding or discharge, occasionally an abnormal Pap smear, or manifestations of distant metastases.

■ Clinical or gross examination typically reveals an exophytic polypoid cervical mass up to 7 cm in diameter. Brown to blue-black pigmentation of the tumor has been observed in one half of the cases. Contiguous or noncontiguous vaginal involvement has been identified in some cases.

■ Metastatic tumor at the time of diagnosis was found in 60% of cases. About 90% of patients with follow-up information have died of tumor, usually within less than 2 years of presentation. The 5-year survival rate for patients with stage I tumors is somewhat better (25%). A difference in the median survival rate between stages IA and IB (48 versus 14.5 months) has also been found.

Pathologic Findings

■ The tumors are microscopically similar to melanomas in other sites, being typically composed of nests and sheets of polygonal to spindle-shaped cells with mitotically active pleomorphic nuclei and fine, brown intracytoplasmic pigment. About 25% of tumors are amelanotic.

■ In situ melanoma (typically the lentiginous type) within the adjacent mucosa has been found in only one third of the reported cases, a finding that provides evidence that the tumor is primary rather than metastatic. In the absence of in situ changes or melanosis in occasional cases, microscopic distinction from metastatic melanoma may be difficult or impossible.

Differential Diagnosis

■ As in other sites, cervical melanomas can mimic a variety of tumors, and the pathologist always should consider melanoma when dealing with a poorly differentiated tumor.

■ Undifferentiated carcinoma. Immunoreactivity for S-100 and HMB-45 antigens and negativity for cytokeratin strongly favor or establish a diagnosis of melanoma over that of undifferentiated carcinoma. The presence of in situ melanoma (in cases of primary melanoma), cytoplasmic pigment, or both are additional supportive features.

■ Leiomyosarcoma (versus melanomas with a prominent spindle cell component). Features that are diagnostic or supportive of spindle cell melanoma include the presence of melanin, in situ melanoma, immunoreactivity for S-100 and HMB-45 antigens, and absence of immunoreactivity for markers of smooth muscle differentiation. Absence of in situ changes helps distinguish melanomas from pigmented malignant schwannomas (page 233).

■ Alveolar soft part sarcomas (see Chapter 9). These tumors, in contrast to melanoma, have uniform, mitotically inactive nuclei and cytoplasm that contains periodic acid–Schiff–positive diastase-resistant granules and crystals.

■ Benign melanotic lesions (see Chapter 4).

Reference

Clark KC, Butz WR, Hapke MR. Primary malignant melanoma of the uterine cervix: case report with world literature review. Int J Gynecol Pathol 18:265–273, 1999.

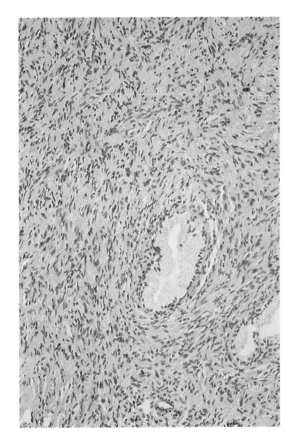

Figure 10–26. Malignant melanoma of the uterine cervix. Malignant spindle cells surround benign endocervical glands. The tumor had an associated in situ component.

UTERINE INVOLVEMENT BY HEMATOPOIETIC AND HISTIOCYTIC DISORDERS

Uterine Involvement as the Initial Site of Malignant Lymphoma

■ Only 0.5% of extranodal non-Hodgkin's lymphoma were considered of uterine origin in one study. There is a dominant mass in the cervix in 90% of cases; the remainder involve the corpus or both the cervix and corpus.

■ The high cure rate with local therapy supports a uterine origin in these cases, but some cases may represent uterine involvement by occult, more widespread lymphomas.

■ The tumors may be misdiagnosed by the pathologist because lymphomas are unexpected at this site and may be confused with other types of malignant neoplasm or an inflammatory process.

Clinical Features

■ The tumors occur over a wide age range (15 to 90 years), with median and mean ages of 41 and 44 years, respectively, in patients with cervical tumors in the two largest series. Three B-cell lymphomas of the endometrium occurred in women in their sixties.

■ The most common symptom is vaginal bleeding; vaginal discharge, dyspareunia, and pain may also occur. Some patients are asymptomatic, with the tumor being detected by a Pap smear or as an incidental microscopic finding.

■ Pelvic examination may reveal a cervical mass, usually nonulcerated, that may result in a diffusely enlarged, barrel-shaped cervix, with or without involvement of local structures (vagina, paracervical tissues, pelvic side walls, lower uterine segment). In cases with corpus involvement, a pelvic mass or an enlarged uterus may be palpable.

Gross Features

- Cervical tumors may be a polypoid exophytic mass, a solitary or multinodular submucosal cervical mass, or a circumferential tumor with a barrel-shaped cervix. Extensive local spread (e.g., parametria, vagina) is common. Corpus tumors may form a polypoid endometrial mass, diffusely coat the endometrium, or grow as one or more myometrial or endomyometrial infiltrative masses.
- The cut surfaces are fleshy, rubbery, or firm, and white to tan to yellow. Areas of hemorrhage, necrosis, or both may be present.

Microscopic Features

- Most uterine lymphomas are B-cell lymphomas of the diffuse large cell type. There are also reports of other subtypes, including small noncleaved cell (non-Burkitt's type), diffuse small cleaved cell type, diffuse mixed small and large cell type, diffuse large cell types (both not otherwise specified and immunoblastic), and follicular lymphomas.
- Rare types have included Burkitt's lymphoma, intravascular lymphoma, B-cell lymphomas of marginal zone type, and T-cell lymphoma.
- A subepithelial band of uninvolved stroma is often present in cervical lymphomas that tend to surround and entrap normal endocervical glands. The cervical tumors are usually deeply invasive, occurring as circumscribed nodules with pushing margins. Perivascular spread is common with follicular lymphomas.
- Prominent sclerosis is common in cases of cervical tumors, resulting in epithelial-like patterns, including single cells, cords, or groups of cells separated by fine fibrils or dense bands of collagen. In the sclerotic areas, the neoplastic cells are frequently spindle shaped, resembling fibroblasts.
- Benign lymphocytes and, often, plasma cells are immediately beneath the epithelium and at the periphery of the neoplastic infiltrate in cervical tumors.
- Endometrial lymphomas do not tend to have the sclerosis that is a feature of many cervical lymphomas and resemble lymphomas as seen elsewhere.

Differential Diagnosis

- Lymphoma-like lesions in the cervix and corpus (see Chapters 4 and 7).
- Secondary lymphomatous involvement of cervix and corpus. This type of involvement is much more common than primary uterine lymphomas and has been documented at autopsy in up to 10% of women with disseminated lymphoma.
  - Clinical manifestations are often absent, but vaginal bleeding or discharge have been the presenting complaint in a few cases.
  - Secondary involvement is usually by one of the more common subtypes of non-Hodgkin's lymphoma, but the uterus rarely is involved by disseminated Burkitt's lymphoma, angiotropic lymphoma, or Hodgkin's disease.

- Small cell carcinomas (SCCs) may be difficult to distinguish from a lymphoma, particularly in a small biopsy specimen, if the tissue is not optimally fixed, processed, or both.
  - SCCs tend to obliterate normal structures, whereas lymphoma tends to infiltrate with relative preservation of the normal glands and typically spares the subepithelial stroma.
  - The carcinoma cells have molded nuclei with finely granular or smudged chromatin, whereas the lymphoma cells lack nuclear molding and have more coarsely clumped chromatin; rosette-like structures or focal squamous or glandular differentiation in the tumor indicate SCC.
  - Immunoreactivity for epithelial markers (cytokeratins) and negativity for leukocyte common antigen and other lymphoid markers favor SCC.
- Lymphoepithelioma-like carcinoma of the cervix (see Chapter 5). Cohesive nests or trabecular arrangements of epithelial cells (with cytokeratin immunoreactivity) and a benign appearance of the lymphoid cells exclude lymphoma.
- Sarcoma, including endometrial stromal sarcoma, in cases of lymphomas with sclerosis and spindled nuclei.
  - Features favoring lymphoma include an admixture of small cleaved cells and large noncleaved cells, a focal nodular pattern, and focal perivascular infiltration.
  - Features favoring a diagnosis of endometrial stromal sarcoma include a network of uniform small vessels, cells that mimic normal endometrial stromal cells, and immunoreactivity for vimentin and actin.

Behavior

- Uterine lymphomas have a favorable prognosis when treated by hysterectomy and postoperative irradiation, chemotherapy, or both.
- Harris and Scully found overall and relapse-free 5-year survival rates of 77% and 70%, respectively, for all stages, and 93% and 84% for stage IE. None of the patients with stage IE disease who received definitive local initial therapy relapsed.

References

Andrews SJ, Hernandez E, Woods J, Cook B. Burkitt's-like lymphoma presenting as a gynecologic tumor. Gynecol Oncol 30:131–136, 1988.

Davey D, Munn R, Smith LW, Cibull ML. Angiotrophic lymphoma: presentation in uterine vessels with cytogenetic studies. Arch Pathol Lab Med 114:879–882, 1990.

Ferry JA, Young RH. Malignant lymphoma of the genitourinary tract. Curr Diagn Pathol 4:145–169, 1997.

Harris NL, Scully RE. Malignant lymphoma and granulocytic sarcoma of the uterus and vagina: a clinicopathologic analysis of 27 cases. Cancer 53:2530–2545, 1984.

Masunaga A, Abe M, Tsujii E, et al. Primary uterine T cell lymphoma. Int J Gynecol Pathol 17:376–379, 1998.

Muntz HG, Ferry JA, Flynn D, et al. Stage 1E primary malignant lymphomas of the uterine cervix. Cancer 68:2023–2032, 1991.

Perren T, Farrant M, McCarthy K, et al. Lymphomas of the cervix and upper vagina: a report of five cases and a review of the literature. Gynecol Oncol 44:87–95, 1992.

Raggio ML, Bostrom SG, Harden EA. Hodgkin's lymphoma of the

uterus presenting as refractory pelvic inflammatory disease. J Reprod Med 33:827–830, 1988.

Stroh EL, Besa PC, Cox JD, et al. Treatment of patients with lymphomas of the uterus or cervix with combination chemotherapy and radiation therapy. Cancer 75:2392–2399, 1995.

van de Rijn M, Kamel OW, Chang PP, et al. Primary low-grade endometrial B-cell lymphoma. Am J Surg Pathol 21:187–194, 1997.

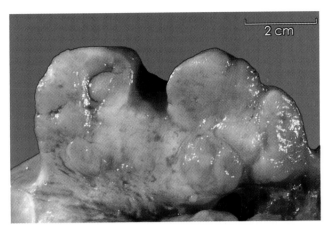

Figure 10–27. Malignant lymphoma of uterine cervix (sectioned surface). Homogeneous, fleshy tumor involves the entire thickness of the cervical wall.

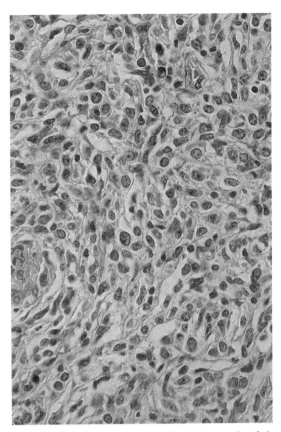

Figure 10–29. Malignant lymphoma of the uterine cervix of the diffuse, large cell type. Some of the tumor cells are spindle shaped. Note intercellular collagen.

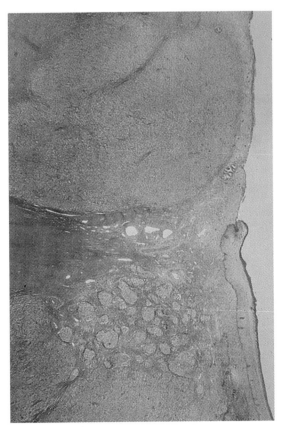

Figure 10–28. Malignant lymphoma of the uterine cervix of the diffuse, large cell type with focal follicular areas (*bottom*).

Uterine Involvement by Leukemia

In Patients With Recognized Leukemia

■ Leukemic cells are found in cervicovaginal smears in as many as 28% of leukemic patients. The uterine involvement is usually unassociated with symptoms, but occasionally there is abnormal bleeding, pain, a cervical mass, or combinations thereof.

■ Uterine involvement is identified at autopsy in 40% of women who die of leukemia. In one autopsy study, the frequency of uterine involvement was 25% (acute lymphoblastic leukemia), 11% (acute myelogenous leukemia), 14% (chronic lymphocytic leukemia), and 4% (chronic granulocytic leukemia).

As Initial Site of Involvement

■ About 15 cases of myelogenous leukemia have presented as granulocytic sarcomas of the uterus in patients 26 to 75 years of age (mean, 47 years). The patients typically have abnormal vaginal bleeding, pain, or in some patients, malignant cells in Pap smears.

■ The cervix has been involved in all but one case in which the corpus only was involved. In 50% of the cervical cases, the vagina, the corpus, the parametrium, or the vulva were also involved.

■ Involvement of sites outside the female genital tract in some cases has included lymph nodes, the gastrointestinal tract, or bone marrow.

■ In most patients, an absence of leukemic cells in the peripheral blood at presentation was eventually followed by acute myelogenous leukemia. About 85% of patients with follow-up have died of their disease.

■ Gross examination of the cervix may reveal nodules, ulcers, or large masses, often extending into the vagina or paracervical tissues. The cut surface varies from gray-tan to gray-blue to green.

■ Microscopic examination reveals infiltration of immature granulocytes around normal structures, with an appearance similar to that of granulocytic sarcoma in other sites.

■ The differential diagnosis includes malignant lymphoma or, occasionally, small cell carcinoma or sarcoma. Granulocytic sarcomas may be difficult or impossible to differentiate from lymphoma without the use of the chloroacetate esterase stain, an immunohistochemical stain for lysozyme, or both.

References

Barcos M, Lane W, Gomez GA, et al. An autopsy study of 1206 acute and chronic leukemias (1958 to 1982). Cancer 60:827–837, 1987.

Ceelen GH, Sakurai M. Vaginal cytology in leukemia. Acta Cytol 6: 370–372, 1962.

Friedman HD, Adelson MD, Elder RC, Lemke SM. Granulocytic sarcoma of the uterine cervix—literature review of granulocytic sarcoma of the female genital tract. Cancer 46:128–137, 1992.

Oliva E, Ferry JA, Young RH, et al. Granulocytic sarcoma of the female genital tract: a clinicopathologic study of 11 cases. Am J Surg Pathol 21:1156–1165, 1997.

Plasmacytoma

■ Uterine involvement occurs in less than 1% of cases of multiple myeloma. One case of myeloma was initially diagnosed on a cervical smear and biopsy of a polypoid endocervical mass.

■ The differential diagnosis includes plasma cell cervicitis (see Chapter 4).

References

Figueroa JM, Huffaker AK, Diehl EJ. Malignant plasma cells in cervical smear. Acta Cytol 22:43–45, 1978.

Smith NL, Baird DB, Strausbauch PH. Endometrial involvement by multiple myeloma. Int J Gynecol Pathol 16:173–175, 1997.

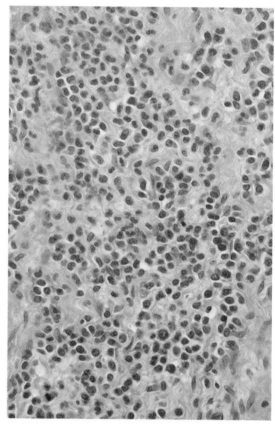

Figure 10–30. Granulocytic sarcoma of the uterine cervix. A tumor with this appearance is difficult to distinguish from a lymphoma without special stains.

Uterine Involvement by Histiocytic Disorders

■ The three reported cases of uterine involvement by Langerhans' cell histiocytosis (LCH; i.e., histiocytosis X, eosinophilic granuloma) have included a 38-year-old woman with endometrial and vulvar involvement who had no evidence of disease 6 years after partial vulvectomy; a 29-year-old woman with vulvar, vaginal, cervical, and endometrial involvement who was lost to follow-up after cervicectomy and irradiation; and a 33-year-old woman with cervical involvement who had no evidence of disease 3 years after cervicectomy.

■ One case of cervical involvment by Rosai-Dorfman disease (sinus histiocytosis with massive lymphadenopathy [SHML]) occurred in a 37-year-old woman who underwent hysterectomy for menorrhagia. There were no abnormal findings on physical examination, including an absence of lymphadenopathy.

■ The differential diagnosis includes uterine involvement by granulomatous or lipogranulomatous inflammation and malakoplakia (see Chapters 4 and 7). The characteristic microscopic features of LCH and SHML facilitate their distinction from these inflammatory lesions.

References

Axiotis CA, Merino MJ, Duray PH. Langerhans cell histiocytosis of the female genital tract. Cancer 67:1650–1660, 1991.

Murray J, Fox H. Rosai-Dorfman disease of the uterine cervix. Int J Gynecol Pathol 10:209–213, 1991.

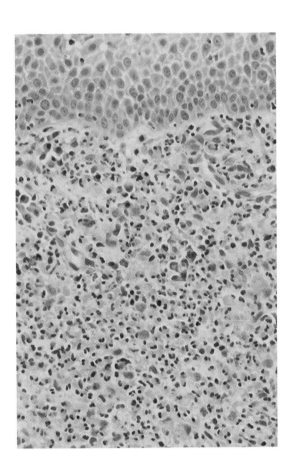

Figure 10–31. Eosinophilic granuloma involving the uterine cervix.

CARCINOMAS METASTATIC TO THE UTERUS

From Genital Tract Carcinomas

■ Uterine involvement by genital tract carcinomas is usually a result of direct extension of vaginal or tubal carcinomas or ingrowth of ovarian carcinomas that have involved the uterine serosa or cul-de-sac. In such cases, the primary tumor is usually clinically apparent.

■ Endocervical implantation metastasis by an endometrial adenocarcinoma is sometimes a complication of a fractional dilatation and curettage procedure. This finding does not alter prognosis or require specific treatment.

■ Spread from an occult ovarian, tubal, or peritoneal carcinoma may be rarely detected as microscopic fragments of tumor within a currettage specimen. An occult ovarian or tubal carcinoma may occasionally be associated with cervical involvement that clinically mimics a primary carcinoma in this site.

From Extragenital Carcinomas

■ Uterine involvement by metastatic carcinoma is usually associated with disseminated spread in a patient with a known primary tumor, and in such cases, the diagnosis is usually straightforward. Misdiagnosis is more likely when the uterine tumor is the presenting manifestation of an extragenital carcinoma.

■ Extragenital carcinomas that most commonly metastasize to the uterus are those arising from the breast, stomach, and colon. Cancers that rarely metastasize to the uterus include carcinomas of lung (e.g., anaplastic small cell carcinoma, adenocarcinoma), pancreas, gallbladder, kidney, renal pelvis, urinary bladder, and thyroid, as well as malignant melanoma, appendiceal carcinoid tumor, and malignant mesothelioma.

■ In surgical material of metastatic carcinomas to the uterus, Takeda found that the cervix only was involved in 60% of cases, the corpus only in 21% of cases, and both sites in 18% of cases.

■ In hysterectomy specimens containing metastatic cancer, Kumar and Hart found the tumor was confined to the myometrium in eight of nine cases and involved the endometrium and myometrium in the ninth case. Rare sites of involvement include leiomyomas and endometrial polyps.

■ Several morphologic features may suggest a possible or probable metastasis:

- An appearance on clinical or macroscopic examination that is atypical for a primary carcinoma
- Tumor confined to the myometrium or endocervical stroma with a normal overlying surface epithelium
- A multinodular growth pattern
- A permeative growth pattern within the endometrial or endocervical stroma with tumor entrapping normal glands
- Unusually prominent involvement of lymphatics or blood vessels
- A lack of associated precancerous changes or an in situ carcinoma

■ Specific extragenital primary tumors should be considered when the microscopic features are atypical for a primary uterine neoplasm such as a prominent signet-ring cell component (breast or stomach), thin cords of tumor cells (breast), copious necrotic debris ("dirty necrosis") within the lumina of the neoplastic glands (colon), and replacement of the normal endometrium or endocervical epithelium by well-differentiated mucinous epithelium with goblet cells (appendix).

References

Abdul-Karim FW, Bennert KW, Macfee M. Accidental detection of nonmetastatic ovarian adenocarcinoma in tissue samples recovered during dilatation and curettage. Int J Gynecol Pathol 12:355–359, 1993.

Fanning J, Alvarez PM, Tsukada Y, Piver MS. Cervical implantation metastasis by endometrial adenocarcinoma. Cancer 68:1335–1339, 1991.

Imachi M, Tsukamoto N, Amagase H, et al. Metastatic adenocarcinoma to the uterine cervix from gastric cancer: a clinicopathologic analysis of 16 cases. Cancer 71:3472–3477, 1993.

Kumar NB, Hart WR. Metastases to the uterine corpus from extragenital cancers: a clinicopathologic study of 63 cases. Cancer 50:2163–2169, 1982.

Lemoine NR, Hall PA. Epithelial tumors metastatic to the uterine cervix: a study of 63 cases and review of the literature. Cancer 57:2002–2005, 1986.

Mazur MT, Hsueh S, Gersell DJ. Metastases to the female genital tract: analysis of 325 cases. Cancer 53:1978–1984, 1984.

McComas BC, Farnum JB, Donaldson RC. Ovarian carcinoma presenting as a cervical metastasis. Obstet Gynecol 63:593–596, 1984.

Moore WF, Bentley RC, Kim K-Y, et al. Goblet-cell mucinous epithelium lining the endometrium and endocervix: evidence of metastases from an appendiceal primary tumor through the use of cytokeratin 7 and 20 immunostains. Int J Gynecol Pathol 17:363–367, 1998.

Takeda M, Diamond SM, DeMarco M, Quinn DM. Cytologic diagnosis of malignant melanoma metastatic to the endometrium. Acta Cytol 22:503–506, 1978.

Yazigi R, Sandstad J, Munoz AK. Breast cancer metastasizing to the uterine cervix. Cancer 61:2558–2560, 1988.

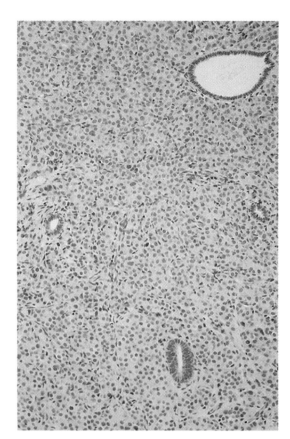

Figure 10–32. Metastatic lobular carcinoma of the breast involving the endometrium. The tumor cells diffusely replace the endometrial stroma and entrap normal endometrial glands.

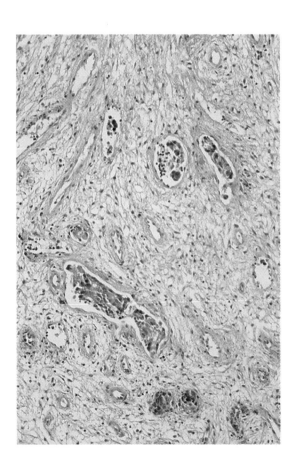

Figure 10–33. Metastatic gastric adenocarcinoma with prominent involvement of myometrial vessels, an appearance common in tumors metastatic to the uterus.

CHAPTER 11

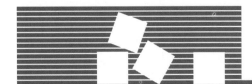

The Fallopian Tube and Broad Ligament

TUMOR-LIKE LESIONS OF THE FALLOPIAN TUBE

Metaplasia

Mucinous Metaplasia

- Mucinous metaplasia of the tubal epithelium is characterized by replacement of the normal epithelium by a single layer of benign-appearing mucinous columnar cells of the endocervical type.
- Mucinous metaplasia may occur in women with Peutz-Jeghers syndrome and may be associated with ovarian mucinous tumors (i.e., cystadenomas or carcinomas) and cervical mucinous tumors. These findings suggest that, in at least some cases, "mucinous metaplasia" of the tubal epithelium may actually represent mucosal spread from a mucinous tumor elsewhere in the female genital tract.

Transitional Cell Metaplasia

- Transitional cell metaplasia of the tubal epithelium, which was detected as an incidental microscopic finding in 3 of 10,000 specimens of fallopian tube, has been suggested as a possible source of tubal carcinoma of the same cell type (page 251).

References

Egan AJM, Russell P. Transitional (urothelial) metaplasia of the fallopian tube mucosa: morphological assessment of three cases. Int J Gynecol Pathol 15:72–76, 1996.

Giles A, Yoon J, Lindley R. Multifocal mucinous neoplasia of the female genital system. Histopathology 25:281–283, 1994.

Seidman JD. Mucinous lesions of the fallopian tube: a report of seven cases. Am J Surg Pathol 18:1205–1212, 1994.

Hyperplasia

- Hyperplasia of the tubal epithelium is an incidental idiopathic finding in up to 18% of fallopian tubes re-

moved with unselected hysterectomy specimens. This finding is often associated with unopposed estrogenic stimulation and serous borderline ovarian tumors but may occur without any known predisposing conditions.
- Epithelial stratification, a papillary or cribriform pattern, mitotic activity, or combinations thereof may be seen, but the cellular atypia is not enough to cause confusion with carcinoma in situ.

Pseudocarcinomatous Hyperplasia

- The most atypical forms of tubal hyperplasia are usually associated with tuberculous or nontuberculous salpingitis and have occasionally been misdiagnosed as carcinoma.
- In tuberculous salpingitis, fusion of tubal plicae can form multiple glandlike spaces, which may have a cribriform pattern and a lining of mildly to moderately atypical epithelium with sporadic mitotic activity. Tubercles in the lamina propria or wall of the tube and a lack of malignant nuclear features of the epithelial cells facilitate the diagnosis.
- More commonly, cases of nontuberculous salpingitis may be associated with striking pseudocarcinomatous changes in addition to those found in tuberculous salpingitis, including pseudoinvasion of the myosalpinx by glandlike structures, intravascular epithelial cells, psammoma bodies, and a marked reactive hyperplasia of the overlying mesothelium, sometimes with pseudoglandular spaces.
- Evidence favoring pseudocarcinomatous proliferation in these cases includes the absence of a gross tumor; the presence of severe chronic salpingitis (although occasional tubal carcinomas may be associated with salpingitis); a paucity of mitotic figures; a lack of severe nuclear atypicality and atypical mitotic figures; and recognition of any serosal proliferation as mesothelial on the basis of the architecture and immunoprofile of the cells (see Chapter 20).

242

References

Cheung ANY, Young RH, Scully RE. Pseudocarcinomatous hyperplasia of the fallopian tube associated with salpingitis: a report of 14 cases. Am J Surg Pathol 8:1125–1130, 1994.

Dougherty CM, Cotten NM. Proliferative epithelial lesions of the uterine tube. I. Adenomatous hyperplasia. Obstet Gynecol 24:849–854, 1964.

Moore SW, Enterline HT. Significance of proliferative epithelial lesions of the uterine tube. Obstet Gynecol 45:385–390, 1975.

Pauerstein CJ, Woodruff JD. Cellular patterns in proliferative and anaplastic disease of the fallopian tube. Am J Obstet Gynecol 96:486–492, 1966.

Robey SS, Silva EG. Epithelial hyperplasia of the fallopian tube: its association with serous borderline tumors of ovary. Int J Gynecol Pathol 8:214–220, 1989.

Stern J, Buscema J, Parmley T, et al. Atypical epithelial proliferations in the fallopian tube. Am J Obstet Gynecol 140:309–312, 1981.

Yanai-Inbar I, Siriaunkgul S, Silverberg SG. Mucosal epithelial proliferation of the fallopian tube: a particular association with ovarian serous tumor of low malignant potential? Int J Gynecol Pathol 14:107–113, 1995.

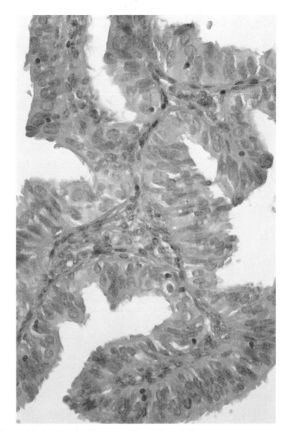

Figure 11–2. Atypical hyperplasia of the tubal mucosa.

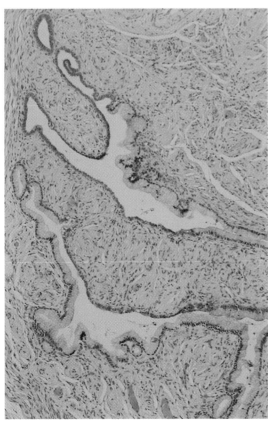

Figure 11–1. Mucinous metaplasia of the tubal mucosa.

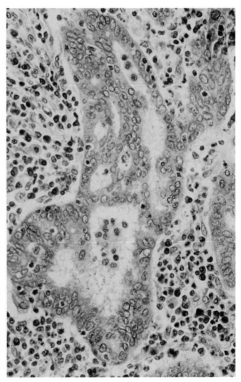

Figure 11–3. Pseudocarcinomatous hyperplasia of the tubal mucosa associated with chronic salpingitis. Notice the cribriform pattern and inflammatory cells.

Salpingitis Isthmica Nodosa

- Salpingitis isthmica nodosa (SIN), which is of uncertain pathogenesis, is usually found in young women (mean age, 26 years) and may cause infertility or predispose to ectopic pregnancy.
- SIN, which is bilateral in about 85% of cases, typically forms a yellow-white nodular swelling up to 2 cm in diameter that usually involves the isthmus; occasionally, it is grossly inconspicuous. Sectioning shows firm, rubbery tissue often with small cystic spaces.
- Variably sized and cystic glands lined by tubal epithelium, usually unaccompanied by endometrial-type stroma, lie within a typically thickened myosalpinx.

The glands are actually diverticula that communicate with the tubal lumen.
- SIN is distinguished from carcinoma by the regular distribution of widely spaced glands, the lack of significant cellular atypia, and the absence of a reactive stromal response.

References

Benjamin CL, Beaver DC. Pathogenesis of salpingitis isthmica nodosa. Am J Clin Pathol 21:212–222, 1951.

Honoré LH. Salpingitis isthmica nodosa in female infertility and ectopic tubal pregnancy. Fertil Steril 29:164–168, 1978.

Majmudar B, Henderson PH III, Sample E. Salpingitis isthmica nodosa: a high-risk factor for tubal pregnancy. Obstet Gynecol 62:73–78, 1983.

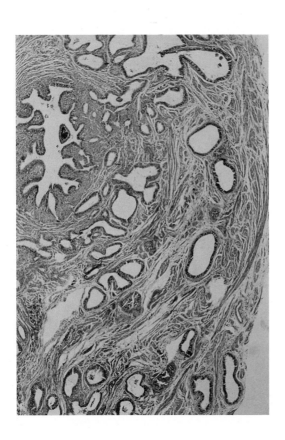

Figure 11–4. Salpingitis isthmica nodosa.

Heat Artifact

- Operative cauterization or heating of the specimen after surgical removal may cause an appearance of cellular pseudostratification with marked elongation and hyperchromatic nuclei.
- Recognition of the distinctive appearance of this change should facilitate its differentiation from carcinoma.

Reference

Cornog JL, Currie JL, Rubin A. Heat artifact simulating adenocarcinoma of fallopian tube. JAMA 214:1118–1119, 1970.

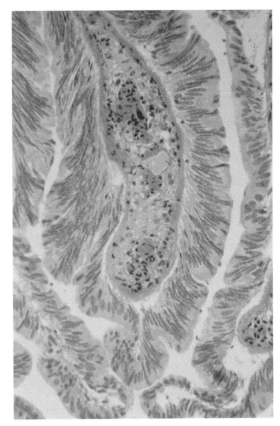

Figure 11–5. Tubal mucosa showing cautery artifact.

Ectopic Pregnancy

- In about 50% of cases of tubal pregnancy, there is focal distention of the ampulla that typically has a thinned wall and a dusky red serosal surface; the tube may be ruptured. Less commonly, the isthmus or, least often, the interstitial portion or fimbriated end are involved. Rarely, a hemorrhagic mass dissects into the broad ligament and even into the contralateral adnexa.
- Microscopic examination may reveal fetal parts, viable or necrotic villi, trophoblast, and blood clot. Evidence of an underlying predisposing lesion (e.g., chronic salpingitis, SIN, endometriosis, a small tumor) may be present.
- Persistence of the tubal pregnancy occurs in some cases after conservative treatment, manifested by acute symptoms postoperatively or a persistence or rising of the beta human chorionic gonadotropin titer.

- Foci of intermediate trophoblast (which may form a placental site nodule) or ghost outlines of chorionic villi within the mucosa, myosalpinx, or even paratubal soft tissue, representing the residue of an old, clinically unrecognized ectopic pregnancy, are an occasional finding in salpingectomy specimens.

References

Budowick M, Johnson TRB, Genadry R, et al. The histopathology of the developing tubal ectopic pregnancy. Fertil Steril 34:169–171, 1980.
Gonzalez FA, Waxman M. Ectopic pregnancy: a retrospective study of 501 consecutive patients. Diagn Gynecol Obstet 3:181–186, 1981.
Jacques SM, Qureshi F, Ramirez NC, Lawrence WD. Retained trophoblastic tissue in fallopian tubes: a consequence of unsuspected ectopic pregnancies. Int J Gynecol Pathol 16:219–224, 1997.
Pauerstein CJ, Croxatto HB, Eddy CA, et al. Anatomy and pathology of tubal pregnancy. Obstet Gynecol 67:301–308, 1986.

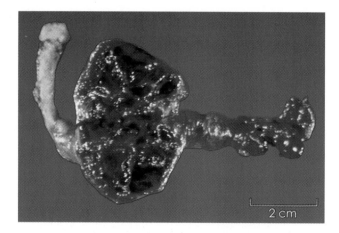

Figure 11–6. Tubal pregnancy. The tube is distended by a hemorrhagic mass.

Pregnancy-Related Changes

Arias-Stella Reaction

■ The Arias-Stella reaction (ASR) in the tube has been observed in 16% of cases of ectopic tubal pregnancy and in some patients with an intrauterine pregnancy.
■ The association with pregnancy, the absence of a mass lesion, the distinctive cytologic features, and lack of invasion differentiate it from the rare clear cell carcinoma of the tube.

Clear Cell Change of Pregnancy

■ One tubal example of clear cell change has been reported in association with a tubal pregnancy. The lesion should be distinguished from clear cell carcinoma, using criteria similar to those applicable for clear cell change in the endometrium (page 136).

Ectopic Decidua

■ Microscopic foci of decidua have been found in the tubal lamina propria in 5% to 8% of pregnant women at term, in one third of cases of ectopic pregnancy, and only rarely in women receiving progestins. Similar foci have also been identified in the serosal connective tissue in approximately 5% of tubal-ligation specimens.

■ The distinctive features of decidual cells should facilitate the diagnosis, but potential confusion with a signet-ring cell carcinoma arises rarely when the decidual cells contain mucin-filled intracytoplasmic vacuoles. The mucin, however, is alcianophilic and periodic acid–Schiff (PAS) negative, unlike the mucin of a signet-ring cell carcinoma.

References

Birch HW, Collins CG. Atypical changes of genital epithelium associated with ectopic pregnancy. Am J Obstet Gynecol 81:1198–1208, 1961.

Clement PB, Young RH, Scully RE. Non-trophoblastic pathology of the female genital tract and peritoneum associated with pregnancy. Semin Diagn Pathol 6:372–406, 1989.

Milchgrub S, Sandstad J. Arias-Stella reaction in fallopian tube epithelium: a light and electron microscopic study with a review of the literature. Am J Clin Pathol 95:892–895, 1991.

Mills SE, Fechner RE. Stromal and epithelial changes in the fallopian tube following hormonal therapy. Hum Pathol 11:583–585, 1983.

Tilden IL, Winstedt R. Decidual reactions in fallopian tubes: histologic study of tubal segments from 144 post-partum sterilizations. Am J Pathol 19:1043–1051, 1943.

Tziortziotis DV, Bouros AC, Ziogas VS, Young RH. Clear cell hyperplasia of the fallopian tube epithelium associated with ectopic pregnancy: report of a case. Int J Gynecol Pathol 16:79–80, 1997.

Zaytsev P, Taxy JB. Pregnancy-associated ectopic decidua. Am J Surg Pathol 11:526–530, 1987.

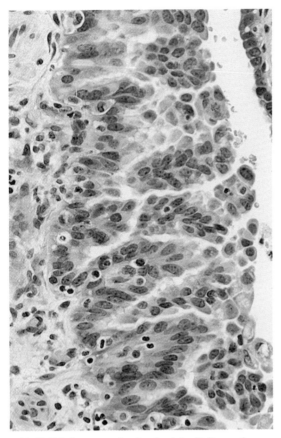

Figure 11-7. Tubal mucosa, showing the Arias-Stella reaction.

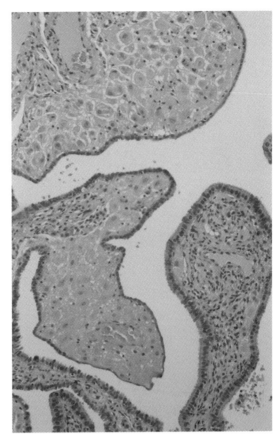

Figure 11-8. Ectopic decidua within the stroma of the tubal plicae.

Endometriosis

- Endometrial tissue extends directly from the uterine cornu and replaces the mucosa of the interstitial and isthmic portions of the tube in up to 25% and 10% of women, respectively, a finding considered a normal variation.
- Luminal occlusion by the ectopic endometrial tissue (i.e., "endometrial colonization" or intraluminal endometriosis), which may be bilateral, accounts for 15% to 20% of cases of infertility. The finding has also been implicated as a cause of tubal pregnancy and may give rise to tubal polyps (page 249).
- Typical or serosal tubal endometriosis is most commonly associated with endometriosis elsewhere in the pelvis; the myosalpinx and mucosa are not usually involved.
- In some cases of pelvic endometriosis, with or without tubal involvement, the plicae are expanded by masses of pseudoxanthoma cells (page 425), so-called pseudo-

xanthomatous salpingitis or pseudoxanthomatous salpingiosis.
- Postsalpingectomy endometriosis occurs at the tip of the proximal tubal stump, usually 1 to 4 years after ligation; it may be associated with SIN. Endometrial glands and stroma extend from the endosalpinx into the muscularis, often to the serosa. Tuboperitoneal fistulas, which may lead to a postligation ectopic pregnancy, are a complication in some cases.

References

Cioltei A, Tasca L, Titiriga L, et al. Nodular salpingitis and tubal endometriosis. I. Comparative clinical study. Acta Eur Fertil 10:135–141, 1979.

De Brux J. The contribution of pathological anatomy to the diagnosis and prognosis of different forms of tubal sterility. Acta Eur Fertil 6:185–195, 1975.

Fortier KJ, Haney AF. The pathologic spectrum of uterotubal junction obstruction. Obstet Gynecol 65:93–98, 1985.

Lisa JR, Gioia JD, Rubin IC. Observations on the interstitial portion of the fallopian tube. Surg Gynecol Obstet 99:159–169, 1954.

Rock JA, Parmley TH, King TM, et al. Endometriosis and the development of tuboperitoneal fistulas after tubal ligation. Fertil Steril 35:16–20, 1981.

Rubin IC, Lisa JR, Trinidad S. Further observations on ectopic endometrium of the fallopian tube. Surg Gynecol Obstet 103:469–474, 1956.

Seidman JD, Oberer S, Bitterman P, Aisner SC. Pathogenesis of pseudoxanthomatous salpingiosis. Mod Pathol 6:53–55, 1993.

Sheldon RS, Wilson RB, Dockerty MB. Serosal endometriosis of fallopian tubes. Am J Obstet Gynecol 99:882–884, 1967.

Stock RJ. Postsalpingectomy endometriosis: a reassessment. Obstet Gynecol 60:560–570, 1982.

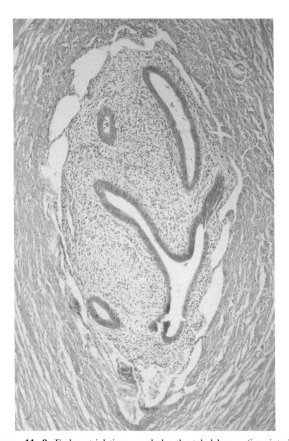

Figure 11–9. Endometrial tissue occludes the tubal lumen (i.e., intraluminal endometriosis or endometrial colonization).

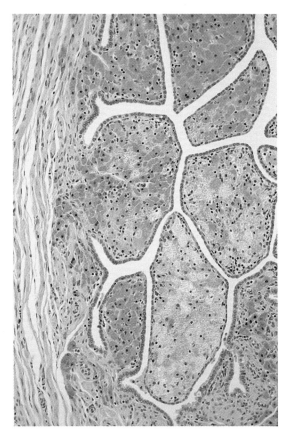

Figure 11–10. Pseudoxanthomatous salpingitis. The stroma of the plicae is infiltrated by numerous foamy and pigmented histocytes in a patient with pelvic endometriosis.

Torsion

■ Tubal torsion may occur as an isolated finding, but it usually accompanies torsion of the adjacent ovary. On gross inspection, the tube is usually swollen and hemorrhagic. Rarely, the torsion is synchronously or metachronously bilateral.

References

Bernardus RE, Van Der Slikke JW, Roex AJM, et al. Torsion of the fallopian tube: some considerations on its etiology. Obstet Gynecol 64:675–678, 1984.

Dunnihoo DR, Wolff J. Bilateral torsion of the adnexa: a case report and a review of the world literature. Obstet Gynecol 64:555–595, 1984.

Prolapse (see Chapter 3)

Walthard Nests (see Chapter 19)

Ectopic Tissue in Fallopian Tube

■ Nests of hilus cells occur in the endosalpinx (especially in the fimbria) and paratubal connective tissue in 0.5% of salpingectomy specimens.

■ A single case of ectopic pancreas in the fallopian tube has been reported.

References

Honoré LH, O'Hara KE. Ovarian hilus cell heterotopia. Obstet Gynecol 53:461–464, 1979.

Lewis JD. Hilus-cell hyperplasia of ovaries and tubes. Obstet Gynecol 24:728–731, 1964.

Mason TE, Quagliarello JR. Ectopic pancreas in the fallopian tube: report of a first case. Obstet Gynecol 48:70s–73s, 1976.

TUMORS OF THE FALLOPIAN TUBE

Benign Epithelial Tumors

Endometrioid Polyp

■ Endometrioid polyp, also referred to as adenomatous polyp, is the most common benign tumor of the fallopian tube.

■ The polyps may result in infertility or ectopic pregnancy by obstructing the tubal lumen and have been demonstrated radiographically in 1.2% to 2.5% of infertile women and pathologically in 11% of hysterectomy specimens that included a fallopian tube.

■ The polyps are usually found within the interstitial portion of the tube and are frequently associated with, and presumably arise from, mucosal endometriosis (page 247).

■ Although most of the lesions are not recognized grossly, they can reach 1.3 cm in the maximal dimension. The polyps are commonly attached to the tubal epithelium by a broad base and resemble intrauterine endometrial polyps.

Papilloma and Cystadenoma

■ Papillomas range up to 3 cm in diameter and are loosely attached to the tubal mucosa and consist of delicate, branching fibrovascular stalks lined by indifferent or tubal-type epithelium.

■ Serous cystadenomas resemble their ovarian counterparts.

Metaplastic Papillary Tumor

■ Metaplastic papillary tumor (MPT) is an uncommon lesion and is an incidental microscopic finding in segments of fallopian tube removed during the postpartum period, although rarely it occurs in nonpregnant women.

■ MPTs consist of papillae and cellular buds composed of epithelial cells with abundant eosinophilic cytoplasm and intracellular and extracellular mucin. Mitotic figures may be seen rarely.

■ Whether MPTs are neoplastic or only proliferative, metaplastic lesions is unsettled, but the latter is favored.

References

Alvarado-Cabrero I, Navani SS, Young RH, Scully RE. Tumors of the fimbriated end of the fallopian tube: a clinicopathologic analysis of 20 cases. Int J Gynecol Pathol 16:189–196, 1997.

Bartnik J, Powell WS, Moriber-Katz S, et al. Metaplastic papillary tumor of the fallopian tube: case report, immunohistochemical features and review of the literature. Arch Pathol Lab Med 113:545–547, 1989.

David MP, Ben-Zwi D, Langer L. Tubal intramural polyps and their relationship to infertility. Fertil Steril 35:526–531, 1981.

Donnez J, Casanas-Roux F, Ferin J, Thomas K. Tubal polyps, epithelial inclusions, and endometriosis after tubal sterilization. Fertil Steril 41: 564–568, 1984.

Glazener CMA, Loveden LM, Richardson SJ, et al. Tubo-cornual polyps: their relevance in subfertility. Hum Reprod 2:59–62, 1987.

Heller DS, Rubinstein N, Dikman S, et al. Adenomatous polyp of the fallopian tube—a case report. J Reprod Med 36:82–84, 1991.

Lisa JR, Gioia JD, Rubin IC. Observations on the interstitial portion of the fallopian tube. Surg Gynecol Obstet 99:159–169, 1954.

Saffos RO, Rhatigan RM, Scully RE. Metaplastic papillary tumor of the fallopian tube—a distinctive lesion of pregnancy. Am J Clin Pathol 74:232–236, 1980.

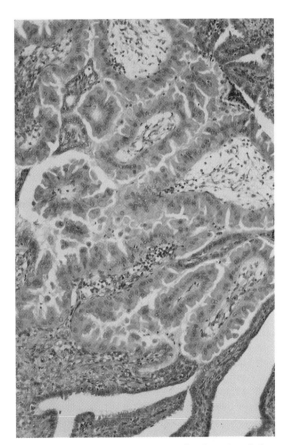

Figure 11–11. Metaplastic papillary tumor involves the tubal mucosa in a pregnant woman.

Borderline Tumors

■ Rare tubal tumors resembling ovarian serous or endometrioid borderline tumors have been described, some of which have arisen from the fimbria.

■ Four "mucinous borderline tumors" of the tube have been reported, three in association with pseudomyxoma peritonei. Although these tumors may have arisen from foci of mucinous metaplasia of the tubal epithelium (page 242), in none of the four cases was the appendix examined microscopically. Secondary spread to the tube from an undetected appendiceal tumor therefore cannot be excluded in these cases.

References

Alvarado-Cabrero I, Navani SS, Young RH, Scully RE. Tumors of the fimbriated end of the fallopian tube: a clinicopathologic analysis of 20 cases. Int J Gynecol Pathol 16:189–196 1997.

Gatto V, Selim MA, Lankerani M. Primary carcinoma of the fallopian tube in an adolescent. J Surg Oncol 33:212–214, 1986.

Seidman JD. Mucinous lesions of the fallopian tube: a report of seven cases. Am J Surg Pathol 18:1205–1212, 1994.

Zheng W, Wolf S, Kramer EE, et al. Borderline papillary serous tumor of the fallopian tube. Am J Surg Pathol 20:30–35, 1996.

Carcinomas

Clinical Features

■ Carcinomas of the tube account for at least 0.3% of all gynecologic cancers, but this figure may be low because carcinomas involving the tube and ovary usually are classified as ovarian. The tubal origin of some such tumors is suggested by a screening study using serum CA-125 assays that detected a ratio of tubal to ovarian carcinomas of 1:6, in contrast to that of 1:150 based on the generally cited frequencies of the two tumors.

■ An increased frequency of tubal carcinoma in cases of ovarian carcinoma may be a result of independent primary tumors reflecting a "field change," or the tubal lesions may represent implants of ovarian tumor. Women with tubal carcinomas may also have an increased frequency of endometrial and breast carcinomas.

■ Women with tubal carcinoma, who range from 14 to 87 years of age (mean, 57 years), usually present with abnormal vaginal bleeding or discharge and abdominal pain. Hydrops tubae profluens (i.e., relief of colicky pain and decrease in size of an abdominal mass associated with the vaginal discharge of watery fluid) occurs in less than 10% of cases and is not specific for tubal carcinoma. Only 3% of tumors are diagnosed preoperatively.

■ Cervical-vaginal cytologic examination is positive in as many as 60% of the cases, but the figure is much lower in most series. Rarely, a fragment of tubal carcinoma in an endocervical or endometrial curettage specimen is the first manifestation of the disease.

■ An elevated serum CA-125 level is common, and its measurement may be useful in monitoring the course of affected patients. Ultrasound examination has also been effective in the diagnosis of tubal carcinoma.

Table 11–1

FIGO STAGING OF CARCINOMA OF THE FALLOPIAN TUBE

Stage 0	Carcinoma in situ (limited to tubal mucosa)
Stage I	Growth is limited to fallopian tubes.
Ia	Growth is limited to one tube with extension into submucosa and/or muscularis but not penetrating serosal surface; no ascites.
Ib	Growth is limited to both tubes with extension into submucosa and/or muscularis but not penetrating serosal surface; no ascites.
Ic	Tumor is stage Ia and Ib but with extensions through or onto tubal serosa or with ascites containing malignant cells or with positive peritoneal washings.
I(F)*	Carcinoma is confined to the fimbria.
Stage II	Growth involves one or both fallopian tubes with pelvic extension.
IIa	Extension and/or metastases to uterus and/or ovaries.
IIb	Extension to other pelvic tissues
Stage III	Tumor involves one or both fallopian tubes with peritoneal implants outside pelvis and/or positive retroperitoneal or inguinal nodes. Superficial liver metastases equal stage III. Tumor appears limited to the true pelvis but with histologically proven extension to small bowel or omentum.
IIIa	Tumor is grossly limited to true pelvis with negative nodes but with histologically confirmed microscopic seeding of abdominal peritoneal surfaces.
IIIb	Tumor involves one or both tubes with histologically confirmed implants of abdominal peritoneal surfaces, with none exceeding 2 cm in diameter. Lymph nodes are negative.
IIIc	Abdominal implants are >2 cm in diameter and/or retroperitoneal or inguinal nodes are positive.
Stage IV	Growth involves one or both fallopian tubes with distant metastases. If pleural effusion is present, cytologic fluid must be positive for malignant cells to be stage IV. Parenchymal liver metastases equals stage IV.

* Category added by the authors.

■ The International Federation of Gynecology and Obstetrics (FIGO) stage (Table 11–1) has varied among series (21% to 56% stage I, 9% to 20% stage II, 16% to 55% stage III, 4% to 12% stage IV), but tubal carcinomas usually are of lower stage than ovarian carcinomas.

Gross Features

■ The tumors have been reported to be bilateral in as many as 20% of the cases, but only 3% of tumors were bilateral in a recent large study. The ratio of ampullary to isthmic tumors is 2:1. About 8% of tumors are confined to the fimbria.

■ Part or all of the tube may be distended by luminal watery fluid or blood, with an external appearance resembling that of hydrosalpinx or hematosalpinx. Any dilated fallopian tube encountered at operation should be opened and examined intraoperatively. Tumor on the tubal serosa or obvious infiltration of the adjacent viscera or the pelvic wall may be seen.

■ Opening the tube usually reveals a localized or diffuse, soft, gray to pink, friable mucosal tumor; occasionally, multiple tumors are present. The sectioned surface is solid or partly cystic. Mural involvement, hemorrhage, and yellow necrotic areas are common.

- Some tumors form a mass that replaces part of the tube and the ipsilateral ovary ("tubo-ovarian carcinoma") (see Differential Diagnosis, below).

Microscopic Features

- The diagnosis of in situ tubal carcinoma should be limited to flat or minimally papillary, grossly inapparent lesions with full-thickness replacement of tubal epithelium by obviously malignant cells. If associated with a carcinoma of similar type in another organ, the tubal lesion may represent an implant rather than a primary tumor.
- Although there is considerable variation in the reported frequency of the various microscopic subtypes of invasive tubal carcinomas, in our experience, about one half of the carcinomas are serous, about one fourth are endometrioid, about one fifth are transitional or undifferentiated, and the remainder are other cell types. In one large series, 8% of all cell types were grade 1, 20% were grade 2, and 72% were grade 3.
- Serous carcinomas resemble their ovarian counterparts, with papillarity, cellular buds, slitlike glandular spaces, solid sheets, and occasionally, tumor giant cells and psammoma bodies. The tumors are usually high grade and may be associated with a contiguous in situ carcinoma. Necrosis and vascular space invasion are common.
- Endometrioid carcinomas resemble their endometrial counterparts. In one series, 5 of 26 tumors were grade 1, 11 were grade 2, and 10 were grade 3. The tumors are usually noninvasive or only superficially invasive. Occasional features include contiguity with and possible origin from endometriosis, squamous differentiation, spindled epithelial cells, oxyphilic cells, and trabecular patterns.
  - A subtype of endometrioid carcinoma resembles the wolffian adnexal tumor (page 261). A mostly solid proliferation of small, oval to spindled cells is punctured by small to cystic glands, many with luminal PAS-positive colloid-like secretions. Foci of typical endometrioid carcinoma are usually present but may be minor. The tumors are usually noninvasive.
- In one large series of cases of tubal carcinoma, the mucinous type accounted for 6% of the cases. One other invasive mucinous carcinoma was bilateral and associated with a mucinous adenocarcinoma of the cervix.
  - One tubal mucinous carcinoma in situ adjacent to an area of mucinous metaplasia occurred in a woman with adenocarcinoma in situ of the cervix and bilateral ovarian mucinous carcinomas with peritoneal spread.
- Undifferentiated large cell carcinomas account for as many as 8% of tubal carcinomas.
- Uncommon to rare subtypes of tubal carcinoma include transitional cell carcinoma, clear cell carcinoma, squamous cell carcinoma, lymphoepithelioma-like carcinoma, hepatoid carcinoma, and glassy cell carcinoma.

Differential Diagnosis

- Ovarian carcinoma with spread to the tube. In such cases, the usual predominance of the ovarian tumor facilitates the diagnosis, but occasionally both organs are fused to form a solid or cystic mass.
  - "In situ carcinoma" adjacent to the tubal tumor is not a helpful differential feature, because this appearance can be mimicked by carcinomas spreading to the tubal epithelium.
  - When the origin of the tumor is not clear, the designation "tubo-ovarian carcinoma" is an appropriate one that may allow a more accurate determination of the relative frequency of tubal and ovarian carcinomas.
- Pseudocarcinomatous hyperplasia (page 242).

Behavior

- Tubal carcinoma spreads most commonly to the peritoneum, adjacent organs, and lymph nodes (i.e., paraaortic and pelvic and occasionally inguinal). Distant metastases occur in almost 50% of the tumors with extratubal spread, a frequency higher than for ovarian carcinomas.
- Recurrences usually are identified within the first 2 or 3 postoperative years but may be as late as 9 years.
- Stage is the most important prognostic factor.
  - The 5-year survival for stage I and II tumors is about 50% and for stage III and IV tumors, 15% to 20%.
  - Subdividing stage Ia tumors into Ia0 (no invasion), Ia1 (invasion only of lamina propria), and Ia2 (deeper invasion but no serosal involvement) indicates a decreasing survival with increasing depth of invasion.
  - The 1(F) tumors (i.e., confined to fimbria) have a similar prognosis to that of stage Ic tumors (i.e., invasive tumors with serosal involvement).
- Adverse prognostic factors in some studies have included increasing age, a patent tubal ostium, vascular invasion, and a high volume of residual tumor.

References

Alvarado-Cabrero I, Navani SS, Young RH, Scully RE. Tumors of the fimbriated end of the fallopian tube: a clinicopathologic analysis of 20 cases. Int J Gynecol Pathol 16:189–196, 1997.

Alvarado-Cabrero I, Young RH, Vamvakakas EC, Scully RE. Carcinoma of the fallopian tube: a clinicopathologic study of 105 cases with observations on staging and prognostic factors. Gynecol Oncol 72:367–379, 1999.

Aoyama T, Mizuno T, Andoh K, et al. Alpha-fetoprotein–producing (hepatoid) carcinoma of the fallopian tube. Gynecol Oncol 63:261–266, 1996.

Baekelandt M, Kockx M, Wesling F, Gerris J. Primary adenocarcinoma of the fallopian tube: review of the literature. Int J Gynecol Cancer 3:65–71, 1993.

Cheung ANY, Ngan HYS, Cheng D, et al. Clinicopathologic study of 16 cases of primary tubal malignancy. Int J Gynecol Cancer 4:111–118, 1994.

Cheung ANY, So KF, Ngan HYS, Wong LC. Primary squamous carcinoma of fallopian tube. Int J Gynecol Pathol 13:92–95, 1994.

Daya D, Young RH, Scully RE. Endometrioid carcinoma of the fallopian tube resembling an adnexal tumor of probable wolffian origin: a report of six cases. Int J Gynecol Pathol 11:122–130, 1992.

Herbold DR, Axelrod JH, Bobowski SJ, et al. Glassy cell carcinoma of the fallopian tube: a case report. Int J Gynecol Pathol 7:384–390, 1988.

Jackson-York GL, Ramzy I. Synchronous papillary mucinous adenocarcinoma of the endocervix and fallopian tubes. Int J Gynecol Pathol 11:63–67, 1992.

Koshiyama M, Konishi I, Yoshidi M, et al. Transitional cell carcinoma of the fallopian tube: a light and electron microscopic study. Int J Gynecol Pathol 13:175–180, 1994.

Navani SS, Alvarado-Cabrero I, Young RH, Scully RE. Endometrioid carcinoma of the fallopian tube: a clinicopathologic analysis of 26 cases. Gynecol Oncol 63:371–378, 1996.

Nordin AJ. Primary carcinoma of the fallopian tube: a 20-year literature review. Obstet Gynecol Surv 49:349–361, 1994.

Rosen A, Klein M, Lahousen M, et al., for the Austrian Cooperative Study Group for Fallopian Tube Carcinoma. Primary carcinoma of the fallopian tube—a retrospective analysis of 115 patients. Br J Cancer 68:605–609, 1993.

Seidman JD. Mucinous lesions of the fallopian tube: a report of seven cases. Am J Surg Pathol 18:1205–1212, 1994.

Uehira K, Hashimoto H, Tsuneyoski M, Enjoji M. Transitional cell carcinoma pattern in primary carcinoma of the fallopian tube. Cancer 72:2447–2456, 1993.

Voet RL, Lifshitz S. Primary clear cell adenocarcinoma of the fallopian tube: light microscopic and ultrastructural findings. Int J Gynecol Pathol 1:292–298, 1982.

Woolas R, Jacobs I, Prys Davies A, et al. What is the true incidence of primary fallopian tube carcinoma? Int J Gynecol Cancer 4:384–388, 1994.

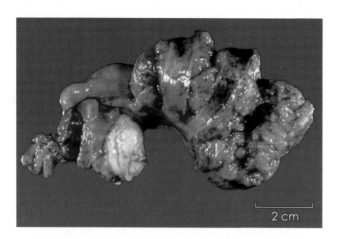

Figure 11–12. Tubal carcinoma. The tubal lumen is distended by a fleshy, lobulated tumor.

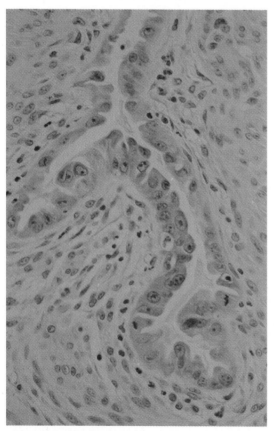

Figure 11–13. Tubal adenocarcinoma in situ. Malignant cells line the tubal lumen.

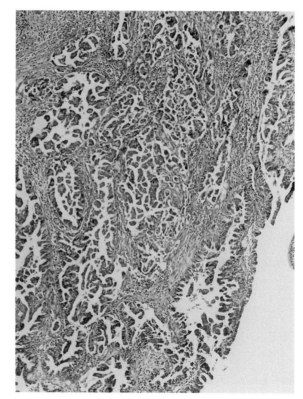

Figure 11–14. Papillary serous carcinoma of the fallopian tube.

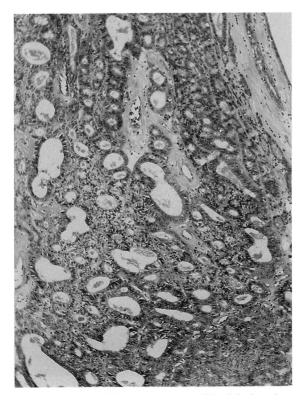

Figure 11–15. Endometrioid adenocarcinoma of the fallopian tube.

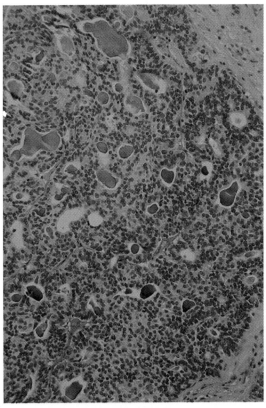

Figure 11–16. Endometrioid adenocarcinoma of the fallopian tube resembling a wolffian adnexal tumor.

Mixed Epithelial-Mesenchymal Tumors

Benign Tumors

- The rare reported examples of tubal adenofibromas and cystadenofibromas have resembled those encountered in the ovary, including rare bilateral cases. They may be intraluminal or attached to the fimbriated end or the serosal surface, have smooth or papillary surfaces, and range up to 3 cm in diameter.
- Most of the tumors have been of the serous type, but some are endometrioid. Rare tumors have borderline features.

References

Alvarado-Cabrero I, Navani SS, Young RH, Scully RE. Tumors of the fimbriated end of the fallopian tube: a clinicopathologic analysis of 20 cases. Int J Gynecol Pathol 16:189–196 1997.

Casasola SV, Mindan JP. Cystadenofibroma of fallopian tube. Appl Pathol 7:256–259, 1989.

Chen KT. Bilateral papillary adenofibroma of the fallopian tube. Am J Surg Pathol 75:229–231, 1981.

De la Fuente AA. Benign mixed müllerian tumour-adenofibroma of the fallopian tube. Histopathology 6:661–666, 1982.

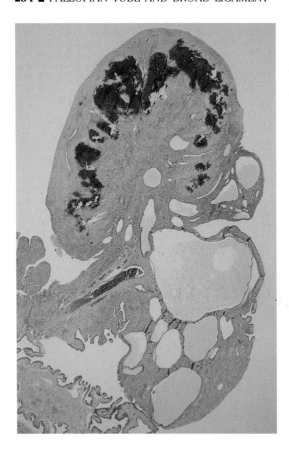

Figure 11–17. Serous cystadenofibroma of the fimbriated end of a fallopian tube. Calcification is prominent within the fibromatous component.

Adenosarcoma

■ Rare tubal examples of adenosarcoma have been reported, including one of fimbrial origin that recurred.

Reference

Gollard R, Kosty M, Bordin G, et al. Two unusual presentations of müllerian adenosarcoma: case reports, literature review, and treatment considerations. Gynecol Oncol 59:412–422, 1995.

Malignant Müllerian Mixed Tumors

■ Patients with malignant müllerian mixed tumors (MMMTs) are almost always postmenopausal (mean age, 60 years) and usually present with a watery or bloody vaginal discharge, abdominal pain, or both.
■ Laparotomy typically reveals distention of a tube by tumor with spread to the pelvis or abdomen or both in most of the cases.
■ On gross examination, the tumor, which may be hemorrhagic and necrotic, usually fills the lumen. The microscopic features are identical to uterine MMMTs (see Chapter 9).

■ The 5-year survival rate is approximately 15%, and the mean length of survival is only 16 to 20 months.
■ The differential diagnosis includes tumors that are rare in the fallopian tube and that are distinguished from MMMTs by criteria discussed elsewhere. These include adenosarcoma (see Chapter 9), endometrioid carcinoma with a prominent spindle cell epithelial component (see Chapter 14), and immature teratoma (see Chapter 15).

References

Carlson JA, Ackerman BL, Wheeler JE. Malignant mixed müllerian tumor of the fallopian tube. Cancer 71:187–192, 1993.
Hellström A-C, Auer G, Silverswärd C, Pettersson F. Prognostic factors in malignant mixed müllerian tumor of the fallopian tube; the Radiumhemmett series 1923–1995. Int J Gynecol Cancer 6:467–472, 1996.
Weber AM, Hewett WF, Gajewski WH, Curry SL. Malignant mixed müllerian tumors of the fallopian tube. Gynecol Oncol 50:239–243, 1993.

Benign Tumors of Soft Tissue Type

■ Leiomyomas are the most common of these. Most are small; they may be submucosal, intramural, or subserosal and may undergo the same degenerative changes as their uterine counterparts. They may predispose the patient to tubal pregnancy.

■ Rarer tubal tumors in this category include neurilemoma, angiomyolipoma, lipoma, lymphangioma, ganglioneuroma, and hemangioma. Several hemangiomas have manifested with hemoperitoneum.

References

Dede JA, Janovski NA. Lipoma of the uterine tube—a gynecologic rarity. Obstet Gynecol 22:461–467, 1963.

Ebrahimi T, Okagaki T. Hemangioma of the fallopian tube. Am J Obstet Gynecol 115:864–865, 1973.

Honoré LH. Parauterine leiomyomas in women: a clinicopathologic study of 22 cases. Eur J Obstet Gynecol Reprod Biol 11:273–279, 1981.

Katz DA, Thom D, Bogard P, Dermer-MS. Angiomyolipoma of the fallopian tube. Am J Obstet Gynecol 148:341–343, 1984.

Mroueh J, Margono F, Feinkind L. Tubal pregnancy associated with ampullary tubal leiomyoma. Obstet Gynecol 81:880–882, 1993.

Okagaki T, Richart RM. Neurilemoma of the fallopian tube. Am J Obstet Gynecol 106:929, 1970.

Sanes S, Warner R. Primary lymphangioma of the fallopian tube. Am J Obstet Gynecol 37:316–321, 1939.

Spanta R, Lawrence WD. Soft tissue chondroma of the fallopian tube: differential diagnosis and histogenetic considerations. Pathol Res Pract 190:174–176, 1995.

Weber DL, Fazzini E. Ganglioneuroma of the fallopian tube: a hitherto unreported finding. Acta Neuropathol (Berl) 16:173–175, 1970.

Malignant Tumors of Soft Tissue Type

■ Primary tubal sarcomas are rare; almost all are leiomyosarcomas, which occur throughout adult life (median age, 47 years). The presenting symptoms are similar to those of other tubal cancers.

■ The tumors are usually large and grossly and microscopically resemble uterine leiomyosarcomas. The survival has been poor in the reported cases, with metastases often detected within 2 years of diagnosis.

■ Rare sarcomas of other types, including embryonal rhabdomyosarcoma and malignant fibrous histiocytoma, also have been reported.

References

Buchwalter CL, Jenison EL, Fromm M, et al. Pure embryonal rhabdomyosarcoma of the fallopian tube. Gynecol Oncol 67:95–101, 1997.

Halligan AWF, McGuinness EPJ. Malignant fibrous histiocytoma of the fallopian tube. Br J Obstet Gynaecol 97:275–276, 1990.

Jacoby A, Fuller A, Thor AD, Muntz HG. Primary leiomyosarcoma of the fallopian tube. Gynecol Oncol 51:404–407, 1993.

Adenomatoid Tumor

General Features

■ The adenomatoid tumor is the most common benign neoplasm of the fallopian tube and is usually an incidental finding in a middle-aged or elderly woman.

Pathologic Features

■ The tumors are usually 2.0 cm or less in diameter, circumscribed, firm, and gray, white, or yellow mural

masses. Rarely, they are bilateral or associated with similar tumors in the uterus.

■ The microscopic features are identical to those occurring in uterine adenomatoid tumors (see Chapter 10).

Differential Diagnosis

■ Other benign tumors, particularly lymphangiomas and leiomyomas. Careful examination of the tumor cells should permit their distinction from endothelial cells, and immunoperoxidase stains for cytokeratin and *Ulex europaeus* facilitate the diagnosis in difficult cases.

■ Malignant mesotheliomas and adenocarcinomas, particularly those of signet-ring cell type. The circumscribed gross appearance, bland cytologic findings, and mitotic inactivity characteristic of adenomatoid tumors are not features of these malignant tumors.

References

Honoré LH, O'Hara KE. Adenomatoid tumor of the fimbrial endosalpinx: report of two cases with discussion of histogenesis. Eur J Obstet Gynecol Reprod Biol 9:335–339, 1979.

Srigley JR, Colgan TJ. Multifocal and diffuse adenomatoid tumor involving the uterus and fallopian tube. Ultrastruct Pathol 12:351–355, 1988.

Youngs LA, Taylor HB. Adenomatoid tumors of the uterus and fallopian tube. Am J Clin Pathol 48:537–545, 1967.

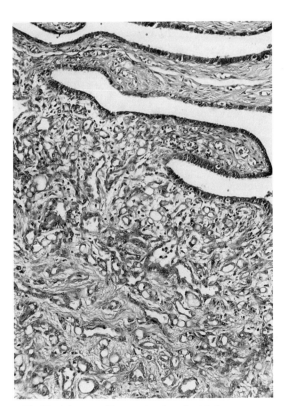

Figure 11–18. Adenomatoid tumor involves the tubal mucosa.

Germ Cell Tumors

- Tubal teratomas, of which about 50 have been reported, are usually attached by a pedicle to the mucosa and have ranged up to 20 cm in diameter. Most of them have been dermoid cysts, but rare solid, mature or immature teratomas have been reported.
- Two tumors composed entirely of thyroid tissue (i. e., struma salpingi) have been reported.

References

Bagainski L, Yazigi R, Sandstad J. Immature (malignant) teratoma of the fallopian tube. Am J Obstet Gynecol 160:671–672, 1989.

Frost RG, Roongpisuthipong A, Cheek BH, Majmudar BN. Immature teratoma of the fallopian tube: a case report. J Reprod Med 34:62–64, 1989.

Hoda SA, Huvos AG. Struma salpingis associated with struma ovarii. Am J Surg Pathol 17:1187–1189, 1993.

Kutteh WH, Albert T. Mature cystic teratoma of the fallopian tube associated with an ectopic pregnancy. Obstet Gynecol 78:984–986, 1991.

Mazzarella P, Okagaki T, Richart RM. Teratoma of the uterine tube: a case report and review of the literature. Obstet Gynecol 39:381–388, 1972.

Trophoblastic Disease

- Hydatidiform moles, placental site trophoblastic tumors, and gestational choriocarcinomas of tubal origin may mimic an ectopic pregnancy on clinical and gross examination. Differentiation of a mole from an ectopic pregnancy with hydropic villi depends on criteria similar to those used in the uterine corpus.

Tubal Choriocarcinoma

- Tubal choriocarcinomas, which have occurred in patients from 16 to 56 years of age (mean 33 years), account for approximately 4% of all choriocarcinomas.
- Intraoperative or gross examination reveals a hemorrhagic, friable mass, often with associated hemoperitoneum. Microscopic examination shows typical features of gestational choriocarcinoma.
- Invasion of the myosalpinx by trophoblast cells having the typical features of choriocarcinoma is essential to exclude the trophoblast of an early ectopic pregnancy in which villi are not found.
- Chemotherapy has resulted in a salvage rate of 94%.

References

Dekel A, van Iddekinge B, Isaacson C, et al. Primary choriocarcinoma of the fallopian tube. Report of a case with survival and postoperative delivery: review of the literature. Obstet Gynecol Surv 41:142–148, 1986.

Muto MG, Lage JM, Berkowitz RS. Gestational trophoblastic disease of the fallopian tube. J Reprod Med 36:57–60, 1991.

Ober WB, Maier RC. Gestational choriocarcinoma of the fallopian tube. Diagn Gynecol Obstet 3:213–231, 1981.

Su Y, Cheng W, Chen C, et al. Pregnancy with primary tubal placental site trophoblastic tumor—a case report and literature review. Gynecol Oncol 73:322–325, 1999.

Malignant Lymphoma and Leukemia

- The fallopian tube is commonly involved when the female genital tract (especially the ovary) is involved by malignant lymphoma or leukemia. We have seen one case of lymphoma that appeared confined to the tube.
- The gross and microscopic features of tubal lymphoma and leukemia are similar to these disorders occurring elsewhere.

References

Cecalupo AJ, Frankel LS, Sullivan MP. Pelvic and ovarian extramedullary leukemic relapse in young girls: a report of four cases and review of the literature. Cancer 50:587–593, 1982.

Osborne BM, Robboy SJ. Lymphomas or leukemia presenting as ovarian tumors: an analysis of 42 cases. Cancer 52:1933–1943, 1983.

Secondary Tumors

From Other Sites in the Female Genital Tract

- Secondary involvement of the tube by direct spread or metastasis is much more common than primary tubal carcinoma. Most such tumors have spread directly from the ovary, a diagnosis usually suggested by the gross pathologic findings. Luminal or serosal tubal involvement is also common in cases of ovarian serous borderline tumors.
- Direct extension and intraluminal spread account for secondary tubal involvement by endometrial carcinoma. Direct extension of cervical carcinoma to the tube is rare, except at autopsy, but occasional cervical carcinomas, some of which are in situ, spread upward to the tube by the endometrium.
- Uterine sarcomas, ovarian and peritoneal serous tumors, and mesotheliomas frequently involve the tubal serosa (and in serous tumors, the lumen) but are rarely the source of diagnostic difficulty.

From Sites Outside the Female Genital Tract

- Only about 6% of metastases to the tube originate outside the genital tract, most commonly from the breast, gastrointestinal tract, or urinary bladder.
- The microscopic features depend on the morphologic features of the primary tumor and the extent and distribution of tubal involvement. Vascular invasion is often seen in the plicae.
- In rare cases of pseudomyxoma peritonei, the tubal epithelium is replaced focally by mucinous epithelium, which is usually at least slightly atypical, a feature distinguishing it from benign mucinous metaplasia (page 242).
- The diagnosis is usually established by the clinical history, the operative findings, or both, in addition to the distinctive microscopic features. Epithelial involvement by secondary carcinoma may be indistingushable microscopically from carcinoma in situ.

References

Finn WF, Javert CT. Primary and metastatic cancer of the fallopian tube. Cancer 2:803–814, 1949.

Honoré LH, O'Hara KE. Ovarian hilus cell heterotopia. Obstet Gynecol 53:461–464, 1979.

Mazur MT, Hsueh S, Gersell DJ. Metastases to the female genital tract: analysis of 325 cases. Cancer 53:1978–1984, 1984.

Pins MR, Young RH, Crum CP, et al. Cervical squamous cell carcinoma in situ with intraepithelial extension to the upper genital tract and invasion of tubes and ovaries: report of a case with human papillomavirus analysis. Int J Gynecol Pathol 16:272–278, 1997.

Seidman JD, Sherman ME, Kurman RJ. Fallopian tube calcifications and chronic salpingitis associated with ovarian serous borderline tumors (SBLT) [Abstract]. Mod Pathol 11:114A, 1998.

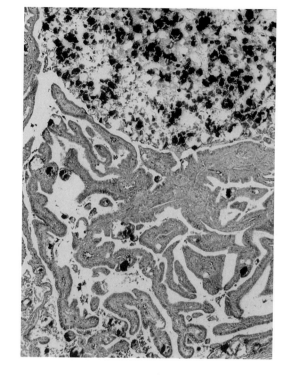

Figure 11–19. Ovarian serous borderline tumor involves the tubal mucosa and lumen.

TUMOR-LIKE LESIONS OF THE BROAD LIGAMENT

Embryonic Rests

- The most common embryonic remnants in the broad ligament are mesonephric remnants: small hollow tubules lined by nonciliated cuboidal cells that are associated with a prominent basement membrane and that are usually surrounded by a cuff of smooth muscle.
- Adrenocortical rests have been identified in about 25% of carefully sectioned broad ligaments. Rarely, these remnants can undergo hyperplasia in response to a corticotropin-secreting pituitary tumor (i.e., in Nelson's syndrome). Collections of hilus cells are occasionally encountered in the broad ligament.

Cysts

- Cysts are of müllerian, mesonephric, or mesothelial origin, although the lining epithelium, especially in the large cysts, may have a nonspecific appearance precluding subclassification. The cysts range from microscopic to rare examples 20 cm or larger. Complications include torsion, infarction, and infection.
- Pedunculated cysts of müllerian origin (i.e., hydatids of Morgagni) that lie near the tubal fimbria are the most common. The cysts are usually lined by tubal-type epithelium that may form folds resembling the tubal plicae, an appearance suggesting origin in an accessory tube.
- Cysts that are sessile but otherwise similar to hydatids of Morgagni are occasionally found within the leaves

of the broad ligament. The distinction of a müllerian cyst from a cystadenoma may be difficult, although the latter usually has a stromal component resembling that of an ovarian serous tumor.

- Some cysts are lined by cuboidal or flattened mesothelial cells, occasionally in the form of a multilocular peritoneal inclusion cyst (page 449).
- Cysts of mesonephric type are lined by cuboidal, usually nonciliated cells and may be associated with a prominent basement membrane like the remnants from which they arise.

Other Tumor-like Lesions

- Endometriosis often involves the broad ligament, usually in association with other pelvic foci of endometriosis.
- Inflammatory lesions caused by bacteria or foreign bodies (usually representing spread from an adjacent pelvic organ), inflammatory pseudotumors, and malacoplakia may involve the broad ligament.
- One case of nodular fasciitis involving the round ligament presented as a small nodule in a labium.

- One case of a uterus-like mass, similar to those occurring in the ovary (see Chapter 12), has been encountered in the broad ligament.

References

Ahmed AA, Swan RW, Owen A, et al. Uterus-like mass arising in the broad ligament: a metaplasia or müllerian duct anomaly? Int J Gynecol Pathol 16:279–281, 1997.

Breen JL, Lukeman JM, Neubecker RD. Nodular fasciitis of the round ligament: report of a case. Gynecol Oncol 19:397–400, 1984.

Falls JL. Accessory adrenal cortex in the broad ligament: incidence and functional significance. Cancer 8:143–150, 1955.

Gardner GH, Greene RR, Peckham BM. Normal and cystic structures of the broad ligament. Am J Obstet Gynecol 55:917–939, 1948.

Genadry R, Parmley T, Woodruff JD. The origin and clinical behavior of the parovarian tumor. Am J Obstet Gynecol 129:873–879, 1977.

Rao NR. Malacoplakia of broad ligament, inguinal region, and endometrium. Arch Pathol 88:85–88, 1969.

Samaha M, Woodruff JD. Paratubal cysts: frequency, histogenesis and associated clinical features. Obstet Gynecol 65:691–694, 1985.

Verdonk C, Guerin C, Lufkin E, Hodgson SF. Activation of virilizing adrenal rest tissues by excessive ACTH production: an unusual presentation of Nelson's syndrome. Am J Med 73:455–459, 1982.

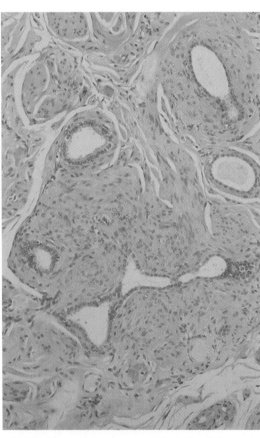

Figure 11–20. Mesonephric remnants within the broad ligament.

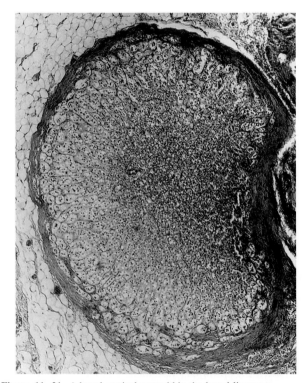

Figure 11–21. Adrenal cortical rest within the broad ligament.

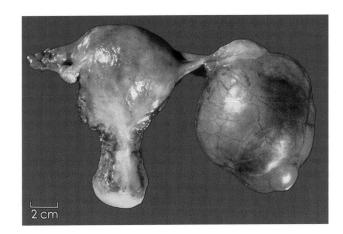

Figure 11–22. A nonneoplastic cyst within the broad ligament abuts a normal ovary.

TUMORS OF THE BROAD LIGAMENT

- These tumors are one fifth as common as ovarian tumors, and only 2% of them are borderline or invasive, in contrast to a frequency of 25% for ovarian tumors.
- The tumors range from 3 to 40 cm, with about 70% between 5 and 12 cm; about 15% are bilateral.
- The clinical manifestations are similar to those of ovarian tumors.

Epithelial Tumors of Müllerian Type

- Serous cystadenomas are the most common epithelial tumors of müllerian type. They can generally be distinguished from nonneoplastic serous cysts by the presence of a thick wall composed of cellular, ovarian-type stroma and an absence of folds or plicae.
- Serous borderline tumors of the broad ligament are the second most common tumor in this site and have clinical and pathologic features identical to their ovarian counterparts. They have been found in women 19 to 67 years of age (mean, 33 years), and all have been unilateral and without evidence of spread.
- Other benign or borderline epithelial tumors occasionally encountered in the broad ligament include mucinous tumors of intestinal type, Brenner tumors, and mixed epithelial–type tumors. One of the latter tumors, a benign papillary tumor that showed endometrioid and serous differentiation, occurred in a patient with von Hippel-Lindau disease.
- Carcinomas of müllerian type include, in approximate order of frequency, endometrioid, clear cell, serous, mucinous, and transitional cell carcinomas.
  - The clinical and pathologic features of these tumors, some of which were associated with spread beyond the broad ligament, are similar to their ovarian counterparts.
  - Some of the endometrioid and clear cell carcinomas were associated with and may have arisen from foci of endometriosis.

References

Altaras MM, Jaffe R, Corduba M, et al. Primary paraovarian cystadenocarcinoma: clinical and management aspects and literature review. Gynecol Oncol 38:268–272, 1990.

Aslani M, Ahn G-H, Scully RE. Serous papillary cystadenoma of borderline malignancy of the broad ligament: a report of 25 cases. Int J Gynecol Pathol 7:131–138, 1988.

Aslani M, Scully RE. Primary carcinoma of the broad ligament: report of four cases and review of the literature. Cancer 64:1640–1645, 1989.

Hampton HL, Huffman HT, Meeks GR. Extraovarian Brenner tumor. Obstet Gynecol 79:844–846, 1992.

Honoré LH, Nickerson KG. Papillary serous cystadenoma arising in a paramesonephric cyst of the parovarium. Am J Obstet Gynecol 125: 870–871, 1976.

Jensen ML, Nielsen MN. Broad ligament mucinous cystadenoma of borderline malignancy. Histopathology 16:89–103, 1990.

Thomason RN, Rush W, Dave H. Transitional cell carcinoma arising within a paratubal cyst: report of a case. Int J Gynecol Pathol 14: 270–273, 1995.

Werness BA, Guccion JG. Tumor of the broad ligament in von Hippel-Lindau disease of probable müllerian origin. Int J Gynecol Pathol 16: 282–285, 1997.

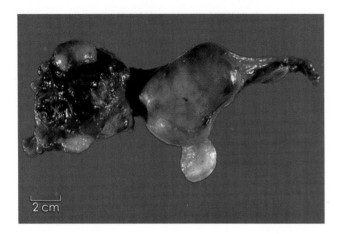

Figure 11–23. Adenocarcinoma arising within the broad ligament.

Epithelial Tumors of Definite or Probable Wolffian Origin

Papillary Cystadenoma

■ Four cases of papillary cystadenoma of the broad ligament have been reported in patients with von Hippel-
Lindau disease; in one case, the tumor was the first
manifestation of the disease. In two cases, the cysts
were bilateral.

■ The tumors were cystic, were less than 3 cm in diameter, and contained papillae lined by cuboidal nonciliated
cells with bland nuclei.

References

Gersell DJ, King TC. Papillary cystadenoma of the mesosalpinx in von
Hippel-Lindau disease. Am J Surg Pathol 12:145–149, 1994.
Korn WT, Schatzki SC, Disciullo AJ, Scully RE. Papillary cystadenoma
of the broad ligament in von Hippel-Lindau disease. Am J Obstet
Gynecol 163:596–598, 1990.

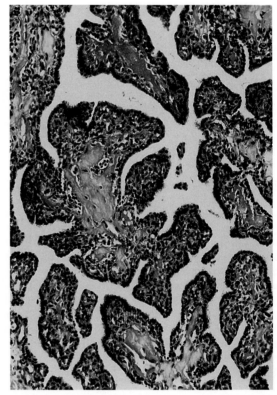

Figure 11–24. Papillary cystadenoma of the broad ligament associated
with von Hippel-Lindau disease.

Female Adnexal Tumor of Probable Wolffian Origin

- About 40 cases of female adnexal tumor of probable wolffian origin (FATWO) have been reported in patients 15 to 81 years of age. The tumors are unilateral, 0.5 to 18 cm in diameter, and usually found within the leaves of the broad ligament or pedunculated from it or the fallopian tube.
- The sectioned surfaces are solid or predominantly solid with small cysts. The solid tissue varies from gray-white to tan or yellow and is typically firm or rubbery. Hemorrhage and necrosis are uncommon.
- The low-power appearance varies from cystic or sievelike (with luminal eosinophilic secretions) to predominantly solid with scattered cysts to solid. The solid areas consist of sheets of cells or closely packed solid or hollow tubules; the latter may require reticulum or PAS stains to demonstrate. A prominent fibrous stroma may separate the tubules or result in a lobulated pattern.
- The cells have scanty eosinophilic cytoplasm and are typically epithelioid but occasionally spindle shaped. The nuclei are usually uniform and pale with no or few mitotic figures. Rare tumors have focal areas with markedly atypical cells with increased mitotic activity.
- Evidence supporting the wolffian origin of these tumors includes:
  - Their typical location in the broad ligament
  - Ultrastructural findings, including the absence or paucity of cilia, Golgi complexes, secretory granules, and glycogen, as well as the presence of a thick peritubular basal lamina
  - Absent immunoreactivity for epithelial membrane antigen, Tag 72, and carcinoembryonic antigen, in contrast to typically opposite findings in müllerian-type tumors
- Four tumors have been clinically malignant with spread at the time of diagnosis or recurrent tumor, which may occur more than 5 years postoperatively. Some of the clinically malignant tumors were focally atypical, but others had a bland appearance.
- All FATWOs should be considered to have a malignant potential, and the follow-up should be prolonged.

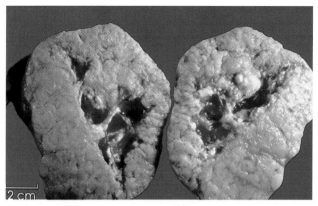

Figure 11–25. Sectioned surface of a female adnexal tumor of probable wolffian origin.

References

Daya D. Malignant female adnexal tumor of probable wolffian origin with review of the literature. Arch Pathol Lab Med 118:310–312, 1994.

Kariminejad MH, Scully RE. Female adnexal tumor of probable wolffian origin: a distinctive pathologic entity. Cancer 31:671–677, 1973.

Rahilly MA, Williams ARW, Krausz T, Al Nafussi AL. Female adnexal tumour of probable wolffian origin: a clinicopathological and immunohistochemical study of three cases. Histopathology 26:69–74, 1995.

Tavassoli FA, Andrade R, Merino M. Retiform wolffian adenoma. In: Fenoglio-Preiser CM, Wolffe M, Rilke R (eds): Progress in Surgical Pathology, vol. 11. New York: Field & Wood Medical Publishers, 1990:121–136.

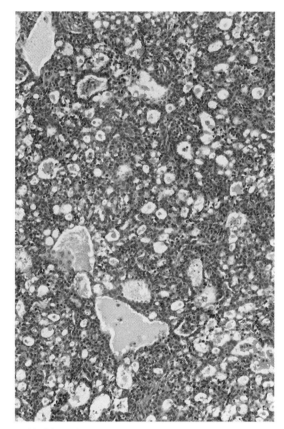

Figure 11–26. A female adnexal tumor of probable wolffian origin with a sievelike pattern.

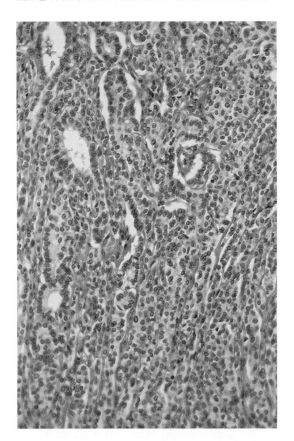

Figure 11–27. Female adnexal tumor of probable wolffian origin. Occasional tubules interrupt a solid growth pattern.

Ependymoma

- Three ependymomas of the broad ligament and one of the uterosacral ligament, which arose in patients 13 to 48 years of age, have varied from 1 cm in diameter to a mass that filled the pelvis.
- The tumors microscopically resemble those of the central nervous system. Cysts with papillae and psammoma bodies may mimic a serous papillary carcinoma, a diagnosis excluded by the presence of perivascular rosettes, immunoreactivity for glial fibrillary acidic protein, or both.
- The tumor had spread at the time of operation in two cases; a third patient had two retroperitoneal recurrences of tumor over a period of 24 years.

References

Bell DA, Woodruff JM, Scully RE. Ependymoma of the broad ligament: a report of two cases. Am J Surg Pathol 8:203–209, 1984.

Duggan MA, Hugh J, Nation JG, et al. Ependymoma of uterosacral ligament. Cancer 64:2565–2567, 1989.

Grody WW, Nieberg RK, Bhuta S. Ependymoma-like tumor of the mesovarium. Arch Pathol Lab Med 109:291–293, 1985.

Mixed Epithelial-Mesenchymal Tumors

- The adenomyoma, which is composed of endometrial-type glands (with or without endometrioid stroma) and proliferating smooth muscle is the most common mixed epithelial-mesenchymal tumor of the broad ligament.
- One high-grade müllerian adenosarcoma of the round ligament was fatal within a year after its discovery.

Reference

Kao GF, Norris HS. Benign and low grade variants of mixed mesodermal tumors (adenosarcoma) of the ovary and adnexal region. Cancer 42:1314–1324, 1978.

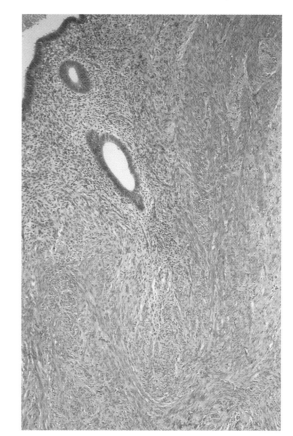

Figure 11–28. Adenomyoma within the broad ligament. Notice the admixture of endometrial epithelium, stroma, and smooth muscle.

Soft Tissue Tumors

Benign Tumors

■ Leiomyomas and lipomas are the most common benign mesenchymal tumors of the broad ligament and round ligament. The tumors are usually small; large tumors may be associated with symptoms.

■ A ligamentous origin can be established only when the tumors are clearly separated from the tube and myometrium.

■ Rare tumors in this category have included a fibroma with heterotopic bone formation and two benign mesenchyomas composed of fat and smooth muscle cells and thin-walled blood vessels.

References

Honoré LH. Parauterine leiomyomas in women: a clinicopathologic study of 22 cases. Eur J Obstet Gynecol Reprod Biol 11:273–279, 1981.

Nuovo MA, Nuovo GJ, Smith D, Lewis SH. Benign mesenchymoma of the round ligament: a report of two cases with immunohistochemistry. Am J Clin Pathol 93:421–424, 1990.

Terada S, Suzuki N, Uchide K, et al. Parovarian fibroma with heterotopic bone formation of probable wolffian origin. Gynecol Oncol 50:115–118, 1993.

Malignant Tumors

■ Leiomyosarcomas, which are the most common sarcoma of the broad ligament, are associated with a poor prognosis.

■ Rare sarcomas arising in this site have included examples of embryonal rhabdomyosarcoma (two cases, both in children and both fatal), endometrial stromal sarcoma arising in endometriosis, malignant fibrous histiocytoma, myxoid liposarcoma, and Ewing's sarcoma.

References

Cheng W-F, Lin H-H, Chen C-K, et al. Leiomyosarcoma of the broad ligament: a case report and literature review. Gynecol Oncol 56:85–89, 1995.

Mai Y-L, Wu M-Y, Lin Y-H, et al. Malignant fibrous histiocytoma of the broad ligament. Gynecol Oncol 54:362–364, 1994.

Ghazali S. Embryonic rhabdomyosarcoma of the urogenital tract. Br J Surg 60:124–128, 1973.

Longway SR, Lind HM, Haghighi P. Extraskeletal Ewing's sarcoma arising in the broad ligament. Arch Pathol Lab Med 110:1058–1061, 1986.

Persad V. Endometrial stromal sarcoma of the broad ligament arising in the area of endometriosis in a paramesonephric cyst. Br J Obstet Gynaecol 84:149–152, 1977.

Singh TT, Hopkins MP, Price J, Schuen R. Myxoid liposarcoma of the broad ligament. Int J Gynecol Cancer 2:220–223, 1992.

Miscellaneous and Secondary Tumors

- A variety of miscellaneous tumors, many of them of ovarian type, have arisen in the broad ligament. Some of them may have originated in an accessory ovary.
- Germ cell tumors have included dermoid cysts, a yolk sac tumor, and a choriocarcinoma; it was not clear if the choriocarcinoma was of germ or gestational origin.
- Sex cord–stromal tumors originating in the broad ligament include granulosa cell tumors and tumors in the thecoma-fibroma category. Some of these tumors were associated with estrogenic manifestations.
- Steroid cell tumors arising in the broad ligament may originate from the common adrenal-cortical rests in this site (page 257). Hormonal manifestations (e.g., sexual precocity, virilism) may occur.
- Rare examples of other tumors arising in the broad ligament have included adenomatoid tumors, pheochromocytomas (one of which was associated with hypertension), and a carcinoid tumor.

- Any cancer arising in the uterus, fallopian tube, or elsewhere may spread to the broad ligament by direct extension, lymphatics, or blood vessels. Intravenous leiomyomatosis and endometrial stromal sarcoma of the uterus may present at operation as a mass within the broad ligament.

References

Al-Jafari MS, Panton HM, Gradwell E. Phaeochromocytoma of the broad ligament: case report. Br J Obstet Gynaecol 92:649–651, 1985.

Clement PB, Young RH, Scully RE. Extraovarian pelvic yolk sac tumors. Cancer 62:620–626, 1988.

Gabbay-Mor M, Ovadia Y, Neri A. Accessory ovaries with bilateral dermoid cysts. Eur J Obstet Gynecol Reprod Biol 14:171–173, 1982.

Jafri NH, Niemann TH, Nicklin JL, Copeland LJ. A carcinoid tumor of the broad ligament. Obstet Gynecol 92:708, 1998.

Kay S, Schneider V, Litt J. Choriocarcinoma of the mesosalpinx masquerading as congestive heart failure: ultrastructural observations of the tumor. Int J Gynecol Pathol 2:72–87, 1983.

Keitoku M, Konishi I, Nanbu K, et al. Extraovarian sex cord–stromal tumor: case report and review of the literature. Int J Gynecol Pathol 16:180–185, 1997.

Roth LM, Davis MM, Sutton GP. Steroid cell tumor of the broad ligament arising in an accessory ovary. Arch Pathol Lab Med 120: 405–409, 1996.

Williamson HO, Moore MP. Ovarian and paraovarian adenomatoid tumors: case reports. Am J Obstet Gynecol 90:388–394, 1964.

CHAPTER 12

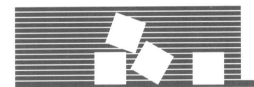

Tumor-like Lesions of the Ovary

LESIONS OF THE FOLLICULAR AND STROMAL ELEMENTS

Follicle Cyst

Clinical Features

- Solitary follicle cysts (FCs) are most common in non-pregnant women of reproductive age, particularly around the times of menarche and menopause; they rarely occur after menopause. In the reproductive era, FCs may be a result of abnormalities of pituitary gonadotropin secretion.
- FCs may cause menstrual irregularities because of estrogen production or may rupture, causing acute abdominal pain with hemoperitoneum and, exceptionally, exsanguination. Palpable FCs can be confused clinically with a neoplasm.
- FCs are uncommon in children in whom they may cause isosexual pseudoprecocity, which regresses after removal or puncture of the cyst or occasionally resolves spontaneously. These cysts probably are autonomous, because they are not associated with elevated gonadotropin levels at the time of diagnosis.
- Some FCs in children may be a component of the McCune-Albright syndrome, and in such cases, there may be one or several cysts, which are occasionally bilateral. Occasionally, ovulation, corpus luteum formation, and the possibility of pregnancy occur. In contrast to isolated FCs, those associated with the syndrome may recur after removal with a return of the precocity.
- FCs develop rarely in utero or during the neonatal period and may undergo torsion, hemorrhage, or rupture. They almost always regress within a few months after birth.

Pathologic Features

- Solitary FCs are usually less than 8 cm in diameter, except during pregnancy or the puerperium (page 277). They usually have smooth surfaces, thin walls, and contain watery fluid or occasionally contain blood.
- FCs are usually lined by granulosa cells and luteinized

theca cells. The granulosa cells also may be luteinized and are often focally denuded. Some simple cysts in women of reproductive age probably represent the end stage of follicle cysts.

Differential Diagnosis With Unilocular Granulosa Cell Tumor

- Unilocular granulosa cell tumors (UGCTs), like FCs, may be lined by an orderly arrangement of granulosa cells and theca cells but are almost always much larger than FCs and have a more disorderly admixture of the two cell types, with obviously neoplastic aggregates of granulosa cells in their walls in many cases.
- The granulosa cells lining a UGCT usually do not have the conspicuous eosinophilic cytoplasm that is often present in the granulosa cells of a FC, Moreover, their nuclei, in contrast to those in FCs, resemble those of typical GCTs.

References

Adelman S, Benson CD, Hertzler JH. Surgical lesions of the ovary in infancy and childhood. Surg Gynecol Obstet 141:219–222, 1975.

Danon M, Robboy SJ, Kim S, et al. Cushing's syndrome, sexual precocity and polyostotic fibrous dysplasia (Albright syndrome) in infancy. J Pediatr 87:917–921, 1975.

DeSa DJ. Follicular ovarian cysts in stillbirths and neonates. Arch Dis Child 50:45–50, 1975.

Liapi C, Evain-Brion D. Diagnosis of ovarian follicular cysts from birth to puberty: a report of twenty cases. Acta Pediatr Scand 76:91–96, 1987.

Nussbaum AR, Sanders RC, Hartman DS, et al. Neonatal ovarian cysts: sonographic-pathologic correlation. Radiology 168:817–821, 1988.

Strickler RC, Kelly RW, Askin FB. Postmenopausal ovarian follicle cyst: an unusual cause of estrogen excess. Int J Gynecol Pathol 3:318–322, 1984.

Widdowson DJ, Pilling DW, Cook RCM. Neonatal ovarian cysts: therapeutic dilemma. Arch Dis Child 63:737–742, 1988.

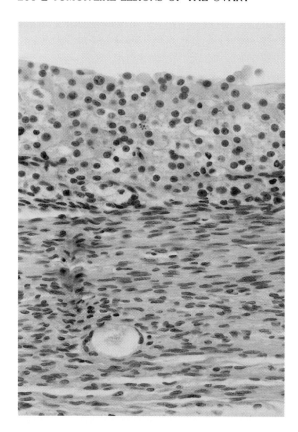

Figure 12–1. Luteinized granulosa cells line a follicle cyst in a girl with McCune-Albright syndrome. The cyst was associated with precocious pseudopuberty.

Corpus Luteum Cyst

- Corpus luteum cyst refers to a cystic corpus luteum greater than 2 cm in diameter. Such cysts may be associated with menstrual irregularities, including amenorrhea, and they may rupture with intraabdominal hemorrhage. Corpora lutea and cysts derived from them rarely occur in neonates or in postmenopausal women.
- The cyst wall and lining are usually yellow and surround a lumen that is typically distended with blood. The wall is composed of a thick, convoluted layer of large luteinized granulosa cells interrupted at its periphery by wedges of much smaller luteinized theca interna cells.

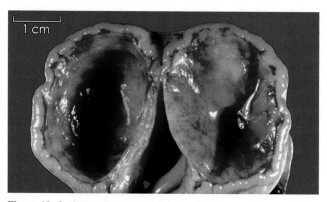

Figure 12–2. Corpus luteum cyst.

References

Hallatt JG, Steele CH Jr, Snyder M. Ruptured corpus luteum with hemoperitoneum: a study of 173 surgical cases. Am J Obstet Gynecol 149:5–9, 1984.

Miles PA, Penney LL. Corpus luteum formation in the fetus. Obstet Gynecol 61:525–529, 1983.

Polycystic Ovarian Disease

Clinical Features

■ Polycystic ovarian disease (PCOD), also called Stein-Leventhal syndrome, typically occurs in young women who present with menstrual disturbances (oligoamenorrhea, menometrorrhagia), infertility, obesity, and hirsutism. The clinical manifestations may simulate an androgenic or estrogenic ovarian tumor.

■ Other endocrine disturbances in some patients include hyperprolactinemia or late-onset congenital adrenal hyperplasia.

■ Patients usually have hyperandrogenemia and an elevated serum estrone level (caused by peripheral conversion of androstenedione) with a reversal of the estradiol-estrone ratio. The follicle-stimulating hormone (FSH) level is usually low to normal, the luteinizing hormone (LH) level is high, and there is an exaggerated response of LH to gonadotropin-releasing hormone.

■ Ovulating women with minor evidence of hyperandrogenism but without menstrual irregularity may also have polycystic ovaries that contain corpora lutea and albicantia, indicating lack of a clear boundary between normality and the clinical syndrome of PCOD.

■ Patients with PCOD may have an endometrium that varies from inactive to hyperplastic or, in fewer than 5% of cases, adenocarcinoma, which is almost always a low-grade endometrioid carcinoma.

Pathologic Features

■ Both ovaries are typically enlarged and rounded, and have multiple small follicle cysts visible beneath a thickened, white, superficial cortex; occasionally, the ovaries are of normal size.

■ Sectioning reveals multiple cortical cysts of approximately equal size and a medulla consisting of homogeneous stroma with no or sparse corpora lutea or corpora albicantia.

■ The follicular cysts are lined by a thin layer of nonluteinized granulosa cells and usually by a thick layer of luteinized theca interna cells, which may also be prominent around atretic follicles (i.e., follicular hyperthecosis).

■ Some luteinized stromal cells can be found in most cases, indicating a morphologic overlap with stromal hyperthecosis. The outer cortex is typically hypocellular, fibrotic, and contains numerous, often thick-walled blood vessels.

■ Coincidental ovarian tumors of diverse types can be an additional finding in occasional patients.

Differential Diagnosis

■ Polycystic ovaries resembling those of PCOD are seen occasionally in normal prepubertal and peripubertal children and in girls in the second decade with primary hypothyroidism.

■ Stromal hyperthecosis is discussed in the next section.

References

Adams J, Polson DW, Franks S. Prevalence of polycystic ovaries in women with anovulation and idiopathic hirsutism. Br Med J 293: 355–358, 1986.

Babaknia A, Calfopoulos P, Jones HW. The Stein-Leventhal syndrome and coincidental ovarian tumors. Obstet Gynecol 47:223–224, 1976.

Barnes R, Rosenfield RL. The polycystic ovary syndrome: pathogenesis and treatment. Ann Intern Med 110:386–399, 1989.

Goldzieher JW. Polycystic ovarian disease. Fertil Steril 35:371–394, 1981.

Hughesdon PE. Morphology and morphogenesis of the Stein-Leventhal ovary and of so-called "hyperthecosis." Obstet Gynecol Surv 37:59–77, 1982.

Lindsay AN, Voorhess ML, Macgillivray MH. Multicystic ovaries detected by sonography in children with hypothyroidism. Am J Dis Child 134:588–592, 1980.

Polson DW, Wadsworth J, Adams J, Franks S. Polycystic ovaries—a common finding in normal women. Lancet 2:870–872, 1988.

Smith KD, Steinberger E, Perloff WH. Polycystic ovarian disease: a report of 301 patients. Am J Obstet Gynecol 93:994–1001, 1965.

Yen SSC. The polycystic ovary syndrome. Clin Endocrinol 12:177–208, 1980.

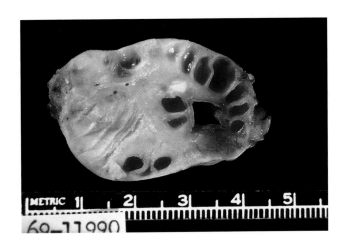

Figure 12–3. Polycystic ovarian disease. Notice the multiple cystic follicles on the sectioned surface of the ovary.

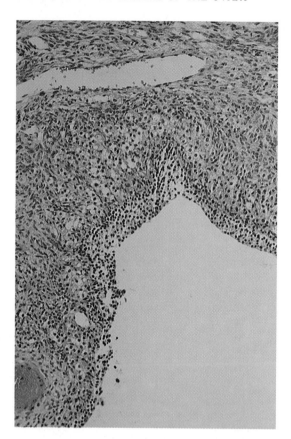

Figure 12–4. Polycystic ovarian disease. A follicle cyst is lined by an inner layer of nonluteinized granulosa cells and a thick outer layer of luteinized theca interna cells.

Stromal Hyperthecosis

Clinical Features

- The clinical manifestations may resemble those of PCOD, but stromal hyperthecosis (SH) more often has a gradual or, less commonly, an abrupt onset of virilization (with elevated serum testosterone levels) in a premenopausal woman who often also exhibits obesity, hypertension, and decreased glucose tolerance.
- As in patients with PCOD, elevated serum estrone levels, which may cause endometrial hyperplasia or carcinoma, may also be present. Estrogenic manifestations usually predominate when SH occurs in postmenopausal women, in whom the disease is usually milder.
- The disorder is occasionally familial. Insulin resistance, sometimes accompanied by diabetes, acanthosis nigricans, and hyperandrogenism (HAIR-AN syndrome) have been described in a small subset of women considered clinically to have SH or PCOD.

Pathologic Features

- Both ovaries may be enlarged to 8 cm, with variable replacement by solid white to yellow stroma, sometimes simulating bilateral tumors; rarely, the involvement is unilateral. In premenopausal women, PCOD-like changes (i.e., white opaque external surface and multiple superficial follicle cysts) may be visible.
- Rarely, there is a synchronous ovarian neoplasm, which occasionally has a hormone-secreting potential.
- Microscopically, lipid-poor or lipid-rich luteinized stromal cells are scattered singly, in small nests, or nodules (i.e., nodular hyperthecosis), typically on a background of stromal hyperplasia. In premenopausal women, follicular hyperthecosis and sclerosis of the outer cortex, characteristic of POD, are also common.
- Hilus cell hyperplasia or a hilus cell tumor may also be present in one or both ovaries.
- Patients with the HAIR-AN syndrome almost always have SH with multiple follicle cysts, which may be

accompanied by superficial cortical sclerosis and stromal edema and fibrosis.

■ Enzymes involved in the conversion of cholesterol to steroid hormones have been demonstrated immunohistochemically in the luteinized stromal cells and the adjacent spindle-shaped stromal cells in cases of SH, consistent with androgen synthesis by these cells.

Differential Diagnosis

■ Stromal luteoma. An arbitrary size criterion (>1 cm) separates these tumors from the nodules of nodular hyperthecosis.

■ Luteinized thecoma (see Chapter 16).

References

See those after Stromal Hyperplasia.

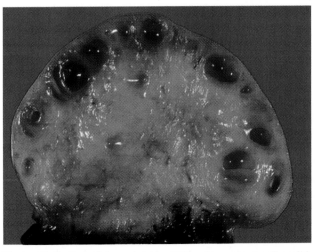

Figure 12–5. Stromal hyperthecosis. Notice the predominantly solid, homogenous, yellow sectioned surface and a few cystic follicles.

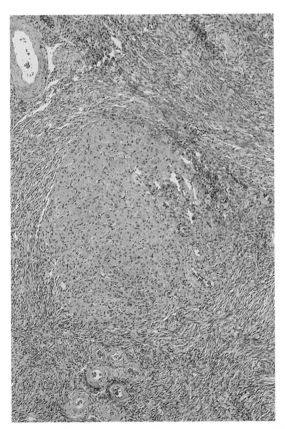

Figure 12–6. Nodular stromal hyperthecosis. A nodule of luteinized stromal cells lies within the ovarian stroma.

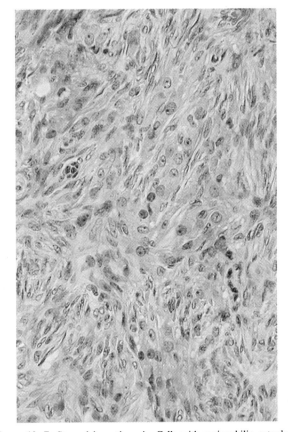

Figure 12–7. Stromal hyperthecosis. Cells with eosinophilic cytoplasm and a rounded nucleus with a prominent nucleolus are admixed with spindled stromal cells.

Stromal Hyperplasia

Clinical Features

▪ This process is a commmon incidental microscopic finding in the ovaries of perimenopausal or postmenopausal women.

▪ Occasionally, there are androgenic or estrogenic manifestations as well as obesity, hypertension, and disorders of glucose metabolism, although these findings are much less frequent or less obtrusive than in stromal hyperthecosis.

Pathologic Features

▪ The ovaries may be normal in size or slightly enlarged by ill-defined, white or pale yellow, occasionally confluent nodules within the stroma of the medulla, cortex, or both.

▪ On microscopic examination, the medulla and, to a lesser extent, the cortex are replaced by a nodular or diffuse, densely cellular proliferation of small stromal cells with scanty, nonluteinized cytoplasm.

▪ Some of the hyperplastic cells contain oxidative enzymes that are important in steroid hormone production, although in some cases hormones may be produced by rare lutein cells not sampled microscopically or by spindle-shaped cells that are transitional morphologically between typical stromal cells and lutein cells.

Differential Diagnosis

▪ Ovarian fibroma (see Chapter 16).

▪ Low-grade endometrioid stromal sarcoma (see Chapter 14). Features favoring or diagnostic of this disorder over that of SH include marked ovarian enlargement, oval rather than spindle-shaped cells, mitotic figures, and regularly distributed arterioles.

References

Barbieri RL, Ryan KJ. Hyperandrogenism, insulin resistance, and acanthosis nigricans syndrome: a common endocrinopathy with distinct pathophysiologic features. Am J Obstet Gynecol 147:90–101, 1983.

Boss JH, Scully RE, Wegner KH, Cohen RB. Structural variation in the adult ovary—clinical significance. Obstet Gynecol 25:747–764, 1965.

Dunaif A, Hoffman AR, Scully RE, et al. Clinical, biochemical, and ovarian morphologic features in women with acanthosis nigricans and masculinization. Obstet Gynecol 66:545–552, 1985.

Hirakawa T, Thor AD, Osawa Y, et al. Stromal hyperthecosis of the ovary: immunohistochemical distribution of steroidogenic enzymes [Abstract]. Mod Pathol 5:65a, 1992.

Judd HL, Scully RE, Herbst AL, et al. Familial hyperthecosis: comparison of endocrinologic and histologic findings with polycystic ovarian disease. Am J Obstet Gynecol 117:976–982, 1973.

Sasano H, Fukunaga M, Rojas M, Silverberg SG. Hyperthecosis of the ovary: clinicopathologic study of 19 cases with immunohistochemical analysis of steroidogenic enzymes. Int J Gynecol Pathol 8:311–320, 1989.

Snowden JA, Harkin PJR, Thornton JG, Wells M. Morphometric assessment of ovarian stromal proliferation—a clinicopathological study. Histopathology 14:369–379, 1989.

Taylor SI, Dons RF, Hernandez E, et al. Insulin resistance associated with androgen excess in women with autoantibodies to the insulin receptor. Ann Intern Med 97:851–855, 1982.

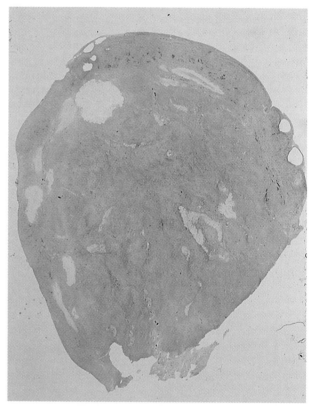

Figure 12–8. Stromal hyperplasia in a 66-year-old woman.

Massive Edema

Clinical Features

■ The patients are between 6 and 33 years old (mean, 21 years). Seventy-five percent of them present with abdominal pain, which may be acute, and abdominal swelling. Other manifestations include disorders of menstruation, evidence of androgen excess, or both.

■ Laparotomy reveals ovarian enlargement, which is bilateral in 10% of cases, and partial or complete torsion of the ovarian pedicle in about 50% of the cases, implicating torsion in the pathogenesis.

Pathologic Features

■ The ovaries are 5.5 to 35 cm in diameter (mean, 11.5 cm), with an opaque, white outer surface through which small follicle cysts may be seen. Abundant watery fluid typically exudes from the sectioned surfaces, which appear edematous or gelatinous.

■ Microscopically, edematous, hypocellular stroma surrounds rather than displaces follicles and their derivatives. The peripheral cortex is typically composed of dense, nonedematous, collagenous tissue.

■ Features in a minority of cases include small foci of a fibromatous stromal proliferation and luteinized stromal cells.

Differential Diagnosis

■ Edematous fibroma (see Chapter 16), luteinized thecoma associated with sclerosing peritonitis (see Chapter 16), and Krukenberg tumor (see Chapter 18). Distinction from a Krukenberg tumor depends on the absence of signet-ring cells in the edematous tissue.

References

Roth LM, Deaton RL, Sternberg WH. Massive ovarian edema: a clinicopathologic study of five cases including ultrastructural observations and review of the literature. Am J Surg Pathol 3:11–21, 1979.

Young RH, Scully RE. Fibromatosis and massive edema of the ovary possibly related entities: a report of 14 cases of fibromatosis and 11 cases of massive edema. Int J Gynecol Pathol 3:153–178, 1984.

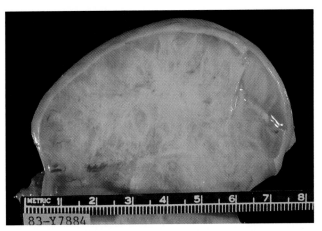

Figure 12–9. Massive edema (sectioned surface).

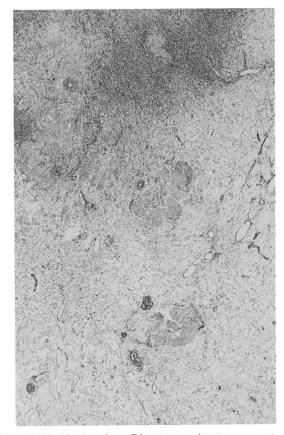

Figure 12–10. Massive edema. Edematous ovarian stroma separates the corpora fibrosa.

Fibromatosis

Clinical Features

■ Patients between 13 and 39 years old (mean, 25 years) usually present with menstrual irregularities or amenorrhea and, rarely, virilization.

■ At operation, the process is found to be bilateral in 20% of the cases; some involved ovaries have twisted on their pedicles.

Pathologic Features

■ The enlarged ovaries are 8 to 14 cm in the maximal dimension and have smooth or lobulated external surfaces. The sectioned surfaces are typically firm and white or grey; small cysts may be visible.

■ Proliferating spindle cells and abundant collagen surround follicular derivatives. The fibromatous proliferation is usually diffuse, but occasionally it predominantly involves the cortex (i.e., cortical fibromatosis).

■ Luteinized stromal cells, foci of stromal edema, and focal nests of sex cord–type cells occur in some cases.

Differential Diagnosis

■ Fibroma (see Chapter 16). Entrapment of follicular derivatives strongly favors the diagnosis of fibromatosis. The distinction between the two lesions in a superficial biopsy may not be possible.

■ Granulosa cell tumor with fibromatous component (see Chapter 16). This tumor enters the differential diagnosis in cases of fibromatosis with sex cord–like nests. Entrapment of normal follicles and bilaterality favor fibromatosis.

■ Brenner tumor (see Chapter 14). This tumor enters the differential diagnosis in cases of fibromatosis with sex cord–like nests. The cells in the latter, however, are easily distinguishable from those of a Brenner tumor in their number, shape, and nuclear features.

Reference

Young RH, Scully RE. Fibromatosis and massive edema of the ovary possibly related entities: a report of 14 cases of fibromatosis and 11 cases of massive edema. Int J Gynecol Pathol 3:153–178, 1984.

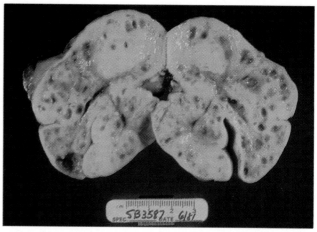

Figure 12–11. Ovarian fibromatosis (sectioned surface). Solid, white tissue surrounds cystic follicles.

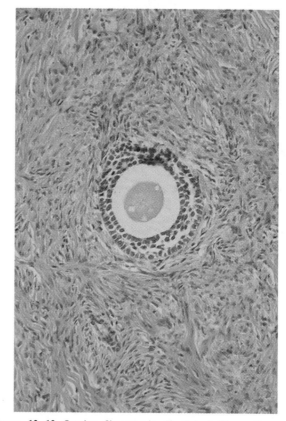

Figure 12–12. Ovarian fibromatosis. Hyalinized fibrous tissue surrounds a follicle.

Hilus Cell Hyperplasia

- Hyperplastic hilus cells (hilar Leydig cells) are typically in a nodular arrangement and may exhibit cellular enlargement, nuclear pleomorphism, hyperchromasia, and multinucleation. Physiologic proliferations of hilus cells may occur during pregnancy or after the menopause.
- Androgenic or estrogenic manifestations and elevated serum testosterone levels occur in some cases. Hilus cell proliferations may account for at least some of the hirsutism that is frequently observed in pregnant women.
- Hilus cell hyperplasia is commonly associated with stromal hyperplasia, stromal hyperthecosis, or hilus cell tumor, or may occur along the hilar border of an ovarian tumor or cyst. Rarely, it is associated with the resistant ovary syndrome or gonadal dysgenesis, disorders associated with elevated LH levels.
- The microscopic distinction between a large hyperplastic nodule of hilus cells and a hilus cell tumor is arbitrary; we diagnose the latter when the nodule is more than 1 cm in diameter.

References

Davidson BJ, Waisman J, Judd HL. Longstanding virilism in a woman with hyperplasia and neoplasia of ovarian lipidic cells. Obstet Gynecol 58:753–759, 1981.

Judd HL, Scully RE, Atkins L, et al. Pure gonadal dysgenesis with progressive hirsutism: demonstration of testosterone production by gonadal streaks. N Engl J Med 282:881–885, 1970.

Meldrum DR, Frumar AM, Shamonki IM, et al. Ovarian and adrenal steroidogenesis in a virilized patient with gonadotropin-resistant ovaries and hilus cell hyperplasia. Obstet Gynecol 56:216–221, 1980.

Sternberg WH. The morphology, androgenic function, hyperplasia, and tumours of the human ovarian hilus cells. Am J Pathol 25:493–521, 1949.

Sternberg WH, Segaloff A, Gaskill CJ. Influence of chorionic gonadotropin on human ovarian hilus cells (Leydig-like cells). J Clin Endocrinol Metab 13:139–153, 1953.

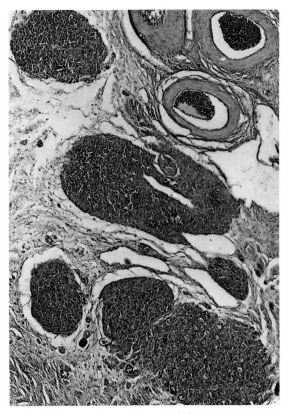

Figure 12–13. Nodular hilus cell hyperplasia in a pregnant woman.

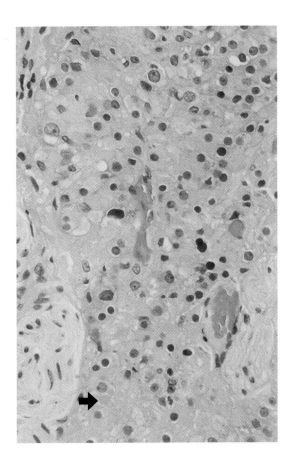

Figure 12–14. Hilus cell hyperplasia in a postmenopausal woman. Notice the focally hyperchromatic and atypical nuclei. No typical Reinke crystals are present, but several rounded, intracellular inclusions (probably crystal precursors) are visible (*arrow*).

Pregnancy Luteoma

Clinical Features

- The patients are typically in their third or fourth decades, 80% are multiparous, and a similar proportion are black. The ovarian enlargement is usually an incidental finding at term during cesarean section or postpartum tubal ligation. Rarely, a pelvic mass is palpable or obstructs the birth canal.

- In about 25% of cases, hirsutism or virilization appears during the latter half of pregnancy; 70% of female infants born to masculinized mothers are also virilized. Levels of plasma androgens, including testosterone, are elevated in virilized patients and occasionally in nonvirilized patients and their infants.

- There is postpartum regression of the lesions, and the size of the ovaries and serum androgen levels normalize within several weeks.

Pathologic Features

- Luteomas range from microscopic to larger than 20 cm in diameter (median diameter of 6.6 cm in one study), with cut surfaces that are solid, fleshy, circumscribed, red to brown, and often focally hemorrhagic. The lesions are multiple in about 50% and bilateral in at least one third of cases.

- Well-circumscribed nodules, which occasionally contain follicles filled with pale fluid or colloid-like material, consist of lutinized cells intermediate in size between the luteinized granulosa cells and luteinized theca cells of adjacent follicles.

- The cells have abundant eosinophilic, lipid-poor cytoplasm, which is typically immunoreactive for inhibin, with central, often slightly pleomorphic and hyperchromatic nuclei and prominent nucleoli. Mitotic figures (up to 7 MF per 10 high-power-fields [HPF]), which may be abnormal, are usually present. The stroma is scanty and reticulin fibrils surround groups of cells.

- Uncommon features include focal ballooning degeneration of the cytoplasm and intracellular colloid droplets.

- Within days to weeks postpartum, the luteomas degenerate, with eventual conversion to brown puckered scars. Microscopic examination reveals shrunken nests of degenerating, lipid-filled luteoma cells with pyknotic nuclei, lymphocytic infiltration, and fibrosis.

Differential Diagnosis

- Metastatic tumor when intraoperative inspection reveals multiple or bilateral nodules. Metastatic cancer can usually be excluded by frozen section examination of one of the nodules.

- A lipid-poor or lipid-free steroid cell tumor (see Chapter 16) and other tumors listed in Appendix 4. An ovarian mass composed entirely of lipid-free steroid type cells in the third trimester should be considered a pregnancy luteoma unless there is good evidence to the contrary.

References

Garcia-Bunuel R, Berek JS, Woodruff JD. Luteomas of pregnancy. Obstet Gynecol 45:407–414, 1975.

Hensleigh PA, Woodruff JD. Differential maternal-fetal response to androgenizing luteoma or hyperreactio luteinalis. Obstet Gynecol Surv 33:262–271, 1978.

Kommoss F, Oliva E, Bhan AK, et al. Inhibin expression in ovarian tumors and tumor-like lesions: an immunohistochemical study. Mod Pathol 11:656–664, 1998.

Norris HJ, Taylor HB. Nodular theca-lutein hyperplasia of pregnancy (so-called "pregnancy luteoma"): a clinical and pathological study of 15 cases. Am J Clin Pathol 47:557–566, 1967.

Rice BF, Barclay DL, Sternberg WH. Luteoma of pregnancy: steroidogenic and morphologic considerations. Am J Obstet Gynecol 104:871–878, 1969.

Sternberg WH, Barclay DL. Luteoma of pregnancy. Am J Obstet Gynecol 95:165–184, 1996.

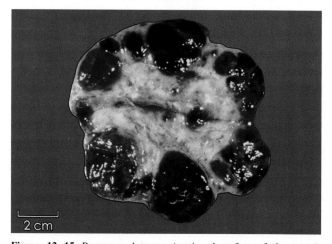

Figure 12–15. Pregnancy luteoma (sectioned surface of the ovary). Notice the multiple reddish brown nodules.

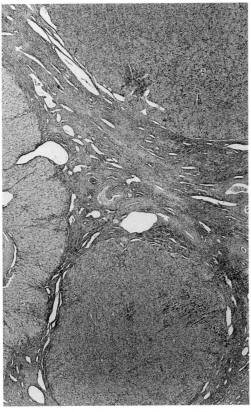

Figure 12–16. Pregnancy luteoma. Parts of two nodules and the convoluted edge of a corpus luteum of pregnancy (*left*) are seen.

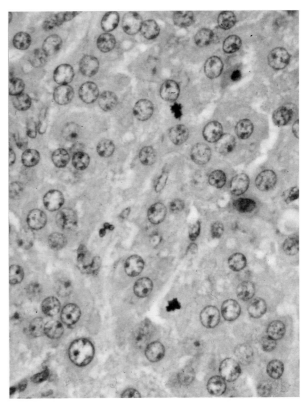

Figure 12–17. Pregnancy luteoma. Notice the mitotic figures.

Hyperreactio Luteinalis

Clinical Features

- Hyperreactio luteinalis (HL) is usually associated with conditions accompanied by elevated hCG levels, such as hydatidiform mole, choriocarcinoma, fetal hydrops, and multiple gestations. The frequency of HL in women with gestational trophoblastic disease (GTD) ranges from 10% (by clinical examination) to 40% (by ultrasonography).
- Sixty percent of cases unassociated with GTD are associated with a normal singleton pregnancy.
- HL presents as a pelvic mass during any trimester, at cesarean section, or rarely, during the puerperium. Symptoms are usually absent, but complications (e.g., intracystic hemorrhage, torsion, rupture, hemoperitoneum) may cause abdominal pain; the hemoperitoneum has been rarely fatal.
- In cases of HL secondary to GTD, ovarian enlargement may be detected at the time of the diagnostic dilatation and curettage or during the postoperative follow-up period.
- In about 15% of cases unassociated with GTD, there has been virilization of the patient but not the female infant. Elevated plasma testosterone levels occur in these patients as well as in nonvirilized patients with GTD.
- Regression of HL typically occurs during the puerperium but occasionally may not be complete until 6 months postpartum. Rarely, HL regresses spontaneously during pregnancy. In cases associated with GTD, regression typically occurs 2 to 12 weeks after uterine evacuation, but occasionally the cysts persist for long periods.
- An iatrogenic form of HL, the ovarian hyperstimulation syndrome (OHS), results from ovulation induction, typically with the use of FSH and human chorionic gonadotropin (hCG), or clomiphene alone. The syndrome occurs only after ovulation and is more severe in patients who conceive.
- In severe cases of OHS, the ovaries can become mas-

sive and may be accompanied by ascites, sometimes with hydrothorax. Elevation of the serum levels of estrogens, progesterone, and testosterone typically occurs. Hemoconcentration with secondary oliguria and thromboembolic phenomena are life-threatening complications.

■ Operative intervention in cases of HL and the OHS is needed only to remove infarcted tissue, control hemorrhage, or diminish androgen production in virilized patients.

Pathologic Features

■ Multiple, almost always bilateral, thin-walled cysts enlarge the ovaries, which may be larger than 35 cm in diameter; the cysts are filled with clear or hemorrhagic fluid.

■ Microscopic examination reveals multiple, large follicle cysts in which the theca interna cells and, to a lesser degree, the granulosa cells are hyperplastic, enlarged, and luteinized. Edema of the theca interna and the interfollicular stroma is common, and the stroma may contain luteinized cells.

■ The changes in OHS are identical, with the additional finding of one or more corpora lutea.

Differential Diagnosis

■ HL may be mistaken at laparotomy for a cystic ovarian tumor, occasionally leading to an unwarranted bilateral oophorectomy. Rarely, a coexistent pregnancy luteoma increases the suspicion of a neoplastic process. Frozen section examination of the cyst wall should facilitate the diagnosis.

References

Caspi E, Schreyer P, Bukovsky J. Ovarian lutein cysts in pregnancy. Obstet Gynecol 42:388–398, 1973.

Curry SL, Hammond CB, Tyrey L, et al. Hydatidiform mole: diagnosis, management, and long-term follow-up of 347 patients. Obstet Gynecol 45:1–8, 1975.

Haning RV Jr, Strawn EY, Nolten WE. Pathophysiology of the ovarian hyperstimulation syndrome. Obstet Gynecol 66:220–224, 1985.

Montz FJ, Schlaerth JB, Morrow CP. The natural history of theca lutein cysts. Obstet Gynecol 72:247–251, 1988.

Wajda KJ, Lucas JG, Marsh WL Jr. Hyperreactio luteinalis: benign disorder masquerading as an ovarian neoplasm. Arch Pathol Lab Med 113:921–925, 1989.

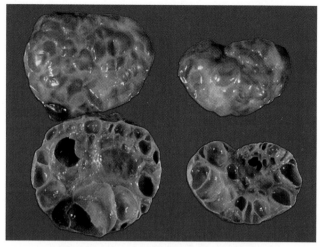

Figure 12–18. Hyperreactio luteinalis. Serosal and sectioned surfaces of both ovaries are shown.

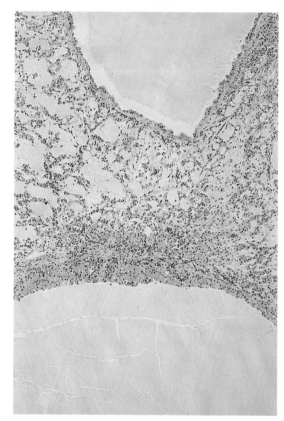

Figure 12–19. Hyperreactio luteinalis. Two follicle cysts are lined by a layer of luteinized cells (i.e., granulosa and theca cells). Luteinized stromal cells lie within the edematous stroma that separates the two cysts.

Large, Solitary, Luteinized Follicle Cyst of Pregnancy and Puerperium

Clinical Features

■ The cyst may cause abdominal swelling, but it is usually an incidental finding at cesarean section or identified on physical examination during the first postpartum visit. No endocrine disturbance has been reported.

Pathologic Features

■ The cysts, which have ranged from 8 to 26 cm (median, 25 cm), are unilocular, are thin walled, and contain watery fluid.
■ One to several layers of luteinized granulosa and theca cells, which frequently appear indistinguishable, form the cyst lining. Nests of luteinized cells may be embedded within the fibrous tissue of the cyst wall.
■ The cells have abundant eosinophilic to, less often, vacuolated cytoplasm. Their size and shape vary considerably, and they exhibit focal marked nuclear pleomorphism and hyperchromasia. Mitotic figures are absent.
■ All the patients have had an uneventful postoperative course.

Differential Diagnosis

■ Unilocular cystic granuloma cell tumors (UGCTs), adult or juvenile type (see Chapter 16). These tumors are grossly indistinguishable from the luteinized cyst but have different microscopic features. The presence of follicles or other epithelial formations in the lining or wall of GCTs is a helpful distinguishing feature.

Reference

Clement PB, Scully RE. Large solitary luteinized follicle cyst of pregnancy and puerperium. Am J Surg Pathol 4:431–438, 1980.

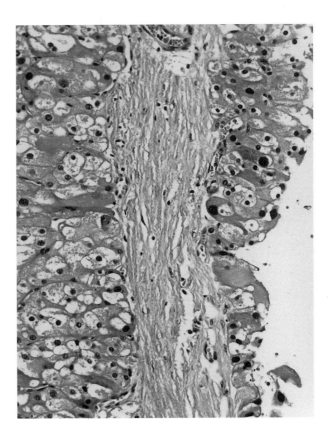

Figure 12–20. Large, solitary luteinized follicle cyst of pregnancy. Large luteinized cells with clear and eosinophilic cytoplasm and focally atypical nuclei line the cyst and occupy its wall.

Granulosa Cell Proliferations of Pregnancy

■ Granulosa cell proliferations of pregnancy have been encountered as incidental findings in the ovaries of pregnant women and rarely in nonpregnant women and newborns.

■ The proliferations are usually multiple and lie within atretic follicles, which are typically enveloped by a thick layer of luteinized theca cells. The granulosa cells may be arranged in solid, insular, microfollicular, or trabecular patterns, and they contain scanty cytoplasm and grooved nuclei.

■ Rarely, the proliferating cells simulate a small Sertoli cell tumor, growing in a solid tubular pattern and containing moderate amounts of finely vacuolated cytoplasm suggesting the presence of lipid.

■ In another rare pattern, the granulosa cells are arranged in nodules and are luteinized with variably sized, round, nongrooved nuclei. The appearance resembles that of a pregnancy luteoma except for the origin from granulosa cells and the larger size of their cells.

Differential Diagnosis

■ Small granulosa or Sertoli cell tumors. Although the granulosa proliferations may be small tumors, their frequency during pregnancy, microscopic size, multifocality, and confinement to atretic follicles suggest a nonneoplastic hormonal response.

References

Clement PB, Young RH, Scully RE. Ovarian granulosa cell proliferations of pregnancy: a report of nine cases. Hum Pathol 19:657–662, 1988.

McKay DG, Hertig AT, Hickey WF. The histogenesis of granulosa and theca cell tumors of the human ovary. Obstet Gynecol 1:125–136, 1953.

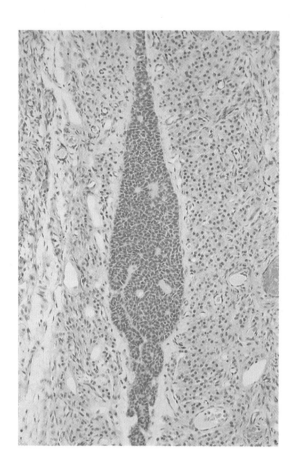

Figure 12–21. Granulosa cell proliferation in pregnancy. A nest of nonluteinized granulosa cells with Call-Exner bodies occupies the center of an atretic follicle, which is surrounded by a thick layer of luteinized theca interna cells.

Ectopic Decidua

- A decidual reaction within the ovary is most commonly a response to the hormonal milieu of pregnancy, may occur as early as the ninth week of gestation, and is present in almost all ovaries at term.
- Less commonly, ovarian decidua is associated with trophoblastic disease, occurs in patients treated with progestins, is adjacent to a corpus luteum, is associated with hormonally active ovarian or adrenal lesions, occurs after pelvic irradiation, or occasionally is an idiopathic finding in premenopausal or postmenopausal women.
- Ovarian decidua is usually an incidental microscopic finding, but careful inspection may reveal tan to often hemorrhagic nodules on the ovarian surface and rarely large, soft, hemorrhagic masses.

- The decidua typically occurs within the superficial cortical stroma and within periovarian adhesions, but it may be seen within the medulla. It resembles eutopic decidua (see Chapter 7) and ectopic decidua occurring in other sites.

References

Bersch W, Alexy E, Heuser HP, Staemmler HJ. Ectopic decidua formation in the ovary (so-called deciduoma). Virchows Arch A (Pathol Anat) 360:173–177, 1973.

Herr JC, Heidger PM Jr, Scott JR, et al. Decidual cells in the human ovary at term. I. Incidence, gross anatomy and ultrastructural features of merocrine secretion. Am J Anat 152:7–28, 1978.

Ober WB, Grady HG, Schoenbucher AK. Ectopic ovarian decidua without pregnancy. Am J Pathol 33:199–217, 1957.

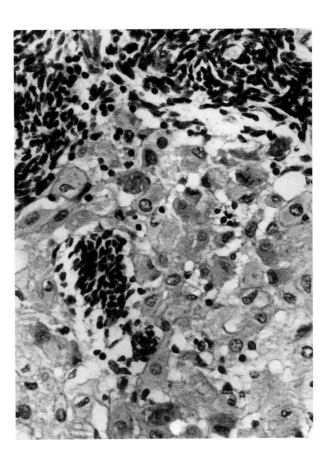

Figure 12–22. Ectopic decidua within the ovarian stroma.

INFLAMMATORY LESIONS

Bacterial Infections

Miscellaneous Bacterial Infections

- Ovarian involvement in pelvic inflammatory disease (PID) usually is caused by spread from salpingitis and typically takes the form of a tubo-ovarian abscess, which is usually bilateral. In some cases, the PID is a complication of the use of an intrauterine device (IUD).
- The usual clinical manifestations include abdominal or pelvic pain, an adnexal mass, fever, vaginal discharge or bleeding, and occasionally, urinary symptoms. No more than 50% of patients have a history of PID, suggesting that subclinical infections are common.
- Tubo-ovarian fibrous adhesions are the usual sequelae. Occasionally, a healed abscess becomes a cyst.
- The rare unilateral or bilateral ovarian abscess without salpingitis usually results from direct or lymphatic spread of an intestinal infection (e.g., diverticulitis, appendicitis) or a postoperative pelvic infection; rarely, it represents a blood-borne infection. The diagnosis in these cases may not be apparent until the organ is sectioned because it is often unremarkable externally.
- Rupture of an ovarian or tubo-ovarian abscess occasionally may lead to peritonitis or fistulas with the colon, urinary bladder, or vagina.
- Rarely, a chronic abscess may result in a solid mass (i.e., xanthogranuloma, xanthogranulomatous oophoritis) composed of foamy histiocytes, multinucleated giant cells, plasma cells, neutrophils, foci of necrosis, and fibrosis. Occasionally, a similar process more diffusely involves the adnexa.

References

Eschenbach DA. Epidemiology and diagnosis of acute pelvic inflammatory disease. Obstet Gynecol 55:142S–152S, 1980.

Kaufman DW, Shapiro S, Rosenberg L, et al. Intrauterine contraceptive device use and pelvic inflammatory disease. Am J Obstet Gynecol 136:159–162, 1980.

Ladefoged C, Lorentzen M. Xanthogranulomatous inflammation of the female genital tract. Histopathology 13:541–551, 1988.

Landers DV, Sweet RL. Current trends in the diagnosis and treatment of tubo-ovarian abscess. Am J Obstet Gynecol 151:1098–1110, 1985.

Wetchler SJ, Dunn LJ. Ovarian abscess: report of a case and a review of the literature. Obstet Gynecol Surv 40:476–485, 1985.

Actinomyocosis

- Pelvic actinomycosis is usually a complication of an IUD, although most cases of IUD-related PID are non-actinomycotic. The lesion typically occurs in women who have had an IUD in place longer than 3 years.
- Abscesses, which are often multiple, involve the ovary and fallopian tube, usually unilaterally. The characteristic actinomycotic (sulfur) granules are rarely grossly visible within the abscess cavities.
- The typical but nonspecific inflammatory response consists of neutrophils and foamy histiocytes, which may be admixed with lymphocytes and plasma cells.

Diagnosis requires finding the sulfur granules within the inflammatory exudate, but they may be sparse.

- The granules are composed of circumscribed rounded masses of basophilic, gram-positive bacteria in branching filaments with a characteristic radial or palisading pattern at the periphery.
- Almost 90% of women with granules in endometrial curettings or cervicovaginal smears are found to have a tubo-ovarian abscess.

References

Bhagavan BS, Gupta PK. Genital actinomycosis and intrauterine contraceptive devices. Hum Pathol 9:567–578, 1978.

Burkman R, Schlesselman S, McCaffrey L, et al. The relationship of genital tract actinomycetes and the development of pelvic inflammatory disease. Am J Obstet Gynecol 143:585–589, 1982.

Keebler C, Chatwani A, Schwartz R. Actinomycosis infection associated with intrauterine contraceptive devices. Am J Obstet Gynecol 145:596–599, 1983.

Muller-Holzner E, Ruth NR, Abfalter E, et al. IUD-associated pelvic actinomycosis: a report of five cases. Int J Gynecol Pathol 14:70–74, 1995.

Schmidt WA, Bedrossian CWM, Ali V, et al. Actinomycosis and intrauterine contraceptive devices. Diagn Gynecol Obstet 2:165–177, 1980.

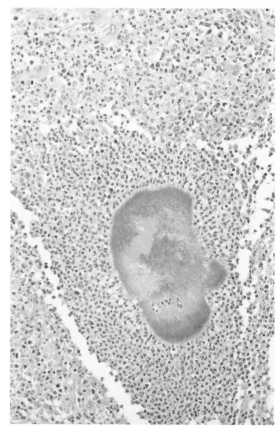

Figure 12–23. Sulfur granule within an actinomycotic tubo-ovarian abscess.

Tuberculosis

- The tubes are almost always involved in tuberculosis of the female genital tract, whereas the ovaries are involved in only 10% of cases. When the ovary is enlarged, granulomas on the adjacent peritoneum may simulate metastatic ovarian cancer at operation.
- The ovaries are typically adherent to the tubal ampullae. Grossly visible caseation is rare. The involvement is typically confined to the cortex.

References

Nogales-Ortiz F, Taracon I, Nogales FF. The pathology of female genital tract tuberculosis. Obstet Gynecol 53:422–428, 1979.

Sutherland AM. Postmenopausal tuberculosis of the female genital tract. Obstet Gynecol 59:54S–57S, 1982.

Malacoplakia

- Only 3 of about 25 reported cases of gynecologic malacoplakia have involved the ovary.
- Friable, yellow, focally hemorrhagic and necrotic masses occupy one or both ovaries, the fallopian tubes, or rarely, contiguous portions of small and large bowel, simulating a malignant ovarian tumor.
- The microscopic features are identical to malacoplakia in other sites.
- The differential diagnosis includes neoplasms composed of cells with abundant eosinophilic cytoplasm, such as a steroid cell tumor. Recognition of the lesional cells as histiocytes and the presence of Michaelis-Guttman bodies facilitate the diagnosis. In rare cases in which Michaelis-Guttman bodies are equivocal, immunostains may be indicated to confirm that the cells are histiocytes.

Reference

Klempner LB, Giglio PG, Niebles A. Malacoplakia of the ovary. Obstet Gynecol 69:537–540, 1987.

Parasitic Infections

Schistosomiasis

- Schistosomiasis in endemic areas is the only common parasitic infestation of the ovary. The fallopian tube is usually also involved. The patients usually have lower abdominal pain, a pelvic mass, and occasionally, irregular menses and infertility.
- The operative findings of enlargement of the tube or ovary or both and scattered peritoneal nodules simulate the implants of a malignant tumor. Microscopically, granulomas, often containing eosinophils, surround schistosoma ova; dense fibrosis is common later in the disease.

Enterobiasis

- Ovarian involvement by *Enterobius vermicularis* is usually an incidental operative finding on the surface or, rarely, within the ovary. In several cases, there has been simultaneous involvement of the pelvic peritoneum, simulating metastatic tumor.
- Granulomas, which may undergo caseation and may contain eosinophils, surround the adult female worms and ova. The worms probably reach the peritoneal cavity by migrating from the perineum through the lumen of the female genital tract.

Echinococcosis

- Rare cases of ovarian echinococcosis have been described. In one of them, a typical hydatid cyst enlarged the ovary to 12 cm in diameter.

References

Arean VM. Manson's schistosomiasis of the female genital tract. Am J Obstet Gynecol 72:1038–1053, 1956.

Azhar H. Primary echinococcal infection of the ovary. Br J Obstet Gynaecol 84:633, 1977.

Hangval H, Habibi H, Moshref A, Rahimi A. Case report of an ovarian hydatid cyst. J Trop Med Hyg 82:34–35, 1979.

McMahon JN, Connolly CE, Long SV, Meehan FB. Enterobius granulomas of the uterus, ovary and pelvic peritoneum: two case reports. Br J Obstet Gynaecol 91:289–290, 1984.

Fungal Infections

- Fungal infections of the ovary are rare, even in patients with disseminated disease. Three examples of tubo-ovarian abscess, caused by *Blastomyces dermatitidis,* have been reported. In one case, the abscesses were bilateral and associated with miliary nodules involving the pelvic peritoneum.
- Seven of 11 patients with coccidioidomycosis of the upper female genital tract had tubo-ovarian and peritoneal involvement.
- One case of tubo-ovarian abscess caused by *Aspergillus* has been reported in an IUD user; rupture of the abscess led to generalized peritonitis.

References

Bylund DJ, Nanfro JJ, Marsh WL Jr. Coccidioidomycosis of the female genital tract. Arch Pathol Lab Med 110:232–235, 1986.

Farber ER, Leahy MS, Meadows TR. Endometrial blastomycosis acquired by sexual contact. Obstet Gynecol 32:195–199, 1968.

Murray JJ, Clark CA, Lands RH, et al. Reactivation blastomycosis presenting as a tuboovarian abscess. Obstet Gynecol 64:828–830, 1985.

Granulomas

Foreign-Body Granulomas

- A variety of foreign materials may evoke a granulomatous reaction on the ovarian and extraovarian peritoneal surfaces (see Chapter 20), mimicking a malignant tumor at operation. Some ovarian granulomas may contain refractile crystalline material of uncertain origin.

Isolated Palisading Granulomas

- These ovarian granulomas are usually encountered as an incidental microscopic finding. In many cases, they appear to be a response to an operation performed on the involved ovary months to years earlier.

■ The granulomas are typically multiple and occasionally bilateral. Central zones of fibrinoid necrosis or hyalinization are usually surrounded by palisading, sometimes multinucleated histiocytes and other inflammatory cells (i.e., lymphocytes, plasma cells, eosinophils); a fibrous pseudocapsule forms in some of the cases.

■ Similar ovarian granulomas, with the additional finding of carbon pigment, may occur as a response to cautery or fulguration.

■ The differential diagnosis of these granulomas is with other ovarian granulomas, including necrotic pseudo-xanthomatous nodules of endometriosis (see Chapter 19).

Granulomas From Systemic Disease

■ In the rare case of ovarian involvement by sarcoidosis, the granulomas are an incidental microscopic finding. In most cases, the patient has systemic sarcoidosis with involvement of other gynecologic sites or paraaortic lymph nodes.

■ Crohn's disease may cause granulomatous oophoritis, usually by direct extension of the inflammatory process from the bowel; the ipsilateral fallopian tube is also involved in most cases.

References

Al Dawoud, Yates R, Foulis AK. Postoperative necrotizing granulomas in the ovary. J Clin Pathol 44:524–529, 1991.

Chalvardjian A. Sarcoidosis of the female genital tract. Am J Obstet Gynecol 132:78–80, 1978.

Herbold DR, Frable WJ, Kraus FT. Isolated non-infectious granuloma of the ovary. Int J Gynecol Pathol 2:380–391, 1984.

Honoré LH. Combined suppurative and noncaseating granulomatous oophoritis associated with distal ileitis (Crohn's disease). Eur J Obstet Gynaecol Reprod Biol 12:91–94, 1981.

Kernohan NM, Best PV, Jandial V, Kitchener HC. Palisading granuloma of the ovary. Histopathology 19:279–280, 1991.

McCluggage WG, Allen DC. Ovarian granulomas: a report of 32 cases. J Clin Pathol 50:324–327, 1997.

Mostafa SAM, Bargeron CB, Flower RW, et al. Foreign body granulomas in normal ovaries. Obstet Gynecol 66:701–702, 1985.

Tatum ET, Beattie JF Jr, Bryson K. Postoperative carbon pigment granuloma: a report of eight cases involving the ovary. Hum Pathol 27:1008–1111, 1996.

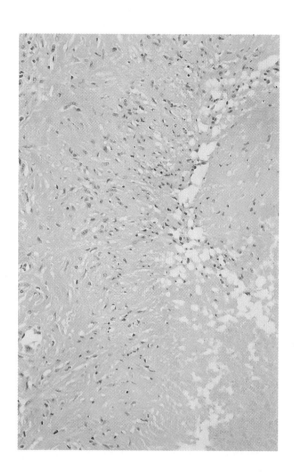

Figure 12–24. Isolated, palisading granuloma within the ovary. Histiocytes surround a central area of necrosis.

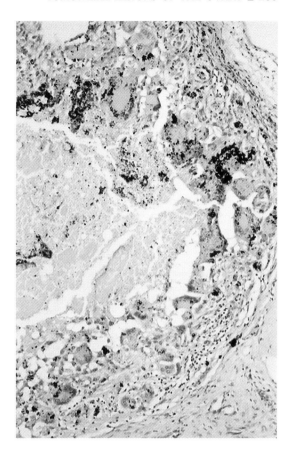

Figure 12–25. Granulomatous response to carbon pigment within the ovary after cautery treatment of endometriosis.

MISCELLANEOUS DISORDERS

Ovarian Pregnancy

- The diagnosis of ovarian pregnancy, which accounts for up to 1% of ectopic pregnancies, is tenable only when there is no involvement of the fallopian tube. There is an increased frequency in patients with IUDs.
- The typical presentation is severe pain with hemoperitoneum, and at laparotomy and on gross examination, the enlarged hemorrhagic ovary may mimic a hemorrhagic neoplasm. Gross identification of an embryo sometimes indicates the diagnosis, and in other cases microscopic examination is diagnostic.
- Distinction between an ovarian pregnancy and the rare examples of primary ovarian gestational trophoblastic disease is made by applying criteria similar to those used in the uterus (see Chapter 10).

References

Gray CL, Ruffolo EH. Ovarian pregnancy associated with intrauterine contraceptive devices. Am J Obstet Gynecol 132:134–139, 1978.

Hallatt JG. Primary ovarian pregnancy: a report of twenty-five cases. Am J Obstet Gynecol 143:55–60, 1982.

Ovarian Remnant Syndrome

- Women with the ovarian remnant syndrome have a history of bilateral oophorectomy, which was often difficult because of dense fibrous adhesions, the latter usually a complication of PID or endometriosis.
- The patient may present weeks to years after oophorectomy with pelvic pain, which may be cyclical, and in about 50% of the cases, a mass is palpable. Rarely, patients have ureteral or small intestinal obstructions. At reoperation, a corpus luteum cyst may be found.
- Microscopic examination discloses ovarian tissue, which may contain cystic follicles or corpora lutea surrounded by fibrous tissue; endometriosis may also be present.

References

Payan HM, Gilbert EF. Mesenteric cyst-ovarian implant syndrome. Arch Pathol Lab Med 111:282–284, 1987.

Pettit PD, Lee RA. Ovarian remnant syndrome: diagnostic dilemma and surgical challenge. Obstet Gynecol 71:580–583, 1988.

Steege JF. Ovarian remnant syndrome. Obstet Gynecol 70:64–67, 1987.

Zaitoon MM. Ureteral obstruction secondary to retained ovarian remnants: a case report and review of the literature. J Urol 137:973–974, 1987.

Mesothelial Proliferation

■ Proliferation of mesothelial cells on the ovarian surface, within periovarian fibrous adhesions, and within the walls of endometriotic or neoplastic ovarian cysts may be confused with a neoplastic process on microscopic examination. This process is discussed in detail in Chapter 20.

References

Clement PB, Young RH. Florid mesothelial hyperplasia associated with ovarian tumors: a potential source of error in tumor diagnosis and staging. Int J Gynecol Pathol 12:51–58, 1993.

McFadden DE, Clement PB. Peritoneal inclusion cysts with mural mesothelial proliferation: a clinicopathological analysis of six cases. Am J Surg Pathol 10:844–854, 1986.

Surface Stromal Proliferations

■ Polypoid stromal proliferations on the ovarian surface may be visible as warty excrescences on gross examination but are commonly incidental microscopic findings in women of late reproductive and postmenopausal ages.

■ The projections are composed of ovarian stroma exhibiting various degrees of hyalinization covered by a single layer of surface epithelium. An arbitrary size limit of less than 1 cm separates these proliferations from serous surface papillomas (see Chapter 13). Unlike the latter, surface stromal proliferations are usually multiple.

Autoimmune Oophoritis

■ About 25 cases of histologically documented autoimmune oophoritis, a subtype of primary ovarian failure, have occurred in women 17 to 48 years old (mean, 31 years). The typical symptoms are oligomenorrhea or amenorrhea or symptoms related to multiple follicle cysts, including pelvic pain and adnexal torsion.

■ Serum antibodies against steroid cells of various types, Addison's disease, Hashimoto's thyroiditis, and a variety of other autoimmune disorders have been identified in some cases.

■ On gross examination, the ovaries may be small or normal in size, but in one third of the cases, one or both are enlarged by multiple follicle cysts. The cysts are more common in the earlier phases of the disease and are probably caused by elevated pituitary gonadotropins.

■ Lymphocytes, plasma cells, eosinophils, and rarely, sarcoid-like granulomas involve developing follicles, with the number of inflammatory cells increasing with the degree of follicular maturation. The theca interna layer is typically more intensely infiltrated than the granulosa layer and may be focally destroyed.

■ In some cases, hilus cells are also destroyed by the inflammatory process.

References

Bannatyne P, Russell P, Shearman RP. Autoimmune oophoritis: a clinicopathologic assessment of 12 cases. Int J Gynecol Pathol 9:191–207, 1990.

Biscotti CV, Hart WR, Lucas JG. Cystic ovarian enlargement resulting from autoimmune oophoritis: Obstet Gynecol 74:492–495, 1989.

Lonsdale RN, Roberts PF, Trowell JE. Autoimmune oophoritis associated with polycystic ovaries. Histopathology 19:77–81, 1991.

Sedmak DD, Hart WR, Tubbs RR. Autoimmune oophoritis: a histopathologic study of involved ovaries with immunologic characterization of the mononuclear cell infiltrate. Int J Gynecol Pathol 6:73–81, 1987.

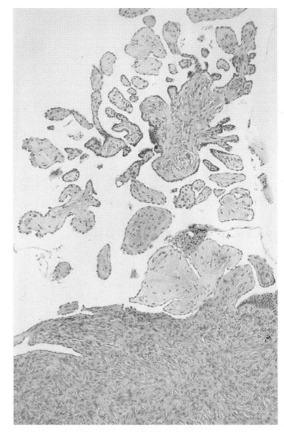

Figure 12–26. Surface papillary stromal proliferation.

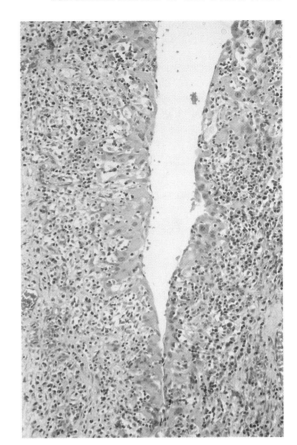

Figure 12–27. Autoimmune oophoritis. Lymphoid cells infiltrate the luteinized cells of a cystic follicle.

Torsion and Infarction

- Ovarian or adnexal torsion is most often a complication of an ovarian or parovarian lesion, usually a nonneoplastic cyst or benign tumor but occasionally a cancer. Torsion of a normal ovary is rare, but it is more common in infants and children, and it may be bilateral. The potential role of torsion in massive edema has been discussed previously (page 271).
- The clinical findings simulate those of acute appendicitis, or there is recurrent abdominal pain; occasionally, an adnexal mass is palpable. Laparotomy reveals a torsed, swollen, hemorrhagic, and in some cases, infarcted tubo-ovarian mass.
- In rare cases of asymptomatic torsion and infarction, autoamputation may result in a mass, which is occasionally calcified and lying free in the peritoneal cavity, or attached to adjacent structures.
- Any hemorrhagic, infarcted ovarian mass should be thoroughly sectioned miscroscopically to exclude a neoplasm. The viable foci are most likely to be found at

the periphery of the lesion, although rarely the entire mass is necrotic, and a definite diagnosis is not possible.

References

Azoury RS, Chehab RM, Mufarrij IK. The twisted adnexa: a clinical pathological review. Diagn Gynecol Obstet 2:185–191, 1980.

Demopoulos RI, Bigelow B, Vasa U. Infarcted uterine adnexa: associated pathology. NY State J Med 78:2027–2029, 1978.

Dunnihoo DR, Wolff J. Bilateral torsion of the adnexa: a case report and a review of the world literature. Obstet Gynecol 64:55S–59S, 1984.

Evans JP. Torsion of the normal uterine adnexa in premenarcheal girls. J Pediatr Surg 13:195–196, 1978.

Hibbard LT. Adnexal torsion. Am J Obstet Gynecol 152:456–461, 1985.

Changes Caused by Metabolic Disease

- Amyloidosis rarely involves the ovaries, typically as an incidental histologic finding in patients with systemic amyloidosis, although a single case of tumor-like amyloidosis apparently confined to the ovary has been reported.

■ Rare cases of ovarian enlargement from involvement by systemic storage disorders have been reported. The stored material is typically within histocytes, allowing distinction from a steroid cell tumor.

References

Copeland W Jr, Hawley PC, Teteris NJ. Gynecologic amyloidosis. Am J Obstet Gynecol 153:555–556, 1985.

Dincsoy HP, Rolfes DB, McGraw CA, Schubert WK. Cholesterol ester storage disease and mesenteric lipodystrophy. Am J Clin Pathol 81: 263–269, 1984.

Salomonowitz E. Tumorformige Amyloidose des Ovars. Geburtshilfe Frauenheilkd 40:644–667, 1980.

Wassman ER, Johnson K, Shapiro LJ, et al. Postmortem findings in the Hurler-Scheie syndrome (mucopolysaccharidosis I-H/S). Birth Defects 18:13–18, 1982.

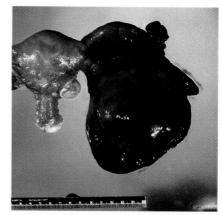

Figure 12–28. Adnexal torsion and hemorrhagic infarction. A benign cyst was found in the ovary.

Simple Cyst

■ Simple cysts are of unknown origin because the lining is atrophic or has been destroyed by desiccation or rubbing after removal. Some are lined by a thin layer of indifferent-appearing cells that resemble epithelial or mesothelial cells. The wall is composed of fibrous tissue.

■ The identification of theca cells in the wall or a serous, endometrioid, or other epithelial lining on careful search may lead to a more specific diagnosis. Even a rare cystic struma ovarii may be misdiagnosed as a simple cyst if inconspicuous follicles in the wall are overlooked.

Rete Cyst (see Chapter 17)

Idiopathic Calcification

■ Extensive, idiopathic calcification may result in stony hard ovaries of normal size. Microscopic examination in the one reported case of this lesion showed numerous spherical, laminated, calcific foci without accompanying epithelial cells.

■ The differential diagnosis includes serous tumors with confluent psammoma bodies, but these tumors contain neoplastic epithelial cells. A "burned-out" calcified gonadoblastoma is suggested by abnormal gonadal development, the presence of a Y chromosome, and residual typical gonadoblastoma in the same or contralateral gonad.

Reference

Clement PB, Cooney TP. Idiopathic multifocal calcification of the ovarian stroma. Arch Pathol Lab Med 116:204–205, 1992.

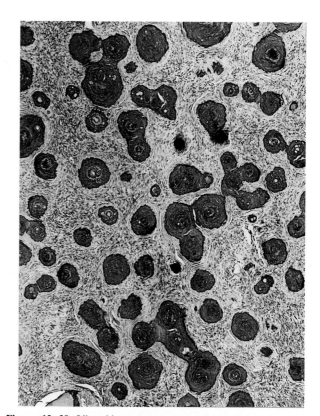

Figure 12–29. Idiopathic psammomatous calcification of the ovarian stroma.

Uterus-like Adnexal Mass

■ Uterus-like adnexal masses consist of a central cavity lined by endometrium surrounded by a thick wall of smooth muscle within an ovary or at the site of an ovary. Two of the seven patients with this finding have had an elevated serum CA-125 level, and two have had a presumably unrelated breast cancer.

■ The pathogenetic mechanism in most cases appears to be prominent smooth muscle metaplasia within ovarian endometriosis (i.e., endomyometriosis) (see Chapter 19). An abnormality of the ipsilateral upper urinary tract in two cases suggests that a congenital müllerian duct anomaly may be an alternate explanation in some cases.

Reference

Pai SA, Desai SB, Borges AM. Uteruslike masses of the ovary associated with breast cancer and raised serum CA-125. Am J Surg Pathol 22:333–337, 1998.

Splenic-Gonadal Fusion

■ Splenic-gonadal fusion is a rare anomaly that results from fusion of the anlage of both organs during embryonic development. The male to female ratio is 9:1. Affected females are usually newborns who may have partially undescended ovaries and other congenital anomalies. In these cases, a cordlike structure connects the spleen to the left ovary; intraovarian splenic nodules may also be present.

■ One case was diagnosed in an adult female who had a septate uterus and a cluster of splenic nodules surrounding an otherwise normal left ovary. The differential diagnosis in this case includes traumatic splenosis (page 451).

References

Almenoff IA. Splenic-gonadal dysgenesis. NY State J Med 66:1679–1691, 1966.

Meneses MF, Ostrowski ML. Female splenic-gonadal fusion of the discontinuous type. Hum Pathol 20:486–488, 1989.

Putschar WGJ, Manion WC. Splenic-gonadal fusion. Am J Pathol 32:15–33, 1956.

Ectopic Prostatic Tissue

■ One case of ectopic prostatic tissue within the ovary arising from hilar mesonephric rests has been reported in a 70-year-old woman.

Reference

Smith CET, Toplis PJ, Nogales FF. Ovarian prostatic tissue originating from hilar mesonephric rests. Am J Surg Pathol 23:232–236, 1999.

Mucicarminophilic Histiocytosis

■ Mucicarminophilic histiocytosis is discussed in Chapter 20. When there is prominent ovarian involvement, features that distinguish it from a Krukenberg tumor include the lack of a mass, the uniformly bland nuclei, and the failure of the signet-ring–like cells to stain with the periodic acid–Schiff stain.

Miscellaneous Tumor-like Alterations Related to Normal Structures

Hydropic Change Within Surface Epithelial Inclusion Glands

■ The cells lining surface epithelial inclusion glands occasionally exhibit striking hydropic swelling, resulting in clear cytoplasm that displaces the nucleus. The appearance can mimic a signet-ring cell carcinoma, especially when the cells proliferate to form solid nests.

■ Awareness of this phenomenon, its relation to inclusion glands, and negative staining for mucin facilitate the diagnosis.

Artifactual Displacement of Granulosa Cells

■ Nonluteinized granulosa cells of normal follicles can be artifactually introduced into tissue spaces or vascular channels during sectioning. When the displaced cells are shrunken or crushed, this finding can be misinterpreted as a small cell carcinoma. Awareness of this artifact, the bland nuclear features of the cells, and their similarity to cells lining nearby follicles are clues to the correct diagnosis.

■ Similarly, granulosa cells deposited on the ovarian surface after follicle rupture may be misinterpreted as mesothelial cells, and when the cells are numerous and luteinized, they may even suggest the diagnosis of a mesothelioma. The granulosa cells typically show only punctate staining for cytokeratin, in contrast to diffuse cytoplasmic staining in mesothelial cells.

Other Findings

■ Granulosa cells and theca interna cells of the normal follicle typically exhibit brisk mitotic activity and may be occasionally misinterpreted as a small cancer if the relation of the cells to the follicle is not appreciated. Similarly, the mitotically active spindled cells of the theca externa can be mistaken for a sarcoma if the rest of the follicle is not in the same plane of section.

■ The corpus luteum of late pregnancy and the puerperium may contain numerous calcific deposits that can be misinterpreted as recurrent or metastatic serous borderline tumor.

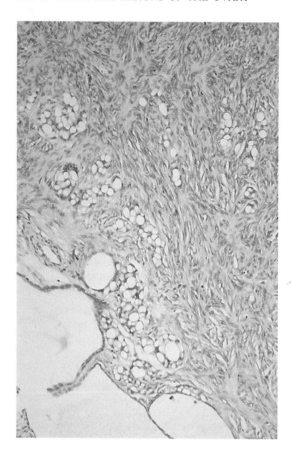

Figure 12–30. Hydropic degeneration of cells lining surface epithelial inclusion cysts. Similar cells form solid nests within the adjacent ovarian stroma.

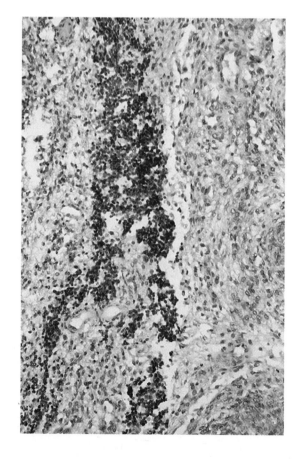

Figure 12–31. Displaced granulosa cells occupy an artifactual cleft within the ovarian stroma. This finding has occasionally suggested the diagnosis of small cell carcinoma.

CHAPTER 13

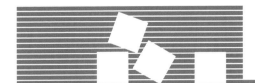

Surface Epithelial-Stromal Tumors: General Features, Serous Tumors, and Mucinous Tumors

GENERAL FEATURES

Terminology and Classification

- Surface epithelial-stromal tumors (SESTs) (Table 13–1) usually arise from the ovarian surface epithelium (or epithelial inclusion glands or cysts derived therefrom) and the adjacent ovarian stroma. Some mucinous and squamous tumors are of germ cell origin, arising from a component of a teratoma.
- The word *stroma* is included in the terminology because stroma is present in variable amounts in all subtypes and is the predominant neoplastic element in some of them. The stroma is derived in most cases from the ovarian stroma.
- SESTs are subclassified by
  - Their epithelial cell types
  - The relative amounts of their epithelial and stromal components
  - The location of their epithelial elements: surface (exophytic), cystic (endophytic), or both
  - Their growth patterns and nuclear features that categorize them as benign (i.e., absent or minimal cellular stratification or atypia; no invasion), borderline tumors or tumors of low malignant potential (i.e., epithelial stratification and atypia; no invasion), or carcinomas (i.e., invasion).
- Aside from the Brenner subtype of transitional cell tumor, which typically contains a predominant stromal component, when the stroma of SESTs occupies an area greater than that of the glands, the suffix *-fibroma* is added (e.g., serous adenofibroma), and when more than a rare cyst larger than 1 cm in diameter is present, the prefix *cyst-* is used (e.g., serous cystadenofibroma).

Grading

- There is no universally accepted grading system for surface epithelial carcinomas. Systems proposed by the International Federation of Gynecology and Obstetrics (FIGO), World Health Organization (WHO), and the Gynecologic Oncology Group (GOG) are based on architectural features that are sometimes combined with nuclear features. Regardless of which of these grading systems is used, many studies have found that grade is an important prognostic factor in these tumors.
- Shimizu and colleagues have recently proposed a grading system modeled on the Nottingham system for breast carcinoma. They found that their system was reproducible and more predictive of prognosis than the FIGO system. Silva and Gershenson, however, have found some aspects of this system problematic.

Clinical Features

- SESTs account for about 50% of all ovarian tumors and for about 90% of ovarian cancers in the Western world.
- The clinical presentation is usually that of pelvic or abdominal pain or abdominal swelling. Some tumors, including carcinomas, may be associated with vague abdominal symptoms, malaise, or gastrointestinal complaints or rarely with other complaints related to metastatic spread. Rare tumors may manifest with paraneoplastic, paraendocrine, or endocrine symptoms.
- Examination usually reveals an adnexal mass or masses; ascites or evidence of peritoneal spread may be present in patients with borderline tumors or carcinomas. Serum levels of certain markers, especially CA-125, are frequently elevated.

Table 13–1

WORLD HEALTH ORGANIZATION HISTOLOGIC CLASSIFICATION OF SURFACE
EPITHELIAL-STROMAL TUMORS

Serous Tumors
  Benign
    Cystadenoma and papillary cystadenoma
      Surface papilloma
      Adenofibroma and cystadenofibroma
  Of borderline malignancy (low malignant potential)
    Cystic tumor and papillary cystic tumor
      Surface papillary tumor
      Adenofibroma and cystadenofibroma
  Malignant
    Adenocarcinoma, papillary adenocarcinoma, and papillary cystadenocarcinoma
      Surface papillary adenocarcinoma
      Adenocarcinofibroma and cystadenocarcinofibroma (malignant adenofibroma and cystadenofibroma)
Mucinous Tumors, Endocervical-like and Intestinal Type
  Benign
    Cystadenoma
    Adenofibroma and cystadenofibroma
  Of borderline malignancy (low malignant potential)
    Cystic tumor
    Adenofibroma and cystadenofibroma
  Malignant
    Adenocarcinoma and cystadenocarcinoma
    Adenocarcinofibroma and cystadenocarcinofibroma (malignant adenofibroma and cystadenofibroma)
Endometrioid Tumors
  Benign
    Cystadenoma
      Cystadenoma with squamous differentiation
      Adenofibroma and cystadenofibroma
      Adenofibroma and cystadenofibroma with squamous differentiation
  Of borderline malignancy (low malignant potential)
    Cystic tumor
      Cystic tumor with squamous differentiation
      Adenofibroma and cystadenofibroma
      Adenofibroma and cystadenofibroma with squamous differentiation
  Malignant
    Adenocarcinoma and cystadenocarcinoma
      Adenocarcinoma and cystadenocarcinoma with squamous differentiation
      Adenocarcinofibroma and cystadenocarcinofibroma (malignant adenofibroma
        and cystadenofibroma)
      Adenocarcinofibroma and cystadenocarcinofibroma with squamous differentiation (malignant adeno-
        fibroma and cystadenofibroma with squamous differentiation)
  Epithelial-stromal and stromal
    Adenosarcoma, homologous and heterologous
    Mesodermal (müllerian) mixed tumor (carcinosarcoma), homologous and heterologous
    Stromal sarcoma
Clear Cell Tumors
  Benign
    Cystadenoma
      Adenofibroma and cystadenofibroma
  Of borderline malignancy (low malignant potential)
    Cystic tumor
      Adenofibroma and cystadenofibroma
  Malignant
    Adenocarcinoma
      Adenocarcinofibroma and cystadenocarcinofibroma (malignant adenofibroma and cystadenofibroma)
Transitional Cell Tumors
  Brenner tumor
  Brenner tumor of borderline malignancy (proliferating)
  Malignant Brenner tumor
  Transitional cell carcinoma (non-Brenner type)
Squamous Cell Tumors
Mixed Epithelial Tumors (specify types)
  Benign
    Of borderline malignancy (low malignant potential)
    Malignant
Undifferentiated Carcinoma

Table 13–2

TUMOR-NODE-METASTASIS AND INTERNATIONAL FEDERATION OF GYNECOLOGY AND
OBSTETRICS STAGING SYSTEMS FOR OVARIAN CANCER

Primary Tumor (T)

TNM	*FIGO*	*DEFINITION*
TX	—	Primary tumor cannot be assessed
T0	—	No evidence of primary tumor
T1	I	Tumor limited to ovaries (one or both)
T1a	IA	Tumor limited to one ovary; capsule intact, no tumor on ovarian surface, no malignant cells in ascites or peritoneal washings
T1b	IB	Tumor limited to both ovaries; capsules intact, no tumor on ovarian surface, no malignant cells in ascites or peritoneal washings
T1c	IC	Tumor limited to one or both ovaries with any of the following: capsule ruptured, tumor on ovarian surface, malignant cells in ascites or peritoneal washings
T2	II	Tumor involves one or both ovaries with pelvic extension
T2a	IIA	Extension and/or implants on the uterus and/or tube(s); no malignant cells in ascites or peritoneal washings
T2b	IIB	Extension to other pelvic tissues; no malignant cells in ascites or peritoneal washings
T2c	IIC	Pelvic extension (IIa or IIb) with malignant cells in ascites or peritoneal washings
T3 and/or N1	III	Tumor involves one or both ovaries with microscopically confirmed peritoneal metastasis outside the pelvis and/or regional lymph node metastasis
T3a	IIIA	Microscopic peritoneal metastasis beyond the pelvis
T3b	IIIB	Macroscopic peritoneal metastasis beyond the pelvis 2 cm or less in greatest dimension
T3c and/or N1	IIIC	Peritoneal metastasis beyond the pelvis more than 2 cm in greatest dimension and/or regional lymph node metastasis
M1	IV	Distant metastasis (excludes peritoneal metastasis)

Note: Liver capsule metastasis is T3/stage III; liver parenchymal metastasis is M1/stage IV. Pleural effusion must have positive cytology for M1/stage IV.

Regional Lymph Nodes (N)

NX	Regional lymph nodes cannot be assessed
N0	No regional lymph node metastasis
N1	Regional lymph node metastasis

Distant Metastasis (M)

TNM	*FIGO*	*DEFINITION*
MX	—	Presence of distant metastasis cannot be assessed
M0	—	No distant metastasis
M1	IV	Distant metastasis (excludes peritoneal metastasis)

Note: The presence of nonmalignant ascites is not classified. The presence of ascites does not affect staging unless malignant cells are present.

pTNM Pathologic Classification

The pT, pN, and pM categories correspond to the T, N, and M categories.

Stage Grouping

AJCC/UICC				*FIGO*
Stage IA	T1a	N0	M0	Stage IA
Stage IB	T1b	N0	M0	Stage IB
Stage IC	T1c	N0	M0	Stage IC
Stage IIA	T2a	N0	M0	Stage IIA
Stage IIB	T2b	N0	M0	Stage IIB
Stage IIC	T2c	N0	M0	Stage IIC
Stage IIIA	T3a	N0	M0	Stage IIIA
Stage IIIB	T3b	N0	M0	Stage IIIB
Stage IIIC	T3c	N0	M0	Stage IIIC
	Any T	N1	M0	
Stage IV	Any T	Any N	M1	Stage IV

AJCC, American Joint Committee on Cancer; UICC, Union Internationale Contre le Cancer.
From Beahrs OH, Henson DE, Hutter RV, Kennedy BJ (eds): Manual for Staging of Cancer, 4th ed. Philadelphia: JB Lippincott, 1992, and from Sobin LH, Wittekind C (eds): TMN Classification of Malignant Tumors, 5th ed. New York: John Wiley & Sons, 1997.

■ The stromal component of these tumors can secrete estrogenic or androgenic hormones with resultant endocrine manifestations; such tumors are said to have "functioning stroma." The steroidogenic stromal cells in such cases typically have a luteinized appearance.

■ The most commonly used staging systems for ovarian cancer are reproduced in Table 13–2.

References

Shimizu Y, Kamoi S, Amada S, et al. Toward the development of a univeral grading system for ovarian epithelial carcinoma: testing of a proposed system in a series of 461 patients with uniform treatment and follow-up. Cancer 82:893–901, 1998.

Shimizu Y, Kamoi S, Amada S, et al. Toward the development of a univeral grading system for ovarian epithelial carcinoma. I. Prognostic significance of histopathologic features—problems involved in the architectural grading system. Gynecol Oncol 70:2–12, 1998.

Silva EG, Gershenson DM. Standardized histologic grading of epithelial ovarian cancer: elusive after all these years [editorial]. Gynecol Oncol 70:1, 1998.

SEROUS TUMORS

- Serous tumors account for about 30% of all ovarian neoplasms in the Western world; of these, about 60% are benign, 10% are borderline (SBLTs), and 30% are carcinomatous. SBLTs and invasive serous tumors together account for 40% to 45% of all ovarian cancers.
- Benign serous tumors may occur at any age but are most common in the reproductive era. SBLTs and carcinomas are rare before the age of 20 years. The average patient ages for borderline tumors and serous carcinomas is 46 years and 56 years, respectively.
- The full spectrum of serous tumors that occur in the ovary can also be encountered as primary peritoneal serous tumors (see Chapter 19).

Benign Serous Tumors

Gross Features

- Serous cystadenomas are composed of one or more thin-walled cysts with watery fluid and a lining that is smooth or with soft to firm, polypoid excrescences composed almost entirely of stroma. The tumors are on average only one half of the size of mucinous cystadenomas and are bilateral in 7% to 20% of cases.
- Serous surface papillomas appear as polypoid excrescences on the outer surface of one or both ovaries.
- Serous adenofibromas and cystadenofibromas are typically hard, white to yellow-white, predominantly solid, fibromatous tumors that contain glands or fluid-filled cysts. The cyst linings may bear polypoid excrescences.
- The excrescences and the hard consistency of the stromal component may prompt an erroneous gross impression of carcinoma.

Microscopic Features

- The cysts and polypoid stromal excrescences, which may be dense and collagenous or markedly edematous, are typically lined by an epithelium similar to that of the fallopian tube, including ciliated cells and less numerous nonciliated, secretory cells.
- Tumors lined entirely by nonspecific, cuboidal or columnar, nonciliated epithelium are also classified as serous.
- Psammoma bodies may be present but usually are inconspicuous.

Differential Diagnosis

- Epithelial inclusion cyst. This distinction is based arbitrarily on size, with the lesion being considered neoplastic if it is larger than 1 cm in diameter.
- Rete cystadenoma (see Chapter 17). Differential features include a hilar location, smooth muscle or a proliferation of hilus cells in their walls, shallow crevices along their inner surfaces, and lining cells with rare or no cilia.
- Cystic struma ovarii (see Chapter 15). Rare follicles with colloid and immunoreactivity for thyroglobulin establish the diagnosis.
- Endometrioid adenofibroma. These tumors have stratified, predominantly nonciliated epithelial cells with endometrioid features; squamous differentiation may be seen. In some equivocal cases, a diagnosis of "adenofibroma, question serous or endometrioid" is justifiable.
- Papillary surface excrescences (see Chapter 12). These, in contrast to surface serous papillomas, are usually multifocal and microscopic; grossly visible lesions, by definition, are less than 1 cm in diameter.

Borderline Serous Tumors

Gross Features

- Polypoid excrescenses accompanied by fine papillae, imparting a velvety appearance, characteristically occupy part or all of the lining of one or more cysts, the outer surface of the ovary (i.e., serous surface papilloma of borderline malignancy), or both.
- Solid areas may result from papillae filling a cyst or, more commonly, from a fibromatous component (i.e., serous cystadenofibroma of borderline malignancy).
- The intracystic fluid in some tumors may be mucoid, potentially resembling that of mucinous tumors.
- SBLTs are bilateral in 25% to 30% of cases.

Microscopic Features of Primary Tumors

- Polypoid stromal excrescences covered by cellular papillae line cysts, involve the outer surface of the ovary, or both. The cellular papillae often appear to be free floating because their point of attachment is not in the plane of section. Psammoma bodies may be present.
- The lining cells typically exhibit mild to moderate (or rarely, marked) nuclear atypicality, rare to occasional mitotic figures, and stratification, with cellular buds that may appear detached.
- The tumor cells typically have scanty cytoplasm but may contain abundant eosinophilic cytoplasm; cells of the latter type are more numerous if the patient is pregnant. The neoplastic cells may secrete abundant mucin, but cytoplasmic mucin is confined to the tips of the cells.
- Absence of invasion (other than microinvasion) is a definitional feature. Several findings that may be confused with invasion:
  - An orderly stromal penetration by glands, tubules, and microcysts with papillae without a stromal reaction that reflects the complexity of the epithelial and stromal proliferation
  - Intracystic or, less commonly, surface patterns, including cribriform growth; a "micropapillary" pattern characterized by filiform cellular papillae, without the hierarchal, arborescent pattern of the usual SBLT,

resulting in a medusa-head appearance; and solid intracystic proliferations. Any of these patterns in a SBLT warrants extensive sampling to exclude invasion. In the absence of the latter, we still categorize tumors with these features as SBLTs.

- "Autoimplantation" characterized by the presence of sharply delimited desmoplastic plaques, usually occurring on the outer surface but occasionally on the inner, cystic surface of the tumor, resembling the noninvasive desmoplastic implants that may occur on the extraovarian peritoneum.
- Florid mesothelial hyperplasia in the wall of the tumor (see Chapter 20).
- Microinvasion of the stroma. This occurs in 10% to 15% of SBLTs and is characterized by one or more discrete foci of tumor cells with borderline features in the stroma, with none of the foci larger than 10 mm².
  a. These foci consist of single epithelial cells, often with abundant eosinophilic cytoplasm, and small clusters or papillary aggregates of such cells, sometimes accompanied by psammoma bodies, usually without a stromal response.
  b. The invasive cells may occupy spaces, some of which result from fluid secretion by the tumor cells, whereas others are lymphatics.

■ We refer to rare, well-sampled borderline tumors with foci of an exclusively intraepithelial proliferation of carcinomatous cells as "SBLTs with intraepithelial carcinoma." More experience with these tumors is needed before knowledge of their behavior is established.

■ Occasionally, foci of SBLT occur in an otherwise benign-appearing serous tumor or, much less often, are admixed with foci of invasive serous carcinoma. In such cases, the proportion of each component should be noted in the pathology report.

Microscopic Features of Implants of Borderline Serous Tumors

■ Extraovarian peritoneal lesions associated with SBLTs include endosalpingiosis (see Chapter 19), the presence of which does not affect the stage of an accompanying ovarian borderline tumor; noninvasive deposits of SBLT; and invasive implants indistinguishable from low-grade serous carcinoma.

■ Although some observers interpret the peritoneal "implants" as independent foci of primary neoplasia instead of true implants, the quantity and microscopic features of the peritoneal lesions and not their site of origin determine management.

■ Noninvasive implants, which account for almost 90% of the implants, are composed predominantly of neoplastic epithelial cells (i.e., epithelial implants) or of desmoplastic stroma (i.e., desmoplastic implants).

■ Noninvasive epithelial implants resemble the papillary proliferations of the primary ovarian tumor. Noninvasive desmoplastic implants form sharply circumscribed plaques or nodules on the surface of the peritoneum, sometimes with extension as septa between omental lobules.

- Necrosis and acute inflammation may be present in the early stages, whereas the late lesions are composed of dense fibrous desmoplastic stroma containing small numbers of disorderly, jagged nests of tumor cells, individual tumor cells, and psammoma bodies.
- If the biopsy specimen does not include underlying tissue, the lesion is considered noninvasive on the assumption that it has been stripped away with ease.

■ Invasive implants, which account for about 10% of the implants, infiltrate underlying tissue in a disorderly fashion. When present in omental tissue, they typically have an irregular border, with replacement of the adipose tissue.

■ Implants should be sampled extensively because noninvasive and invasive implants may coexist at different sites and some implants of serous carcinoma may be noninvasive. The epithelial component of the latter, in contrast to that of a noninvasive desmoplastic implant of a borderline tumor, usually occupies more than 25% of the tumor and has higher-grade nuclei.

■ Involvement of the fallopian tube lumen or mucosa by psammoma bodies, often accompanied by neoplastic epithelial cells, is common in SBLTs.

Differential Diagnosis

■ Endocervical-like mucinous borderline tumors (page 308). These tumors contain cells with abundant intracellular mucin and have other distinctive features.

■ Retiform Sertoli-Leydig cell tumors (see Chapter 16).

■ Extraovarian SBLTs (see Chapter 19).

■ Noninvasive implants of serous carcinoma and foci of florid mesothelial hyperplasia (see Chapter 20) may be confused with the implants of serous borderline tumors.

■ The differential diagnosis of metastatic SBLT to lymph nodes includes two other lesions, which may partly account for the high frequency of metastatic SBLT in certain instances:
  - Primary intranodal SBLT. In some cases, intranodal SBLT merges with intranodal endosalpingiosis (see Chapter 19), suggesting origin from the latter.
  - Intranodal hyperplastic mesothelial cells (see Chapter 20).

Behavior

■ SBLTs are confined to one or both ovaries in approximately 70% of cases, with spread at the time of presentation within the pelvis in about 10%; to the upper abdomen, lymph nodes, or both in about 20%; and more distantly in less than 1%, with the latter figure indicating the rarity of hematogenous spread of SBLTs.

■ Segal and Hart found that the risk of extraovarian implants is much higher in SBLTs that have an exophytic (serosal) component than in those that have no serosal involvement (62% versus 4%).

■ Sampling of pelvic lymph nodes, paraaortic lymph nodes, or both revealed involvement in 23% of cases in one study and a corresponding figure of 50% in another investigation that included all types of ovarian borderline tumor (70% were serous) and in which both pelvic and paraaortic lymph nodes were sampled.

- Tan and associates have found that SBLTs extend rarely to extraabdominal lymph nodes (including cervical nodes), that the lymph node involvement may not be detected until years after removal of the primary tumor, and that in some cases the nodes may be replaced by poorly differentiated serous neoplasia.
- The 5-year survival figures for patients with stages I, II, and III serous borderline tumors are between 90% and 95%. Aure and coworkers, however, found that the survival rate for patients with extraovarian spread dropped from 97% to 76% in the follow-up interval between 5 and 20 years.

Prognostic Factors in Serous Borderline Tumors

Stage: SBLTs have a low recurrence rate (10% to 15%), and almost all of those that recur are stage II or higher.

- In a small study of recurrent stage I tumors (Silva and colleagues), the only difference between tumors that recurred and those that did not was a much higher frequency of associated endosalpingiosis (72.7% versus 12.5%) in the former.
- That at least some of the "recurrences" in the above study represented new primary tumors is suggested by the long interval between oophorectomy and recurrence (mean, 16 years) and the observation that most of the recurrences were serous carcinomas.

Macroscopic Residual Disease: This is an important predictor of recurrence and survival in most studies.

Type of Implant: In most studies, patients with noninvasive peritoneal implants, whether predominantly epithelial or desmoplastic, have an excellent prognosis, whereas patients with invasive implants have a poor prognosis.

- Gershenson and coworkers found, in contrast to the foregoing, that progressive or recurrent tumor developed in about 30% of women with *noninvasive* implants (mean follow-up, 10.3 years). All patients dying of disease had invasive low-grade serous carcinomas in the recurrent tumor; no patients with BLT in the recurrence died of tumor.
- Other features of implants (i.e., severe nuclear atypicality, mitotic activity, aneuploidy) may also worsen the prognosis but require additional investigation.

Unusual Growth Patterns Within the Primary Tumors: Solid, cribriform, and micropapillary patterns have not been encountered in a sufficient number of cases with long-term follow-up to be certain of their significance.

- Burks and associates found that the micropapillary pattern is associated with a poorer prognosis for stage II and III tumors.
- Katzenstein and coworkers and Eichhorn and associates, however, found no prognostic significance associated with micropapillary and other unusual patterns.

These patterns, however, appear to be associated with an increased likelihood of invasive implants.

Microinvasion: Follow-up of patients with SBLTs with microinvasion of the stroma indicates that these tumors are associated with a prognosis similar to that of tumors lacking microinvasive foci.

Lymph Node Involvement: The prognostic significance of lymph node involvement in SBLTs is still unclear, but the limited experience has not demonstrated any effect on survival.

Associated Serous Carcinoma: One study has found that, not surprisingly, borderline serous tumors associated with focal areas (<50%) of serous carcinoma are aggressive with a prognosis similar to that of serous carcinoma.

References

Bell DA, Scully RE. Ovarian serous borderline tumors with stromal microinvasion: a report of 21 cases. Hum Pathol 21:397–403, 1990.

Bell DA, Scully RE. Clinicopathologic features of lymph node involvement with ovarian serous borderline tumors [Abstract]. Mod Pathol 5:61A, 1992.

Bell DA, Weinstock MA, Scully RE. Peritoneal implants of ovarian serous borderline tumors: histologic features and prognosis. Cancer 62:2212–2222, 1988.

Burks RT, Sherman ME, Kurman RJ. Micropapillary serous carcinoma of ovary: a distinctive low-grade carcinoma related to serous borderline tumors. Am J Surg Pathol 20:1319–1330, 1996.

Eichhorn JH, Bell DA, Young RH, Scully RE. Ovarian serous borderline tumors of solid, micropapillary and cribriform types: a study of 42 cases. Am J Surg Pathol 23:397–409, 1999.

Gershenson DM, Silva EG, Levy L, et al. Ovarian serous borderline tumors with invasive peritoneal implants. Cancer 82:1096–1103, 1998.

Gershenson DM, Silva EG, Tortolero-Luna G, et al. Serous borderline tumors of the ovary with noninvasive peritoneal implants. Cancer 83:2157–2163, 1998.

Katzenstein A-L A, Mazur MT, Morgan TE, Kao M-S. Proliferative serous tumors of the ovary. Am J Surg Pathol 2:339–355, 1978.

Kennedy AW, Hart WR. Ovarian papillary serous tumors of low malignant potential (serous borderline tumors): a long term follow-up study, incuding patients with microinvasion, lymph node involvement, and transformation to invasive serous carcinoma. Cancer 78:278–286, 1996.

Kurman RJ, Trimble CL. The behavior of serous tumors of low malignant potential: are they ever malignant? Int J Gynecol Pathol 12:120–127, 1993.

Leake JF, Rader JS, Woodruff JD, Rosenshein NB. Retroperitoneal lymphatic involvement with epithelial ovarian tumors of low malignant potential. Gynecol Oncol 42:124–130, 1991.

McCaughey WTE, Kirk ME, Lester W, Dardick I. Peritoneal epithelial lesions associated with proliferative serous tumours of ovary. Histopathology 8:195–208, 1984.

Mooney J, Silva E, Tornos C, Gershenson D. Unusual features of serous neoplasms of low malignant potential during pregnancy. Gynecol Oncol 65:30–35, 1997.

Nayar R, Siriaunkgul S, Robbins KM, et al. Microinvasion in low malignant potential tumors of the ovary. Hum Pathol 27:521–527, 1996.

Rice LW, Berkowitz RS, Mark SD, et al. Epithelial ovarian tumors of borderline malignancy. Gynecol Oncol 39:195–198, 1990.

Segal GH, Hart WR. Ovarian serous tumors of low malignant potential (serous borderline tumors): the relationship of exophytic surface tumor to peritoneal "implants." Am J Surg Pathol 16:577–583, 1992.

Seidman JD, Kurman RJ. Subclassification of serous borderline tumors of the ovary into benign and malignant types: a clinicopathologic study of 65 advanced stage cases. Am J Surg Pathol 20:1331–1335, 1996.

Seidman JD, Sherman ME, Kurman RJ. Fallopian tube calcifications and chronic salpingitis associated with ovarian serous borderline tumors [Abstract]. Mod Pathol 11:114A, 1998.

Silva EG, Tornos CS, Malpica A, Gershenson DM. Ovarian serous neoplasms of low malignant potential associated with focal areas of serous carcinoma. Mod Pathol 10:663–667, 1997.

Silva EG, Tornos C, Zhuang Z, et al. Tumor recurrence in stage I ovarian serous neoplasms of low malignant potential. Int J Gynecol Pathol 17:1–6, 1998.

Tan LK, Flynn SD, Carcangiu ML. Ovarian serous borderline tumors with lymph node involvement: clinicopathologic and DNA content study of seven cases and review of the literature. Am J Surg Pathol 18:904–912, 1994.

Tavassoli FA. Serous tumor of low malignant potential with early stromal invasion (serous LMP with microinvasion). Mod Pathol 1:407–414, 1988.

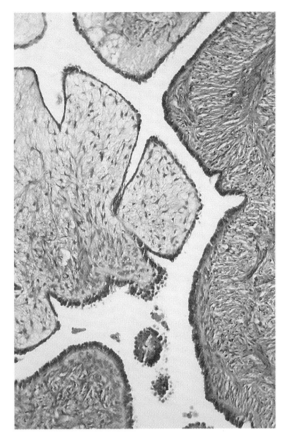

Figure 13–3. Papillary serous cystadenoma. The minimal cellular stratification (*bottom*) is at least partly caused by tangential sectioning.

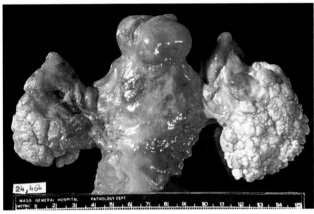

Figure 13–1. Bilateral, surface serous papillomas.

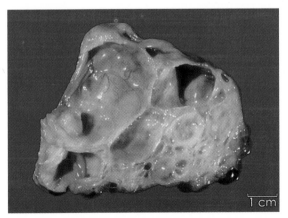

Figure 13–2. Serous cystadenofibroma (sectioned surface).

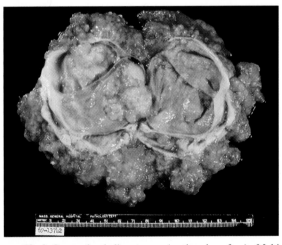

Figure 13–4. Serous borderline tumor (sectioned surface). Multiple, velvety papillae, some with a hydropic appearance, cover the serosa and focally line a cyst lumen.

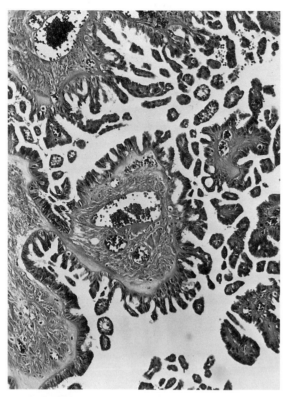

Figure 13–5. Typical low-power appearance of a serous cystic borderline tumor.

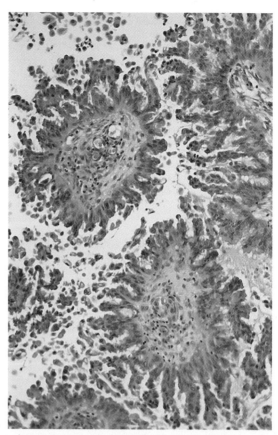

Figure 13–7. Serous borderline tumor with a micropapillary pattern.

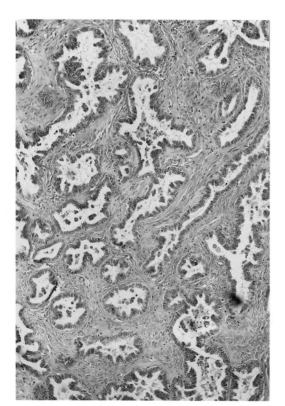

Figure 13–6. Serous borderline tumor. Orderly pattern of invagination with small glandlike spaces separated by a fibromatous stroma, an appearance that should not be mistaken for stromal invasion.

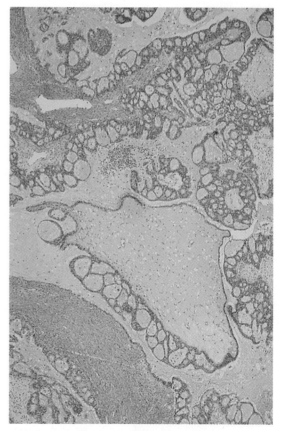

Figure 13–8. Serous borderline tumor with a cribriform pattern.

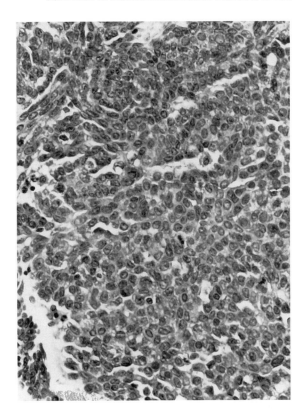

Figure 13–9. Serous borderline tumor. A striking intracystic proliferation of cells results in an almost solid growth pattern. The cells have bland nuclear features.

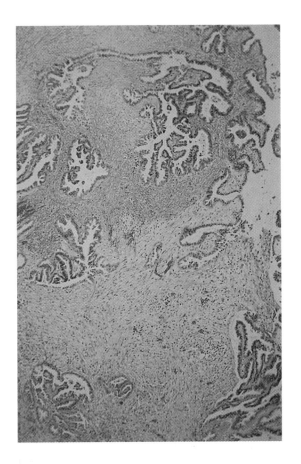

Figure 13–10. Autoimplant (*bottom*) in an otherwise typical serous borderline tumor (*top*). The autoimplant has an appearance similar to an extraovarian noninvasive desmoplastic implant.

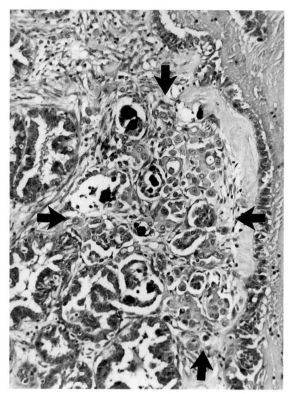

Figure 13–11. Serous borderline tumor with microinvasion (*arrows*).

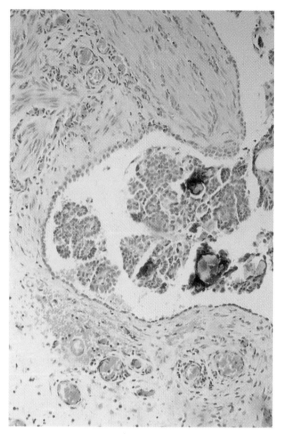

Figure 13–12. Noninvasive epithelial implant of a serous borderline tumor.

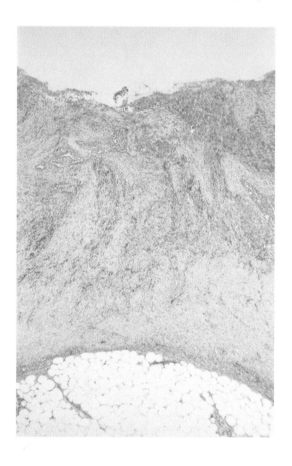

Figure 13–13. Noninvasive desmoplastic implant of a serous borderline tumor. Notice the sharply circumscribed border with the underlying omental adipose tissue.

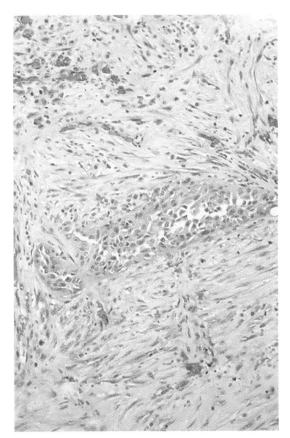

Figure 13–14. Noninvasive desmoplastic implant of a serous borderline tumor (higher-power view of Figure 13–13). A single focus of tumor is surrounded by abundant cellular desmoplastic stroma.

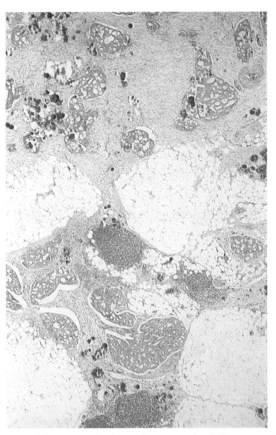

Figure 13–15. Invasive implants of a serous borderline tumor. The omentum is infiltrated by nests of tumor with a cribriform pattern. Note the numerous tumor nests resulting in a greater cellularity than seen in noninvasive desmoplastic implants (compare with Fig. 13–14).

Figure 13–16. Serous borderline tumor involving a pelvic lymph node. The tumor merges with benign endosalpingiotic glands (*top*), suggesting origin in the node.

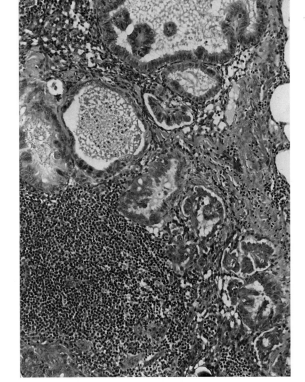

Serous Carcinomas

Gross Features

- Serous carcinomas range from predominantly cystic papillary tumors to entirely solid, soft or hard masses, often having papillary surfaces.
- Rarely, the tumor is entirely exophytic (serous surface carcinoma) with soft, white to red, velvety patches or hard plaques on the ovarian surface.
- Most serous carcinomas cannot be distinguished grossly from other types of poorly differentiated ovarian cancer.
- Serous carcinomas are bilateral in about two thirds of all the cases but in only about one fourth of stage I cases.

Microscopic Features

- There is almost always stromal invasion (with the exception of some serous surface papillary carcinomas), more extensive cellular budding, more confluent cellular growth, and usually greater nuclear atypicality than encountered in serous borderline tumors. The rare intracystic papillary serous carcinoma that lacks obvious stromal invasion should not be confused with a SBLT, with the former having obviously malignant nuclear features.
- Stromal invasion is defined as either disorderly penetration of the cyst wall or the stromal component of a predominantly fibrous tumor by carcinoma cells, with or without a stromal reaction; or confluence of carcinoma in the cyst wall or in the stromal component of a predominantly fibromatous tumor
- If the area of invasion is less than 10 mm², it can be designated *microinvasive*. Microinvasive carcinoma should be distinguished from microinvasive borderline tumor (described earlier), in which a distinctive pattern is present and the invasive cells are not carcinomatous.
- The extent of papillarity varies from those with only rare papillae to those that are predominantly or exclusively papillary. The papillae are typically small but are occasionally large with prominent vessels in their stromal cores.
- Tumors that are moderately or poorly differentiated architecturally generally consist of solid sheets of cells with or without glands or, more commonly, with irregular, slitlike spaces. Anaplastic giant cells may be seen. Another pattern consists of small nests of moderately differentiated epithelial cells or tubules lined by similar cells within a collagenous stroma.
- The cells in most serous carcinomas have nonspecific features. Confusing features that are present in some tumors are foci of hobnail cells or cells with abundant eosinophilic cytoplasm. The tumors are graded by their nuclear features.
- Laminated psammoma bodies occur in variable numbers and may coalesce to form larger, amorphous, calcific aggregates.
- Psammocarcinomas are invasive, highly differentiated serous tumors characterized by destructive stromal invasion; no more than moderate nuclear atypicality; no solid areas of epithelial proliferation except for rare nests of less than 15 cells in diameter; and more than 75% of the papillae and nests containing psammoma bodies. Thorough sampling is important because areas resembling psammocarcinoma may be admixed with typical serous carcinoma.
- Serous surface carcinomas range from highly papillary to those with an almost solid architecture; they may invade the underlying ovarian stroma. Their distinction from peritoneal papillary serous carcinomas with ovarian involvement is discussed in Chapter 19.
- Rare features in serous carcinomas include foci resembling adenoid cystic carcinoma, focal squamous differentiation, and foci of syncytiotrophoblastic giant cells.
- Mural nodules of homologous or heterologous sarcoma or anaplastic carcinoma have been described rarely in association with benign, borderline, or carcinomatous serous cystic tumors.

Differential Diagnosis

- Endometrioid adenocarcinoma. Features favoring this diagnosis include an orderly glandular or villoglandular pattern, squamous differentiation, no or rare psammoma bodies, and various patterns more typical of endometrioid carcinoma (see Chapter 14). Poorly differentiated adenocarcinomas with intermediate or overlapping features between serous and endometrioid are considered to be serous because they behave like the latter.
- Papillary clear cell carcinoma. Features favoring this diagnosis include a tubulocystic pattern; clear, hobnail, or oxyphilic cells; and hyalinization of papillary cores.
- Retiform Sertoli-Leydig cell tumor (see Chapter 16). Features favoring this diagnosis include an age younger than 30 years, androgenic manifestations, and the presence in most cases of more familiar patterns of Sertoli-Leydig cell tumor. Retiform tubules are usually lined by cells that are better differentiated than those of a serous carcinoma.
- Ependymoma (see Chapter 15). The diagnosis is established by the presence of perivascular pseudorosettes and immunoreactivity for glial fibrillary acidic protein.
- Ovarian involvement by malignant epithelial mesothelioma (see Chapter 20). Features favoring this diagnosis include a tubulopapillary pattern, uniformly cuboidal cells with eosinophilic cytoplasm, absence of high-grade nuclear features, few or no psammoma bodies, absence of staining with periodic acid–Schiff after diastase digestion, and absence of immunostaining with a variety of "epithelial" antigens (see Chapter 20).
- Secondary involvement by extraovarian serous carcinoma. Features favoring metastasis from an endometrial serous carcinoma when such a tumor is present include deep myometrial and myometrial vascular space invasion and prominent involvement of lymphatics within the ovary and its hilus.
  - In some cases, it may be impossible to decide if the ovarian tumor is metastatic, is an independent primary tumor, or is the sole primary tumor with endometrial spread.

- The distinction between high-stage ovarian serous carcinomas and serous carcinomas arising from the extraovarian peritoneum is discussed in Chapter 19.
■ Metastatic breast carcinoma that is focally papillary. A history of breast carcinoma and comparison of its microscopic features with those of the ovarian tumor facilitate the diagnosis. Staining for gross cystic disease fluid protein strongly favors metastatic breast carcinoma.

Spread and Behavior

■ Serous carcinomas are confined to one or both ovaries in 16% of cases, with spread at the time of presentation within the pelvis in 11%; to the upper abdomen, lymph nodes, or both in 55%; and more distantly in 18% of the cases.
■ Sampling of pelvic lymph nodes, paraaortic lymph nodes, or both has shown involvement in up to 63% of cases of serous carcinoma.
■ FIGO 5-year survival figures for patients with serous carcinoma are 76% (stage I), 56% (stage II), 25% (stage III), and 9% (stage IV). Even incidentally detected microscopic serous carcinomas are associated with a guarded prognosis.
■ Carey and associates found architectural grading to be a strong independent indicator of prognosis.

References

Aure JC, Hoeg K, Kolstad P. Clinical and histologic studies of ovarian carcinoma: long-term follow-up of 990 cases. Obstet Gynecol 37:1–9, 1971.

Baergen RN, Rutgers JL. Mural nodules in common epithelial tumors of the ovary. Int J Gynecol Pathol 13:62–72, 1994.

Bell DA, Scully RE. Early de novo ovarian carcinoma: a study of fourteen cases. Cancer 73:1859–1864, 1994.

Carey MS, Dembo AJ, Simm JE, et al. Testing the validity of a prognostic classification in patients with surgically optimal ovarian carcinoma: a 15-year review. Int J Gynecol Cancer 3:24–35, 1993.

Gilks CB, Bell DA, Scully RE. Serous psammocarcinoma of the ovary and peritoneum. Int J Gynecol Pathol 9:110–121, 1990.

Goldberg GL, Scheiner J, Friedman A, et al. Lymph node sampling in patients with epithelial ovarian carcinoma. Gynecol Oncol 47:143–145, 1992.

Longacre TA, Kempson RL, Hendrickson MR. Well-differentiated serous neoplasms of the ovary. In State of the Art Reviews: Pathology. Philadelphia: Hanley & Belfus, 1992: 255–306.

Ulbright TM, Roth LM, Sutton GP. Papillary serous carcinoma of the ovary with squamous differentiation. Int J Gynecol Pathol 9:86–94, 1990.

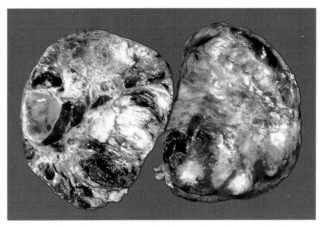

Figure 13–17. Serous carcinoma (serosal and sectioned surfaces).

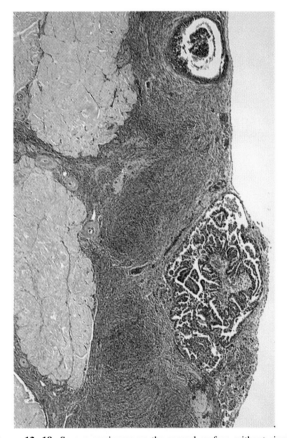

Figure 13–18. Serous carcinoma on the serosal surface without significant parenchymal involvement.

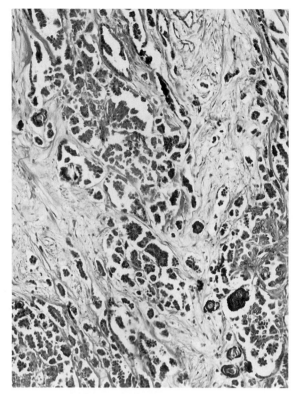

Figure 13–19. Serous carcinoma. There is obvious stromal invasion by small cellular papillae and nests within a desmoplastic stroma.

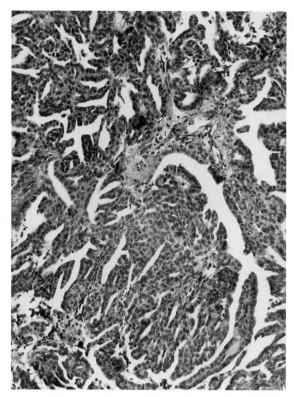

Figure 13–20. Serous carcinoma with papillae and slitlike spaces.

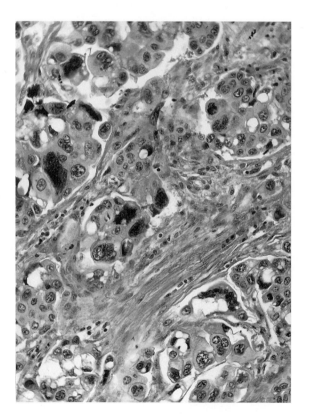

Figure 13–21. Serous carcinoma. Notice the striking nuclear pleomorphism and tumor giant cells.

MUCINOUS TUMORS

General Features

- Mucinous tumors account for 12% to 15% of all ovarian tumors in the Western world. Mucinous cystadenomas account for about 10% of benign ovarian tumors and mucinous carcinomas for about 10% of ovarian cancers.
- About 75% of mucinous tumors are benign. The proportion of the remainder that are borderline (MBLTs) or carcinomas has varied in the literature, but by current criteria, MBLTs are much more common than invasive mucinous carcinomas. Misclassification of MBLTs and mucinous carcinomas metastatic to the ovary likely accounts for a greater proportion of primary mucinous carcinomas in some studies.
- That some mucinous tumors may be of germ cell origin is suggested by an association with dermoid cysts in about 5% of mucinous tumors and the presence in many mucinous tumors of intestinal-type cells. The frequent presence of mucinous epithelium within Brenner tumors and the rare occurrence of small Brenner tumors in the walls of mucinous cystic tumors suggest that the Brenner tumor may also rarely give rise to mucinous tumors.
- Mucinous cystadenomas occur at any age but are most common in the third and fourth decades of life. MBLTs and carcinomas generally occur in older women, with mean ages in both groups in the first half of the sixth decade. Although rare in the first 2 decades, mucinous tumors of all types are more common in this period than analogous serous tumors.
- Mucinous ovarian tumors may be accompanied by hormonal manifestations caused by the secretion of steroid hormones, usually derived from cells within the stroma of the tumor. Less common manifestations are the Zollinger-Ellison syndrome, caused by gastrin production by neuroendocrine cells in the lining epithelium of the cysts, and the carcinoid syndrome.
- The CA-125 level is elevated in up to 67% of cases of mucinous carcinoma, carcinoembryonic antigen (CEA) in up to 88%, and carbohydrate antigen (CA19-9) in up to 83% of cases. The serum level of inhibin is elevated in almost 90% and 80% of mucinous BLTs and carcinomas, respectively.
- Excluding mucinous tumors associated with pseudomyxoma peritonei (page 311), MBLTs of the usual (intestinal) type are almost always stage I, as are 80% to 90% of primary ovarian mucinous carcinomas. An occult extraovarian mucinous adenocarcinoma with secondary ovarian spread should be therefore excluded in ovarian mucinous adenocarcinomas that are stage II or higher.
- Mucinous ovarian tumors may coexist with mucinous adenocarcinomas of the cervix, particularly adenoma malignum (page 116), an association that may occur in patients with the Peutz-Jeghers syndrome. In such cases, it may be difficult or impossible to determine whether the ovarian tumor is an independent primary tumor or metastatic from the cervical tumor.

Gross Features

- Mucinous neoplasms tend to be the largest of all ovarian tumors. Diameters of 30 cm and weights of several kilograms are not uncommon.
- Mucinous cystadenomas may be unilocular but are more often multilocular, with thin walls and a content of mucinous fluid. Borderline tumors and carcinomas much more often contain papillae, soft and mucoid to firm solid areas, and especially in carcinomas, areas of hemorrhage and necrosis.
- Mucinous tumors of the intestinal type frequently contain benign, borderline, and carcinomatous areas within the same tumor, necessitating careful inspection and judicious sampling for microscopic examination. Ruptured locules should be sampled and designated separately.
- Benign mucinous tumors are bilateral in 2% to 5% and intestinal borderline tumors and carcinomas in about 6% of stage I cases. In contrast, 40% of endocervical MBLTs are bilateral. Bilateral ovarian mucinous adenocarcinomas should raise the possibility of an extraovarian tumor with secondary ovarian spread.

Microscopic Features of Benign Tumors

- Glands and cysts, which occasionally contain papillae with fibrovascular cores, are lined by mucinous epithelium consisting of a single row of uniform, mucin-filled columnar cells with basal nuclei.
- The common finding of goblet cells, argyrophil cells, serotonin-containing cells, peptide hormone–containing cells, and occasionally, argentaffin and Paneth cells suggests a gastrointestinal rather than endocervical nature of the neoplastic cells in some cases.
- The stroma of the tumors usually resembles collagenized ovarian stroma. In mucinous adenofibromas, the predominant stromal component has an appearance similar to that of a fibroma.
- Other, mostly uncommon, findings in the stroma include pools of mucin (often with a histiocytic or foreign-body inflammatory response), luteinized cells (particularly during pregnancy), calcified spicules, bands of smooth muscle, a desmoplastic response to areas of necrosis, and mural nodules of various types (see page 310).

Microscopic Features of Borderline Tumors and Carcinomas

- Most borderline mucinous cystic tumors have more obvious and extensive intestinalization of their epithelial linings than their benign counterparts (intestinal mucinous borderline tumors [IMBLTs]), whereas about 10% of them lack obviously intestinal-type epithelium and are designated "endocervical-like" (EMBLTs) or of "müllerian type."
- IMBLTS lack papillae or have filiform papillae. The cysts and papillae are lined by epithelium with vari-

Table 13–3

DIFFERENTIAL MICROSCOPIC FEATURES BETWEEN TWO SUBTYPES OF INTESTINAL-TYPE MUCINOUS BORDERLINE TUMORS

Characteristic	Usual Type	With Intraepithelial Carcinoma
Tumor cells	Atypical nuclear features usually with abundant cytoplasmic mucin	Malignant nuclear features, often with sparse or no cytoplasmic mucin
Intracystic growth patterns	1. Papillae short and blunt to filiform, often branching, with at least minimal stromal support	1. Stroma-free cellular papillae
	2. Secondary gland formation with at least minimal stromal support	2. Cribriform (no stromal support)
	3. Cellular stratification, usually with a height of three or fewer cells	3. Cellular stratification, usually with a height of four or more cells

Adapted from Scully RE, Young RH, Clement PB. Tumors of the Ovary, Maldeveloped Gonads, Fallopian Tube, and Broad Ligament, AFIP fascicle, third series. Washington, DC: Armed Forces Institute of Pathology,

able numbers of goblet cells and other intestinal cell types.

■ The epithelium varies from atypical (IMBLT of usual type) to carcinomatous (IMBLT with intraepithelial carcinoma) (Table 13–3). Benign areas are also commonly present in IMBLTs. Some pathologists prefer to group IMBLTS with intraepithelial carcinoma as a subtype of mucinous carcinoma, using designations such as "intraglandular mucinous carcinoma" or "noninvasive mucinous carcinoma" to indicate an absence of invasion.

■ By definition, extensive stromal invasion is absent in both types of IMBLTs, but microinvasion (each focus of invasion <10 mm²) may occur (i.e., microinvasive IMBLT, microinvasive IMBLT with intraepithelial carcinoma).

■ The diagnosis of mucinous carcinoma requires invasion (page 300) exceeding that allowable in microinvasive tumors. The stroma may be desmoplastic, extensively infiltrated by inflammatory cells, or both, or it may resemble ovarian stroma and contain clusters of lutein cells. Benign and borderline areas are also frequently present, underscoring the need for thorough histologic sampling in ovarian mucinous tumors.

■ Hoerl and Hart found that extensive stromal invasion was always associated with a component of intraepithelial (intraglandular) carcinoma and was always present in stage I mucinous carcinomas that metastasized.

■ Mucinous carcinomas are usually composed of mucinous cells that are not specifically of endocervical or intestinal-type mucinous cells and that may be composed of cells that are uniformly rich in mucin or that contain minimal intracytoplasmic mucin. Cells of the latter type focally may resemble those of a well-differentiated endometrioid adenocarcinoma.

■ "Dirty" necrosis is present in some primary mucinous carcinomas of the ovary, although this finding is more common in metastatic colonic carcinomas to the ovary. Unusual findings in mucinous carcinomas include a focal component of a signet-ring cell or colloid carcinoma.

■ Borderline and malignant mucinous tumors contain stromal pools of escaped mucin from the glands and cysts in about 25% of cases, often associated with histiocytes and a foreign-body giant cell reaction.

■ Less commonly, dissection of mucin into the stroma (i.e., pseudomyxoma ovarii) is associated with pseudomyxoma peritonei (PP). In pseudomyxoma ovarii, the mucin is typically unassociated with a brisk inflammatory cell or foreign-body giant cell response and often contains or is partly lined by neoplastic epithelial cells.

Differential Diagnosis

■ Serous and endometrioid carcinomas with abundant luminal mucin (versus mucinous carcinoma).
  • Mucinous carcinomas, in contrast to the other two tumors, contain at least occasional goblet cells with mucin-rich cytoplasm. Very small foci of benign-appearing endocervical-type epithelium, however, may be encountered in endometrioid carcinomas.
  • Vimentin-immunoreactivity favors the diagnosis of serous or endometrioid carcinoma, whereas cytoplasmic CEA-positivity favors a diagnosis of mucinous carcinoma.

■ Sertoli-Leydig cell tumors (SLCTs) with heterologous mucinous epithelium (see Chapter 16). These tumors contain, in addition to the mucinous elements, foci of typical SLCT, usually of intermediate type.

■ Mucinous carcinoid tumors (see Chapter 15).

■ Metastatic adenocarcinomas from the gastrointestinal tract, biliary tract, pancreas, and uterine cervix (see Chapter 18).

■ Metastatic low-grade mucinous tumor from the appendix (see Pseudomyxoma Peritonei, page 311).

Behavior and Prognosis

■ The 5-year survival rate for patients with stage I IMBLTs, including those with microinvasion, is 100% in most studies, 90% to 100% for stage II, and 50% for stage III. Most of the reported tumors that are more advanced than stage I, however, have been associated with pseudomyxoma peritonei and probably are metastatic from the appendix (see Pseudomyxoma Peritonei, page 311).

■ The survival rates for patients with mucinous carcinomas are 83% (stage I), 55% (stage II), 21% (stage III), and 9% (stage IV). Recent studies have found even higher (>90%) survival rates for stage I tumors. By far the most important prognostic parameter in cases of mucinous carcinomas is stage.

■ The behavior of IMBLTs with intraepithelial carcinoma, with or without microinvasion, has been similar to that of the usual IMBLTs in some studies, whereas others have found that the former patients have presented at a higher stage or have been associated with a poorer survival when stage I.

■ Architectural grading of mucinous carcinomas in some studies has had independent prognostic significance.

References

Bell DA. Mucinous adenofibromas of the ovary: a report of 10 cases. Am J Surg Pathol 15:227–232, 1991.

Chaitin BA, Gershenson DM, Evans HL. Mucinous tumors of the ovary: a clinicopathologic study of 70 cases. Cancer 55:1958–1962, 1985.

Hart WR. Ovarian epithelial tumors of borderline malignancy (carcinomas of low malignant potential). Hum Pathol 8:541–549, 1977.

Hart WR, Norris HJ. Borderline and malignant mucinous tumors of the ovary: histologic criteria and clinical behavior. Cancer 31:1031–1044, 1973.

Hendrickson MR, Kempson RL. Well-differentiated mucinous neoplasms of the ovary. In State of the Art Reviews: Pathology: Surface Epithelial Neoplasms of the Ovary. Philadelphia: Hanley and Belfus, 1992:1–27.

Hoerl HD, Hart WR. Primary ovarian mucinous cystadenocarcinomas: a clinicopathologic study of 49 cases with long-term follow-up. Am J Surg Pathol 12:1449–1462, 1998.

Khunamornpong S, Russell P, Dalrymple C. Proliferating mucinous tumors of the ovaries with microinvasion: morphological assessment of 13 cases. Int J Gynecol Pathol 18:238–246, 1999.

Lee KR, Scully RE. Mucinous tumors of the ovary [Abstract]. Mod Pathol 11:107A, 1998.

Riopel MA, Ronnett BM, Kurman RJ. Evaluation of diagnostic criteria and behavior of mucinous ovarian intestinal-type mucinous tumors: Atypical proliferative (borderline) tumors and intraepithelial, microinvasive, invasive and metastatic carcinomas. Am J Surg Pathol 23:617–635, 1999.

Siriaunkgul S, Robbins KM, McGowan L, Silverberg SG. Ovarian mucinous tumors of low malignant potential: a clinicopathologic study of 54 tumors of intestinal and müllerian type. Int J Gynecol Pathol 14:198–208, 1995.

Sumithran E, Susil BJ, Looi L-M. The prognostic significance of grading in borderline mucinous tumors of the ovary. Hum Pathol 19:15–18, 1988.

Watkin W, Silva EG, Gershenson DM. Mucinous carcinoma of the ovary: pathologic prognostic factors. Cancer 208–212, 1992.

Young RH, Scully RE. Mucinous ovarian tumors associated with mucinous adenocarcinoma of the cervix. Int J Gynecol Pathol 7:99–111, 1988.

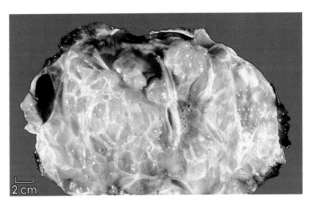

Figure 13–22. Mucinous cystadenoma (sectioned surface). An intestinal mucinous borderline tumor would have a similar appearance.

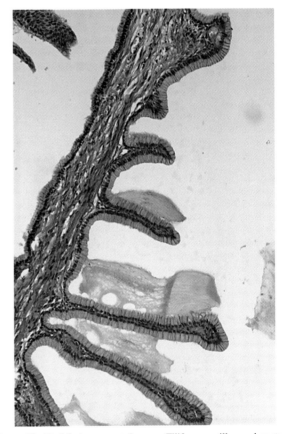

Figure 13–23. Mucinous cystadenoma. Filiform papillae and cysts are lined by a single layer of benign mucinous epithelium.

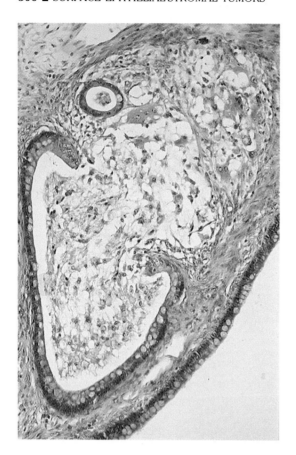

Figure 13–24. Mucinous cystadenoma. Gland rupture has resulted in a histiocytic response to extravasated mucin.

Figure 13–25. Mucinous intestinal borderline tumor of the usual type. Notice the cellular stratification, atypia, and mitotic figures. Although only a single goblet cell is present (*arrow*), numerous argentaffin cells with subnuclear reddish brown granules are present.

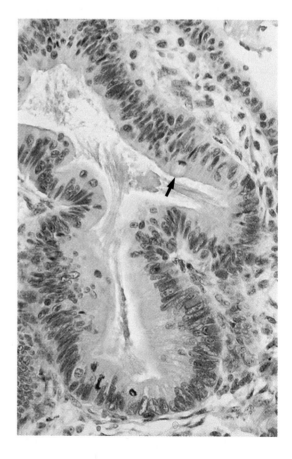

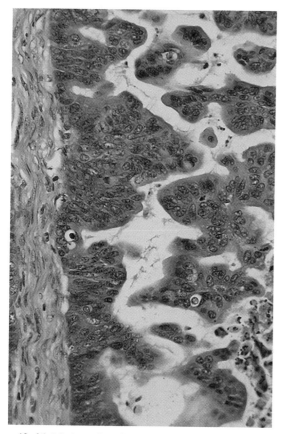

Figure 13–26. Mucinous intestinal borderline tumor with intraepithelial carcinoma. There was no obvious tumor invasion.

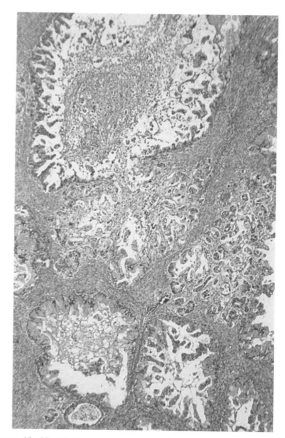

Figure 13–28. Mucinous carcinoma. Notice the areas of stromal invasion (*center*).

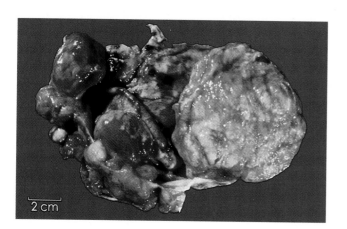

Figure 13–27. Mucinous carcinoma (sectioned surface) with cysts and solid fleshy areas.

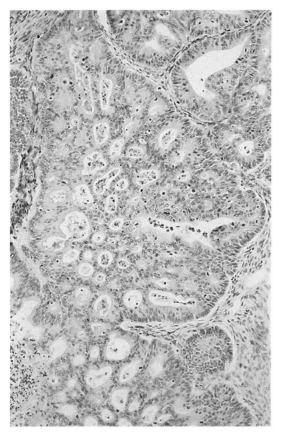

Figure 13–29. Mucinous carcinoma with a cribriform pattern. Obvious stromal invasion was present in other areas.

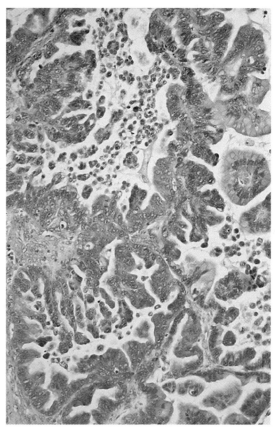

Figure 13–30. Mucinous carcinoma. Notice the striking cellular stratification and marked nuclear atypicality. Obvious stromal invasion was present in other areas.

Endocervical Mucinous Borderline Tumors

- EMBLTs account for only 15% of mucinous BLTs. EMBLTs tend to be smaller and more often unilocular or with fewer locules than those of intestinal type. They may arise within an endometriotic cyst.
- EMBLTs architecturally resemble SBLTs with bulbous stromal papillae and smaller cellular papillae and cellular buds composed of mildly to moderately atypical epithelial cells, which may reach more than 20 cells high.
- Many neoplastic cells in EMBLTs contain abundant cytoplasmic mucin, but some are usually mucin free and have abundant eosinophilic cytoplasm.
- Numerous neutrophils are almost always present in the stroma, among the neoplastic epithelial cells, and in the luminal mucin.
- Foci of microinvasion are seen in rare cases.

- EMBLTs are associated with ipsilateral ovarian endometriosis in 20% of cases and with endometriosis anywhere in the pelvis in 30% of cases.
- Differential diagnosis
  - EMBLTs of mixed cell type (see Chapter 14), which contain tubal, endometrioid, or squamous elements, alone or in combination, in addition to mucinous epithelium.
  - Serous BLTs resemble EMBLTs on low-power microscopic examination and may contain eosinophilic cells like those in EMBLTs but lack endocervical-like mucinous epithelium.
- Isolated peritoneal implants or lymph node metastases have been reported in approximately 20% of EMBLTs, but there have been no fatalities. Based on a few cases, microinvasion does not appear to be an adverse prognostic feature. Long-term follow-up data on a large number of cases of EMBLTs are needed to more clearly assess their behavior.

References

Riopel MA, Ronnett BM, Kurman RJ. Diagnostic criteria and behavior of seromucinous ovarian tumors: borderline, microinvasive, and invasive [Abstract]. Mod Pathol 11:113A, 1998.

Rutgers JL, Scully RE. Ovarian müllerian mucinous papillary cystadenomas of borderline malignancy: a clinicopathologic analysis. Cancer 61:340–348, 1988.

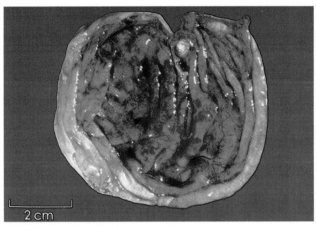

Figure 13–31. Endocervical mucinous borderline tumor. The specimen consists of an opened unilocular cyst. Several excrescences are seen within the cyst lining.

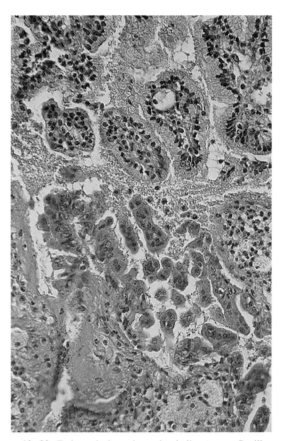

Figure 13–33. Endocervical mucinous borderline tumor. Papillae with stromal cores are lined by endocervical-type cells. Notice the atypical stratified epithelial cells with eosinophilic cytoplasm.

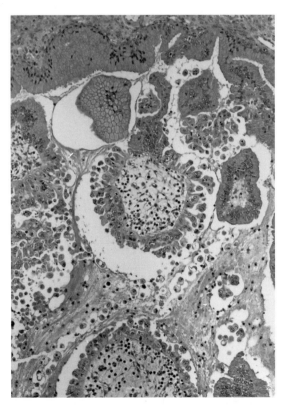

Figure 13–32. Endocervical mucinous borderline tumor. Notice the lining of endocervical-type cells (*top*) and papillae containing inflammatory cells (mostly neutrophils) and lined by stratified cells that were eosinophilic.

Mural Nodules in Mucinous Tumors

- Rare mucinous cystic tumors contain mural nodules that may be anaplastic carcinoma, sarcomas of various types, carcinosarcoma, sarcoma-like nodules, mixed nodules, or leiomyomas.

- The nodules of anaplastic carcinoma consist of solid sheets of large, rounded epithelial cells with high-grade nuclei and often with abundant eosinophilic cytoplasm, poorly differentiated spindle-shaped epithelial cells, or both; focal glandular differentiation may be seen. The nodules are typically ill defined, and the tumor cells may invade vessels.

- Sarcomatous nodules have included fibrosarcoma, rhabdomyosarcoma, and undifferentiated sarcoma, all of which tend to be ill defined and may invade vessels. A carcinosarcomatous nodule in the wall of a mucinous cystadenocarcinoma has been reported.

- Sarcoma-like nodules are single or multiple, soft or firm, and are usually reddish-brown.

  - Sharply circumscribed nodules are typically composed of various numbers of pleomorphic cells with bizarre nuclei, typical and atypical mitotic figures (as many as 10 per 10 high-power fields), spindle cells, epulis-type giant cells, and acute and chronic inflammatory cells.

  - Hemorrhage and necrosis are common, but vascular invasion is absent.

  - These nodules are considered reactive because of their associated benign clinical course. Perplexing features are focal staining of the pleomorphic cells for cytokeratin and the occasional finding of adenocarcinoma or anaplastic carcinoma within the nodule (i.e., mixed nodule).

- All of the reported patients with sarcoma-like mural nodules have had a benign clinical course, whereas most patients with mural nodules of anaplastic carcinoma have had a malignant course. Too few cases of sarcomatous nodules have been published to warrant a conclusion regarding their prognosis.

References

Baergen RN, Rutgers JL. Mural nodules in common epithelial tumors of the ovary. Int J Gynecol Pathol 13:62–72, 1994.

Prat J, Scully RE. Ovarian mucinous tumors with sarcoma-like mural nodules: a report of seven cases. Cancer 44:1332–1344, 1979.

Prat J, Scully RE. Sarcomas in ovarian mucinous tumors: a report of two cases. Cancer 44:1327–1331, 1979.

Prat J, Young RH, Scully RE. Ovarian mucinous tumors with foci of anaplastic carcinoma. Cancer 50:300–304, 1982.

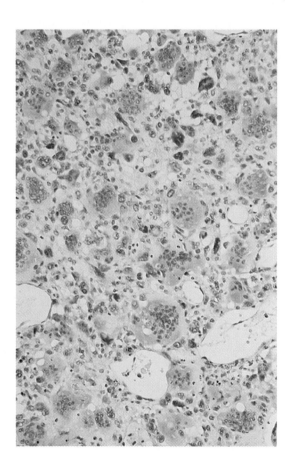

Figure 13–34. Mucinous cystic tumor with a pseudosarcomatous mural nodule. Many of the numerous giant cells resemble osteoclastic-type giant cells.

Pseudomyxoma Peritonei

Origin

- When pseudomyxoma peritonei (PP) (i.e., masses of jelly-like mucus in the pelvis and often in the abdomen) is associated with a cystic ovarian mucinous tumor (OMT), the disease has been traditionally interpreted as stage II or III ovarian borderline tumor or carcinoma. Most later studies, however, have concluded that the PP and the OMT are secondary to spread from an appendiceal mucinous tumor (AMT) in most cases.
- Several arguments support the spread of a primary AMT to the ovary and peritoneum in cases of PP:
  - The common finding of an AMT in association with OMTs in cases of PP in which the appendix has been investigated microscopically in contrast to its far lower frequency in the absence of peritoneal involvement
  - The usual histologic similarity of the AMT and OMT when both are adequately sampled
  - The much higher frequency of bilaterality of OMTs in the presence of appendiceal and peritoneal involvement than in its absence, correlating with the much greater frequency of bilaterality of metastatic than primary OMTs in general
  - The higher frequency of involvement of the right ovary when the OMT is unilateral in cases of appendiceal and peritoneal involvement, in contrast to a similar frequency of involvement of both ovaries in its absence
  - Differences in the microscopic appearance of OMTs in the presence of appendiceal and peritoneal involvement compared to in its absence—specifically, the common finding of unusually tall mucinous epithelium and extensive pseudomyxoma ovarii in the former and their usual absence in the latter
  - When an OMT coexists with an AMT in cases of PP, the tumors usually have an identical immunoprofile, including negative results for HAM 56 and CK 7, findings typical for intestinal primary tumors in contrast to opposite reactions for OMTs unassociated with PP
  - When an OMT coexists with an AMT in cases of PP, the tumors have an identical *K-ras* mutation
  - The finding of a "normal" appendix in association with the OMT does not exclude an appendiceal origin for the PP unless the appendix has been well sampled because appendiceal tumors may be small and rupture sites may require thorough microscopic sampling to identify
  - Differences in the microscopic appearance or immunoprofile of the appendiceal and ovarian tumors may reflect tumor heterogeneity, inadequate sampling of either tumor, or the frequently higher degree of differentiation in metastatic tumor to the ovary than in the primary tumor
- Some arguments have been advanced for the independent primary nature of the OMT still favored by some investigators:
  - Reports of a normal appendix or an unruptured AMT in some cases of PP associated with OMTs

- Differences in the observed degree of malignancy of the AMTs and OMTs on microscopic examination
- Immunohistochemical differences between the two tumors in many cases
- Reports of the occasional coexistence of an OMT and an AMT in the absence of peritoneal involvement

Microscopic Features of Pseudomyxoma Peritonei

- Extraovarian, intraabdominal mucus associated with OMTs may be of several types, all of which have been included in studies of PP, and there is no consensus on how many of these types of intraabdominal mucus warrant the designation of PP:
  - Free mucin in the abdominal cavity (mucinous ascites)
  - Small or large deposits of mucin adherent to peritoneal surfaces, containing inflammatory and mesothelial cells and sometimes organizing capillaries and fibroblasts, but usually lacking neoplastic epithelial cells
  - Masses composed of pools of mucin, which may or may not contain neoplastic cells, surrounded by dense collagenous tissue (i.e., dissecting mucin)

Intraoperative Management and Reporting of Cases

- Prospective study of new cases of PP should include as extensive sampling of all the lesions as technically feasible in addition to further studies with special immunohistochemical and molecular biology techniques. The appendix should be removed for complete histologic examination, even if its intraoperative appearance is normal.
- The ovarian and appendiceal tumors, which show the same range of histologic and cytologic features, should be designated by the degree of atypicality of the epithelium as benign, borderline (atypical), or malignant. We do not regard dissection of mucin containing only benign or atypical cells as true invasion.
- Until generally accepted methods for determining whether the ovarian cystic tumors are independent primary tumors or metastatic from the appendix are available, those that are associated with PP should continue to be staged as ovarian tumors, with the realization that their clinical behavior may not reflect accurately that of mucinous tumors of unquestionable ovarian origin.
- PP, which is a clinical and surgical designation, should not appear as a diagnosis in the pathology report. The report should contain the following information:
  - An accurate appraisal of the ovarian and appendiceal tumors as benign, borderline, or malignant, with a notation about the presence or absence of rupture
  - Assessment of the peritoneal lesions as mucinous ascites (i.e., free fluid in abdomen), organizing mucinous fluid, or mucin dissection with fibrosis
  - The presence or absence of neoplastic cells and whether they appear benign, borderline (atypical), or malignant

Behavior

■ The peritoneal lesions of PP most commonly contain benign to borderline mucinous epithelium. The clinical course in such cases is typically a slowly progressive one over a period of many years.

■ Several studies have found that patients with PP in which the peritoneal deposits were free of neoplastic epithelial cells had a more favorable prognosis than those with cell-containing deposits.

■ Ronnett and coworkers have shown the importance of distinguishing between peritoneal deposits containing carcinomatous cells ("peritoneal mucinous carcinomatosis" [PMC]) and those containing only benign or borderline epithelium ("peritoneal adenomucinosis" [PAM]). Tumors with intermediate features or in which the primary and metastatic tumor have discordant features (PAM in primary, PMC in metastases) behave more like PMC.

  • PMC usually arises from a mucinous adenocarcinoma of the appendix or large or small bowel, whereas PAM usually arises from a benign or low-grade mucinous tumor of the appendix.

  • PMC, unlike PAM, often metastasizes to lymph nodes and invades parenchymal organs.

  • PMC is associated with a much poorer survival than PAM (10% at 5 years versus 80% at 10 years).

References

Chuaqui RF, Zhuang Z, Emmert-Buck MR, et al. Genetic analysis of synchronous mucinous tumors of the ovary and appendix. Hum Pathol 27:165–171, 1996.

Costa MJ. Psuedomyxoma peritonei: histologic predictors of patient survival. Arch Pathol Lab Med 118:1215–1219, 1994.

Cuatrecasas M, Matias-Guiu X, Prat J. Synchronous mucinous tumors of the appendix and the ovary associated with pseudomyxoma peritonei: a clinicopathologic study of six cases with comparative analysis of c-Ki-ras mutations. Am J Surg Pathol 20:739–746, 1996.

Guerrieri C, Franlund B, Fristedt S, et al. Mucinous tumors of the vermiform appendix and ovary, and pseudomyxoma peritonei: histogenetic implications of cytokeratin 7 expression. Hum Pathol 28:1039–1045, 1997.

Michael H, Sutton G, Roth LM. Ovarian carcinoma with extracellular mucin production: reassessment of "pseudomyxoma ovarii et peritonei." Int J Gynecol Pathol 6:298–312, 1987.

Prayson RA, Hart WR, Petras RE. Pseudomyxoma peritonei: a clinicopathologic study of 19 cases with emphasis on site of origin and nature of associated ovarian tumors. Am J Surg Pathol 18:591–603, 1994.

Ronnett BM, Kurman RJ, Zahn CM, et al. Pseudomyxoma peritonei in women: a clinicopathologic analysis of 30 cases with emphasis on site of origin, prognosis, and relationship to ovarian mucinous tumors of low malignant potential. Hum Pathol 56:509–524, 1995.

Ronnett BM, Shmookler BM, Diener-West M, et al. Immunohistochemical evidence supporting the appendiceal origin of pseudomyxoma peritonei in women. Int J Gynecol Pathol 16:1–9, 1997.

Ronnett BM, Shmookler BM, Sugarbaker PH, Kurman RJ. Pseudomyxoma peritonei: new concepts in diagnosis, origin, nomenclature, and relationship to mucinous borderline (low malignant potential) tumors of the ovary. Anat Pathol 2:198–226, 1997.

Ronnett BM, Szych C, Staebler A, et al. Molecular genetic evidence supporting the appendiceal origin of pseudomyxoma peritonei in women [Abstract]. Mod Pathol 12:123A, 1999.

Seidman JD, Elsayed AM, Sobin LH, Tavassoli FA. Association of mucinous tumors of the ovary and appendix: a clinicopathologic study of 25 cases. Am J Surg Pathol 17:22–34, 1992.

Young RH, Gilks CB, Scully RE. Mucinous tumors of the appendix associated with mucinous tumors of the ovary and pseudomyxoma peritonei: a clinicopathological analysis of 22 cases supporting an origin in the appendix. Am J Surg Pathol 15:415–429, 1991.

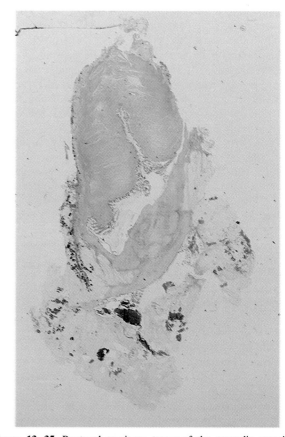

Figure 13–35. Ruptured mucinous tumor of the appendix associated with pseudomyxoma peritonei. The appendiceal lumen is dilated and lined by neoplastic mucinous epithelium. A rupture site is present at the 2-o'clock position. The serosal surface is covered by masses of mucin.

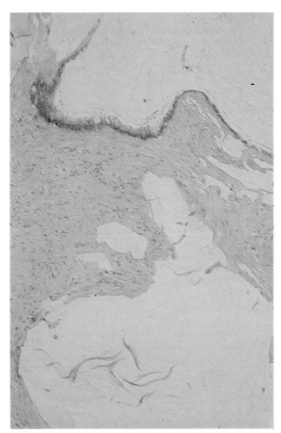

Figure 13-36. Pseudomyxoma peritonei. The omentum is infiltrated by implants of borderline mucinous epithelium and pools of acellular mucin that elicit a fibrotic stromal reaction.

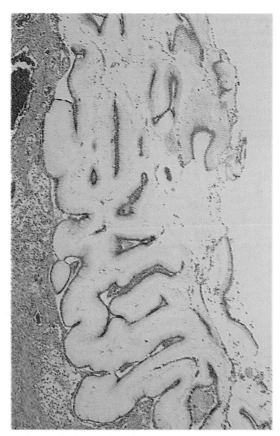

Figure 13-37. Ovarian cystic mucinous tumor in a woman with a low-grade mucinous tumor of the appendix and pseudomyxoma peritonei. Notice the unusually tall mucinous cells with a benign appearance.

CHAPTER14

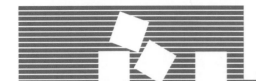

Surface Epithelial-Stromal Tumors: Endometrioid, Clear Cell, Transitional, Squamous, Undifferentiated, and Mixed Cell Types

ENDOMETRIOID TUMORS

General Features

- Endometrioid tumors resemble closely tumors that are encountered more commonly in the endometrium, including endometrioid carcinomas, stromal sarcomas, müllerian adenosarcomas, and malignant müllerian mixed tumors.
- An origin from endometriosis is demonstrable in a minority of cases. Most endometrioid tumors probably arise directly from surface epithelial inclusions, the ovarian stroma, or both.
- Some pathologists regard endometriosis as a neoplasm, a view supported by the finding of a monoclonal X-chromosome inactivation pattern in some endometriotic cysts. Endometriosis, putative precancerous changes in endometriosis, and neoplasms derived from endometriosis are discussed in Chapter 19.

Epithelial Tumors

General Features

- Endometrioid epithelial tumors account for 2% to 4% of all ovarian tumors. Most endometrioid tumors are carcinomas, which account for 10% to 20% of ovarian carcinomas. Fewer than 1% of benign ovarian neoplasms are endometrioid, and only 2% to 3% of borderline epithelial tumors are endometrioid; most of these tumors are adenofibromas.
- Benign, borderline, and malignant endometrioid epithelial tumors occur most commonly in women in the older reproductive and postmenopausal age groups, with mean ages in the sixth decade.
- Endometrioid tumors are accompanied by endometriosis in the same ovary or elsewhere in the pelvis in as many as 38% of cases. In almost 25% of cases of endometrioid carcinoma in one study, there was ipsilateral atypical endometriosis. A transition to endometriotic epithelium has been reported in 5% to 10% of ovarian endometrioid carcinomas.
- Between 15% and 20% of endometrioid carcinomas of the ovary are associated with a synchronous or, rarely, a metachronous endometrial carcinoma. Criteria for distinguishing among ovarian endometrioid carcinoma with spread to the uterus, vice versa, and independent primary neoplasia of both organs are discussed on pages 316 and 317.
- The association of ovarian endometrioid carcinomas with endometriosis, endometrial carcinoma, or both and the known response of endometriotic tissue to steroid hormones suggest that some endometrioid carcinomas of the ovary may have the same risk factors for their development as endometrial carcinomas.
- The clinical manifestations of ovarian endometrioid carcinomas are similar in general to those of other ovarian cancers, including elevation of the serum CA-125 level in most cases and the occasional presence of endocrine manifestations caused by steroid hormone secretion.

Gross Features

- Endometrioid tumors have no features that distinguish them from other surface epithelial-stromal tumors (except clear cell tumors) other than the more frequent presence in the same ovary of endometriosis from which the tumor may have arisen.

- Endometrioid adenofibromas, including those of borderline malignancy, are predominantly solid but may contain occasional cysts. Benign and borderline tumors are almost always unilateral.
- Carcinomas range from soft, friable, or fibrous, solid tumors (resembling adenofibromas) to cystic tumors with a thin, soft papillary lining or with a fungating intracystic mass. The cysts may contain chocolate-colored fluid or mucus. Seventeen percent of stage I endometrioid carcinomas are bilateral.

Microscopic Features of Benign Tumors

- The rare endometrioid cystadenomas are lined by stratified, typically nonciliated epithelium devoid of mucin. Endometriotic stroma or pigmented histiocytes characteristic of an endometriotic cyst should be excluded by thorough sampling. In rare cases, intracystic polypoid and papillary proliferations of bland endometrioid epithelium are found.
- Endometrioid adenofibromas contain glands lined by stratified non-mucin–containing epithelium and, in some cases, squamous morules (occasionally with central necrosis) separated by a predominant fibromatous stromal component. Foci with simple columnar, cuboidal, or flat epithelium result in a morphologic overlap with a serous adenofibroma (see Chapter 13).
- Some benign, borderline, or malignant adenofibromatous tumors have an unusually cellular, mitotically active stroma; frankly malignant features, however, are not present. This finding appears to have no adverse prognostic significance.

Microscopic Features of Borderline Tumors

- Most of these tumors have an adenofibromatous pattern in which atypical to cytologically malignant, endometrioid-type cells forming nests or lining glands or cysts are separated by a fibromatous stroma; obvious stromal invasion is absent.
- If the epithelium is carcinomatous, the tumor is designated "borderline tumor with intraepithelial carcinoma," and the tumor is graded 1 to 3 according to criteria used for grading endometrioid carcinoma of the uterine corpus (see Chapter 8).
- If stromal invasion is present, we distinguish between microinvasion (one or more foci 10 mm² or less in area) and more extensively invasive carcinoma, which may coexist with a benign or borderline adenofibroma (i.e., carcinoma in an adenofibroma).
- The reported cases of borderline endometrioid adenofibromas with or without microinvasion have been clinically benign. Recognition of features that may predict a malignant behavior requires additional experience with these tumors.
- Rarely, an intracystic villoglandular tumor is lined by endometrioid epithelium that is atypical (i.e., borderline endometrioid tumor with epithelial atypia) or malignant (i.e., borderline endometrioid tumor with intraepithelial carcinoma).

Typical Microscopic Features of Endometrioid Carcinoma

- Most ovarian endometrioid carcinomas resemble closely the common subtypes of endometrioid carcinoma of the uterine corpus. Grade 1 tumors and the well-differentiated areas of higher-grade tumors have invasive round, oval, or tubular glands lined by stratified non-mucin–containing epithelium. Adenofibromatous foci are often admixed.
- Other common patterns include a cribriform pattern and a villoglandular pattern. Rarely, the tumor cells are confined to the lining of a cyst.
- Squamous differentiation occurs in 33% to 50% of endometrioid carcinomas as morules of small, immature but benign-appearing squamous cells or as nests or diffuse areas of cytologically malignant squamous epithelium.
  - "Endometrioid adenocarcinoma with squamous differentiation" is used to designate these tumors, which should be graded exclusively on the basis of the glandular component.
  - Keratinization in these tumors may elicit a foreign-body giant cell reaction and calcification.
- Abundant luminal or apical cytoplasmic mucin warrants the appellation "mucin-rich" endometrioid carcinoma. Minor foci of mucinous epithelium in rare endometrioid carcinomas should not lead to an erroneous diagnosis of mucinous carcinoma. Occasionally, glands with luminal eosinophilic colloid-like material may simulate struma ovarii.

Uncommon and Rare Variants of Endometrioid Carcinoma

- Sex cord–like foci occur in endometrioid carcinomas and are occasionally extensive, potentially resulting in a misdiagnosis of sex cord–stromal tumor.
  - Areas can resemble Sertoli cell and Sertoli-Leydig cell neoplasia, including small, well-differentiated glands in a lobular arrangement and solid, tubular structures containing cells with pale, oval nuclei and a central, pale, cytoplasmic pseudosyncytium.
  - In some tumors, the cytoplasm is vacuolated and lipid rich, the appearance simulating that of a lipid-rich Sertoli cell tumor (see Chapter 16). Rarely, thin cords resembling sex cords are present.
  - Luteinized stromal cells in some of these cases may be mistaken for Leydig cells and cause virilization, increasing the likelihood of misdiagnosis.
  - Some tumors have solid areas sometimes punctured by tubular, round, or tiny rosette-like glands, the latter simulating the microfollicular pattern of an adult granulosa cell tumor. Occasionally, an insular or trabecular pattern of solid or microglandular aggregates enhances the resemblance.

■ Focal to extensive aggregates of spindle-shaped epithelial cells are an occasional finding in endometrioid carcinomas.
- The spindle cells may appear to transform into fibroblasts with collagen production within the aggregates and at their periphery.
- Occasionally, spindle cell nests undergo transition to clearly recognizable squamous cells, suggesting that the former represents abortive squamous differentiation.

■ Oxyphilic endometrioid adenocarcinomas are characterized by tumor cells with abundant oxyphilic cytoplasm.

■ Secretory endometrioid adenocarcinomas are characterized by glandular lining cells that are vacuolated, resembling the glandular cells of a 16-day secretory endometrium.

■ In ciliated cell endometrioid adenocarcinomas, which usually have a cribriform pattern, most of the glandular lining cells bear cilia.

■ Rare endometrioid carcinomas have scattered balloon-like, presumably hydropic, vacuoles or similar vacuoles occupying the basal portion of the cytoplasm, with apical displacement of the nuclei.

■ About 10% of endometrioid carcinomas contain argyrophil cells of the neuroendocrine type. Rare endometrioid carcinomas are admixed with undifferentiated carcinomas that have neuroendocrine features (see Chapter 17).

Differential Diagnosis

■ Serous and mucinous neoplasms (pages 300 and 304).

■ Brenner tumor (versus an endometrioid adenofibroma with morules). Features favoring a diagnosis of Brenner tumor include a mucinous (or rarely serous) glandular component and the presence of nuclear grooves.

■ Clear cell adenocarcinoma (versus secretory endometrioid carcinoma). Features favoring secretory carcinoma include glands with basal and supranuclear vacuoles and absence of cells with completely vacuolated cytoplasm and eccentric nuclei. Rare carcinomas are composed of secretory endometrioid carcinoma and clear cell carcinoma.

■ MMMT (versus endometrioid carcinoma with spindled epithelial cells) (see page 322).

■ Sertoli-stromal cell tumors. Features favoring a diagnosis of endometrioid carcinoma include a postmenopausal age, bilaterality, foci of typical endometrioid carcinoma, luminal mucin, squamous differentiation, an adenofibromatous component, immunoreactivity for epithelial membrane antigen (EMA) and cytokeratin 7, and an absence of immunoreactivity for inhibin.

■ Granulosa cell tumor.
- This differential diagnosis is based on the coexistence of other characteristic patterns of either tumor, on the different appearances of the microglands of an endometrioid carcinoma and Call-Exner bodies, and the different nuclear features of the two tumors.
- Immunoreactivity for EMA and cytokeratin 7 favors endometrioid carcinoma, whereas positivity for inhibin strongly favors granulosa cell tumor.

Table 14–1.
ENDOMETRIOID TUMORS OF OVARY AND ENDOMETRIUM: ENDOMETRIAL PRIMARY AND OVARIAN SECONDARY TUMORS

1. Histologic similarity of the tumors
2. Large endometrial tumor—small ovarian tumor(s)
3. Atypical endometrial hyperplasia also present
4. Deep myometrial invasion
   a. Direct extension into adnexa
   b. Vascular space invasion in myometrium
5. Spread elsewhere in typical pattern of endometrial carcinoma
6. Ovarian tumors, bilateral and/or multinodular
7. Hilar location, vascular space invasion, surface implants, or combination in ovary
8. Ovarian endometriosis absent
9. Aneuploidy with similar DNA indices or diploidy of both tumors*
10. Similar molecular genetic or karyotypic abnormalities in both tumors

* The possibility of tumor heterogeneity must be taken into account in the evaluation of the ploidy findings.

■ Metastatic endometrial carcinoma from the uterine corpus.
- Features that favor synchronous primary neoplasia of both organs or metastasis from one organ to the other are listed in Tables 14–1 through 14–3; in some cases, however, interpretation of the relation of the two tumors is difficult or impossible.
- The excellent prognosis in cases in which the tumor is confined to both organs indicates that, at least in this situation, the neoplasms are usually independent primary tumors. The major prognostic determinant in such cases is the depth of myoinvasion by the endometrial tumor.

■ Extragenital metastatic carcinomas, particularly those arising in the intestine (page 410).

■ Endometrioid-like yolk sac tumor (YST) (see Chapter 15)
- Features favoring this diagnosis include an age younger than 30 years, the presence of more common patterns of YST, and immunoreactivity for alpha-fetoprotein (AFP)

Table 14–2.
ENDOMETRIOID TUMORS OF OVARY AND ENDOMETRIUM: OVARIAN PRIMARY AND ENDOMETRIAL SECONDARY TUMORS

1. Histologic similarity of the tumors
2. Large ovarian tumor—small endometrial tumor
3. Ovarian endometriosis present
4. Location in ovarian parenchyma
5. Direct extension from ovary predominantly into outer wall of uterus
6. Spread elsewhere in typical pattern of ovarian carcinoma
7. Ovarian tumor unilateral (80% to 90% of cases) and forming single mass
8. No atypical hyperplasia in endometrium
9. Aneuploidy with similar DNA indices or diploidy of both tumors*
10. Similar molecular genetic or karyotypic abnormalities in both tumors

* The possibility of tumor heterogeneity must be taken into account in the evaluation of the ploidy findings.

Table 14–3.
ENDOMETRIOID TUMORS OF OVARY AND
ENDOMETRIUM: INDEPENDENT OVARIAN AND
ENDOMETRIAL PRIMARY TUMORS

1. Histologic dissimilarity of the tumors
2. No or only superficial myometrial invasion of endometrial tumor
3. No vascular space invasion of endometrial tumor
4. Atypical endometrial hyperplasia also present
5. Absence of other evidence of spread of endometrial tumor
6. Ovarian tumor unilateral (80% to 90% of cases)
7. Ovarian tumor located in parenchyma
8. No vascular space invasion, surface implants, or predominant hilar location in ovary
9. Absence of other evidence of spread of ovarian tumor
10. Ovarian endometriosis present
11. Different ploidy or DNA indices, if aneuploid, of the tumors*
12. Dissimilar molecular genetic or karyotypic abnormalities in the tumors

* The possibility of tumor heterogeneity must be taken into account in the evaluation of the ploidy findings.

- This differential diagnosis is complicated by the rare YST that arises in an endometrioid carcinoma. In such cases, features diagnostic of endometrioid carcinoma, which may be accompanied by endometriosis, are also present in the specimen, which is usually from an older woman.
- Ovarian tumor of probable wolffian origin (see Chapter 17).
  - These tumors, in contrast to endometrioid carcinomas, are devoid of luminal mucin and squamous differentiation. Other characteristic patterns of endometrioid carcinomas or wolffian tumors are usually also present, facilitating the diagnosis.
  - Immunoreactivity for epithelial membrane antigen and TAG-72 strongly favors a diagnosis of endometrioid carcinoma in this differential.
- Ovarian ependymoma (see Chapter 15). Features confirming this diagnosis include perivascular pseudorosettes, occasional true rosettes, and the basal fibrillary cytoplasm of the cells, which is immunoreactive for glial fibrillary acidic protein (GFAP). Endometrioid carcinomas, however, are occasionally GFAP positive.

Spread

- The spread of endometrioid carcinomas is similar to that of other ovarian carcinomas, although they usually present at a lower stage than serous carcinoma. Thirty-one percent are stage I, 20% are stage II, 38% are stage III, and 11% are stage IV.
- The peritoneal lesions associated with endometrioid adenocarcinomas with squamous differentiation are discussed in Chapter 20.

Prognosis

- The 5-year survival rate is 78% for patients with stage I carcinomas, 63% for stage II, 24% for stage III, and 6% for stage IV.

- In one study, grade 1 and 2 tumors, which had similar survival rates, were associated with a higher survival rate than grade 3 tumors. Another study, however, found a survival difference between grade 1 and grade 2 tumors, although not between grade 2 and grade 3 tumors.
- We grade endometrioid carcinomas using the system adopted by the World Health Organization (WHO) for grading endometrioid carcinomas of the endometrium, although the prognostic significance of this grading system in ovarian endometrioid carcinomas has not been established.

References

Aguirre P, Thor AD, Scully RE. Ovarian endometrioid carcinomas resembling sex cord–stromal tumors: an immunohistochemical study. Int J Gynecol Pathol 8:364–373, 1989.

Bell DA, Scully RE. Atypical and borderline endometrioid adenofibromas of the ovary: a report of 27 cases. Am J Surg Pathol 9:205–214, 1985.

Eifel P, Hendrickson M, Ross J, et al. Simultaneous presentation of carcinoma involving the ovary and the uterine corpus. Cancer 50:163–170, 1982.

Fu YS, Stock RJ, Reagan JW, et al. Significance of squamous component in endometrioid carcinoma of the ovary. Cancer 44:614–621, 1979.

Guerrieri C, Frånlund B, Malmström H, Boeryd B. Ovarian endometrioid carcinomas simulating sex cord-stromal tumors: a study using inhibin and cytokeratin 7. Int J Gynecol Pathol 17:266–271, 1998.

Hughesdon PE. Benign endometrioid tumours of the ovary and the mülerian concept of ovarian epithelial tumours. Histopathology 8:977–990, 1984.

Kline RC, Wharton JT, Atkinson EN, et al. Endometrioid carcinoma of the ovary: retrospective review of 145 cases. Gynecol Oncol 39:337–346, 1990.

Nogales FF, Bergeron C, Carvia RE, et al. Ovarian endometrioid tumors with yolk sac component, an unusual form of ovarian neoplasm: analysis of six cases. Am J Surg Pathol 20:1056–1066, 1996.

Norris HJ. Proliferative endometrioid tumors and endometrioid tumors of low malignant potential of the ovary. Int J Gynecol Pathol 12:134–140, 1993.

Pitman MB, Young RH, Clement PB, et al. Oxyphilic endometrioid carcinoma of the ovary and endometrium: a report of nine cases. Int J Gynecol Pathol 13:290–301, 1994.

Roth LM, Czernobilsky B, Langley FA. Ovarian endometrioid adenofibromatous and cystadenofibromatous tumors: benign, proliferating, and malignant. Cancer 48:1838–1845, 1981.

Roth LM, Liban E, Czernobilsky B. Ovarian endometrioid tumors mimicking Sertoli and Sertoli-Leydig cell tumors: sertoliform variant of endometrioid carcinoma. Cancer 50:1322–1331, 1982.

Snyder RR, Norris JH, Tavassoli F. Endometrioid proliferative and low malignant potential tumors of the ovary: a clinicopathologic study of 46 cases. Am J Surg Pathol 12:661–671, 1988.

Tornos C, Silva EG, Ordonez NG, et al. Endometrioid carcinoma of the ovary with a prominent spindle-cell component, a source of diagnostic confusion: a report of 14 cases. Am J Surg Pathol 19:1343–1353, 1995.

Ueda G, Yamasaki M, Inoue M, et al. Argyrophil cells in the endometrioid carcinoma of the ovary. Cancer 54:1569–1573, 1984.

Ulbright TM, Roth LM. Metastatic and independent cancers of the endometrium and ovary: a clinicopathologic study of 34 cases. Hum Pathol 16:28–34, 1985.

Young RH, Prat J, Scully RE. Ovarian endometrioid carcinomas resembling sex cord–stromal tumors: a clinicopathological analysis of thirteen cases. Am J Surg Pathol 6:513–522, 1982.

Zaino R, Whitney C, Brady MF. Simultaneously detected endometrial and ovarian carcinomas [Abstract]. Mod Pathol 11:118A, 1998.

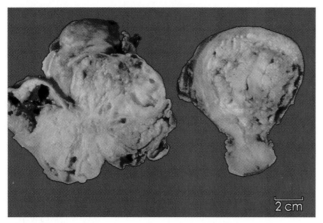

Figure 14–1. Endometrioid carcinoma of ovary (*left*). A synchronous endometrioid carcinoma involves the uterine corpus (*right*).

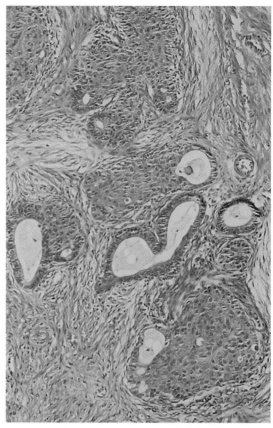

Figure 14–3. Endometrioid adenofibroma of borderline malignancy. Atypical endometrioid glands are separated by a fibromatous stroma. Note squamous morules.

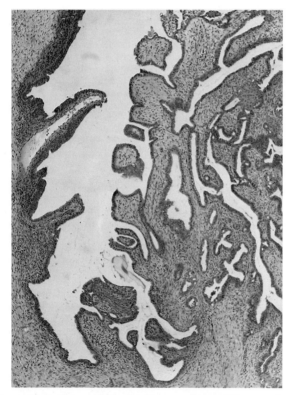

Figure 14–2. Endometrioid adenofibroma arising within an endometriotic cyst, the lining of which is seen at the left.

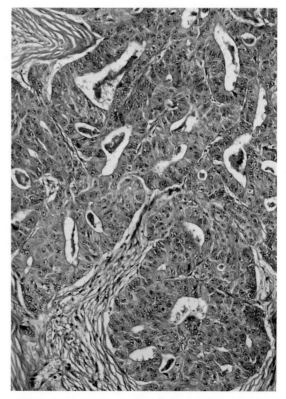

Figure 14–4. Endometrioid adenocarcinoma.

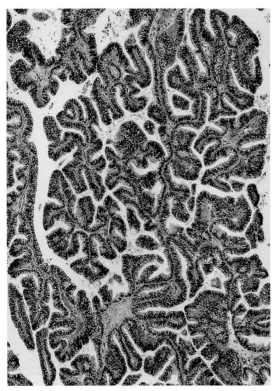

Figure 14–5. Endometrioid adenocarcinoma with a villoglandular pattern.

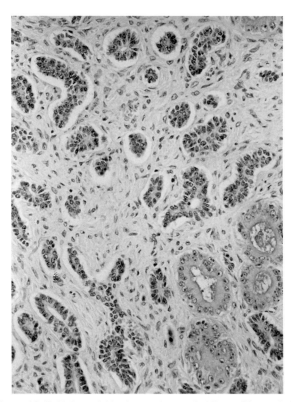

Figure 14–7. Endometrioid adenocarcinoma. Small sertoliform tubules lie within a fibrous stroma. Notice the luminal mucin within a few of the tubules (*bottom right*).

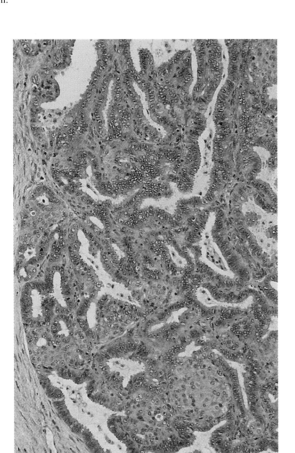

Figure 14–6. Endometrioid adenocarcinoma with squamous differentiation. Squamous morules partly or completely obliterate gland lumens.

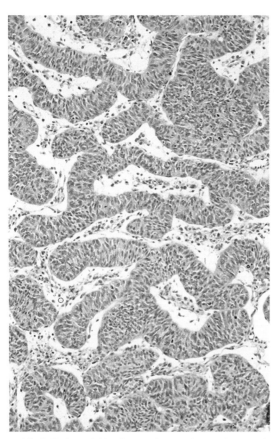

Figure 14–8. Endometrioid adenocarcinoma. A prominent trabecular pattern mimics a sex cord stromal tumor.

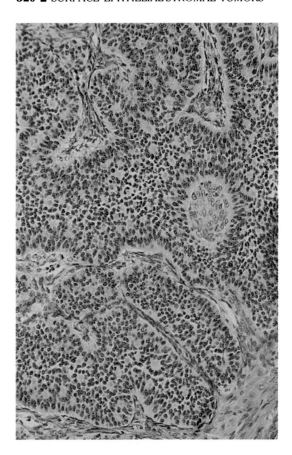

Figure 14–9. Endometrioid adenocarcinoma. The appearance, including small spaces resembling Call-Exner bodies, simulates a granulosa cell tumor.

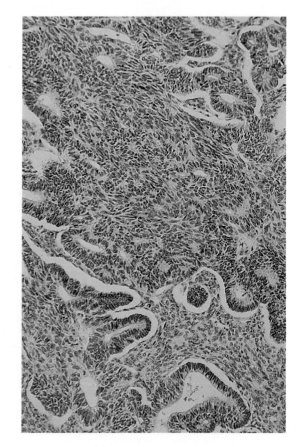

Figure 14–10. Endometrioid adenocarcinoma with a prominent spindle cell component.

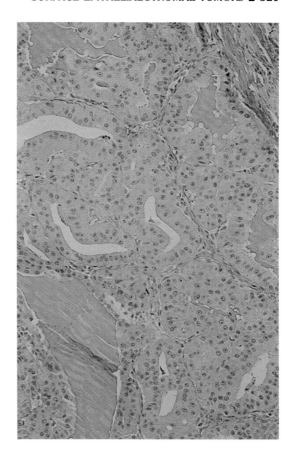

Figure 14-11. Oxyphilic endometrioid adenocarcinoma.

Malignant Mesodermal Mixed Tumors

General Features

■ Malignant mesodermal mixed tumors (MMMTs) account for less than 1% of all ovarian cancers; about 250 cases have been reported. MMMTs occur in the sixth to eighth decades in 75% of the cases and are rare before the age of 40 years.

Gross Features

■ The tumors are typically large, are predominantly solid or cystic, and are commonly necrotic and hemorrhagic. Rarely, they arise within an endometriotic cyst.

■ If tumors of all stages are included, about one third of tumors are bilateral.

Microscopic Features

■ The obviously epithelial component is most commonly serous, endometrioid, or undifferentiated carcinoma.

Squamous cell or clear cell carcinoma is less common, and mucinous carcinoma is rare.

■ The sarcomatous component has the appearance of fibrosarcoma, malignant fibrous histiocytoma, a myxosarcoma, or high-grade endometrial stromal sarcoma in the homologous form of the tumor, which accounts for about 50% of the cases.

■ Heterologous tumors most commonly contain chondrosarcoma, skeletal muscle, or both and occasionally contain malignant-appearing osteoid, bone, or adipose tissue.

■ An unusual but nonspecific feature of MMMTs is the common presence, especially in the sarcomatous component, of hyaline bodies that are periodic acid–Schiff (PAS) positive after diastase.

■ Nonmesodermal types of tissue in some tumors have included glial and neuronal differentiation (with foci occasionally resembling primitive neuroectodermal tumor), well-differentiated hepatic-type cells, and trophoblastic differentiation. Rare tumors have been associated with an increased serum level of AFP.

Differential Diagnosis

■ Immature teratomas (page 347). Features favoring or indicating immature teratoma include an age of less than 30 years, elements derived from all three germ layers, a predominant component of immature neuroectodermal tissue, an embryonal (versus carcinomatous) epithelial component, and immature or mature (versus malignant) cartilage.

■ Moderately and poorly differentiated Sertoli-stromal cell tumors with or without heterologous elements.
  • These tumors usually contain better-differentiated Sertoli-stromal cell elements, almost always occur in young women, and may be virilizing.
  • Surface epithelial-like elements, if present, are mucinous (which usually appear benign or borderline) or retiform.
  • Immunoreactivity for inhibin and absence of EMA staining strongly favor a Sertoli-stromal tumor, whereas the converse favors an MMMT.

■ Endometrioid stromal sarcomas containing sex cord–like elements. These tumors are better differentiated than MMMTs, and the sex cord–like elements have a greater resemblance to the sex cord components of sex cord–stromal tumors than to the müllerian epithelial components of MMMTs.

■ Sarcomatoid carcinomas and carcinomas with an unusually cellular, mitotically active stroma.
  • A diagnosis of MMMT is appropriate when the stromal component has features that if seen in pure form would warrant a diagnosis of sarcoma.
  • We diagnose sarcomatoid carcinoma when the sarcoma-like elements blend with obvious carcinomatous elements, in contrast to the sharp demarcation between the two components that is usually seen in MMMTs. Sarcomatoid carcinomas tend to be lower grade than MMMTs.

Spread and Prognosis

■ More than 90% of MMMTs have extraovarian spread at diagnosis, with 60% being stage III and 10% being stage IV. The metastatic deposits most commonly contain carcinomatous and sarcomatous components but may be purely one or the other.

■ The prognosis is very poor, but an occasional patient survives more than 5 years after removal of the tumor and combination chemotherapy.

References

Al-Nafussi AI, Hughes DE, Williams ARW. Hyaline globules in ovarian tumours. Histopathology 23:563–566, 1993.

Costa MJ, Khan R, Judd R. Carcinosarcoma (malignant mixed müllerian [mesodermal] tumor) of the uterus and ovary: correlation of clinical, pathologic, and immunohistochemical features in 29 cases. Arch Pathol Lab Med 115:583–590, 1991.

Costa MJ, Morris RJ, Wilson R, Judd R. Utility of immunohistochemistry in distinguishing ovarian Sertoli–stromal cell tumors from carcinosarcomas. Hum Pathol 23:787–797, 1992.

DeBrito PA, Silverberg SG, Orenstein JM. Carcinosarcoma (malignant mixed müllerian [mesodermal] tumor) of the female genital tract: immunohistochemical and ultrastructural analysis of 28 cases. Hum Pathol 24:132–142, 1993.

Dictor M. Malignant mixed mesodermal tumor of the ovary: a report of 22 cases. Obstet Gynecol 65:720–724, 1985.

Ehrmann RL, Weidner N, Welch WR, Gleiberman I. Malignant mixed müllerian tumor of the ovary with prominent neuroectodermal differentiation (teratoid carcinosarcoma). Int J Gynecol Pathol 9:272–282, 1990.

Morrow CP, d'Abaing G, Brady LW, et al. A clinical and pathologic study of 30 cases of malignant mixed müllerian epithelial and mesenchymal ovarian tumors: a Gynecologic Oncology Group study. Gynecol Oncol 18:278–292, 1984.

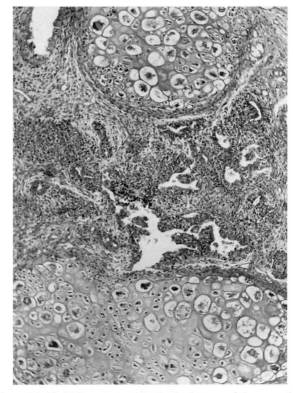

Figure 14–12. Malignant mesodermal mixed tumor of the ovary. Notice the admixture of adenocarcinoma and chondrosarcoma.

Adenosarcoma

■ Most adenosarcomas occur in the fifth and sixth decades.
■ All of the tumors have been unilateral. They may be predominantly solid or cystic, with the solid tissue usually being firm but occasionally soft, depending on its cellularity. Some tumors may be exophytic polypoid masses.

Microscopic Features

■ The stromal component usually resembles a low- to moderate-grade fibrosarcoma or endometrial stromal sarcoma and typically exhibits periglandular condensation, at least focally. Polypoid stromal tissue often projects into dilated gland lumens.
■ The stroma may be focally hypocellular and fibrotic or edematous. Heterologous stromal elements, sex cord–like elements, and sarcomatous overgrowth are occasionally present.
■ Various degrees of stromal nuclear atypicality are present. The mitotic rate of the stromal cells ranges from 2 to more than 40 mitotic figures (MF) per 10 high-power-fields (HPF)
■ The glandular epithelium may be endometrioid, serous, mucinous, or of clear cell type. The epithelium usually has a benign appearance but may exhibit various degrees of nuclear atypicality, occasionally fulfilling the criteria for carcinoma in situ.

Differential Diagnosis

■ Adenofibromas. Criteria for distinguishing adenosarcomas from cellular adenofibromas of uterine type are not well established. On the basis of our experience with uterine adenosarcomas, we diagnose ovarian adenosar-

coma if the stroma is unusually cellular, if there is more than minimal stromal nuclear atypicality, or if the mitotic count is 2 MF or more per 10 HPF.
■ Polypoid endometriosis. This lesion lacks the architectural features (i.e., intracystic polypoid projections of cellular stroma, periglandular cuffing), the mitotic activity, and the stromal nuclear atypicality of adenosarcomas.

Spread and Prognosis

■ Adenosarcomas have spread beyond the ovary into the pelvis or abdomen or both in about one third of cases.
■ These tumors are clinically malignant more often than their counterparts in the uterine corpus. Of 16 patients with follow-up in one study, 3 died of tumor and 8 were alive after one or two recurrences.

References

Clement PB, Scully RE. Extrauterine mesodermal (müllerian) adenosarcoma: a clinicopathologic analysis of five cases. Am J Clin Pathol 69: 276–283, 1978.

Eichhorn JH, Clement PB, Young RH, Scully RE. Mesodermal adenosarcoma of the ovary: a study of 37 cases [Abstract]. Mod Pathol 12: 116A, 1999.

Kao GF, Norris HJ. Benign and low grade variants of mixed mesodermal tumor (adenosarcoma) of the ovary and adnexal region. Cancer 42:1314–1324, 1978.

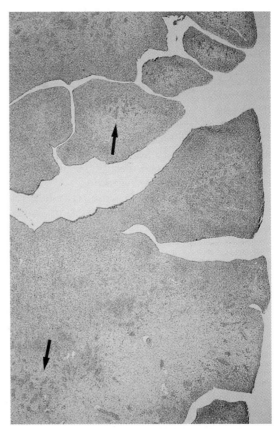

Figure 14–14. Mesodermal adenosarcoma of the ovary. Polypoid masses of sarcomatous stroma project into a cyst lumen. Discrete nests, which represent sex-cord–like aggregates, are just discernible (*arrows*) at this low magnification.

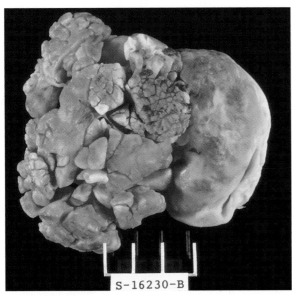

S-16230-B

Figure 14–13. Mesodermal adenosarcoma of the ovary. A polypoid, cauliflower-like mass projects from the serosal surface of the ovary.

Endometrioid Stromal Sarcoma

General Features

- About 55 cases of endometrioid stromal sarcoma (ESS) involving the ovary have been reported. Approximately 50% of them have abutted areas of endometriosis.
- Thirty percent of ovarian ESSs in one study were accompanied by a similar tumor in the uterus diagnosed from 30 years before to 6 years after the discovery of the ovarian tumor, an association suggesting that some ovarian ESSs are metastatic from a uterine ESS.
- The tumors occur over a wide age range (11 to 76 years), with a mean age of 56 years.

Pathologic Features

- Eighty percent of the tumors are unilateral. The mean diameter is 9.5 cm. They are predominantly solid or solid and cystic, with the solid areas having a tan to yellow sectioned surface, often with focal necrosis or hemorrhage.
- A typically diffuse proliferation is composed of small cells with scanty cytoplasm and round to oval nuclei that resemble endometrial stromal cells to some degree. Numerous small arteries resembling the spiral arteries of the normal late secretory endometrium are also typical.
- One half of the tumors, in contrast to most uterine ESSs, contain fibromatous areas that may predominate and exhibit a storiform pattern. Less common findings include sex cord-like elements (i.e., cords and nests of cells and small tubules), foci of smooth muscle, and rare benign endometrioid glands.
- Mitotic activity ranges from less than 1 to more than 30 MF per 10 HPF. Some pathologists have divided the tumors into low grade (<10 MF per 10 HPF) and high grade (≥10 MF per 10 HPF).
- Other findings include foam cells, hyaline plaques and bands, extensive collagen deposition, and a transition between the tumor and endometriosis.
- Reticulin staining discloses a dense pericellular reticulin pattern, and lipid stains may reveal large numbers of fine droplets in the tumor cells and the foam cells.

Differential Diagnosis

- Diffuse adult granulosa cell tumor.
  - Features favoring ESS include a lack of endocrine manifestations, bilaterality, numerous arterioles, reticulin fibrils investing single cells, a tonguelike pattern of infiltration (particularly in any extraovarian tumor), lack of nuclear grooves, inhibin negativity, and association with endometriosis.
  - Foam cells in ESSs, unlike Leydig or lutein cells, contain fine lipid vacuoles and eccentric nuclei without prominent nucleoli.
  - Sex cord-like elements, if present in an ESS, are often a minor component and usually lack the pale grooved nuclei of granulosa cells and lack the distinctive patterns of the Sertoli cell components of a Sertoli-stromal cell tumor.
- MMMT. The differentiation of these tumors from ovarian ESSs with sex cord-like differentiation is discussed on page 322.
- Stromal hyperplasia. This lesion is rarely associated with significant ovarian enlargement and lacks the marked cellularity, arteriolar content, and resemblance to endometrial stroma of ovarian ESSs.
- Ovarian fibroma or thecoma. Estrogenic manifestations and the abundant lipid-rich cytoplasm in the tumor cells of a thecoma are lacking in ovarian ESSs. The cellular areas mimicking normal endometrial stroma with numerous arterioles are absent in a fibroma.
- Metastatic uterine ESS.
  - When an ovarian ESS is associated with a uterine ESS, general features that aid in differentiating primary and metastatic tumors of the ovary in general must be evaluated (see Chapter 18).
  - The relative sizes of the uterine and ovarian tumors, their extent, and the presence or absence of vascular space invasion are important.
  - The pathology slides from any previous hysterectomy specimen must be reviewed; if a hysterectomy has not been performed, it may be impossible to exclude a synchronous uterine ESS.
  - Chang and associates regard ESSs as primary in the ovary only when they are confined to this site and the uterus is free of tumor on pathologic examination. We also accept continuity with ovarian endometriosis as evidence of ovarian origin.
- Other small cell malignant tumors that may involve the ovary (see Appendix 5). Other than their content of small cells, these tumors have significant microscopic differences, including usually a greater degree of nuclear atypia than in ovarian ESSs. Each of these tumors is discussed elsewhere under the respective tumor type.

Spread and Prognosis

- About 75% of ovarian ESSs have spread beyond the ovary at the time of diagnosis to the pelvis, the upper abdomen, or both, and tumors rarely spread distantly, most commonly to the lung.
- In one study of 18 patients with follow-up, 6 were alive and free of disease at 2 to 20 years, 5 were alive with recurrent disease, 5 died of disease at 2 to 22 years, and 2 died of unrelated causes.

References

Chang KL, Crabtree GS, Lim-Tan SK, et al. Primary extrauterine endometrial stromal neoplasms: a clinicopathological study of 20 cases and a review of the literature. Int J Gynecol Pathol 12:282–286, 1993.

Oliva E, Young RH, Scully RE. Primary endometrioid stromal sarcoma of the ovary: a clinicopathological study of 36 cases [Abstract]. Mod Pathol 11:110A, 1998.

Young RH, Prat J, Scully RE. Endometrioid stromal sarcomas of the ovary: a clinicopathologic analysis of 23 cases. Cancer 53:1143–1155, 1984.

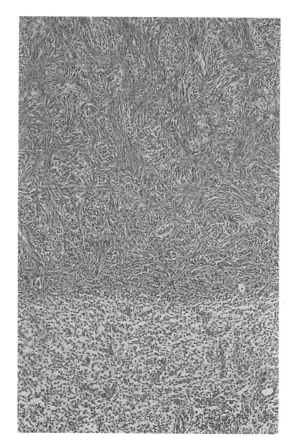

Figure 14–15. Endometrioid stromal sarcoma of the ovary. Tumor with a typical appearance (*bottom*) abuts tumor with a fibromatous appearance.

CLEAR CELL TUMORS

General Features

- Benign clear cell tumors are rare, and borderline forms, almost all of which are adenofibromatous, account for less than 1% of ovarian borderline tumors. Clear cell carcinomas account for 6% of surface epithelial carcinomas. Almost 90% of clear cell carcinomas are diagnosed during the fifth to seventh decades, and 10% are diagnosed in the fourth decade.
- Clear cell carcinomas have clinical manifestations similar in general to those of other epithelial cancers (page 289). However, clear cell carcinomas have the highest association among all epithelial-stromal cancers with ovarian and pelvic endometriosis and with paraendocrine hypercalcemia.
- Although clear cell carcinomas were initially called mesonephromas and subsequently mesonephric and mesonephroid carcinomas, their müllerian nature is now accepted.

Gross Features

- Clear cell adenofibromas (benign or borderline) have a nonspecific adenofibromatous appearance; occasionally, the glands are dilated, giving the sectioned surface a spongy appearance.
- Clear cell carcinomas may be predominantly solid or take the form of unilocular or multilocular cysts with polypoid masses protruding into the lumens.
- The cyst lumens may contain serous or mucinous fluid; in cases in which the tumor has arisen in an endometriotic cyst, the fluid may be chocolate colored, with patchy brown discoloration of the cyst lining.
- Benign and borderline clear cell tumors are almost invariably unilateral; clear cell carcinomas are bilateral in only 2% of stage I cases.

Microscopic Features

- Clear cell adenofibromas are characterized by benign epithelial cells that are of the clear or flattened type, whereas borderline adenofibromas contain atypical epithelium (i.e., borderline adenofibroma) or carcinomatous epithelium without invasion (i.e., borderline adenofibroma with intraepithelial carcinoma).

■ Microinvasion or larger areas of invasion, if present, are defined as for endometrioid tumors (page 315). The epithelial cell types in the borderline tumors are similar to those encountered in clear cell carcinomas.

■ Clear cell carcinomas have a variety of patterns, often admixed, including papillary, tubulocystic, and solid. The stroma, including the cores of the papillae, often contains abundant basement membrane material.

■ The tubules and cysts frequently contain mucin, but intracellular mucin is not a feature of the lining cells. Occasionally, the cysts contain colloid-like material, imparting a struma-like appearance.

■ The usual cell types are the clear cell and the hobnail cell, with the former arranged in solid nests or lining cysts, tubules, and papillae; hobnail cells invariably line lumens and their papillae. The clear cells are rounded or polyhedral and have eccentric nuclei typically without prominent nucleoli. The hobnail cells contain bulbous, usually dark nuclei that protrude into lumens.

■ Less common cell types include
  • Flat or cuboidal cells. The flat cells (sometimes with slightly bulging nuclei) line small cysts, often imparting a deceptively benign appearance, but careful sampling usually reveals areas more easily diagnostic of carcinoma.
  • Oxyphilic cells with abundant eosinophilic cytoplasm. These cells, which sometimes are the predominant cell type, may line glands but more often grow in nests and masses.
  • Signet-ring cells containing mucin (inspissated eosinophilic material within a vacuole). Signet-ring cells, when present, are usually encountered in small foci, but occasionally these cells form a prominent component of the tumor, and they are rarely the only cell type.
  • Undifferentiated epithelial cells. These cells may be found in poorly differentiated areas of clear cell carcinoma.

■ Benign and borderline adenofibromatous components are often present in clear cell carcinomas, and tumors that initially appear to be clear cell adenofibromas must be sampled carefully to exclude areas of carcinoma.

■ A rare clear cell carcinoma contains an extensive infiltrate of round cells, a large number of which are plasma cells; lymphocytes and polymorphonuclear leukocytes may also be present in the infiltrate.

■ Psammoma bodies are occasionally present, especially in papillary clear cell carcinomas.

■ Special staining reveals abundant glycogen within the clear cells, which may also contain lipid. Mucin is typically located in the lumens and in the apex of the cytoplasm of the lining cells but is abundant within the cytoplasm of the signet-ring cells.

■ Rare clear cell carcinomas are immunoreactive for AFP (see differential diagnosis with YST).

Differential Diagnosis

■ Serous carcinoma and the secretory form of endometrioid carcinoma (pages 300 and 316).

■ Dysgerminoma (versus solid clear cell carcinoma). Features favoring clear cell carcinoma include age of more than 40 years, other patterns inconsistent with dysgerminoma, eccentric hyperchromatic nuclei and nonprominent nucleoli (versus central nuclei with one or more prominent nucleoli in dysgerminomas), plasma cell infiltrate (versus lymphocytes in dysgerminomas), and EMA immunoreactivity.

■ YST. Features favoring clear cell carcinoma include patient age of more than 40 years, absence of elevated levels of serum AFP, a reticular pattern, complex papillae with hyalinized cores, immunoreactivity for Leu-M1, and negative staining for AFP. Because rare clear cell carcinomas are AFP positive, a positive reaction does not exclude this diagnosis.

■ Juvenile granulosa cell tumor (JGCT). Features favoring or establishing this diagnosis over that of clear cell carcinoma include a young patient age, associated estrogenic manifestations, the absence of patterns of clear cell carcinoma inconsistent with JGCT, and immunoreactivity for inhibin.

■ Krukenberg tumor (versus clear cell carcinoma with signet-ring–type cells). Features favoring a diagnosis of Krukenberg tumor include a known extraovarian primary mucinous tumor, bilaterality, and uniform distribution of signet-ring cells and small mucinous glands in a cellular fibromatous stroma.

■ Primary and metastatic ovarian tumors with oxyphilic cells (versus oxyphilic clear cell carcinoma). The distinctive features of all the tumors listed in Appendix 4 are described elsewhere in the text.

Spread

■ Forty-three percent of clear cell carcinomas are stage I, 19% are stage II, 29% are stage III, and 9% are stage IV at diagnosis.

Prognosis

■ Clear cell borderline tumors, including those with microinvasion of the stroma, almost always have a benign course. In one case, however, a tumor in the latter category that was incompletely resected was fatal.

■ The 5-year survival rate is 69% for patients with stage I carcinomas, 55% for stage II, 14% for stage III, and 4% for stage IV. These survival rates are poorer than those for epithelial cancers of other cell types, being closer to those of undifferentiated carcinoma.

■ There is no consensus in the literature about the value of pattern, cell type, mitotic index, or grade as prognostic indicators.

References

Bell DA, Scully RE. Benign and borderline clear cell adenofibromas of the ovary. Cancer 56:2922–2931, 1985.

Brescia RJ, Dubin N, Demopoulos RI. Endometrioid and clear cell carcinoma of the ovary: factors affecting survival. Int J Gynecol Pathol 8:132–138, 1989.

Crozier MA, Copeland LJ, Silva EG, et al. Clear cell carcinoma of the ovary: a study of 59 cases. Gynecol Oncol 35:199–203, 1989.

Imachi M, Tsukamoto N, Shimamoto T, et al. Clear cell carcinoma of the ovary: a clinicopathologic analysis of 34 cases. Int J Gynecol Cancer 1:113–119, 1991.

Kao GF, Norris HJ. Unusual cystadenofibromas: endometrioid, mucinous, and clear cell types. Obstet Gynecol 54:729–736, 1979.

Kennedy AW, Biscotti CV, Hart WR, Webster KD. Ovarian clear cell adenocarcinoma. Gynecol Oncol 32:342–349, 1989.

Klemi PJ, Meurman L, Grönroos M, Talerman A. Clear cell (mesonephroid) tumors of the ovary with characteristics resembling, endodermal sinus tumor. Int J Gynecol Pathol 1:95–100, 1982.

Mikami Y, Hata S, Melamed J, et al. Basement membrane material in ovarian clear cell carcinoma: correlation with growth pattern and nuclear grade. Int J Gynecol Pathol 18:52–56, 1999.

Montag AG, Jenison EL, Griffiths CT, et al. Ovarian clear cell carcinoma: a clinicopathologic analysis of 44 cases. Int J Gynecol Pathol 8:85–96, 1989.

O'Brien MER, Schofield JB, Tan S, et al. Clear cell epithelial ovarian cancer (mesonephroid): bad prognosis only in early stages. Gynecol Oncol 49:250–254, 1993.

Roth LM, Langley FA, Fox H, et al. Ovarian clear cell adenofibromatous tumors: benign, of low malignant potential, and associated with invasive clear cell carcinoma. Cancer 53:1156–1163, 1984.

Young RH, Scully RE. Oxyphilic clear cell carcinoma of the ovary: a report of nine cases. Am J Surg Pathol 11:661–667, 1987.

Zirker TA, Silva EG, Morris M, Ordonez NG. Immunohistochemical differentiation of clear-cell carcinoma of the female genital tract and endodermal sinus tumor with the use of alpha-fetoprotein and Leu-M1. Am J Clin Pathol 91:511–514, 1989.

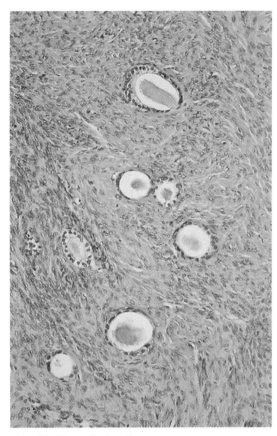

Figure 14–17. Clear cell adenofibroma.

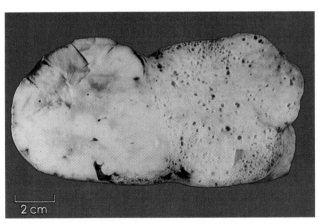

Figure 14–16. Clear cell adenofibroma of a borderline malignancy (*right*) abuts a clear cell carcinoma (*left*). The adenofibroma has a spongy sectioned surface with cysts, contrasting with the solid, fleshy appearance of the clear cell carcinoma.

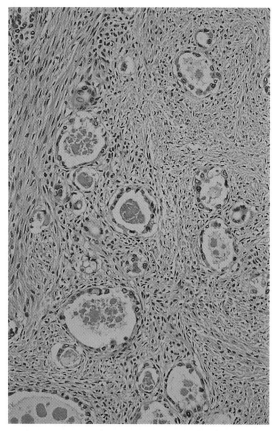

Figure 14–18. Borderline clear cell adenofibroma with microinvasion. Small, solid nests or single cells lie between the noninvasive tubules lined by atypical cells.

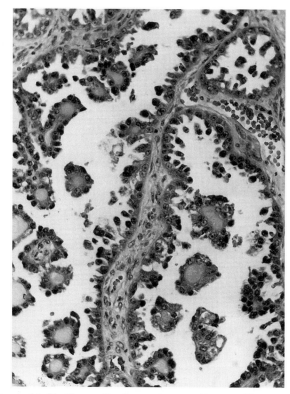

Figure 14–20. Clear cell adenocarcinoma with a papillary pattern. Some of the papillae have hyalinized cores.

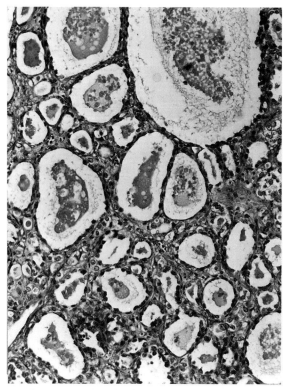

Figure 14–19. Clear cell adenocarcinoma with a tubulocystic pattern.

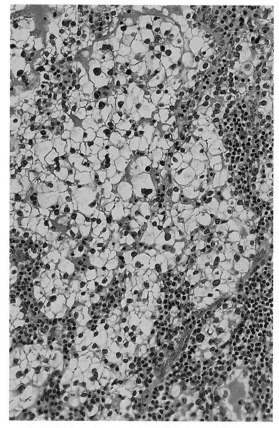

Figure 14–21. Clear cell carcinoma with a solid pattern. Notice the admixed plasma cells.

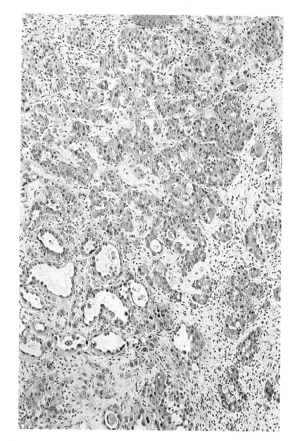

Figure 14–22. Clear cell carcinoma with oxyphilic cells. Typical clear cell carcinoma with a tubulocystic pattern (*bottom left*) merges with nests of cells with abundant eosinophilic cytoplasm.

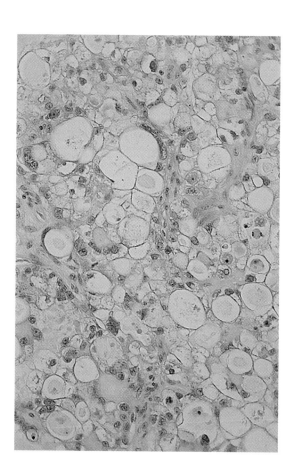

Figure 14–23. Clear cell carcinoma with signet-ring cells.

TRANSITIONAL CELL TUMORS

General Features

- Transitional cell tumors, most of which are benign Brenner tumors, account for 1% to 2% of all ovarian tumors, and for 4% to 5% of benign tumors in the surface epithelial-stromal category.
- Borderline Brenner tumors have accounted for 3% to 5% and malignant Brenner tumors for 5% of all Brenner tumors in some series; Hendrickson and Longacre, however, estimate that each of these types accounts for only 0.5% of transitional cell tumors.
- Silva and colleagues found that pure transitional cell carcinomas (TCCs) accounted for 1% of carcinomas in the surface epithelial-stromal category; in another 5% of cases, TCC was the predominant element; and in another 3%, it was a minor component within a mixed surface epithelial tumor.
- About 95% of Brenner tumors are diagnosed between the ages of 30 and 70 years (most between 40 and 60 years). More than 50% of borderline Brenner tumors, more than 65% of malignant Brenner tumors, and 75% of TCCs are diagnosed in women 50 to 70 years of age.
- Although most transitional cell tumors are considered to be of surface epithelial-stromal origin, the occasional association of Brenner tumors with a dermoid cyst, struma ovarii, or carcinoid tumor suggests a germ cell origin in rare cases. The rare juxtaposition of a hilar Brenner tumor to the rete ovarii supports an origin from the latter, which is of celomic-epithelial or mesonephric origin.
- Brenner tumors are occasionally associated with endocrine manifestations of estrogenic or less often androgenic type, apparently as a result of steroid hormone secretion by their stromal component.

Gross Features of Benign Brenner Tumor

- The tumors are typically small, usually representing an incidental finding: about 50% are less than 2 cm in diameter, and about 30% are detectable only microscopically; 10% are larger than 10 cm. Between 7% and 8% are bilateral.
- The tumors are typically well circumscribed and firm, with a smooth to bosselated serosal surface and a white to pale yellow sectioned surface. Focal calcification is common, and some tumors are extensively calcified. Small or large cysts may be present, and rare tumors are large and multicystic.
- In about 25% of cases, a different type of tumor is present, usually in contact with the Brenner tumor, and contributes to its gross appearance. Two thirds of these tumors are mucinous cystic tumors, which are almost always benign; the remainder are mostly serous cystadenomas and dermoid cysts.

Gross Features of Other Transitional Cell Tumors

- Borderline Brenner tumors, which are almost always unilateral, typically have solid and cystic compo-nents, with the former resembling benign Brenner tumor and the latter usually containing papillae or polyps.
- Malignant Brenner tumors typically have solid and cystic areas, with the latter containing papillary or polypoid masses or mural nodules. Twelve percent are bilateral. Calcification occurs in 50%.
- TCCs resemble grossly other carcinomas of the epithelial-stromal type; the calcification frequently seen in malignant Brenner tumors is absent. The tumors are bilateral in about 15% of cases.

Microscopic Features of Benign Brenner Tumor

- Round or oval nests and occasionally trabeculae composed of transitional cells are admixed with a prominent fibrous stromal component. The nests may be solid or have a central cavity filled with dense eosinophilic secretion.
- The transitional cells contain pale to rarely clear cytoplasm and oval, often grooved nuclei. Rarely, the cells in the center of the nests have squamous features. The cells lining the cavities are usually mucinous, but they occasionally are ciliated-serous or indifferent glandular epithelium. Pure mucinous glands and cysts may also be present. Mixed Brenner and mucinous tumors are discussed on page 335.
- The stromal component usually resembles an ovarian fibroma but rarely has thecomatous features with plump cells that may contain abundant lipid-rich cytoplasm; nests of lutein cells may be present. Stromal spicules of calcification occur in about one third of cases.
- The ultrastructural features of Brenner tumors are similar to those of transitional cell tumors of the urinary tract.
- Immunohistochemical findings are not important for diagnosis, but argyrophilic granules are present in about one third of cases. The granules are frequently immunoreactive for serotonin but rarely stain for peptide hormones.

Microscopic Features of Borderline Brenner Tumor

- These tumors usually resemble papillary TCCs of the urinary tract with a background of a benign Brenner tumor. Invasion is absent (using WHO criteria). Mitotic figures may be numerous.
- TCCs should be graded as in the urinary tract: grade 1 atypia indicates a "borderline Brenner tumor with atypia," whereas grade 2 or 3 TCC warrants a diagnosis of "borderline Brenner tumor with intraepithelial carcinoma."

Microscopic Features of Malignant Brenner Tumor

- The diagnosis of malignant Brenner tumor requires stromal invasion, usually with a background of borderline or benign Brenner tumor.

- The invasive tumor is usually exclusively or predominantly TCC or squamous cell carcinoma. Mucinous carcinoma may also be present, but the rare mucinous adenocarcinoma associated with a benign Brenner tumor should be designated as such rather than as a malignant Brenner tumor.
- The invasive elements are typically grade 2 or higher but occasionally take the form of crowded, irregularly shaped islands of grade 1 TCC.

Microscopic Features of Transitional Cell Carcinoma

- TCC, not otherwise specified, lacks benign and borderline Brenner elements. It is characterized by an undulating cyst lining, an intracystic papillary pattern (i.e., papillary type), or nests of epithelial cells in a fibrous stroma (i.e., malignant Brenner-like type), or both patterns.
- The malignant transitional cells in most cases are grade 2 or 3 but usually lack the bizarre nuclear features often present in serous carcinomas. In more than 50% of the tumors, mucin, sometimes surrounded by glandular epithelium, is present.
- In most cases, the tumor is admixed with other types of surface epithelial carcinoma, usually serous.

Differential Diagnosis

- Of benign Brenner tumor:
  - Endometrioid adenofibroma with squamous differentiation (page 316).
  - Insular granulosa cell tumors and insular carcinoid tumors. These tumors are distinguished from the Brenner tumor by the different features of the neoplastic cells in each of the tumors.
  - Mucinous cystic tumors (versus cystic Brenner tumors). These tumors lack transitional cells at the periphery of the mucinous cells, although the former cells may be compressed and difficult to recognize in some cases.
- Of Brenner tumors of borderline malignancy, malignant Brenner tumors, and TCCs:
  - Metastatic TCCs of urothelial origin (see Chapter 18).
  - Undifferentiated carcinomas (UCs). The tumor cells in UCs usually have scantier cytoplasm than those in TCCs. UCs may contain pseudopapillae secondary to necrosis, but they lack the thick papillae with smooth luminal borders characteristic of TCCs. UCs usually lack the nesting pattern and the mucin of TCCs.
  - GCT of the juvenile or adult type. GCTs rarely have a papillary-cystic pattern simulating that of a borderline Brenner tumor or a TCC. A young age (in JGCTs), the frequent endocrine manifestations, and the usual presence of other more typical patterns of GCT facilitate the diagnosis.

Spread

- No borderline Brenner tumor has as yet been documented to spread beyond the ovary, but only small numbers of cases with long follow-up have been reported.

- Malignant Brenner tumors present with extraovarian spread in about 20% of cases. In contrast, about 70% of TCCs have spread to the abdomen or beyond at the time of diagnosis.

Prognosis

- Austin and Norris found that TCCs have a poorer prognosis than malignant Brenner tumors, stage for stage, with an overall 5-year survival rate of 35%. Survival for stage Ia TCCs is only 43%, compared with 88% for malignant Brenner tumors.
- Silva and coworkers found that when the metastases of ovarian carcinomas are pure TCC or TCC predominant, the tumors are more chemosensitive and patients have a higher 5-year survival rate than patients with other forms of high-stage epithelial ovarian cancer (56% versus 7%).
- The findings of Silva and colleagues, however, were not confirmed in two other studies (Hollingsworth and coworkers; Costa and associates).

References

Aguirre P, Scully RE, Wolfe HJ, DeLellis RA. Argyrophil cells in Brenner tumors: a histochemical and immunohistochemical analysis. Int J Gynecol Pathol 5:223–234, 1986.

Austin RM, Norris HJ. Malignant Brenner tumor and transitional cell carcinoma of the ovary: a comparison. Int J Gynecol Pathol 6:29–39, 1987.

Costa MJ, Jansen C, Dickerman A, Scudder SA. Clinicopathologic significance of transitional cell carcinoma pattern in nonlocalized ovarian epithelial tumors (stages 2–4). Am J Clin Pathol 109:173–180, 1998.

Ehrlich CE, Roth LM. The Brenner tumor: a clinicopathologic study of 57 cases. Cancer 27:332–342, 1971.

Hallgrimsson J, Scully RE. Borderline and malignant Brenner tumours of the ovary: a report of 15 cases. Acta Pathol Microbiol Scand A 80(Suppl 233):56–66, 1972.

Hendrickson MR, Longacre TA. Classification of surface epithelial neoplasms of the ovary. In State of the Art Reviews: Pathology. Philadelphia: Hanley & Belfus, 1993:189–254.

Hollingsworth HC, Steinberg SM, Silverberg SG, Merino MJ. Advanced stage transitional cell carcinoma of the ovary. Hum Pathol 27:1267–1272, 1996.

Miles PA, Norris HJ. Proliferative and malignant Brenner tumors of the ovary. Cancer 30:174–186, 1972.

Pins MR, Scully RE. Malignant Brenner tumors and Brenner tumors of borderline malignancy: a report of 53 cases [Abstract]. Mod Pathol 11:111A, 1998.

Roth LM, Czernobilsky B. Ovarian Brenner tumors. II. Malignant. Cancer 56:592–601, 1985.

Roth LM, Dallenbach-Hellweg G, Czernobilsky B. Ovary Brenner tumors. I. Metaplastic, proliferating, and of low malignant potential. Cancer 56:582–591, 1985.

Silva EG, Robey-Cafferty SS, Smith TL, Gershenson DM. Ovarian carcinomas with transitional cell carcinoma pattern. Am J Clin Pathol 93:457–465, 1990.

Silverberg SG. Brenner tumor of the ovary: a clinicopathologic study of 60 tumors in 54 women. Cancer 28:588–596, 1971.

Trebeck CE, Friedlander ML, Russell P, Baird RI. Brenner tumors of the ovary: a study of the histology, immunochemistry, and cellular DNA content in benign, borderline, and malignant ovarian tumors. Pathology 19:241–246, 1987.

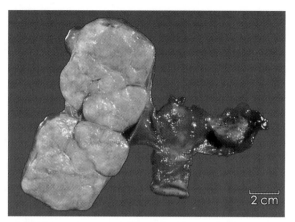

Figure 14–24. Brenner tumor (sectioned surface). There are small, calcified flecks.

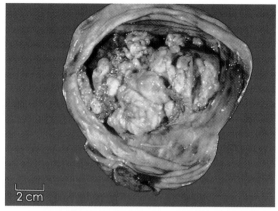

Figure 14–25. Borderline Brenner tumor. An opened cystic tumor is focally lined by polypoid masses.

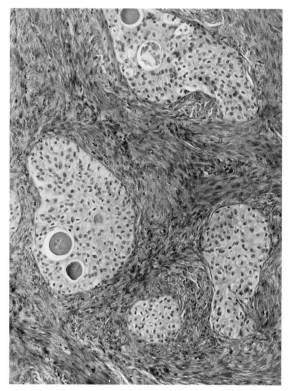

Figure 14–26. Benign Brenner tumor.

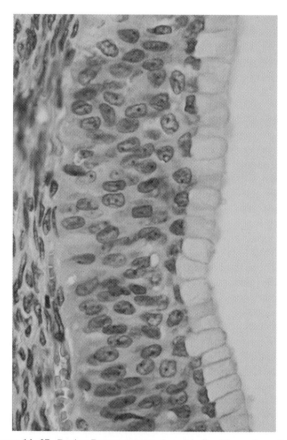

Figure 14–27. Benign Brenner tumor. A cyst is lined by an inner layer of endocervical-type mucinous cells and an outer layer of stratified transitional cells, a few of which have grooved nuclei.

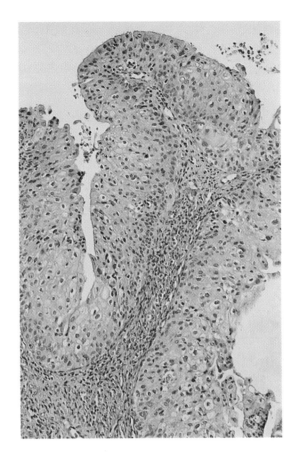

Figure 14–28. Borderline Brenner tumor.

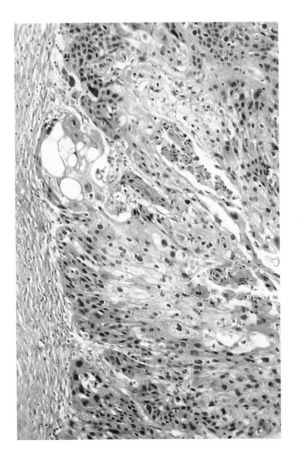

Figure 14–29. Malignant Brenner tumor. The malignant component is squamous cell carcinoma. Benign Brenner tumor was present elsewhere in the tumor.

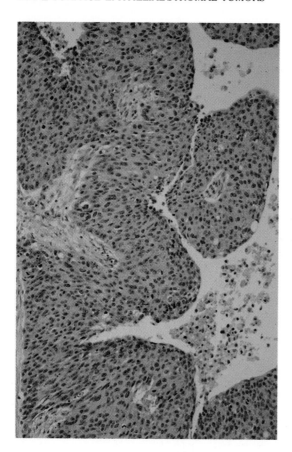

Figure 14–30. Transitional cell carcinoma. Note papillae and undulating lining.

SQUAMOUS CELL TUMORS

Epidermoid Cyst

- Epidermoid cysts and some pure squamous cell carcinomas (SCCs) are included here even though an origin from surface epithelium has not been established conclusively in all the cases.
- The cysts are almost always unilateral and within the ovarian medulla. They have ranged from 0.2 to 4.6 cm in diameter. The cysts are usually filled with yellow-white, creamy material.
- Microscopic examination reveals a lining of keratinizing squamous epithelium. In some cases, Walthard nests or nests resembling benign Brenner tumor have been found in the walls of the cyst.
- Origins from surface epithelial inclusion glands, Walthard nests, and the rete ovarii have been proposed. The presence of hair or a cartilaginous nodule in two cysts associated with Walthard nests suggests a teratomatous origin in some cases.

Squamous Cell Carcinomas

- SCCs of the ovary arise most commonly from the lining of a dermoid cyst (see Chapter 15), less commonly as a component of a Brenner tumor (see Malignant Brenner Tumor, page 330), from endometriosis (SCCE), or in pure form (SCCP).
- Only SCCE and SCCP are classified as SCCs in the surface epithelial-stromal category. The data provided here are derived from the study by Pins and associates.

Clinical Findings

- The seven patients with SCCE were 29 to 70 years old (mean, 49 years), and one, three, one, and two tumors were stages I, II, III, and IV, respectively. One was associated with SCC in situ (SCIS) of the cervix.
- The 11 patients with SCCP were 27 to 73 years old (mean, 56 years), and one, four, five, and one of the tumors were stages I, II, III, and IV, respectively. Three patients had cervical SCIS.

Pathologic Features

- The tumors in both groups tended to be predominantly solid, with multiple small cysts resulting from necrosis, although some tumors were predominantly cystic.
- Microscopically, SCCE and SCCP grew in a variety of patterns categorized as papillary or polypoid, cystic, insular, diffusely infiltrative, verruciform, and sarcomatoid, often with one pattern predominating. All SCCEs were grade 3; 1 and 10 SCCPs were grades 2 and 3, respectively.

Follow-up

- SCCEs and SCCPs have a poorer survival than SCCs arising in dermoid cysts.
- Five of 6 patients with SCCE and adequate follow-up and 5 of 5 similar patients in the literature died of disease, with a mean survival of only 4.5 months. Six of 9 patients with SCCP and follow-up died of disease (mean survival, 11 months), and 5 of 11 similar patients in the literature died of disease.
- For SCCE and SCCP, the stage of the tumor and its grade correlated with overall survival.

Differential Diagnosis

- Endometrioid adenocarcinoma with extensive squamous differentiation. This diagnosis depends on the identification of small foci of the glandular component of the endometrioid carcinoma.
- Secondary SCCs originating in the uterine cervix and possibly other sites. The finding of juxtaposed benign squamous epithelium, endometriosis, or a Brenner tumor indicates probable origin within the ovary.

Prognosis

- After a follow-up period of at least 1 year, the survival for SCCPs in the literature was 0%, and survival for SCCEs was 38%.

References

Fan L-D, Zang H-Y, Zhang X-S. Ovarian epidermoid cyst: report of eight cases. Int J Gynecol Pathol 15:69–71, 1996.

Pins MR, Young RH, Daly WJ, Scully RE. Primary squamous cell carcinoma of the ovary: a report of 37 cases. Am J Surg Pathol 20:823–833, 1996.

Tetu B, Silva EG, Gershenson DM. Squamous cell carcinoma of the ovary. Arch Pathol Lab Med 111:864–866, 1987.

Young RH, Prat J, Scully RE. Epidermoid cyst of the ovary: a report of three cases with comments on histogenesis. Am J Clin Pathol 73:272–276, 1980.

MIXED EPITHELIAL TUMORS

- The mixed epithelial designation refers to surface epithelial-stromal tumors in which different tumor types are recognizable on gross examination or those in which one or more components in addition to the predominant component account for at least 10% of the tumor on microscopic examination.
- Almost all combinations of mixed epithelial neoplasia have been encountered, but only the most noteworthy are listed here.
- Brenner tumor with a mucinous cystic tumor. A diagnosis of mixed mucinous-Brenner tumor is made if both components are grossly detectable or if the minor component (Brenner tumor or pure mucinous tumor) accounts for more than 10% of the neoplasm. Mucinous epithelium within Brenner epithelial nests does not warrant a diagnosis of a mixed epithelial tumor.
- Endocervical-like mucinous cystic tumor of borderline malignancy of the mixed cell type. These tumors resemble endocervical-like mucinous tumors of the typical type clinically and pathologically (see page 308) except for the presence of one or more additional cell types—serous, endometrioid, or squamous.
- Endometrioid carcinoma admixed with a clear cell carcinoma. Because endometrioid carcinomas and clear cell carcinomas are associated with a similar prognosis, this combination would not be expected to have a significant effect on survival.
- TCC with another type of carcinoma (page 331).
- Endometrioid carcinoma with a serous or undifferentiated component. The presence of a serous or undifferentiated carcinomatous component in a stage III or IV endometrioid carcinoma reduced the 5-year and 10-year survival rates from 63% to 8% and from 45% to 0%, respectively, in one study.

References

Brescia RJ, Dubin N, Demopoulos RI. Endometrioid and clear cell carcinoma of the ovary. Int J Gynecol Pathol 8:132–138, 1989.

Czernobilsky B, Silverman BB, Enterline HT. Clear-cell carcinoma of the ovary: a clinicopathologic analysis of pure and mixed forms and comparison with endometrioid carcinoma. Cancer 25:762–772, 1970.

Kurman RJ, Craig JM. Endometrioid and clear cell carcinoma of the ovary. Cancer 29:1653–1664, 1972.

Rutgers JL, Scully RE. Ovarian mixed-epithelial papillary cystadenoma of borderline malignancy of mullerian type: a clinicopathologic analysis. Cancer 61:546–554, 1988.

Tornos C, Silva EG, Khorana SM, Burke TW. High-stage endometrioid carcinoma of the ovary: prognostic significance of pure versus mixed histologic types. Am J Surg Pathol 18:687–693, 1994.

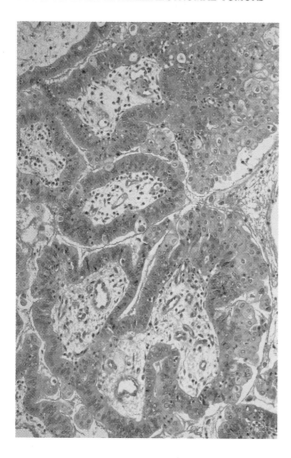

Figure 14–31. Mixed epithelial papillary müllerian cystadenoma of borderline malignancy. Note endometrioid and squamous epithelial elements.

UNDIFFERENTIATED CARCINOMA

General Features

- Applying WHO criteria, 5% or fewer ovarian cancers of epithelial type belong in the undifferentiated category. The corresponding figure from the annual FIGO report, however, is 14%.
- Twelve percent of the tumors are stage I (of which about 20% are bilateral), 11% are stage II, 51% are stage III, and 26% are stage IV. The respective 5-year survival rates are 68%, 40%, 17%, and 6%.

Pathologic Features

- UCs lack gross features that allow their distinction from other poorly differentiated ovarian carcinomas.
- A UC, according to the WHO, is one that shows no differentiation or contains only rare, minor areas of differentiation.
- There is a uniform or almost uniform population of cells with high-grade nuclear features. The tumor cells are usually polygonal but occasionally may be focally

or predominantly spindled, resulting in the appearance of a sarcomatoid carcinoma.

- Rare, minor foci of differentiation into glands, mucin-filled cells, and psammoma bodies may be present. Such differentiation is nonspecific, occurring with various degrees of frequency in many subtypes in the epithelial-stromal cell category.
- Rare UCs are of the small cell type. Some of these tumors have neuroendocrine features (i.e., small cell carcinoma of pulmonary type; see Chapter 17), but they more commonly are small cell carcinomas of the hypercalcemic type, a tumor of unknown lineage (see Chapter 17).
- Rare UCs exhibit focal syncytiotrophoblastic, including choriocarcinomatous, differentiation.

Differential Diagnosis

- TCCs (page 331).
- Diffuse adult GCTs. Features favoring or establishing a diagnosis of UC over that of GCT include advanced stage, nuclear hyperchromatism, and pleomorphism

(that is not of the bizarre, degenerative type; page 365), atypical mitotic figures, EMA positivity and inhibin negativity, and absence of associated endocrine manifestations.

■ Poorly differentiated sarcomas (see Chapter 17), malignant mesodermal mixed tumors (page 321), and lymphomas (see Chapter 17).

■ Metastatic undifferentiated carcinoma. The differential diagnosis of these tumors is based on the general criteria for distinguishing ovarian primary from metastatic tumors (see Chapter 18).

References

Kuwashima Y, Uehara T, Kishi K, et al. Immunohistochemical characterization of undifferentiated carcinomas of the ovary. J Cancer Res Clin Oncol 120:672–677, 1994,

Oliva E, Andrada E, Pezzica E, Prat J. Ovarian carcinomas with choriocarcinomatous differentiation. Cancer 72:2441–2446, 1993.

Pettersson F. Annual Report of the Results of Treatment in Gynecological Cancer. Stockholm: International Federation of Gynecology and Obstetrics, 1991.

Silva EG, Tornos C, Bailey MA, Morris M. Undifferentiated carcinoma of the ovary. Arch Pathol Lab Med 115:377–381, 1991.

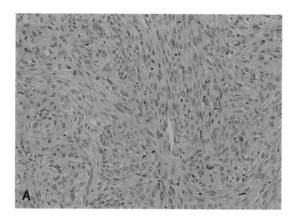
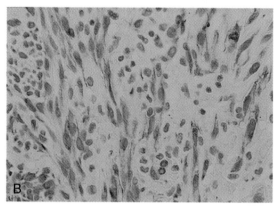

Figure 14–33. *A,* Undifferentiated carcinoma with spindle cells (i.e., sarcomatoid carcinoma). *B,* A cytokeratin stain reveals immunoreactivity of the spindle cells for cytokeratin.

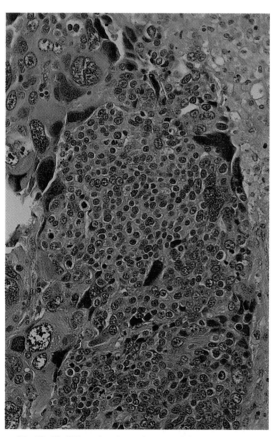

Figure 14–32. Undifferentiated carcinoma with syncytiotrophoblastic-like giant cells.

CHAPTER 15

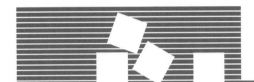

Germic Cell Tumors
of the Ovary

- Germ cell tumors account for about 30% of primary ovarian tumors and are classified as in Table 15–1. Ninety-five percent are benign dermoid cysts (i.e., mature cystic teratomas).
- Malignant germ cell tumors account for 1% to 3% of ovarian cancers in Western countries. In the first 2 decades of life, germ cell tumors account for 60% of all ovarian tumors, one third of which are malignant, accounting for two thirds of ovarian cancers in that age group.
- Approximately 90% of germ cell tumors are pure and 10% mixed with two or more types within the same specimen.
- Most malignant germ cell tumors are of the so-called primitive type. Rare malignant germ cell tumors arising from the somatic tissues of a teratoma (e.g., a squamous cell carcinoma) are of the so-called adult type.

NONTERATOMATOUS GERM CELL TUMORS

Dysgerminoma

Clinical Features

- Dysgerminomas account for nearly 50% of malignant primitive germ cell tumors, for 1% of all ovarian cancers, and for 5% to 10% of ovarian cancers in the first 3 decades.
- Eighty percent of the tumors are encountered in the second and third decades. The tumors are rare before 5 years and after 50 years of age.
- The presenting signs and symptoms are usually related to an abdominal mass. The serum level of lactate dehydrogenase (usually isoenzymes 1 and 2) is elevated in almost all cases.
- The serum level of chorionic gonadotropin (hCG) is elevated in about 3% of cases. These patients often have hormonal manifestations that are typically estro-

genic (e.g., isosexual precocity, menstrual irregularities), but occasionally androgenic.
- Dysgerminomas are occasionally encountered in phenotypic females with gonadal dysgenesis, and in these patients, the tumors usually arise from a gonadoblastoma.
- Extraovarian spread (peritoneum, retroperitoneal lymph nodes) is found at presentation in one third of cases.

Gross Pathologic Findings

- The tumors are usually solid, with a median diameter of 15 cm, a smooth or bosselated serosal surface, and soft, fleshy, lobulated, and cream-colored, gray, pink, or tan sectioned surfaces.
- Cystic degeneration, necrosis, and hemorrhage are present in occasional pure dysgerminomas, but such foci should be sampled to exclude other, more malignant germ cell elements. Calcification suggests an underlying gonadoblastoma.
- Dysgerminomas are bilateral in about 20% of the cases. In one half of these cases, the involvement of the contralateral ovary is microscopic.

Microscopic Findings

- The tumors are composed of cells resembling primordial germ cells in diffuse, insular, trabecular, cordlike, and rarely, tubular patterns. Areas of caseation-like necrosis are common.
- Uniform, rounded tumor cells have discrete cell membranes in well-preserved specimens, clear to occasionally eosinophilic cytoplasm (which is almost always glycogen rich), and a central, large, rounded or flattened nucleus with coarse chromatin and one or several prominent nucleoli. Mitotic figures are usually numerous.
- The stroma of thin to broad fibrous bands almost invariably contains mature lymphocytes, occasionally with lymphoid follicles.

Table 15–1

WORLD HEALTH ORGANIZATION CLASSIFICATION
OF GERM CELL TUMORS OF THE OVARY

Dysgerminoma
    Variant—with syncytiotrophoblastic cells
Yolk sac tumor (endodermal sinus tumor)
    Variants
        Polyvesicular vitelline tumor
        Hepatoid
        Glandular*
Embryonal carcinoma
Polyembryoma
Choriocarcinoma
Teratomas
    Immature
    Mature
        Solid
        Cystic (dermoid cyst)
        With secondary tumor (specify type)
        Fetiform (homunculus)
    Monodermal
        Struma
            Variant—with secondary tumor (specify type)
        Carcinoid
            Insular
            Trabecular
        Strumal carcinoid
        Mucinous carcinoid
        Neuroectodermal tumors (specify type)
        Sebaceous tumors
        Others
Mixed (specify types)

*Some glandular yolk sac tumors resemble endometrioid adenocarcinoma and have been called endometrioid-like tumors.

- A granulomatous stromal reaction, which may be ill defined or sarcoid-like, occurs in 20% of tumors, and if extensive, it may obscure the tumor cells. A similar granulomatous response may occur in lymph nodes harboring metastatic dysgerminoma.
- Syncytiotrophoblastic giant cells (SGCs) that are immunoreactive for hCG occur in 3% of the tumors. Unlike choriocarcinoma, the SGCs are unassociated with cytotrophoblast. Rare hCG-secreting dyserminomas lack SGCs, and in such cases, the dysgerminoma cells may be immunoreactive for hCG.
- Luteinized stromal cells may be admixed with the neoplastic cells or at the periphery of the tumor in some cases, especially those with hCG production. The luteinized cells are the source of the excess estrogens or androgens found in some cases.

Differential Diagnosis

- Solid pattern of yolk sac tumor (YST). Differential features favoring or diagnostic of YST include hyaline bodies, absence of stromal lymphocytes, immunoreactivity for alpha-fetoprotein (AFP), and the presence of other distinctive patterns of YST elsewhere in the tumor.
- Solid pattern of embryonal carcinoma. Differential features favoring or diagnostic of embryonal carcinoma include glandular and papillary patterns, darker cytoplasm, nuclei that are larger and more hyperchromatic

and variable than those of the dysgerminoma, and an absence of a lymphocytic or granulomatous stromal infiltrate with rare exceptions.

- Solid pattern of clear cell carcinoma. Differential features favoring or diagnostic of clear cell carcinoma include postmenopausal age, tubulocystic and papillary patterns, luminal and intracellular mucin, and conspicuous stromal plasma cells.
- Large cell lymphomas. The differing nuclear features of the two tumors, the almost invariable absence of glycogen in lymphomas, and a variety of distinctive immunohistochemical reactions facilitate the differential diagnosis.

Prognosis

- The 5-year survival rate is almost 100% for stage I tumors and 80% to 90% for patients with higher-stage or recurrent tumor.

References

Bjorkholm E, Lundell M, Gyftodimos A, Silfversward C. Dysgerminoma: the Radiumhemmet series, 1927–1984. Cancer 65:38–44, 1990.

Gordon A, Lipton D, Woodruff D. Dysgerminoma: a review of 158 cases from the Emil Novak Tumor Registry. Obstet Gynecol 58:497–504, 1981.

Pressley RH, Muntz HG, Falkenberry S, Rice LW. Serum lactic dehydrogenase as a tumor marker in dysgerminoma. Gynecol Oncol 44:281–283, 1991.

Rutgers JL, Scully RE. Functioning ovarian tumors with peripheral steroid cell proliferation: a report of twenty-four cases. Int J Gynecol Pathol 5:319–337, 1986.

Zaloudek CJ, Tavassoli FA, Norris HJ. Dysgerminoma with syncytiotrophoblastic giant cells: a histologically and clinically distinctive subtype of dysgerminoma. Am J Surg Pathol 5:361–367, 1981.

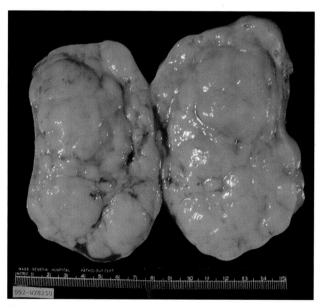

Figure 15–1. Dysgerminoma. The sectioned surface is tan and lobulated.

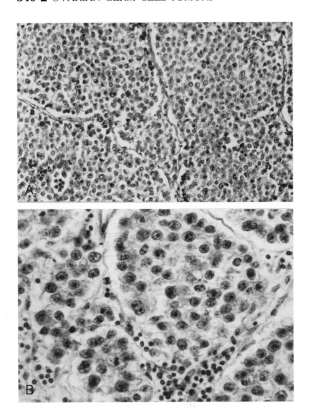

Figure 15–2. Dysgerminoma at medium (*A*) and high (*B*) magnifications.

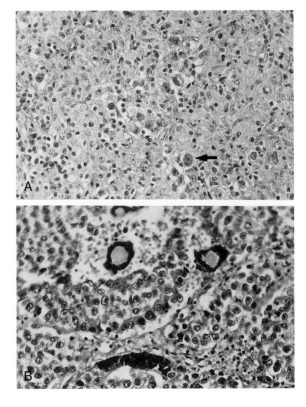

Figure 15–3. Dysgerminoma. *A*, A prominent granulomatous response separates rare, individually disposed tumor cells (one indicated by arrow). *B*, A dysgerminoma contains isolated syncytiotrophoblastic giant cells.

Yolk Sac Tumor

Clinical Features

- YSTs account for about 20% of malignant primitive germ cell tumors. They are most common in the second and third decades (median age, 16 to 19 years) and are rare after 40 years of age. Rare YSTs in elderly women have arisen from surface epithelial tumors. Some YSTs occur in patients with gonadal dysgenesis.
- The patients usually present with abdominal pain and a large abdominal or pelvic mass. The serum level of AFP is elevated preoperatively in almost all patients.
- Extraovarian spread (peritoneum, retroperitoneal lymph nodes) is found at presentation in 30% to 70% of cases.

Gross Features

- YSTs, which have a median diameter of 15 cm, typically have solid and cystic sectioned surfaces. The solid tissue is soft, friable, yellow to gray and is often hemorrhagic and necrotic. Capsular tears are present in 25% of tumors.
- A honeycomb appearance (i.e., many small cysts) is often associated with a polyvesicular-vitelline component.
- Other germ cell elements, most commonly a dermoid cyst, are grossly recognizable in 15% of cases.
- YSTs are almost never bilateral unless the opposite ovary is involved as part of generalized peritoneal spread.

Microscopic Features

- A reticular pattern consisting of a loose meshwork of spaces and cysts occurs at least focally in most YSTs. The spaces are lined by primitive-appearing cells, typically with clear cytoplasm and nuclei that are usually hyperchromatic and irregular and have a prominent nucleolus. Mitotic figures are usually numerous.
- Schiller-Duval bodies (typically within reticular areas) are present in a variable proportion of cases.
  - The Schiller-Duval bodies consist of a rounded or elongated papilla with a fibrovascular core and a lining of primitive columnar cells.
  - The papillae occupy spaces lined by cuboidal, flat, or hobnail cells. Schiller-Duval bodies are usually sparsely distributed, but when numerous and closely packed, a distinctive papillary pattern is created.
- Other patterns are papillary, solid, and festoon (i.e., undulating cords of cells).
- Eosinophilic, periodic acid–Schiff–positive, diastase-resistant, intracellular and extracellular hyaline bodies are present in most YSTs and are most numerous in reticular or hepatoid patterns. Their presence, however, is not specific for YSTs, because they are encountered in a variety of ovarian tumors.
- Stromal changes include:
  - "Parietal" differentiation in more than 90% of tumors: small, usually linear, extracellular accumula-

tions of basement membrane material usually within reticular and solid foci
  - A myxoid or myxomatous pattern in some tumors
  - A mesenchyme-like component of a loose or collagenous stroma containing stellate or spindle-shaped cells, thin-walled blood vessels, and occasionally, skeletal muscle and cartilage
- Cytoplasmic immunoreactivity for AFP is present in almost all tumors (including the variants discussed below), but the staining is often focal.

Variants

- Polyvesicular-vitelline. Cysts, which may exhibit eccentric constrictions, are lined by columnar, cuboidal, or flattened cells. The cysts are often separated by a dense spindle-cell stroma.
- Hepatoid. Large polygonal cells with prominent cell borders, abundant eosinophilic cytoplasm, and round central nuclei with prominent single nucleoli grow in compact masses separated by thin fibrous bands. Hyaline bodies are often numerous. The immunoprofile is similar to that of hepatocellular carcinoma, including carcinoembryonic antigen (CEA) positivity in a canalicular pattern.
- Glandular.
  - The intestinal glandular variant is composed predominantly of large nests of primitive epithelial cells arranged as discrete glands or in a cribriform pattern. The cells show intestinal features on ultrastructural examination.
  - The endometrioid-like variant is composed of tubular glands and villi resembling those of endometrioid carcinoma and often lined by cells with subnuclear or supranuclear vacuoles, simulating the secretory variant of endometrioid carcinoma.
    a. Nests of hepatoid cells within the gland lumens may mimic squamous morules.
    b. An abundant fibrous stroma or a densely cellular stroma with mitotically active spindle cells may create an adenofibromatous or carcinosarcomatous appearance.

Differential Diagnosis

- Other primitive germ cell tumors (see Dysgerminoma and Embryonal Carcinoma, pages 339 and 344).
- Clear cell carcinoma (Table 15–2).
- Endometrioid adenocarcinoma (versus endometrioid-like YST). Features favoring or diagnostic of endometrioid-like YST include a young age, elevated serum AFP level, primitive appearance of the nuclei lining the glands, immunoreactivity for AFP, an absence of squamous metaplasia, and admixture of other patterns of YST or other types of germ cell tumor.
  - Complicating this differential diagnosis are rare tumors composed of an admixture of endometrioid carcinoma and YST (see Chapter 14). These tumors usually occur in women older than those with endometrioid-like YSTs.

Table 15–2

DIFFERENTIAL DIAGNOSIS BETWEEN YOLK
SAC TUMOR AND CLEAR CELL CARCINOMA

Feature	YST	CCC
Age	Typically <30 y	Typically >40 y
Elevated serum AFP	Typical	Absent
Papillae	SDB with vessel	Hyalinized
Hyaline bodies	Typical	Uncommon
AFP immunoreactivity	Typical	Uncommon
Leu-M1 immunoreactivity	Uncommon	Typical
Other germ cell elements	Common	Absent

AFP, alpha-fetoprotein; CCC, clear cell carcinoma; SDB, Schiller-Duval body; YST, yolk sac tumor.

■ Tumors composed of cells with abundant eosinophilic cytoplasm (versus hepatoid YST). These tumors include the tumors listed in Appendix 4, such as steroid cell tumors (see Chapter 16), the oxyphilic variant of clear cell carcinoma (see Chapter 14), hepatoid carcinoma (see Chapter 17), and metastatic hepatocellular carcinoma (see Chapter 18).

Prognosis

■ The postchemotherapy survival rates for stage I tumors are 70% to 90% and 30% to 50% for higher-stage tumors. Serial determination of serum AFP levels is useful in monitoring the effects of therapy and detecting recurrent tumor.

■ Adverse prognostic factors include stage II or greater, gross residual tumor after cytoreductive surgery, and liver involvement.

References

Clement PB, Young RH, Scully RE. Endometrioid-like variant of ovarian yolk sac tumor: a clinicopathological analysis of eight cases. Am J Surg Pathol 11:767–778, 1987.

Devouassoux-Shisheboran M, Schammel DP, Tavassoli FA. Ovarian hepatoid yolk sac tumours: morphological, immunohistochemical and ultrastructural features. Histopathology 34:462–469, 1999.

Gershenson DM, Del Junco G, Herson J, Rutledge FN. Endodermal sinus tumor of the ovary: the M. D. Anderson experience. Obstet Gynecol 61:194–202, 1983.

Kim CR, Hsiu J, Given FT. Intestinal variant of ovarian endodermal sinus tumor. Gynecol Oncol 33:379–381, 1989.

Kurman RJ, Norris HJ. Endodermal sinus tumor of the ovary: a clinical and pathologic analysis of 71 cases. Cancer 38:2404–2419, 1976.

Langley FA, Govan ADT, Anderson MC, et al. Yolk sac and allied tumours of the ovary. Histopathology 5:389–401, 1981.

Michael H, Ulbright TM, Brodhecker CA. The pluripotential nature of the mesenchyme-like component of yolk sac tumor. Arch Pathol Lab Med 113:1115–1119, 1989.

Nogales FF, Bergeron C, Carvia RE, et al. Ovarian endometrioid tumors with yolk sac component, an unusual form of ovarian neoplasm: analysis of six cases. Am J Surg Pathol 20:1056–1066, 1996.

Nogales FF Jr, Matilla A, Nogales-Ortiz F, Galera-Davidson HL. Yolk sac tumors with pure and mixed polyvesicular vitelline patterns. Hum Pathol 9:553–566, 1978.

Prat J, Bhan AK, Dickersin GR, et al. Hepatoid yolk sac tumor of the ovary (endodermal sinus tumor with hepatoid differentiation): a light microscopic, ultrastructural and immunohistochemical study of seven cases. Cancer 50:2355–2368, 1982.

Ulbright TM, Roth LM, Brodhecker CA. Yolk sac differentiation in germ cell tumors: a morphologic study of 50 cases with emphasis on hepatic, enteric, and parietal yolk sac features. Am J Surg Pathol 10:151–164, 1986.

Young RH, Scully RE. Unusual patterns, subtypes, and differential diagnosis of gonadal yolk sac tumors. In Nogales FF (ed): The Human Yolk Sac and Yolk Sac Tumors. Heidelberg: Springer, 1993:309–342.

Zirker TA, Silva EG, Morris M, Ordonez NG. Immunohistochemical differentiation of clear-cell carcinoma of the female genital tract and endodermal sinus tumor with the use of alpha-fetoprotein and Leu-M1. Am J Clin Pathol 91:511–514, 1989.

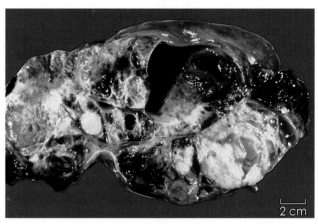

Figure 15–4. Yolk sac tumor. The sectioned surface is solid and cystic with focal hemorrhage and necrosis.

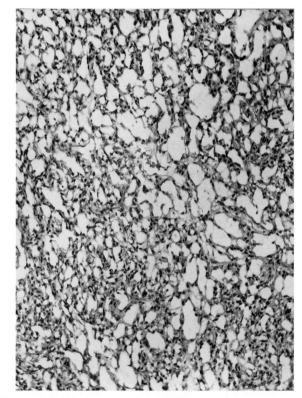

Figure 15–5. Yolk sac tumor with a reticular pattern.

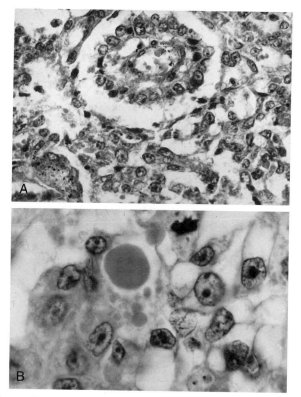

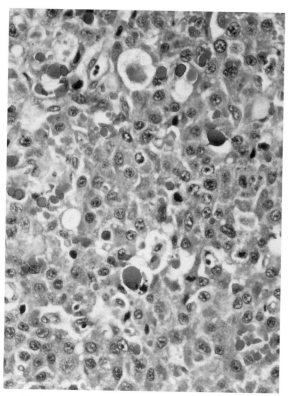

Figure 15–6. Yolk sac tumor. *A,* Reticular pattern with a Schiller-Duval body is seen. *B,* Malignant nuclear features, a mitotic figure, and hyaline bodies are seen.

Figure 15–8. Hepatoid variant of a yolk sac tumor. Notice the hyaline bodies and abundant cytoplasm that was eosinophilic.

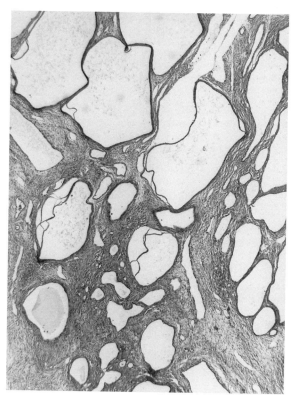

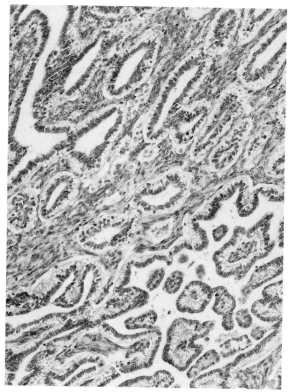

Figure 15–7. Polyvesicular vitelline variant of yolk sac tumor.

Figure 15–9. Glandular (endometrioid-like) variant of yolk sac tumor. Notice the villoglandular pattern and subnuclear vacuolization.

Embryonal Carcinoma

Clinical Features

- Embryonal carcinomas (ECs) are much rarer in the ovary than in the testis, accounting for at most 3% of primitive ovarian germ cell tumors.
- The patients range in age from 4 to 28 years (median, 12 years). The presentation includes an adnexal mass and, in one half of the cases, endocrine manifestations. The latter may take the form of isosexual pseudoprecocity, irregular bleeding, amenorrhea, and hirsutism, alone or in combination. The serum hCG and AFP levels are typically elevated.
- Peritoneal spread, sometimes with involvement of pelvic or intraabdominal viscera, occurs in approximately one half of the cases.

Pathologic Features

- ECs are typically large (median diameter, 17 cm) and have smooth external surfaces. No bilateral cases have been reported. The cut surfaces are predominantly solid and variegated, with white, tan-grey, and yellow soft tissue alternating with cysts containing mucoid material. Foci of hemorrhage and necrosis are common.
- Low-power examination reveals solid sheets and nests of cells, often with central necrosis, and glandlike spaces and papillae.
- The large primitive tumor cells have amphophilic, variably vacuolated cytoplasm, well-defined cell membranes, and round vesicular nuclei with coarse, irregular membranes and one or more prominent nucleoli. Mitotic figures are usually numerous.
- Eosinophilic intracellular hyaline droplets are present in almost all cases. The neoplastic cells are immunoreactive for AFP in some cases.
- SGCs have been in all of the reported tumors. The SGCs are usually individually disposed within or at the periphery of the tumor nests or within the stroma. The SGCs are immunoreactive for hCG.
- Mature teratomatous elements (e.g., squamous epithelium, cartilage, enteric glands) are present in occasional cases.

Differential Diagnosis

- Dysgerminoma (page 339).
- YST. Features favoring or diagnostic of YST include reticular pattern, Schiller-Duval bodies, variant YST patterns (e.g., polyvesicular vitelline, endometrioid-like, hepatoid), and absence of SGCs.
- Poorly differentiated adenocarcinoma or undifferentiated carcinoma. Features favoring or diagnostic of these tumors include late reproductive and postmenopausal age, absence of AFP immunoreactivity (except for the rare hepatoid carcinoma [see Chapter 17]), and an absence of SGCs.
- Juvenile granulosa cell tumors (JGCTs). Features favoring or diagnostic of JGCTs include follicle-like spaces, luteinized neoplastic cells, an absence of SGCs, immunoreactivity for inhibin, and an absence of AFP immunoreactivity.
- Sertoli-Leydig cell tumors (SLCTs). Poorly differentiated areas in SLCTs may focally resemble ECs, with the correct diagnosis resting on the presence of diagnostic patterns of SLCTs (see Chapter 16). Immunoreactivity for inhibin strongly favors a diagnosis of SLCT.

Prognosis

- There was a 50% 5-year survival rate for patients with stage I disease in the only reported series, but most of those patients did not receive chemotherapy.
- In contrast, postoperative chemotherapy was curative in some cases in that series and in other reported cases, including some with extraovarian spread.

References

Kurman RJ, Norris HJ. Embryonal carcinoma of the ovary: a clinicopathologic entity distinct from endodermal sinus tumor resembling embryonal carcinoma of the adult testis. Cancer 38:2420–2433, 1976.
Ueda G, Abe Y, Yoshida M, Fujiwara T. Embryonal carcinoma of the ovary: a six-year survival. Int J Gynecol Obstet 31:287–292, 1990.

Polyembryoma

- Polyembryomas are rare primitive germ cell tumors, with fewer than 10 reported cases.
- The patients are usually children or women of early reproductive age who have manifestations related to a pelvic mass. Elevated serum levels of AFP, hCG, or both are found at presentation in some cases. Extraovarian tumor is found at presentation in some cases.
- Gross examination usually reveals bulky tumors with sectioned surfaces that are typically soft, reddish-brown, spongy or microcystic, and hemorrhagic.
- Polyembryomas are characterized on microscopic examination by myriad small structures resembling early embryos scattered in a collagenous stroma. These embryoid bodies typically consist of two cavities (i.e., amniotic cavity and a yolk sac) separated by an embryonic disk and are typically immunoreactive for AFP.
- hCG-positive syncytiotrophoblastic cells and mature and immature teratomatous elements (especially intestinal tissue or adult or embryonal hepatic tissue) are common.
- Several patients reported in the earlier literature who were not treated with adjuvant chemotherapy died of tumor less than 1 year after presentation. In contrast, other patients, including some with extraovarian spread, have been treated successfully with combination chemotherapy.

References

Chapman DC, Grover R, Schwartz PE. Conservative management of an ovarian polyembryoma. Obstet Gynecol 83:879–882, 1994.
King ME, Hubbell MJ, Talerman A. Mixed germ cell tumor of the ovary with a prominent polyembryoma component. Int J Gynecol Pathol 10:88–95, 1991.

Nakashima N, Murakami S, Fukatsu T, et al. Characteristics of "embryoid body" in human gonadal germ cell tumors. Hum Pathol 19: 1144–1154, 1988.

Prat J, Matias-Guiu X, Scully RE. Hepatic yolk sac differentiation in an ovarian polyembryoma. Surg Pathol 2:147–150, 1989.

Takeda A, Ishizuka T, Goto T, et al. Polyembryoma of ovary producing alpha-fetoprotein and HCG: immunoperoxidase and electron microscopic study. Cancer 14:1878–1889, 1982.

Takemori M, Nishimura R, Yamasaki M, et al. Ovarian mixed germ cell tumor composed of polyembryoma and immature teratoma. Gynecol Oncol 69:260–263, 1998.

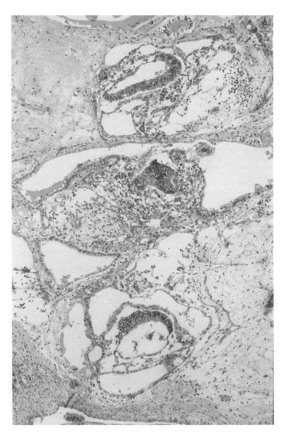

Figure 15–11. Polyembryoma. Two well-developed embryoid bodies are seen with a rudimentary embryoid body between them.

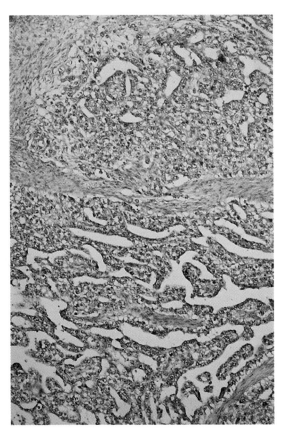

Figure 15–10. Embryonal carcinoma. Solid sheets of cells are interrupted by cleftlike spaces, some of which contain papillae. Syncytiotrophoblastic giant cells were present in other areas of the tumor.

Choriocarcinoma

- Choriocarcinoma in pure form accounts for less than 1% of primitive ovarian germ cell tumors. It is most common as a component of a mixed germ cell tumor, encountered in 20% of the latter in one series.
- A germ cell (versus gestational) origin is confirmed by a prepubertal patient age or the presence of other germ cell elements.
- Ovarian choriocarcinoma typically occurs in children and young adults who present with an adnexal mass, pain, and in occasional cases, hemoperitoneum.
- The serum hCG level is typically elevated, with resultant isosexual pseudoprecocity in children and menstrual abnormalities, breast enlargement, androgenic changes, or combinations thereof in adults.
- The tumors are characteristically solid, hemorrhagic, and friable. Bilateral involvement is rare.
- There is a typical admixture of cytotrophoblast (i.e., large, rounded cells with clear cytoplasm) and hCG-positive syncytiotrophoblast. The syncytiotrophoblastic cells contain cytoplasmic vacuoles, many dark nuclei, and may form syncytial knots. Poorly differentiated areas with a nonspecific appearance are present in some tumors.
- Dilated vascular sinusoids, which are the source of the massive hemorrhage, are common within the tumors. Vascular invasion is prominent in some cases.

Differential Diagnosis

- Malignant germ cell tumors in which isolated syncytiotrophoblastic cells may be encountered, such as embryonal carcinoma, dysgerminoma, and YST. These tumors lack the characteristic admixture of cytotrophoblast and syncytiotrophoblast of choriocarcinoma.
- Rare, poorly differentiated adenocarcinomas of surface epithelial origin, usually occurring in older women, that exhibit trophoblastic differentiation (see Chapter 14).

Prognosis

- Treatment with salpingo-oophorectomy and combination chemotherapy has resulted in apparent cures or prolonged remissions in some patients, including those with extraovarian spread.
- Choriocarcinomas of germ cell origin may be less responsive to chemotherapy than gestational choriocarcinomas.

References

Axe SR, Klein VR, Woodruff JD. Choriocarcinoma of the ovary. Obstet Gynecol 66:111–114, 1985.
Jacobs AJ, Newland JR, Green RK. Pure choriocarcinoma of the ovary. Obstet Gynecol Surv 37:603–609, 1982.

Mixed Malignant Germ Cell Tumors

- These tumors, which contain mixtures of two or more types of germ cell neoplasia, account for 8% to 10% of malignant primitive ovarian germ cell tumors.

- Careful gross examination and judicious sampling of germ cell tumors are important. Each component should be named specifically in the diagnosis in the order of the decreasing quantity of each, and the appended description should quantify the components as accurately as possible.
- The approximate frequencies of germ cell elements in mixed germ cell tumors are dysgerminoma in 75%, YST in 64%, immature teratoma in 58%, embryonal carcinoma in 15%, and choriocarcinoma in 14%. There are two components (most commonly dysgerminoma and YST) in most tumors, with others containing three to five tumor types.
- A rare pattern of mixed germ cell tumor is the *diffuse embryoma,* which is composed of a distinctive necklace-like pattern created by the intermingling of embryonal carcinoma and YST.

References

Cardoso de Almeida PC, Scully RE. Diffuse embryoma of the testis: a distinctive form of mixed germ cell tumor. Am J Surg Pathol 7:633–642, 1983.
Kurman RJ, Norris HJ. Malignant mixed germ cell tumors of the ovary: a clinical and pathologic analysis of 30 cases. Obstet Gynecol 48:579–589, 1976.
Schwartz PE, Chambers SK, Chambers JT, et al. Ovarian germ cell malignancies: the Yale University experience. Gynecol Oncol 45:26–31, 1992.

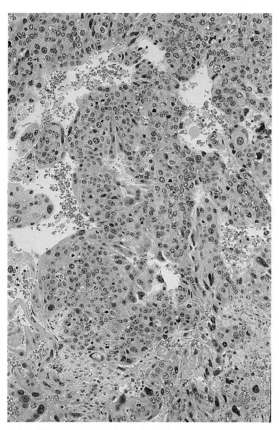

Figure 15–12. Primary ovarian choriocarcinoma. The tumor was associated with a dermoid cyst.

TERATOMAS

Immature Teratoma

Clinical Features

■ Immature teratomas account for only 3% of ovarian teratomas but for almost 20% of primitive germ cell tumors and for 10% to 20% of ovarian cancers in the first 2 decades, the age group in which these tumors usually occur.

■ The clinical presentation is usually that of a palpable abdominal or pelvic mass, frequently accompanied by pain.

■ The serum level of AFP is elevated in two thirds of the patients at presentation, although the levels are usually much lower than those associated with yolk sac tumors. An elevated serum level of hCG occurs in occasional patients, sometimes associated with sexual pseudoprecocity.

■ Immature teratomas are rarely preceded by an ipsilateral dermoid cyst that was resected months to years previously. The risk of an immature teratoma in such patients may be increased if the dermoid cysts are bilateral, multiple, or associated with rupture.

■ Extraovarian spread at the time of operation occurs in one third of patients, usually in the form of peritoneal implants, less commonly nodal metastases, and rarely as hematogenous metastases.

Pathologic Features

■ The tumors have a median diameter of 18 cm, with capsular rupture in almost one half of the cases. The predominantly solid sectioned surfaces are soft, fleshy, and gray to pink; focal hemorrhage and necrosis may be present. Bone and cartilage are visible or palpable in some cases.

■ Small cysts with mucinous, serous, or bloody fluid or hair may be present, and rarely, one or more large cysts occupy most of the specimen. Dermoid cysts are grossly evident in about 25% of the cases.

■ Immature teratomas are only rarely bilateral in the absence of extraovarian spread, but the opposite ovary harbors a dermoid cyst or, less often, another benign tumor in about 10% of the cases.

■ The sine qua non is the presence of some embryonic-appearing tissue that is predominantly neuroectodermal: neuroepithelial rosettes and tubules, cellular foci of mitotically active glia, and rarely, small areas resembling glioblastoma or neuroblastoma.

■ Other common immature tissues are immature or embryonal epithelium of various types (ectodermal and endodermal), including hepatic tissue, and immature mesenchymal elements, such as cartilage and skeletal muscle. However, the diagnosis of "immature" teratoma requires the presence of embryonic tissue rather than simply immature fetal-type tissue.

■ Mature tissues identical to those encountered in mature teratomas are commonly admixed with the immature tissues.

■ Primary and metastatic immature teratoma can be graded by the amount of immature tissue, which is usually neural, that is present.
  • Grade 1 tumors contain rare foci of immature neural tissue (<1 low-power-field [LPF] per slide), grade 2 tumors contain more than 1 but 3 or fewer LPFs of immature neural tissue per slide, and grade 3 tumors contain 4 or more LPFs of immature neural tissue per slide.
  • A two-grade system has been proposed: low grade (grade 1) and high grade (grades 2 and 3).

■ Implants (or nodal metastases) are usually immature but rarely consist exclusively or mainly of mature (i.e., grade 0) glial tissue (i.e., peritoneal gliomatosis). Mature epithelial elements or mature cartilage or foci of endometriosis are occasionally admixed with the glial implants.

■ Generous sampling of the implants by the surgeon and pathologist is important because immature implants may coexist with mature implants.

Differential Diagnosis

■ Mature solid teratomas. These tumors are excluded by the identification of even minor foci of immature tissue. The presence of occasional microscopic immature foci in an otherwise typical dermoid cyst (page 350), however, should not lead to a diagnosis of immature teratoma.

■ Ovarian neuroectodermal tumors (see page 360).

■ Malignant mesodermal mixed tumors. These tumors, in contrast to immature teratomas, typically occur in older women, only rarely contain neuroectodermal elements, and contain foci of obvious adenocarcinoma. Cartilage, if present, usually resembles chondrosarcoma.

Prognosis

■ Almost all patients treated with combination chemotherapy achieve a sustained remission. Chemotherapy is typically associated with a disappearance of high-grade implants; the remaining implants are usually composed exclusively of mature teratoma or necrotic or fibrous tissue.

■ In some cases, continued growth (and rarely local invasion) of the mature implants requires reoperation (so-called growing teratoma syndrome).

■ Almost all patients with peritoneal gliomatosis have a benign clinical course, even without postoperative treatment, but rare cases of glioblastomatous transformation of mature peritoneal gliomatosis have been reported.

References

Anteby EY, Ron M, Revel A, et al. Germ cell tumors of the ovary arising after dermoid cyst resection: a long term follow-up study. Obstet Gynecol 83:605–608, 1994.

Bonazzi C, Peccatori F, Colombo N, et al. Pure ovarian immature teratoma, a unique and curable disease: 10 years' experience of 32 prospectively treated patients. Obstet Gynecol 84:598–604, 1994.

Dadmanesh F, Miller D, Swenerton KD, Clement PB. Gliomatosis peritonei with malignant transformation. Mod Pathol 10:597–601, 1997.

Geisler JP, Goulet R, Foster RS, Sutton GP. Growing teratoma syndrome after chemotherapy for germ cell tumors of the ovary. Obstet Gynecol 84:719–721, 1994.

Gershenson DM, Del Junco G, Silva EG, et al. Immature teratoma of the ovary. Obstet Gynecol 68:624–629, 1986.

Nogales FF Jr, Favara BE, Major FJ, Silverberg SG. Immature teratoma of the ovary with a neural component ("solid" teratoma): a clinicopathologic study of 20 cases. Hum Pathol 7:625–642, 1976.

Norris HJ, Zirkin HJ, Benson WL. Immature (malignant) teratoma of the ovary: a clinical and pathologic study of 58 cases. Cancer 37: 2359–2372, 1976.

O'Connor DM, Norris HJ. The influence of grade on the outcome of stage I ovarian immature (malignant) teratomas and the reproducibility of grading. Int J Gynecol Pathol 13:283–289, 1994.

Perrone T, Steeper TA, Dehner LP. Alpha-fetoprotein localization in pure ovarian teratoma: an immunohistochemical study of 12 cases. Am J Clin Pathol 88:713–717, 1987.

Robboy SJ, Scully RE. Ovarian teratoma with glial implants on the peritoneum. Hum Pathol 1:643–653, 1970.

Yanai-Inbar I, Scully RE. Relation of ovarian dermoid cysts and immature teratomas: an analysis of 350 cases of immature teratoma and 10 cases of dermoid cyst with microscopic foci of immature tissue. Int J Gynecol Pathol 6:203–212, 1987.

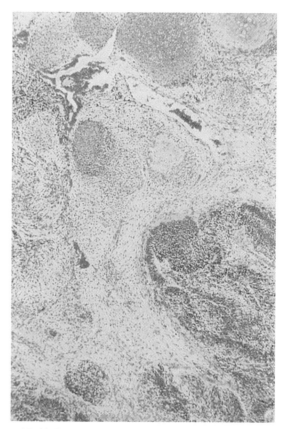

Figure 15–14. Immature teratoma. Darkly staining immature neuroectodermal tissue (*bottom*) and nests of fetal-type cartilage are shown.

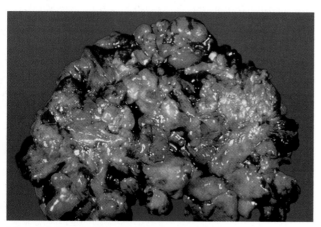

Figure 15–13. Immature teratoma. The sectioned surface is predominantly solid with white brainlike tissue.

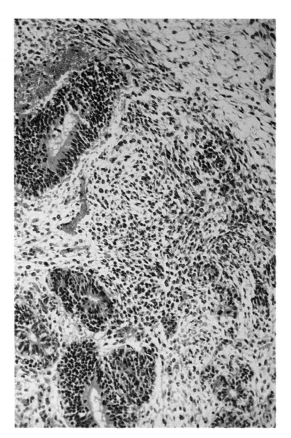

Figure 15–15. Immature teratoma. Immature neural tissue consists of neuroepithelial tubules and cellular glial tissue.

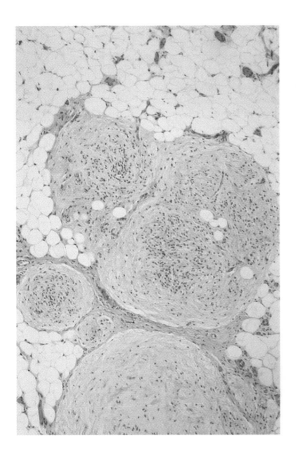

Figure 15–16. Peritoneal gliomatosis in a patient with an ovarian immature teratoma. Glial nodules abut omental adipose tissue.

Mature Solid Teratoma

■ These tumors, which account for 15% to 20% of solid teratomas, occur in the same age distribution as the immature teratoma, and in contrast to dermoid cysts, they rarely occur postmenopausally.

■ Mature peritoneal glial implants are found at presentation in some cases.

■ The macroscopic appearance is similar to that of the immature teratoma, except that soft, necrotic, and hemorrhage foci are much less common.

■ The tumors are characterized by mature tissues representing all three germ layers; mature glial tissue may be the predominant element. Mitotic figures are absent or rare.

■ All of the reported, well-sampled tumors, including those with mature implants, have been associated with a benign clinical course.

■ The differential diagnosis with immature teratomas is discussed under the latter heading.

References

Calame JJ, Schaberg A. Solid teratomas and mixed mullerian tumors of the ovary: a clinical, histological, and immunocytochemical comparative study. Gynecol Oncol 33:212–221, 1989.

diZerega G, Acosta A, Kaufman RH, Kaplan AL. Solid teratoma of the ovary. Gynecol Oncol 3:93–102, 1975.

Peterson WF. Solid, histologically benign teratomas of the ovary: a report of four cases and review of the literature. Am J Obstet Gynecol 72:1094–1102, 1956.

Steeper TA, Mukai K. Solid ovarian teratomas: an immunocytochemical study of thirteen cases with clinicopathologic correlation. Pathol Annu 19(1):81–92, 1984.

Dermoid Cyst

Clinical Features

■ Dermoid cysts (mature cystic teratomas) are the most common ovarian tumor, accounting for up to 44% of them and for up to 58% of benign ovarian tumors.

■ Dermoid cysts occur during the reproductive years in more than 80% of cases but are also found in children, accounting for up to one half of ovarian neoplasms in the first 2 decades. Some tumors are not detected until years after menopause.

■ Dermoid cysts may be associated with the typical symptoms and signs of benign ovarian tumors, but up to 60% are asymptomatic. A radiologic diagnosis can be made in a high proportion of the cases because of the presence of teeth.

■ Complications of dermoid cysts include:
  • Torsion with one or more of the following: infarction, perforation, hemoperitoneum, and autoamputation
  • Bacterial infection of the cyst
  • Perforation into the peritoneal cavity or a hollow viscus; a sudden rupture may lead to an acute abdomen, whereas a slow leak may lead to a granuloma-

tous peritonitis that can mimic metastatic carcinoma or tuberculosis at operation.
  • "Peritoneal melanosis," characterized by tan to black, peritoneal staining or tumor-like nodules (see Chapter 20)
  • Hemolytic anemia that disappears after removal of the tumor

Pathologic Features

■ The tumors are bilateral in about 15% of the cases and are occasionally multiple in one ovary.

■ The typical gross features include contents of yellow to brown sebaceous material and hair, a lining that resembles skin, and one or more rounded, polypoid masses (i.e., mamillae or Rokitansky's protuberances) that are usually composed predominantly of fat.

■ Teeth occur in one third of the cases in the cyst wall or cavity and occasionally within a rudimentary mandible or maxilla. Bone, cartilage, mucinous cysts, adipose tissue, thyroid, and soft brain tissue are visible grossly in some cases.

■ Microscopic examination reveals adult-type tissues, usually representing all three germ layers, sometimes arranged in an organoid fashion. Microscopic foci of immature fetal-type tissues, however, have been encountered rarely in otherwise typical dermoid cysts and appear to have no prognostic significance.

■ There is a predominance of ectodermal derivatives in almost all the cases, including keratinized epidermis, sebaceous and sweat glands, hair follicles, and neuroectodermal elements (glial and peripheral nervous tissue, cerebrum, cerebellum, and choroid plexus).

■ Mesodermal derivatives include smooth muscle, bone, teeth, cartilage, and fat. Endodermal derivatives include respiratory and gastrointestinal epithelium and thyroid and salivary gland tissue. Rare tissues include retina, pancreas, thymus, adrenal, pituitary, kidney, lung, breast, and prostate.

■ Escaped cyst contents elicit a characteristic lipogranulomatous response in the wall of the cyst or the surrounding ovarian tissue, resulting in a sievelike pattern. This finding may be the sole microscopic evidence of a dermoid cyst in rare cases.

Differential Diagnosis

■ The diagnosis is usually straightforward. Markedly cellular cerebellar and retinal tissue should not lead to a diagnosis of immature teratoma.

References

Comerci JT Jr, Licciardi F, Bergh PA, et al. Mature cystic teratoma: a clinicopathologic evaluation of 517 cases and review of the literature. Obstet Gynecol 84:22–28, 1994.

Pantoja E, Noy MA, Axtmayer RW, et al. Ovarian dermoids and their complications: comprehensive historical review. Obstet Gynecol Surv 30:1–20, 1975.

Payne D, Muss HB, Homesley HD, et al. Autoimmune hemolytic anemia and ovarian dermoid cysts: case report and review of the literature. Cancer 48:721–724, 1981.

Peterson WF, Prevost EC, Edmund FT, et al. Benign cystic teratomas of the ovary. Am J Obstet Gynecol 70:368–382, 1955.

Rubin A, Papadaki L. Multicystic structures appearing in mature cystic teratomas of the ovary: an immunohistochemical and ultrastructural study. Histopathology 17:359–363, 1990.

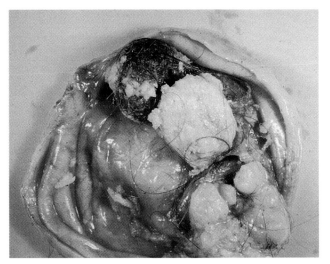

Figure 15–17. Mature cystic teratoma (dermoid cyst). The opened cyst is lined by tissue resembling squamous mucosa; teeth are also present. The cyst contents consist of yellow sebaceous material and hair.

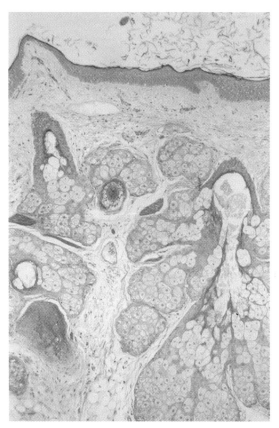

Figure 15–18. Dermoid cyst lining. Epidermis with exfoliating keratin (*top*) is subtended by sebaceous glands and hair follicles.

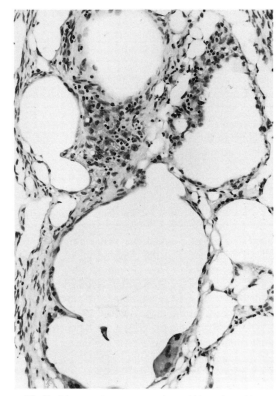

Figure 15–19. Lipogranulomatous reaction within a dermoid cyst wall, so-called sieve-like pattern.

Mature Teratomas With Secondary Tumor

- Cancerous change in a component of a mature teratoma, which has been documented in up to 2% of tumors, typically occurs in women who are between 40 and 60 years of age.
- The clinical presentation ranges from that of a typical dermoid cyst to that of an advanced ovarian cancer, depending on the extent of the secondary tumor. An elevated squamous cell carcinoma antigen is present in some patients in whom the secondary tumor is a squamous cell carcinoma.
- Laparotomy may reveal adherence to surrounding structures, areas of nodularity, thickening of the wall, hemorrhage, or necrosis. In many cases, the tumor has spread throughout the abdomen or to adjacent organs by the time of operation.

Pathologic Features

- The tumors are usually larger than typical dermoid cysts, with more than 90% of them between 10 and 20 cm in maximal dimension.
- Gross examination may reveal cauliflower-like masses protruding into the cavity of the cyst, a mural nodule or plaque, or if extensive, a solid tumor mass obliterating the dermoid cyst. Foci of hemorrhage and necrosis within the malignant component are common.
- The secondary cancer in 80% of cases is squamous cell carcinoma, which is almost always invasive, but rarely in situ.
- Other tumors, including carcinoid tumors, thyroid-type tumors, neuroectodermal tumors, and sebaceous tumors are considered under the heading of Monodermal Teratomas (page 353).
- Rare cancers include adenocarcinomas (including Paget's disease), adenosquamous carcinomas, undifferentiated carcinomas (including small cell carcinoma), sarcomas, and malignant melanomas.
- Rare benign tumors have included corticotropin- and prolactin-secreting pituitary adenomas.

Prognosis

- Five-year survival rates for patients with squamous cell carcinoma have been 77% (stage I) and 11% (stage II or higher). Stage I squamous cell carcinomas that are well differentiated and that lack vascular invasion have a more favorable prognosis than poorly differentiated tumors or those associated with vascular invasion.
- The behavior of adenocarcinomas is similar to that of squamous cell carcinomas. Almost all sarcomas are fatal. The survival rate for patients with malignant melanomas is approximately 50%.

References

Axiotis CA, Lippes HA, Merino MJ, et al. Corticotroph cell pituitary adenoma within an ovarian teratoma: a new cause of Cushing's syndrome. Am J Surg Pathol 11:218–224, 1987.

Davis GL. Malignant melanoma arising in mature ovarian cystic teratoma (dermoid cyst): report of two cases and literature analysis. Int J Gynecol Pathol 15:356–362, 1996.

Hirakawa T, Tsuneyoshi M, Enjoji M. Squamous cell carcinoma arising in mature cystic teratoma of the ovary: clinicopathologic and topographic analysis. Am J Surg Pathol 13:397–405, 1989.

Palmer PE, Bogojavlensky S, Bhan AK, Scully RE. Prolactinoma in wall of ovarian dermoid cyst with hyperprolactinemia. Obstet Gynecol 75:540–543, 1990.

Peterson WF. Malignant degeneration of benign cystic teratomas of the ovary: a collective review of the literature. Obstet Gynecol Surv 12: 793–830, 1957.

Pins MR, Young RH, Daly WJ, Scully RE. Primary squamous cell carcinoma of the ovary: report of 37 cases. Am J Surg Pathol 20: 823–833, 1996.

Tseng C, Chou H, Huang K, et al. Squamous cell carcinoma arising in mature cystic teratoma of the ovary. Gynecol Oncol 63:364–370, 1996.

Fetiform Teratoma

- Fetiform teratoma refers to rare teratomas in which an ovarian cyst contains a structure resembling a malformed human fetus (i.e., homunculus). Most have been diagnosed in the third or fourth decade.
- A homunculus should be distinguished from the fetus-in-fetu, a parasitic monozygotic twin that develops within the upper retroperitoneal space of its partner. Most cases of fetus-in-fetu have occurred in infants younger that 1 year of age, and no examples have been reported in the ovary.

References

Abbott TM, Hermann WJ Jr, Scully RE. Ovarian fetiform teratoma (homunculus) in a 9-year-old girl. Int J Gynecol Pathol 2:392–402, 1984.

Lord JM. Intra-abdominal foetus-in-fetu. J Pathol Bacteriol 72:627–641, 1956.

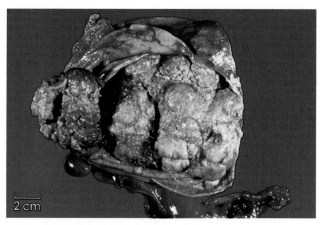

Figure 15–20. Dermoid cyst with a secondary tumor. Polypoid masses of squamous cell carcinoma fill the cyst lumen, and hair is visible.

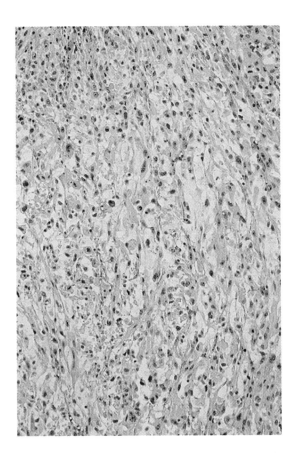

Figure 15–21. Squamous cell carcinoma arising in a dermoid cyst. The tumor cells are spindled and are separated by a myxoid stroma, an appearance potentially mimicking a sarcoma. Typical squamous cell carcinoma was seen in other areas of the tumor.

Monodermal Teratomas

Struma Ovarii

Clinical Features

- The term *struma* is reserved for tumors in which thyroid tissue is the predominant or sole component or forms a grossly recognizable component of a teratoma.
- The peak frequency is in the fifth decade, but some cases occur in prepubertal and postmenopausal females. The usual clinical presentation is related to a mass.
- Ascites is present in about one third of cases and occasionally is accompanied by Meigs' syndrome. Rare cases have clinical evidence of hyperthyroidism.

Pathologic Features

- Struma grossly usually appears as red, brown or greenish-brown, predominantly solid, soft tissue. The struma may be pure but is more commonly associated with another tumor, usually a dermoid cyst and less commonly a mucinous tumor, a carcinoid tumor (strumal carcinoid), or a Brenner tumor.

- Occasionally, struma may form a unilocular or multilocular cyst with mucoid or gelatinous contents; a green to brown color of the cyst contents or lining is a clue to the correct diagnosis.
- Microscopic examination reveals normal thyroid tissue or tissue resembling a thyroid neoplasm, usually an adenoma. Microfollicular, pseudotubular, trabecular, or solid nests or sheets occur alone or in combination. Oxyphil cells or clear cells occasionally predominate.
- The nuclear features are usually bland or mildly atypical. Mitotic figures are usually rare, but as many as 5 mitotic figures per 10 high-power-fields are present in some cases.
- The cysts of cystic strumas are often lined by indifferent flat to cuboidal epithelial cells. Occasional typical thyroid follicles in fibrous septa may be the only clue to the correct diagnosis.
- The presence of birefringent calcium oxalate crystals within the colloid and immunoreactivity of the cell cytoplasm and colloid for thyroglobulin are helpful in establishing the diagnosis, especially in cases with unusual patterns or cell types.
- Rare cases have microscopic evidence of carcinoma,

including a papillary pattern with typical nuclear characteristics of papillary thyroid carcinoma, similar nuclear features in tumors with a follicular pattern, or a follicular carcinoma. Tumors with these features are usually clinically benign (see Behavior, below).

Differential Diagnosis

◼ Surface epithelial tumors (versus cystic struma). Features indicating cystic struma include a green to brown color, occasional thyroid follicles in the septa, the presence of typical struma in some cases, an associated dermoid cyst, calcium oxalate crystals, and immunoreactivity for thyroglobulin.

◼ Steroid cell tumors, Sertoli cell tumors, granulosa cell tumors, paragangliomas, primary or metastatic clear cell carcinomas, hepatoid carcinoma, metastatic hepatocellular carcinoma, and metastatic malignant melanoma (versus oxyphil and clear cell strumas with insular, solid or pseudotubular patterns).
  • Features favoring or diagnostic of struma include an association with a dermoid cyst, the presence of typical thyroid follicles, the presence of calcium oxalate crystals, and immunoreactivity for thyroglobulin.

◼ Carcinoid tumor, hepatoid yolk sac tumor, and primary malignant melanoma (versus oxyphilic struma).
  • Features indicating carcinoid include its distinctive nuclear features and immunoreactivity for chromogranin
  • Features indicating YST include malignant nuclear features, hyaline globules, and AFP immunoreactivity.
  • Features favoring or diagnostic of melanoma include malignant nuclear features and immunoreactivity for S-100 protein and HMB-45.

◼ Clear cell carcinomas, endometrioid carcinomas, Sertoli-Leydig cell tumors, pregnancy luteomas, and potentially rare other lesions that contain struma-like patterns (i.e., spaces filled with material resembling thyroid colloid). Other features of such tumors and an absence of immunoreactivity for thyroglobulin facilitate the diagnosis.

Behavior

◼ Strumas are clinically malignant only rarely. Even strumas with atypical or malignant features on microscopic examination (Devaney and colleagues) have a clinically benign course in almost all cases.

◼ The converse is that some clinically malignant strumas have an innocuous microscopic appearance and may recur more than 10 or 20 years after oophorectomy.

◼ Some cases of struma are associated with benign appearing peritoneal implants (i.e., strumosis).

References

Devaney K, Snyder R, Norris HJ, Tavassoli FA. Prolferative struma ovarii and histologically malignant struma ovarii—a clinicopathologic study of 54 cases. Int J Gynecol Pathol 12:333–343, 1993.

Kempers RD, Dockerty MB, Hoffman DL, Bartholomew LG. Struma ovarii—ascitic, hyperthyroid, and asymptomatic syndromes. Ann Intern Med 72:883–893, 1970.

Nieminen U, Von Numers C, Widholm O. Struma ovarii. Acta Obstet Gynecol Scand 42:399–424, 1963.

Szyfelbein WM, Young RH, Scully RE. Cystic struma ovarii: a frequently unrecognized tumor. A report of 20 cases. Am J Surg Pathol 18:785–788, 1994.

Szyfelbein WM, Young RH, Scully RE. Struma ovarii simulating ovarian tumors of other types: a report of 30 cases. Am J Surg Pathol 19:21–29, 1995.

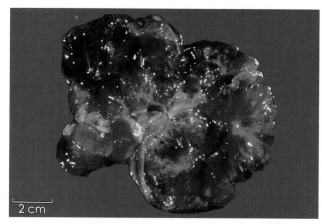

Figure 15–22. Struma ovarii.

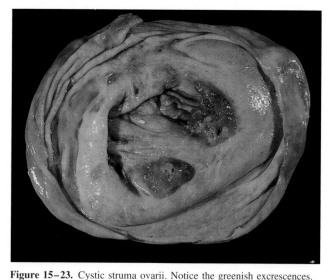

Figure 15–23. Cystic struma ovarii. Notice the greenish excrescences.

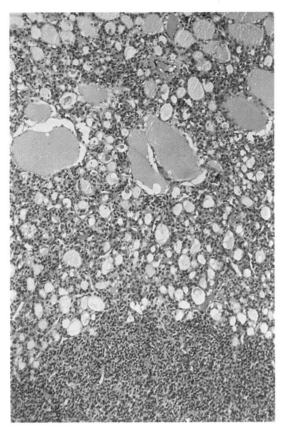

Figure 15–24. Struma ovarii. Macrofollicular, microfollicular, and solid patterns are seen.

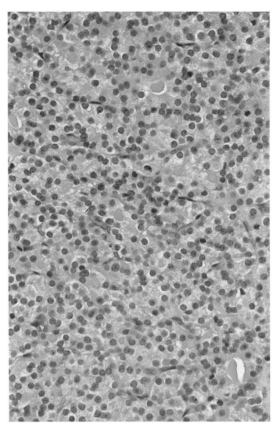

Figure 15–25. Struma ovarii. A solid pattern is composed of oxyphilic cells. A few follicular spaces filled with colloid are also present.

Figure 15–26. Cystic struma. The cells lining a locule are flattened and have a nonspecific appearance (*arrow*). The wall contains occasional small follicles widely separated by edematous tissue.

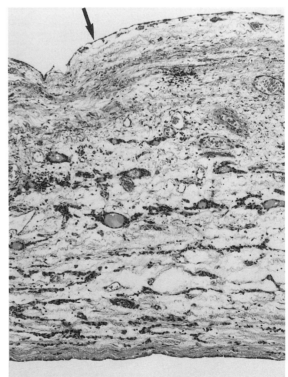

Insular Carcinoid

Clinical Features

■ This is the most common type of primary ovarian carcinoid tumor and occurs in patients in their fourth to eighth decades who usually present with manifestations of a slowly growing ovarian tumor. The tumors are almost always confined to the ovary at the time of laparotomy. Some patients have ascites.

■ About one third of patients have preoperative clinical evidence of the carcinoid syndrome, which usually occurs in patients who are older than 50 years of age and have tumors larger than 7 cm in maximal dimension.

  • The syndrome typically occurs in the absence of extraovarian spread (because the ovarian venous drainage bypasses the liver) and is usually relieved by oophorectomy.

  • Some patients develop progressive tricuspid insufficiency in the absence of persistent tumor.

Pathologic Features

■ The tumor usually appears as a small nodule that protrudes into the lumen or thickens the wall of a dermoid cyst or, rarely, a cystic mucinous tumor. Less commonly, the tumor arises within a mature solid teratoma or forms a large homogeneous mass that replaces the ovary. All of the reported tumors have been unilateral.

■ The sectioned surface is usually predominantly solid, firm, tan to yellow, and variably fibrous. A few small cysts may be present, and the tumor rarely is predominantly cystic.

■ Microscopic examination reveals discrete cellular nests, sometimes punctured by small round acini and separated by a scanty to abundant fibromatous stroma. Eosinophilic secretions, which may undergo psammomatous calcification, are often found in the acini.

■ The tumor cells usually have eosinophilic cytoplasm, which is most abundant in cells lining the acini and at the periphery of the nests, often with reddish-brown argentaffin granules. The nuclei are round and uniform, with stippled chromatin and no or rare mitotic figures.

■ The tumor cells are typically immunoreactive for chromogranin and serotonin, and in fewer than 10% of cases, neurohormonal peptides (see Trabecular Carcinoid, page 357).

Differential Diagnosis

■ Metastatic insular carcinoid (when teratomatous elements are absent). Features of metastatic carcinoid include a definite or probable carcinoid tumor elsewhere (usually the intestine), bilateral involvement, intraovarian growth as multiple nodules, extraovarian metastases (mesenteric lymph nodes, liver), and postoperative clinical or laboratory evidence of the carcinoid syndrome.

■ Microfollicular granulosa cell tumor (GCT). Differential features of this tumor include Call-Exner bodies; tumor cells with scanty cytoplasm; angular, haphazardly oriented, pale, grooved nuclei; and inhibin immunoreactivity.

■ Brenner tumor (BT). Features favoring or diagnostic of BT include transitional cells, absence of prominent argentaffin granules, and the presence of grooved nuclei.

■ Strumal carcinoid. Exclude thyroid tissue by extensive sampling.

Behavior

■ Insular carcinoids usually have a benign clinical course, although there have been rare deaths from intraabdominal recurrent tumor.

References

Robboy SJ. Insular carcinoid of ovary associated with malignant mucinous tumors. Cancer 54:2273–2276, 1984.

Robboy SJ, Norris HJ, Scully RE. Insular carcinoid primary in the ovary: a clinicopathologic analysis of 48 cases. Cancer 36:404–418, 1975.

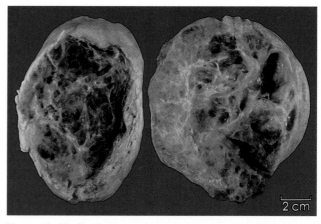

Figure 15–27. Carcinoid tumor (sectioned surface). Solid, yellow-tan tissue and cysts are seen.

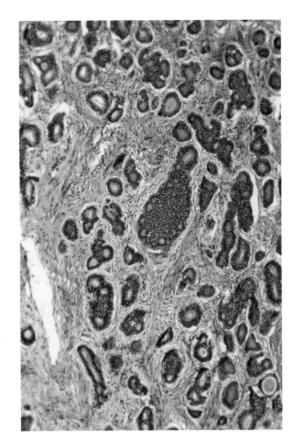

Figure 15–28. Insular carcinoid tumor. Small nests and acini lie within a fibrous stroma.

Trabecular Carcinoid

Clinical Features and Behavior

- These tumors, which are one third as common as insular carcinoids and occur in the third to sixth decades, are usually associated with the clinical manifestations of a slowly growing ovarian tumor.
- None of the patients has had the carcinoid syndrome, but rare patients have had severe chronic constipation due to peptide YY secretion by tumor relieved by oophorectomy.
- There have been no tumor-related deaths. In one case, a peritoneal implant was found 2 years after oophorectomy.

Pathologic Features

- The gross appearances are similar to those of insular carcinoid, with teratomatous elements present in almost all the cases. All the tumors have been unilateral.
- Microscopic examination reveals long, wavy, parallel ribbons of columnar cells with oblong nuclei oriented perpendicular to the axis of the ribbon. The ribbons are separated by a scanty to abundant fibromatous stroma. A minor insular pattern is present in 20% of the cases.
- The tumor cells have moderately abundant, usually argyrophilic, occasionally argentaffinic, eosinophilic cytoplasm and nuclei with finely dispersed chromatin and occasional mitotic figures.
- One or more neurohormonal polypeptides can be demonstrated in about 50% of the tumors: somatostatin, glucagon, pancreatic polypeptide, vasoactive intestinal polypeptide, neurotensin, enkephalin, calcitonin, corticotropin, and peptide YY.

Differential Diagnosis

- Metastatic trabecular carcinoid. The differential features are the same as those used for distinguishing metastatic from primary insular carcinoids (described earlier).
- Strumal carcinoid. Rule out by extensive sampling to exclude thyroid tissue.
- SLCT. The sex cords in SLCTs are usually shorter and less regular than the trabeculae of trabecular carcinoids,

and the neoplastic cells lack argyrophilic cytoplasm and immunoreactivity for neurohormonal peptides. Additionally, most SLCTs are inhibin positive.

References

Motoyama T, Katayama Y, Watanabe H, et al. Functioning ovarian carcinoids induce severe constipation. Cancer 70:513–518, 1992.

Robboy SJ, Scully RE, Norris HJ. Primary trabecular carcinoid of the ovary. Obstet Gynecol 49:202–207, 1977.

Sporrong B, Falkmer S, Robboy SJ, et al. Neurohormonal peptides in ovarian carcinoids: an immunohistochemical study of 81 primary carcinoids and of intraovarian metastases from six mid-gut carcinoids. Cancer 49:68–74, 1982.

Talerman A, Evans MI. Primary trabecular carcinoid tumor of the ovary. Cancer 50:1403–1407, 1982.

Strumal Carcinoid

Clinical Features and Behavior

■ Strumal carcinoid tumors, which have a frequency similar to that of insular carcinoids, occur over a wide age range (20 to 78 years).

■ The clinical presentation is usually related to the presence of an adnexal mass. Extraovarian spread (benign-appearing thyroid tissue) has been found at presentation in only one case.

■ The carcinoid syndrome has been found in only one case, but manifestations suggesting function of the thyroid component have been present in 10%. Chronic contipation relieved by removal of the tumor has been a symptom in rare cases (see Trabecular Carcinoid, page 357).

■ The tumors are almost always clinically benign. The patient with extraovarian tumor at presentation was alive with tumor 1 year after oophorectomy. Only one reported patient has died from tumor, 2.5 years postoperatively.

Pathologic Features

■ The tumors may be pure and form a solid mass not readily distinguishable from other ovarian tumors or may be associated with a teratoma; in the latter, a solid nodule may protrude into the cavity of a dermoid cyst or thicken its wall. Uncommonly, strumal carcinoid predominates in a mature, solid teratoma or is a microscopic focus within a mature teratoma.

■ The sectioned surface is usually homogeneous, yellow or tan, and solid, but it may be variably cystic. The strumal and carcinoid components are each grossly recognizable in some cases.

■ On microscopic examination, the tumors consist of two components, which are usually admixed but occasionally only contiguous, with one being a trabecular or mixed trabecular-insular carcinoid and the other being struma that resembles typical struma ovarii.

■ Glands or cysts lined by mucinous epithelium are seen in one half of the cases and may be conspicuous. These tumors should not be diagnosed as mucinous carcinoid unless the distinctive features of that tumor are seen.

■ The tumors are usually immunoreactive (particularly in the carcinoid component) for chromogranin, synaptophysin, serotonin, prostatic acid phosphatase, and in 40%, neurohormonal peptides (see Trabecular Carcinoid, page 357), including peptide YY in patients with constipation.

■ Both the strumal component and occasionally foci within the carcinoid component are immunoreactive for thyroglobulin.

Differential Diagnosis

■ Trabecular carcinoid (see page 357).

References

Matias-Guiu X, Forteza J, Prat J. Mixed strumal and mucinous carcinoid tumor of the ovary. Int J Gynecol Pathol 14:179–183, 1995.

Motoyama T, Katayama Y, Watanabe H, et al. Functioning ovarian carcinoids induce severe constipation. Cancer 70:513–518, 1992.

Robboy SJ, Scully RE. Strumal carcinoid of the ovary: an analysis of 50 cases of a distinctive tumor composed of thyroid tissue and carcinoid. Cancer 46:2019–2034, 1980.

Snyder RR, Tavassoli FA. Ovarian strumal carcinoid: immunohistochemical, ultrastructural, and clinicopathologic observations. Int J Gynecol Pathol 5:187–201, 1986.

Sporrong B, Falkmer S, Robboy SJ, et al. Neurohormonal peptides in ovarian carcinoids: an immunohistochemical study of 81 primary carcinoids and of intraovarian metastases from six mid-gut carcinoids. Cancer 49:68–74, 1982.

Stagno PA, Petras RE, Hart WR. Strumal carcinoids of the ovary: an immunohistologic and ultrastructural study. Arch Pathol Lab Med 111:440–446, 1987.

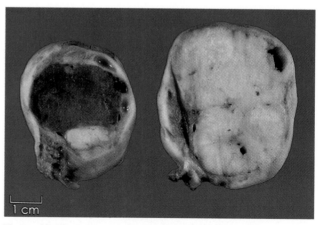

Figure 15–29. Strumal carcinoid tumor (sectioned surface). Strumal (*brown area*) and carcinoid (*white areas*) components are seen.

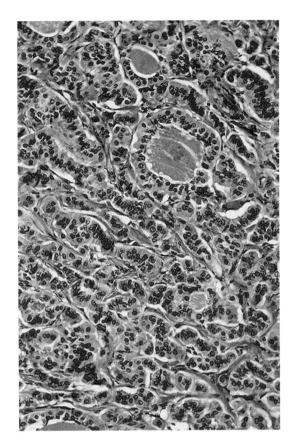

Figure 15–30. Strumal carcinoid tumor. Most of the tumor consists of trabecular carcinoid, with only occasional thyroid follicles.

Mucinous Carcinoid

Clinical Features

- Mucinous carcinoids are rare compared with other ovarian carcinoid tumors.
- The age of the patients and the clinical presentation are similar to those of patients with other types of ovarian carcinoid tumors.

Pathologic Features

- Mucinous carcinoids resemble other ovarian carcinoid tumors on gross examination. They occur in pure form or are associated with a mature teratoma or an epidermoid cyst.
- Microscopic examination reveals small nests scattered through a scanty to abundant fibrous stroma that may contain pools of mucin.
- The nests are composed of various numbers of goblet cells and argyrophil cells, some of which may also be argentaffinic, with uniform, small, and round to oval nuclei.
- The tumors cells are variably immunoreactive for chromogranin, CEA, pancreatic polypeptide, serotonin, and gastrin.

Differential Diagnosis

- Mucinous carcinoid tumors metastatic from the appendix or elsewhere. These tumors are differentiated by the operative and pathologic criteria used for distinguishing metastatic from primary insular carcinoids (page 356). If an ovarian mucinous carcinoid is diagnosed intraoperatively, the appendix should be removed to exclude a primary appendiceal mucinous carcinoid tumor.
- Mucinous carcinomas with argentaffin cells. These tumors may be otherwise typical mucinous tumors with neuroendocrine cells (but without the distinctive nests of mucinous carcinoid) or tumors that resemble a Kru-

kenberg tumor. Rare tumors may be in part mucinous carcinoid and in part mucinous carcinoma, and the various components should be separately diagnosed.

References

Alenghat E, Okagaki T, Talerman A. Primary mucinous carcinoid tumor of the ovary. Cancer 58:777–783, 1986.
Wolpert HR, Fuller AF, Bell DA. Primary mucinous carcinoid tumor of the ovary: a case report. Int J Gynecol Pathol 8:156–162, 1989.

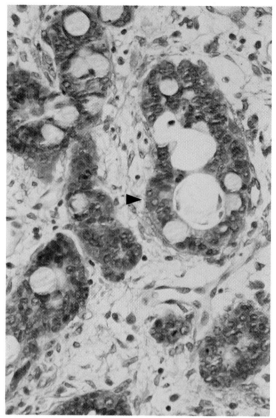

Figure 15–31. Mucinous carcinoid tumor. Notice the goblet cells and cells with red, subnuclear argentaffin granules (*arrowhead*).

Rare Ovarian Carcinoid Tumors

■ These ovarian carcinoid tumors include those of the spindle cell type, resembling their pulmonary counterparts, and those with nonspecific, sometimes poorly differentiated patterns that may merge morphologically with ovarian small cell carcinomas of the pulmonary type.

Reference

Czernobilsky B, Segal M, Dgani R. Primary ovarian carcinoid with marked heterogeneity of microscopic features. Cancer 54:585–589, 1984.

Neuroectodermal Tumors

Clinical and Pathologic Features

■ Neuroectodermal tumors are rare, closely resemble neoplasms of the central nervous system, and occur over a wide age range. The presenting symptoms are usually those of a pelvic mass. More than one half of the patients have extraovarian spread, usually in the form of peritoneal implants at laparotomy.

■ The gross appearance varies from cystic to solid and the maximal dimension from 4 to 20 cm (mean, 14 cm). Intracystic or surface papillary excrescences are present in some cases. Rare tumors are bilateral; in several other cases, the opposite ovary has contained a dermoid cyst.

■ The neoplastic tissue is typically soft and gray-tan to gray-pink to yellow, often with areas of hemorrhage and necrosis.

■ The tumors are categorized as differentiated (ependymomas), primitive (resembling neuroblastoma, medulloepithelioma, medulloblastoma, or ependymoblastoma), and anaplastic (resembling glioblastoma multiforme).

■ Immunoreactivity for glial fibrillary acidic protein (GFAP) is identified in some cases. One primitive tumor stained for MIC2 protein (CD 99) and contained a chromosomal translocation specific for primitive neuroectodermal tumor/Ewing's sarcoma and EWS/FLI-1 chimeric RNA.

Differential Diagnosis

- Immature teratomas. These tumors, in contrast to neuroectodermal tumors, usually show a greater spectrum and diversity of neuroepithelial differentiation and an extensive and varied admixture of endodermal, mesodermal, and other ectodermal tissues, often in an orderly arrangement and without overgrowth of the neuroepithelial elements.
- Serous and endometrioid borderline tumors and carcinomas, sex cord–stromal tumors (SLCTs and GCTs), and ovarian wolffian tumors. Ependymomas are distinguished from these tumors by the characteristic long fibrillary cytoplasmic processes, the perivascular rosettes, and GFAP immunoreactivity.
- Other small cell malignant ovarian tumors, including small cell carcinoma of the hypercalcemic type, malignant lymphoma and leukemia, primary and metastatic small cell carcinoma of the neuroendocrine type, metastatic melanoma, metastatic round cell sarcomas, metastatic neuroblastoma, and the desmoplastic small round cell tumor.
  - Clinical information, thorough sampling of the tumor, and immunohistochemical staining, especially for GFAP, facilitate the differential diagnosis to various degrees in individual cases.

Behavior

- Ependymomas are characterized by an indolent behavior even when extraovarian spread has occurred. Only one tumor, which was stage III, has been fatal.
- The primitive and anaplastic tumors have a generally poor prognosis if extraovarian spread has occurred.

References

Guerrieri C, Jarlsfelt I. Ependymoma of the ovary: a case report with immunohistochemical, ultrastructural, and DNA cytometric findings, as well as histogenetic considerations. Am J Surg Pathol 17:623–632, 1993.

Kawauchi S, Fukuda T, Miyamoto S, et al. Peripheral primitive neuroectodermal tumor of the ovary confirmed by CD99 immunostaining, karyotypic analysis, and RT-PCR for EWS/FLI-1 chimeric mRNA. Am J Surg Pathol 22:1417–1422, 1998.

Kleinman GM, Young RH, Scully RE. Primary ovarian neuroectodermal tumors: a report of 25 cases. Am J Surg Pathol 17:764–778, 1993.

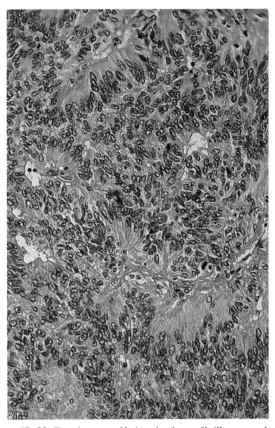

Figure 15–32. Ependymoma. Notice the long, fibrillary cytoplasmic processes abutting the fibrous tissue. The cells were immunoreactive for glial fibrillary acidic protein.

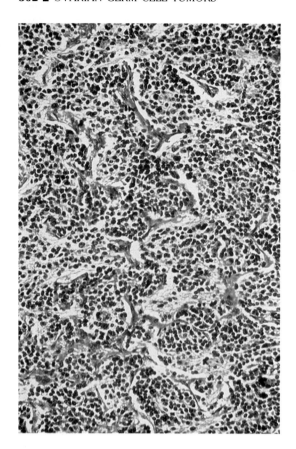

Figure 15–33. Primitive neuroectodermal tumor resembling a neuroblastoma.

Sebaceous Tumors

■ Sebaceous tumors are rare and occur over a wide age range (31 to 79 years). They usually arise within a dermoid cyst. The symptoms are usually those caused by a pelvic mass.

■ Gross examination typically reveals a predominantly cystic tumor, with solid, yellow to tan, nodular or papillary masses projecting into the lumen. All of the tumors have been unilateral, although the opposite ovary may contain a dermoid cyst.

■ The tumors microscopically resemble cutaneous sebaceous neoplasms, including sebaceous adenoma, basal cell carcinoma with sebaceous differentiation, and sebaceous carcinoma. Abundant eosinophilic necrobiotic material with ghost outlines of mature sebaceous cells is a common finding.

■ Only one tumor, a basal cell carcinoma with sebaceous differentiation, recurred.

References

Chumas JC, Scully RE. Sebaceous tumors arising in ovarian dermoid cysts. Int J Gynecol Pathol 10:356–363, 1991.

Papadopoulos AJ, Ahmed H, Pakarian FB, et al. Sebaceous carcinoma arising within an ovarian cystic mature teratoma. Int J Gynecol Cancer 5:76–79, 1995.

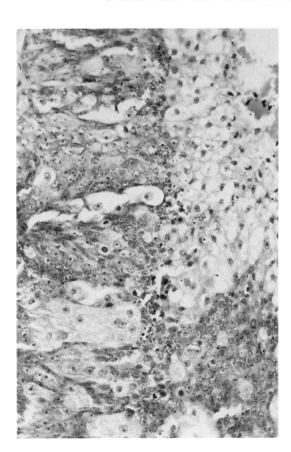

Figure 15–34. Sebaceous carcinoma.

Other Monodermal Teratomas

- This category includes rare ovarian tumors resembling retinal anlage tumor, cysts lined predominantly or exclusively by mature glial tissue, ependymal epithelium, respiratory epithelium, or melanotic epithelium.
- Epidermoid cysts, lined exclusively by mature squamous epithelium may be monodermal teratomas but are more likely of surface epithelial origin (page 334).

References

Anderson MC, McDicken IW. Melanotic cyst of the ovary. J Obstet Gynecol Br Commonw 78:1047–1049, 1971.

Clement PB, Dimmick JE. Endodermal variant of mature cystic teratoma of the ovary: report of a case. Cancer 43:383–385, 1979.

Fogt F, Vortmeyer AO, Ahn G, et al. Neural cyst of the ovary with central nervous system microvasculature. Histopathology 24:477–480, 1994.

King ME, Mouradian JA, Micha JP, et al. Immature teratoma of the ovary with predominant malignant retinal anlage component: a parthenogenically derived tumor. Am J Surg Pathol 9:221–231, 1985.

Nogales FF, Silverberg SG. Epidermoid cysts of the ovary: a report of five cases with histogenetic considerations and ultrastructural findings. Am J Obstet Gynecol 124:523–528, 1976.

Tiltman AJ. Ependymal cyst of the ovary. S Afr Med J 68:424–425, 1985.

Young RH, Prat J, Scully RE. Epidermoid cyst of the ovary: a report of three cases with comments on histogenesis. Am J Clin Pathol 73:272–276, 1980.

CHAPTER 16

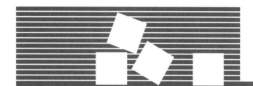

Sex Cord–Stromal and Steroid Cell Tumors

SEX CORD–STROMAL TUMORS

- Sex cord–stromal tumors, which account for 6% of all primary ovarian tumors, are classified on the basis of the constituent cell types (Table 16–1): granulosa cells, theca cells, and their luteinized derivatives, Sertoli cells, Leydig cells, and fibroblasts.

Granulosa Cell Tumors

- Granulosa cell tumors (GCTs) account for 12% of sex cord–stromal tumors and for most clinically malignant examples.

Adult Granulosa Cell Tumor

General Features

- Adult granulosa cell tumors (AGCTs), which account for 1% to 2% of all ovarian tumors and 95% of all GCTs, occur at all ages but peak between 50 and 55 years.
- The usual presentation is related to an adnexal mass, endocrine manifestations, or both. Acute abdominal symptoms from tumor rupture and hemoperitoneum occur in 10% of cases.
- This is the most common ovarian tumor with estrogenic manifestations, which include menometrorrhagia, postmenopausal bleeding, amenorrhea, isosexual pseudoprecocity, endometrial hyperplasia, and in fewer than 5% of cases, endometrial adenocarcinoma, which is almost always a low-grade endometrioid adenocarcinoma.
- Progestational or androgenic manifestations occur rarely; a disproportionate number of androgenic GCTs have been cystic.
- Eighty percent to 90% of the tumors are stage I. The remainder are mostly stage II, but rare tumors are stage III.

Gross Features

- AGCTs have a mean diameter of 12 cm. More than 95% of the tumors are unilateral, and 10% to 15%

rupture preoperatively. The sectioned surfaces are typically solid and cystic, with fluid- or blood-filled cysts separated by solid yellow to white, soft to firm tissue.
- Less common gross appearances include an entirely solid, white to yellow sectioned surface, often with focal hemorrhage and occasionally with areas of necrosis, or multilocular or unilocular, fluid-filled, usually thin-walled cysts.

Typical Microscopic Features

- Granulosa cells are arranged in a wide variety of patterns, frequently admixed, including solid (diffuse), trabecular, insular, follicular, watered silk, and gyriform.
  - Microfollicular: numerous small cavities (Call-Exner bodies) that may contain eosinophilic fluid, degenerating nuclei, hyalinized basement membrane material, or rarely, basophilic fluid
  - Macrofollicular: cysts lined by well-differentiated granulosa cells and occasionally by an outer layer of theca cells
  - Watered-silk (moiré-silk) and gyriform: undulating parallel rows and zigzag cords of granulosa cells, respectively
- Granulosa cells usually have scanty cytoplasm and pale, uniform, angular to oval, often grooved nuclei arranged haphazardly in relation to one another and to the Call-Exner bodies.
- The mitotic rate is variable but less than 3 mitotic figures (MF) per 10 high-power-fields (HPF) in 75% of cases. A diagnosis of GCT should be made with caution in the presence of numerous or abnormal mitotic figures.
- The stromal component is usually scanty but occasionally extensive and may be fibromatous or fibrous but more commonly contains theca externa–like cells or occasionally contains luteinized theca interna–like cells. Granulosa cells usually lack surrounding reticulin, whereas reticulin invests theca cells individually or in small groups.
- The tumor cells are usually immunoreactive for vi-

364

Table 16–1

MODIFIED WORLD HEALTH ORGANIZATION
CLASSIFICATION OF SEX CORD–STROMAL AND
STEROID CELL TUMORS OF THE OVARY

Granulosa–Stromal Cell tumors
  Granulosa cell tumor
    Adult
    Juvenile
  Tumors in the thecoma–fibroma group
    Thecoma
      Typical
      Luteinized*
    Fibroma
    Cellular fibroma
    Fibrosarcoma
    Stromal tumor with minor sex cord elements
    Sclerosing stromal tumor
    Unclassified
    Others†
Sertoli–Stromal Cell Tumors
  Well differentiated
    Sertoli cell tumor
    Sertoli–Leydig cell tumor
  Of intermediate differentiation
    Variant—with heterologous elements (specify type)
  Poorly differentiated (sarcomatoid)
    Variant—with heterologous elements (specify type)
  Retiform
    Variant—with heterologous elements (specify type)
  Sex cord tumor with annular tubules
  Gynandroblastoma
  Unclassified
Steroid (Lipid) Cell Tumors
  Stromal luteoma
  Leydig cell tumor
    Hilus cell tumor
    Leydig cell tumor, nonhilar type
  Unclassified (not otherwise specified)

*A rare tumor has the features of luteinized thecoma and Reinke crystals in the steroid cell component. This tumor has been called stromal-Leydig cell tumor.
†This category includes the rare signet-ring cell stromal tumor and the myxoma.

mentin, cytokeratin (punctate pattern), S-100 protein, smooth muscle actin, and inhibin, but they lack staining for epithelial membrane antigen (EMA). The stromal component may be immunoreactive for desmin.

Uncommon or Rare Features

- Hollow or solid tubular patterns indistinguishable from those of well-differentiated Sertoli cell tumors may be found. If more than 10% of the tumor is tubular, a diagnosis of gynandroblastoma is warranted (see page 383).
- Occasional tumors focally contain luteinized granulosa cells with moderate to abundant eosinophilic cytoplasm and rounded nuclei with a prominent nucleolus; these cells predominate in 2% of tumors.
- Pregnancy-related changes may be found in the last trimester of pregnancy and include prominent edema and extensive luteinization, findings that may obscure the usual features of the tumor.
- Cells with bizarre, enlarged hyperchromatic nuclei, in-

cluding multinucleated forms, occur in 2% of cases. Such cells are typically focal but may be numerous and divert attention from more characteristic areas.
- Rare tumors exhibit hepatic cell differentiation (distinguished from luteinized or Leydig cells by inhibin negativity), sarcomatous transformation, or areas resembling a poorly differentiated carcinoma with highly atypical cells.

Differential Diagnosis

- Undifferentiated carcinoma (page 336).
- Small cell carcinoma of the hypercalcemic type. Features favoring or diagnostic of this tumor include hypercalcemia, absent estrogenic manifestations, hyperchromatic nuclei with lack of grooves, a high mitotic rate, absence of inhibin immunoreactivity, and lack of characteristic patterns of the AGCT.
- Endometrioid stromal sarcoma (page 324).
- Thecomas and cellular fibromas. Cellular fibromas have constituent cells that resemble fibroblasts, and thecomas have constituent cells with appreciable amounts of pale, lipid-rich cytoplasm. These tumors, in contrast to diffuse AGCTs, have a dense pericellular reticulum.
- Large, solitary, luteinized follicle cyst of pregnancy and the puerperium. This cyst is characterized, in contrast to cystic AGCTs, by large, uniformly luteinized cells, some of which contain large, bizarre nuclei.
- Endometrioid carcinomas with sex cord–like patterns (page 315).
- Steroid cell tumor. The diagnosis of luteinized AGCT is made by the focal presence of areas with the architectural and cytologic features of typical (i.e., nonluteinized) AGCT.
- Carcinoid tumors. Features favoring or diagnostic of carcinoid tumor include cells with abundant cytoplasm surrounding lumens containing densely eosinophilic, sometimes calcified secretion, nongrooved nuclei with coarse chromatin, argentaffinic cytoplasm, and chromogranin positivity.
- Gonadoblastomas and sex cord tumors with annular tubules (SCTATs).
  - Hyaline deposits in these tumors are typically larger than Call-Exner bodies, are often calcified, and often merge with thickened basement membranes. Gonadoblastomas contain germ cells and usually arise in the background of intersex.
  - SCTATs typically exhibit prominent ring-shaped simple and complex tubules, and if bilateral or microscopic in size, they are usually associated with the Peutz-Jeghers syndrome.
- Metastatic malignant melanoma. Features favoring or establishing this diagnosis include the history of an extraovarian melanoma, melanin pigment, and HMB-45 immunoreactivity. Obviously malignant nuclear features and a high mitotic rate favor a diagnosis of melanoma, although these features are not present in every case.
- Metastatic breast carcinomas (especially the lobular type). This tumor is distinguished from AGCT by the absence of the typical cytologic features of granulosa

cells, the presence of intracellular mucin, and immunoreactivity for EMA and gross cystic disease fluid protein.

Behavior

- AGCTs may extend beyond the ovary or recur after apparently complete removal, usually within the pelvis and lower abdomen. Distant metastases are rare.
- Recurrences appear more than 5 years after oophorectomy in one half of the cases that recur. Rarely, the interval to first recurrence is several decades. The serum inhibin level may be helpful in detecting recurrent disease.
- The 10-year survival figures in the literature are highly variable (<60% to >90%). Series with poor survival rates are suspect for the inclusion of cases that are not AGCTs by current criteria. There is typically a progressive decline in survival after longer follow-up periods.

Prognostic Factors

- The 10-year survival for stage I tumors is 86% to 96%, compared with 26% to 49% for higher-stage tumors.
- The 25-year survival for intact stage I tumors is 86%, compared with 60% for ruptured stage I tumors.
- Increasing tumor size is associated with a decreased survival in some series, but these differences are not significant if corrected for stage.
- Histologic pattern, grade, mitotic activity, and ploidy have not been consistently shown to have prognostic significance in stage I tumors.
- There is no evidence that tumors with bizarre nuclei are associated with a worse prognosis.

References

Ahmed R, Young RH, Scully RE. Adult granulosa cell tumor of the ovary with foci of hepatic-cell differentiation: a report of four cases and comparison with two cases of granulosa cell tumor with Leydig cells. Am J Surg Pathol 23:1089–1093, 1999.

Bjorkholm E, Silfversward C. Prognostic factors in granulosa cell tumors. Gynecol Oncol 11:261–274, 1981.

Costa MJ, Ames PF, Walls J, Roth LM. Inhibin immunohistochemistry applied to ovarian neoplasms: a novel, effective, diagnostic tool. Hum Pathol 28:1247–1254, 1997.

Costa MJ, DeRose PB, Roth LM, et al. Immunohistochemical phenotype of ovarian granulosa cell tumors: absence of epithelial membrane antigen has diagnostic value. Hum Pathol 25:60–66, 1994.

Fox H, Agrawal K, Langley FA. A clinicopathological study of 92 cases of granulosa cell tumor of the ovary with special reference to the factors influencing prognosis. Cancer 35:231–241, 1975.

Kommoss F, Oliva E, Bhan A, et al Inhibin expression in ovarian neoplasms. Mod Pathol 11:656–664, 1998.

Malmstrom H, Högberg T, Bjorn R, Simonsen E. Granulosa cell tumors of the ovary: prognostic factors and outcome. Gynecol Oncol 52:50–55, 1994.

Nakashima N, Young RH, Scully RE. Androgenic granulosa cell tumors of the ovary: a clinicopathological analysis of seventeen cases and review of the literature. Arch Pathol Lab Med 108:786–791, 1984.

Pelkey TJ, Frierson HF Jr, Mills SE, Stoler MH. The diagnostic utility of inhibin staining in ovarian neoplasms. Int J Gynecol Pathol 17:97–105, 1998.

Riopel MA, Perlman EJ, Seidman JD Jr, et al. Inhibin and epithelial membrane antigen immunohistochemistry assist in the diagnosis of sex cord–stromal tumors and provide clues to the histogenesis of hypercalcemic small cell carcinomas. Int J Gynecol Pathol 17:46–53, 1998.

Rishi M, Howard LN, Bratthauer GL, Tavassoli FA. Use of monoclonal antibody against human inhibin as a marker for sex cord–stromal tumors of the ovary. Am J Surg Pathol 21:583–589, 1997.

Stenwig J, Hazekamp JT, Beecham JB. Granulosa cell tumors of the ovary: a clinicopathological study of 118 cases with long-term follow-up. Gynecol Oncol 7:136–152, 1979.

Susil BJ. Sumithran E. Sarcomatous change in granulosa cell tumor. Hum Pathol 18:397–399, 1987.

Young RH, Dudley AG, Scully RE. Granulosa cell, Sertoli-Leydig cell and unclassified sex cord–stromal tumors associated with pregnancy: a clinicopathological analysis of thirty-six cases. Gynecol Oncol 18:181–205, 1984.

Young RH, Oliva E, Scully RE. Luteinized adult granulosa cell tumors of the ovary: a report of four cases. Int J Gynecol Pathol 13:302–310, 1994.

Young RH, Scully RE. Ovarian sex cord–stromal tumors with bizarre nuclei: a clinicopathologic analysis seventeen cases. Int J Gynecol Pathol 1:325–335, 1983.

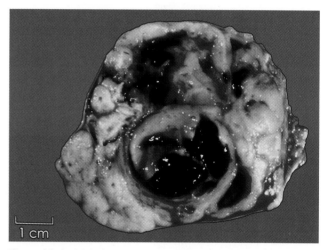

Figure 16–1. Adult-type granulosa cell tumor (sectioned surface). Notice the intracystic hemorrhage.

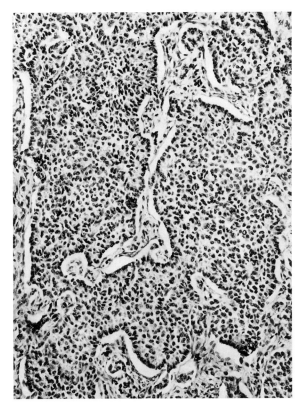

Figure 16–2. Adult-type granulosa cell tumor. Sheets and broad columns of cells are separated by a scanty fibrous stroma.

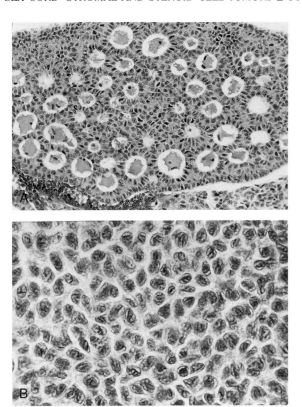

Figure 16–4. Adult-type granulosa cell tumor. *A,* A microfollicular pattern with numerous Call-Exner bodies. *B,* The neoplastic cells have scanty cytoplasm and uniform, grooved nuclei.

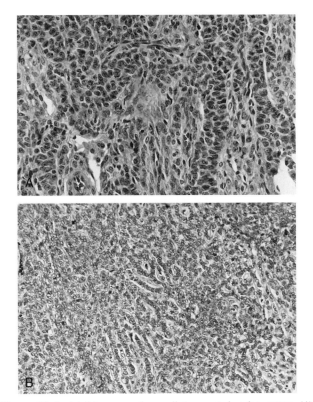

Figure 16–3. Adult-type granulosa cell tumor: trabecular pattern (*A*) and cord-like pattern (*B*).

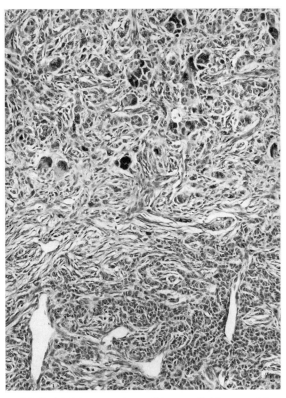

Figure 16–5. Adult-type granulosa cell tumor with bizarre nuclei.

Juvenile Granulosa Cell Tumor

General Features

- Almost all juvenile granulosa cell tumors (JGCTs) occur in the first 3 decades of life. The presentation in postpubertal cases includes abdominal pain or swelling, menstrual irregularities, amenorrhea, or combinations thereof. Isosexual pseudoprecocity occurs in 80% of prepubertal patients.
- Uncommon manifestations include acute abdominal symptoms caused by tumor rupture and hemoperitoneum, androgenic manifestations, and an occasional association with Ollier's disease (enchondromatosis) and Maffucci's syndrome (enchondromatosis and hemangiomatosis).
- Uncommon findings at operation include tumor rupture (10% of cases), ascites (10% of cases), and extraovarian spread (2% of cases) that is usually confined to the pelvis.

Pathologic Features

- The gross features are similar to those of AGCTs. The maximal tumor dimensions have ranged from 3 to 32 cm (mean, 12.5 cm). Only 2% of tumors are bilateral.
- The most common pattern is that of sheets of cells interrupted by occasional follicles of variable size and shape with luminal eosinophilic to basophilic fluid that may be mucicarminophilic. A uniformly solid ("afollicular") pattern is occasionally encountered.
- The follicles are lined by granulosa cells, sometimes with an outer mantle of theca cells, but more commonly, the lining granulosa cells blend into the intervening diffusely cellular areas.
- Granulosa cells typically predominate, but an admixture of granulosa and theca cells or a predominance of theca cells, including foci resembling typical thecoma, are encountered rarely.
- The granulosa cells typically have abundant eosinophilic or vacuolated (luteinized) cytoplasm and generally rounded, nongrooved, euchromatic or hyperchromatic nuclei that have minimal to severe nuclear atypicality, with the latter found in about 5% of cases.
- The theca cells have moderate to large amounts of intracytoplasmic lipid, may be spindle shaped and may have hyperchromatic nuclei.
- Solid areas occasionally contain nodules that may be separated by fibrothecomatous septa, or occasionally the granulosa cells lie in clusters in a fibrous stroma or are scattered within a basophilic fluid.
- Small foci more characteristic of AGCT occur in some cases.
- The neoplastic cells are typically immunoreactive for inhibin.

Differential Diagnosis

- AGCT. Features favoring JGCT include follicles that are irregular in size and shape, numerous luteinized cells, rounded hyperchromatic nuclei that lack grooves, and an absence of Call-Exner bodies.
- Yolk sac tumor (YST) or embryonal carcinoma (versus JGCT with nuclear atypia). Features favoring or diagnostic of these tumors include highly primitive nuclei, absence of follicles, Schiller-Duval bodies (in YSTs), syncytiotrophoblastic elements, positivity for alpha-fetoprotein (AFP) or human chorionic gonadotropin (hCG), and association with other germ cell elements, such as a dermoid cyst.
- Thecoma (versus JGCTs with absent or rare follicles). Tissues should be sampled well to demonstrate follicles or cellular cluster of granulosa cells. Reticulin stains help identify the focal presence of granulosa cells (sparse or absent reticulin). An age younger than 30 years of age and more than slight mitotic activity favor JGCT.
- Steroid cell tumor and pregnancy luteoma (the latter may have follicle-like spaces). These lesions, unlike JGCTs, have patterns and cytologic features that tend to be uniform throughout. The pregnancy luteoma is frequently multiple, bilateral, or both.
- Clear cell, undifferentiated, and transitional cell carcinomas. These carcinomas are exceedingly rare in the age group in which JGCTs almost always occur, and although focally they may exhibit features that overlap with JGCTs, they lack the characteristic features of JGCTs previously described.
- Small cell carcinoma of the hypercalcemic type. Features favoring or diagnostic of small cell carcinoma include hypercalcemia, an absence of estrogenic manifestations, cells with scanty cytoplasm, absence of theca cells, immunoreactivity for EMA, and absent immunoreactivity for inhibin.
- Metastatic malignant melanoma. Features favoring or diagnostic of metastatic melanoma include an age older than 20 years, a history of a primary melanoma, bilaterality, and immunoreactivity for HMB-45.

Behavior

- The survival rate for patients with stage I tumors is 97%. Higher-stage tumors are often fatal; recurrences in these cases almost always occur within the first 3 postoperative years.
- The presence or absence of rupture, the mitotic rate, the degree of nuclear atypicality, DNA ploidy, and S-phase fraction have not been prognostically useful for stage I tumors.

References

Biscotti CV, Hart WR. Juvenile granulosa cell tumors of the ovary. Arch Pathol Lab Med 113:40–46, 1989.

Lack EE, Perez-Atayde AR, Murthy ASK, et al. Granulosa theca cell tumors in premenarchal girls: a clinical and pathological study of 10 cases. Cancer 48:1846–1854, 1981.

Matias-Guiu X, Pons C, Prat J. Mullerian inhibiting substance, alpha-inhibin, and CD99 expression in sex cord stromal tumors and endometrioid ovarian carcinomas resembling sex cord–stromal tumors. Hum Pathol 29:840–845, 1998.

Tanaka Y, Sasaki Y, Nishihura H, et al. Ovarian juvenile granulosa cell tumor associated with Maffucci's syndrome. Am J Clin Pathol 97: 523–527, 1992.

Vassal G, Flamant F, Caillaud JM, et al. Juvenile granulosa cell tumor of the ovary in children: a clinical study of 15 cases. J Clin Oncol 6: 990–995, 1988.

Young RH, Dickersin GR, Scully RE. Juvenile granulosa cell tumor of the ovary: a clinicopathologic analysis of 125 cases. Am J Surg Pathol 8:575–596, 1984.

Zaloudek C, Norris HJ. Granulosa tumors of the ovary in children: a clinical and pathologic study of 32 cases. Am J Surg Pathol 6:503–512, 1982.

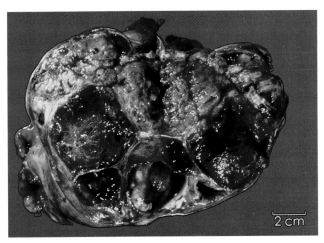

Figure 16–6. Juvenile granulosa cell tumor (sectioned surface).

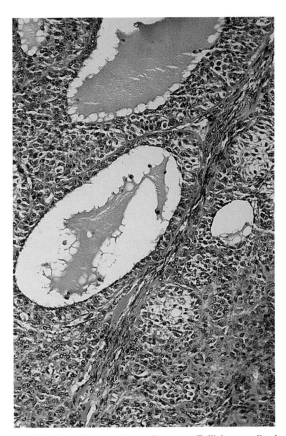

Figure 16–8. Juvenile granulosa cell tumor. Follicles are lined and separated by luteinized cells with clear to eosinophilic cytoplasm.

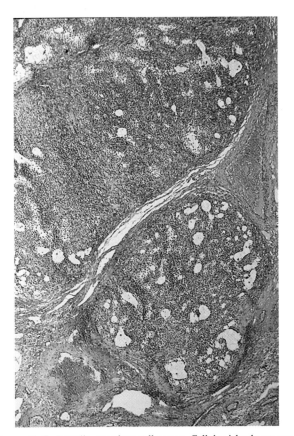

Figure 16–7. Juvenile granulosa cell tumor. Cellular islands are punctured by irregular follicles.

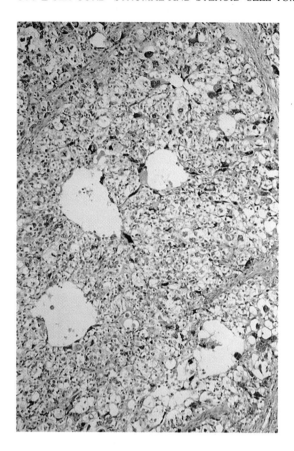

Figure 16–9. Juvenile granulosa cell tumor. Notice the nuclear pleomorphism. Numerous mitotic figures are also present but not clearly seen at this magnification.

Tumors in the Thecoma-Fibroma Group

Thecoma

Clinical Features of Typical Thecomas

- Thecomas, which are about one third as common as granulosa cell tumors, typically occur in postmenopausal women (mean age, 63 years). Only 10% occur before the age of 30 years, and the tumors are rare before puberty. Extensively calcified thecomas tend to occur in young women.
- Thecomas are often associated with estrogenic changes, including uterine bleeding, which occurs in 60% of postmenopausal women with thecomas.
- Twenty percent of postmenopausal women with thecomas have an associated endometrial adenocarcinoma or rarely have a müllerian mixed tumor or endometrial stromal sarcoma.

Clinical Features of Luteinized Thecomas

- Luteinized thecomas (LTs) occur in a younger age group than typical thecomas. Although most common in women older than 50 years of age, 30% occur in those younger than 30 years.
- LTs are associated with a lower frequency of estrogenic changes (50%) and a higher frequency of androgenic changes (11%) than typical thecomas.
- LTs in which the steroid-type cells contain crystals of Reinke are referred to as *stromal-Leydig cell tumors;* 50% of such tumors are virilizing.
- LTs with distinctive features have a rare association with sclerosing peritonitis (page 445).

Pathologic Features

- Most thecomas are 5 to 10 cm in maximal dimension. Only 3% are bilateral.
- The sectioned surfaces are typically solid and yellow or are occasionally predominantly white with only focal tinges of yellow. Secondary changes in some cases include cysts, hemorrhage, necrosis, and focal calcification. Rare tumors are extensively calcified.
- Microscopic examination reveals sheets of oval or rounded cells will ill-defined borders, usually abundant and dense to vacuolated or pale, lipid-rich cytoplasm,

and round to spindle-shaped nuclei with usually little or no atypia.

- Rare tumors contain large bizarre nuclei with a degenerative appearance. Mitotic figures are absent or infrequent in these tumors. However, rare typical or luteinized thecomas with nuclear atypicality and mitotic activity have metastasized.
- *Thecoma with minor sex cord elements* refers to tumors in which granulosa cells, indifferent sex cord–type cells, or sertoliform tubules account for less than 10% of the tumor. This designation is appropriate because the appearance and behavior of these tumors is much more like that of a thecoma than a sex cord tumor.
- Individual tumor cells are usually surrounded by reticulin fibrils. The stroma often contains conspicuous hyaline plaques and may exhibit calcification.
- Luteinized thecomas contain single cells, nests, or rarely, large nodules of luteinized cells. In such cases, the background cells are often purely fibroblastic rather than thecomatous.
- The neoplastic cells are typically immunoreactive for inhibin.

Differential Diagnosis

- Fibromas. Because the distinction between thecomas and fibromas is imprecise and arbitrary, the designation *fibrothecoma* has been used. We prefer to avoid this term, regarding the tumor as a fibroma in the absence of appreciable numbers of the typical large, lipid-laden cells of thecoma.
- Granulosa cell tumors (page 365).
- Steroid cell tumor (versus luteinized thecoma). A diagnosis of steroid cell tumor is appropriate when an associated fibromatous or thecomatous component accounts for less than 10% of the tumor.
- Stromal hyperthecosis (versus luteinized thecoma). This lesion is almost always bilateral, and in addition to lutein cells, the background cells are small stromal cells with minimal collagen, in contrast to the plump, lipid-laden theca cells or large spindle cells of a luteinized thecoma.
- Pregnancy luteomas (versus luteinized thecoma). Pregnancy luteomas, unlike thecomas, are multiple in one half of the cases, contain little or no lipid, and lack a background of fibroma or typical thecoma.

References

Bjorkholm E, Silfversward C. Theca-cell tumors: clinical features and prognosis. Acta Radiol Oncol Radiat Phys Biol 19:241–244, 1980.

Costa MJ, Ames PF, Walls J, Roth LM. Inhibin immunohistochemistry applied to ovarian neoplasms: a novel, effective, diagnostic tool. Hum Pathol 28:1247–1254, 1997.

Kommoss F, Oliva E, Bhan A, et al. Inhibin expression in ovarian neoplasms. Mod Pathol 11:656–664, 1998.

Roth LM, Sternberg WH. Partly luteinized theca cell tumor of the ovary. Cancer 51:1697–1704, 1983.

Sternberg WH, Roth LM. Ovarian stromal tumors containing Leydig cells. 1. Stromal-Leydig cell tumor and non-neoplastic transformation of ovarian stroma to Leydig cells. Cancer 32:940–951, 1973.

Waxman M, Vuletin JC, Urcuyo R, Belling CG. Ovarian low-grade stromal sarcoma with thecomatous features: a critical reappraisal of the so-called "malignant thecoma." Cancer 44:2206–2217, 1979.

Young RH, Clement PB, Scully RE. Calcified thecomas in young women: a report of four cases. Int J Gynecol Pathol 7:343–350, 1988.

Young RH, Scully RE. Ovarian sex-cord–stromal tumors with bizarre nuclei: a clinicopathologic analysis of seventeen cases. Int J Gynecol Pathol 1:325–335, 1983.

Young RH, Scully RE. Ovarian stromal tumors with minor sex cord elements: a report of seven cases. Int J Gynecol Pathol 2:227–234, 1983.

Zhang J, Young RH, Arseneau J, Scully RE. Ovarian stromal tumors containing lutein or Leydig cells (luteinized thecomas and stromal Leydig cell tumors): a clinicopathological analysis of fifty cases. Int J Gynecol Pathol 1:270–285, 1982.

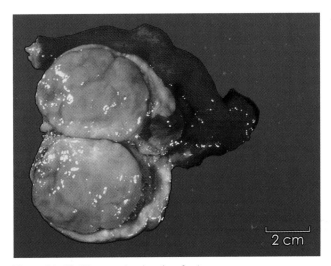

Figure 16–10. Thecoma (sectioned surface).

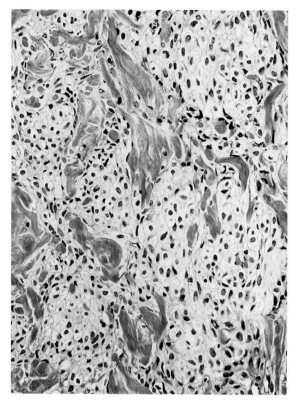

Figure 16–11. Thecoma. The cells have abundant, pale (lipid-rich) cytoplasm and are focally separated by hyaline plaques.

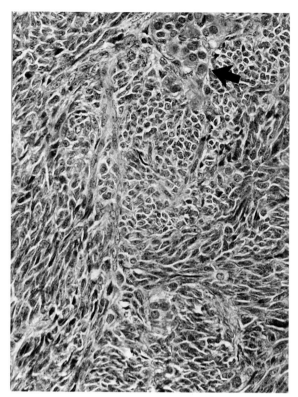

Figure 16–12. Luteinized thecoma. Small nests (*arrow*) and singly disposed luteinized cells lie within intersecting fascicles of spindled cells.

Luteinized Thecoma With Sclerosing Peritonitis

■ Eighteen reported cases of an ovarian lesion, typically interpreted as a variant of luteinized thecoma, have been enigmatically associated with a peritoneal lesion that has been usually interpreted as sclerosing peritonitis (the peritoneal lesion is discussed in Chapter 20).

■ In some cases, the ovarian lesions have been interpreted as ovarian edema and stromal hyperthecosis, fibromatosis, or sarcoma-like nodules, and the peritoneal lesions as fibroma-like proliferations, fibromatosis, or retractile mesenteritis.

■ Twelve patients were 30 years of age or younger, and only two were older than 50 years of age. The usual presentation was that of abdominal swelling from ascites and adnexal masses. Some patients presented with symptoms of bowel obstruction.

■ Gross examination has revealed bilateral ovarian tumors in most cases, with an appearance ranging from large masses to normal-sized or slightly enlarged ovaries with prominent nodular or cerebriform surfaces. The sectioned surfaces in some tumors have edematous areas and cysts.

■ The tumors are typically composed of a dense proliferation of spindle cells with foci of luteinized cells that are typically smaller than those in the usual luteinized thecoma. The spindle cells exhibit striking mitotic activity in some tumors. Edema with microcyst formation occurs in some cases.

■ Postoperative intermittent small bowel obstruction occurred in some cases. Several patients have died of complications related to the peritoneal lesions, but there has been no evidence of recurrence or metastasis of the ovarian lesions.

■ Differential diagnosis of this variant of luteinized thecoma includes a number of lesions, none of which are associated with sclerosing peritonitis:

• Stromal hyperthecosis. Differences include absence of ascites, absence of marked ovarian enlargement, and absence of mitotic activity.

• Massive edema and fibromatosis. These are diffusely hypocellular lesions with marked edema or collagen deposition.

- Edematous cellular fibromas and sclerosing stromal tumors (SSTs). These tumors are typically unilateral, are unassociated with peritonitis, generally are mitotically inactive, and in the case of SSTs, have other distinctive features (page 375).

References

Clement PB, Young RH, Hanna W, Scully RE. Sclerosing peritonitis associated with luteinized thecomas of the ovary: a clinicopathological analysis of six cases. Am J Surg Pathol 18:1–13, 1994.

Iwasa Y, Minamiguchi S, Konishi I, et al. Sclerosing peritonitis associated with luteinized thecoma of the ovary. Pathol Int 46:510–514, 1996.

Scurry J, Allen D, Dobson P. Ovarian fibromatosis, ascites and omental fibromatsis. Histopathology 28:81–84, 1996.

Spiegel GW, Swiger FK. Luteinized thecoma with sclerosing peritonitis presenting as an acute abdomen. Gynecol Oncol 61:275–281, 1996.

Werness BA. Luteinized thecoma with sclerosing peritonitis. Arch Pathol Lab Med 120:303–306, 1996.

Fibroma

Clinical Features

- Fibromas, which account for 4% of all ovarian tumors, occur at all ages but are most frequent during middle age (mean, 48 years); fewer than 10% occur before 30 years of age.
- Meigs' syndrome, which occurs in 1% of patients with these tumors, is defined as the presence of ascites and pleural effusion accompanying a fibrous ovarian tumor, usually a fibroma, with the effusions disappearing after removal of the tumor. Ascites alone occurs in 10% to 15% of ovarian fibromas larger than 10 cm in diameter.
- Fibromas are rarely associated with the nevoid basal cell carcinoma syndrome (NBCCS), also called Gorlin's syndrome; these tumors frequently differ from typical fibromas, as discussed later.

Gross Features

- Fibromas have a mean maximal dimension of 6 cm. Eight percent of tumors are bilateral, most of which are in patients with the NBCCS.
- Gross examination reveals typically hard, chalky-white sectioned surfaces. Areas of edema, occasionally with cyst formation, are common, and some tumors are predominantly edematous or cystic. Hemorrhage and less often necrosis are present in occasional tumors, especially those that are cellular.
- Focal or diffuse calcification occurs in fewer than 10% of the cases. Calcification is almost always identified in patients with the NBCCS.

Microscopic Features

- Sparsely to moderately cellular proliferations of spindle cells with scanty cytoplasm are arranged in intersecting fascicles or occasionally in a storiform pattern.
- The cells may contain small quantities of lipid, rarely have eosinophilic hyaline droplets, and usually have uniform nuclei and only rare mitotic figures.
- The spindle cells are separated by variable amounts of collagen, which is frequently focally hyalinized. Intercellular edema occurs in some tumors.
- About 10% of tumors are densely cellular and are referred to as *cellular fibromas.* These tumors contain an average of 3 MF or fewer per 10 HPF and exhibit no more than mild atypia.
- A minor component of sex cord elements (see page 371) is found in some tumors.
- Only a minority of tumors are immunoreactive for inhibin.

Differential Diagnosis

- Thecoma (page 370).
- Massive edema, fibromatosis, and stromal hyperplasia. Features favoring one of these lesions over fibroma is bilaterality (although only stromal hyperplasia is typically bilateral), entrapment of follicles and their derivatives (massive edema and fibromatosis), proliferation of closely packed, small stromal cells with minimal collagen formation (stromal hyperplasia).
- Primary endometrioid or metastatic endometrial stromal sarcoma (page 371).
- Krukenberg tumor (see Chapter 18).

Prognosis

- Cellular fibromas as defined have a low malignant potential, occasionally recurring in the pelvis or upper abdomen, particularly if they were adherent or ruptured.

References

Dockerty MB, Masson JC. Ovarian fibromas: a clinical and pathologic study of two hundred and eighty-three cases. Am J Obstet Gynecol 47:741–752, 1944.

Kommoss F, Oliva E, Bhan A, et al. Inhibin expression in ovarian neoplasms. Mod Pathol 11:656–664, 1998.

Meigs JV. Fibroma of the ovary with ascites and hydrothorax: Meigs' syndrome. Am J Obstet Gynecol 67:962–987, 1954.

Prat J, Scully RE. Cellular fibromas and fibrosarcomas of the ovary: a comparative clinicopathologic analysis of seventeen cases. Cancer 47:2663–2670, 1981.

Samanth KK, Black WC. Benign ovarian stromal tumors associated with free peritoneal fluid. Am J Obstet Gynecol 107:538–545, 1970.

Young RH, Scully RE. Ovarian stromal tumors with minor sex cord elements: a report of seven cases. Int J Gynecol Pathol 2:227–234, 1983.

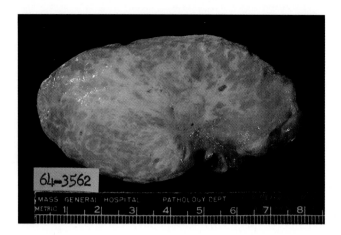

Figure 16–13. Focally edematous fibroma (sectioned surface).

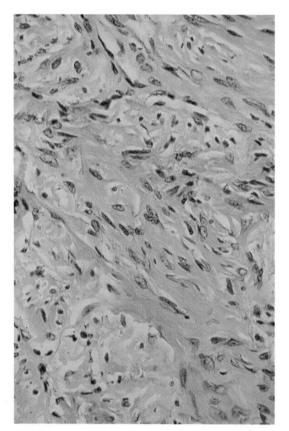

Figure 16–14. Fibroma.

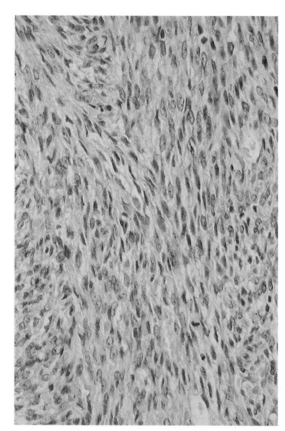

Figure 16–15. Cellular fibroma.

Fibrosarcoma

- Fibrosarcomas, which are the most common ovarian sarcoma, may occur at any age but usually are found in older women. The tumors are rarely associated with Maffucci's syndrome and the nevoid basal cell carcinoma syndrome. Most ovarian fibrosarcomas are clinically malignant.
- Gross examination typically reveals a unilateral, large tumor with a solid sectioned surface, often with focal hemorrhage and necrosis.
- The tumors are densely cellular, with moderate to severe nuclear atypicality and an average mitotic count of 4 MF or more per 10 HPF; abnormal mitotic figures are common.
- The differential diagnosis includes cellular fibroma (no more than mild atypia, usually fewer than 4 MF per 10 HPF) and primary or metastatic endometrial stromal sarcomas (ESSs). ESSs have smaller, less atypical cells with round nuclei and scanty cytoplasm and a characteristic network of arterioles.

References

Christman JE, Ballon SC. Ovarian fibrosarcoma associated with Maffucci's syndrome. Gynecol Oncol 37:290–291, 1990.

Kraemer BB, Silva EG, Sneige N. Fibrosarcoma of ovary: a new component in the nevoid basal-cell carcinoma syndrome. Am J Surg Pathol 8:231–236, 1984.

Prat J, Scully RE. Cellular fibromas and fibrosarcomas of the ovary: a comparative clinicopathologic analysis of seventeen cases. Cancer 47:2663–2670, 1981.

Sclerosing Stromal Tumor

General Features

- Eighty percent of sclerosing stromal tumors (SSTs) are encountered in the first 3 decades (mean age, 27 years). Evidence of estrogen or androgen secretion has been found in a few cases.
- The tumors have been clinically benign in all of the reported cases.

Pathologic Features

- SSTs are typically unilateral, discrete, and sharply demarcated, with a sectioned surface that is predominantly solid and white, sometimes with yellow areas. Areas of edema and cyst formation are common, and rare tumors are unilocular cysts.
- Low-power examination reveals a pseudolobular pattern with cellular nodules separated by paucicellular areas of densely collagenous or edematous connective tissue. Various degrees of sclerosis also occur within the nodules.
- Prominent, thin-walled vessels, which may be dilated and resemble those of a hemangiopericytoma, are typical.
- The nodules are composed of a disorganized admixture of fibroblasts and rounded, vacuolated cells. The latter cells often have shrunken, occasionally eccentric nuclei,

with the appearance sometimes resembling that of signet-ring cells, although in contrast to the latter, the vacuoles contain lipid.
- Lutein cells resembling those in luteinized thecomas are encountered in some functioning SSTs. Occasionally, typical lutein cells with abundant eosinophilic cytoplasm are also prominent in nonfunctioning tumors.
- Only a minority of tumors are immunoreactive for inhibin.

Differential Diagnosis

- Fibromas and thecomas. SSTs have a more heterogeneous appearance than either of these tumors, which lack the pseudolobular pattern, the intimate admixture of fibroblasts and rounded vacuolated cells, and vascularity of SSTs. Rarely the features of an SST are seen in a tumor that is predominantly a fibroma.
- Krukenberg tumor. This tumor may be suggested by the signet-ring–like cells in SSTs, but these cells in SSTs contain lipid rather than mucin.
- Hemangiopericytoma. This tumor may be suggested by the ectatic vessels in SSTs, but hemangiopericytomas lack the other distinctive features of SSTs.

References

Chalvardjian A, Scully, RE. Sclerosing stromal tumors of the ovary. Cancer 31:664–670, 1973.

Gee DC, Russell P. Sclerosing stromal tumours of the ovary. Histopathology 3:367–376, 1979.

Hsu C, Ma L, Mak L. Sclerosing stromal tumor of the ovary: case report and review of the literature. Int J Gynecol Pathol 2:192–200, 1983.

Kommoss F, Oliva E, Bhan A, et al. Inhibin expression in ovarian neoplasms. Mod Pathol 11:656–664, 1998.

Suit PF, Hart WR. Sclerosing stromal tumor of the ovary: an ultrastructural study and review of the literature to evaluate hormonal function. Cleve Clin J Med 55:189–194, 1988.

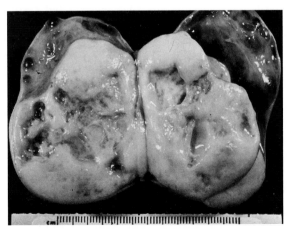

Figure 16–16. Sclerosing stromal tumor (sectioned surface). Note the cystic spaces.

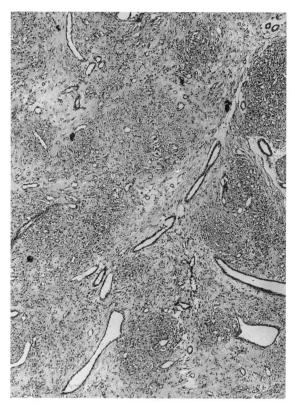

Figure 16–17. Sclerosing stromal tumor. Cellular islands are separated by paucicellular fibrous tissue, creating a pseudolobular pattern. Notice the prominent vascularity.

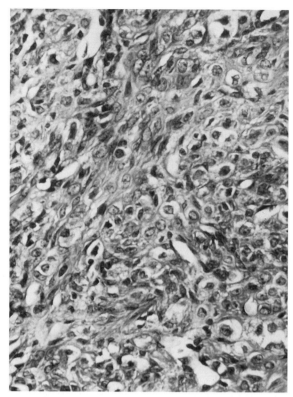

Figure 16–18. Sclerosing stromal tumor. Notice the admixture of polygonal cells with clear cytoplasm and spindled cells.

Signet-Ring Stromal Tumor

- Only five examples of signet-ring stromal tumor, all in adults, have been reported. None has been associated with hormonal manifestations.
- The tumors are uniformly solid or solid and cystic on gross examination.
- Spindle cells merge with rounded cells that have eccentric nuclei and single large vacuoles that are negative for mucin and lipid. The signet-ring cell component may be diffuse or occupy only a portion of an otherwise typical fibroma.
- The differential diagnosis includes Krukenberg tumor (mucin stains facilitate this distinction) and SST, which in contrast to the signet-ring stromal tumor, has pseudolobulation and lipid-rich cells.

References

Dickersin GR, Young RH, Scully RE. Signet-ring stromal and related tumors of the ovary. Ultrastruct Pathol 19:401–419, 1995.

Ramzy I. Signet-ring stromal tumor of ovary: histochemical, light, and electron microscopic study. Cancer 38:166–172, 1976.

Suarez A, Palacios J, Burgos E, Gamallo C. Signet-ring stromal tumor of the ovary: a histochemical and ultrastuctural study. Virchows Arch A 422:333–336, 1993.

Myxoma

- The 10 reported myxomas occurred in patients of reproductive age who had an asymptomatic unilateral adnexal mass.
- That myxoid areas can be found in tumors in the thecoma-fibroma group and SSTs suggests that at least some myxomas are of ovarian stromal origin.
- The mean diameter of the tumors is 11 cm, and they typically have soft sectioned surfaces, often with focal cystic degeneration.
- Microscopically, the tumors have abundant, pale blue to pink intercellular matrix, with the degree of eosinophilia reflecting the amount of collagen present, and a prominent plexus of small blood vessels. The intercellular material stains with colloidal iron and alcian blue and is sensitive to pretreatment with hyaluronidase.
- The bland tumor cells vary from spindle shaped to stellate, with long, tapering cytoplasmic processes. Ul-

trastructural and immunohistochemical findings indicate that the cells are myofibroblasts.

Differential Diagnosis

■ Low-grade sarcomas with myxoid features. Features favoring myxoma include bland cytologic features and rare to absent mitotic figures. The diagnosis of myxoma should be made with caution in the presence of even slight cytologic atypia and occasional mitoses.

■ Massive edema. The typical features of a myxoma, including its alcianophilic matrix and the absence of follicles and their derivatives within the tumor, facilitate this differential.

References

Costa MJ, Morris R, DeRose PB, Cohen C. Histologic and immunohistochemical evidence for considering ovarian myxoma as a variant of the thecoma-fibroma group of ovarian stromal tumors. Arch Pathol Lab Med 117:802–808, 1993.

Costa MJ, Thomas W, Majmudar B, Hewan-Lowe K. Ovarian myxoma: ultrastructural and immunohistochemical findings. Ultrastruct Pathol 16:429–438, 1992.

Eichhorn JH, Scully RE. Ovarian myxoma: clinicopathologic and immunocytologic analysis of five cases and a review of the literature. Int J Gynecol Pathol 10:156–169, 1991.

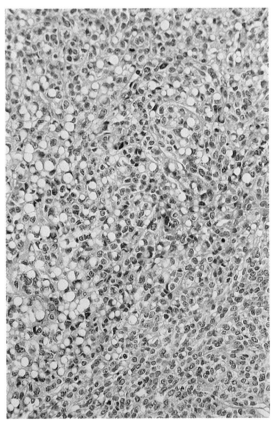

Figure 16–19. Signet-ring stromal tumor.

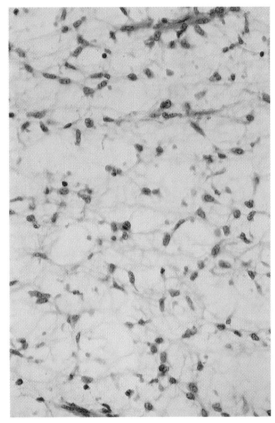

Figure 16–20. Myxoma.

Sertoli–Stromal Cell Tumors

Sertoli Cell Tumor

General Features

- These tumors, which account for 4% of Sertoli–stromal cell tumors (see Table 16–1), occur at any age (mean, 30 years).
- The tumors are usually nonfunctioning but may be estrogenic, less often androgenic, and rarely progestagenic. Rare tumors (most or all of the lipid-rich type) have resulted in isosexual pseudoprecocity. Hypertension results from renin production by the tumor in rare cases.
- The tumors are rarely associated with the Peutz-Jeghers syndrome (PJS). These tumors have had unusual histologic features (lipid-rich or oxyphilic variants).
- The clinical course is usually benign, but one tumor was malignant with distant metastases.

Pathologic Features

- The tumors are unilateral, with an average diameter of 9 cm, and have lobulated, solid, yellow or brown sectioned surfaces.
- The microscopic pattern is characterized by at least focal tubular differentiation, and usually tubules are conspicuous. The tubules may be round or elongated, hollow or solid. The tubules are often arranged in lobules separated by a typically fibrous stroma, which may be hyalinized. Diffuse nondiagnostic foci are seen in some tumors.
- The tubules are lined by cuboidal cells with moderate to abundant cytoplasm, which may be dense and eosinophilic or pale and vacuolated. The solid tubules often contain large cells with abundant cytoplasmic lipid (i.e., lipid-rich Sertoli cell tumor).
- There is usually little or no nuclear atypia or mitotic activity, but rare tumors exhibit significant degrees of each. The single fatal tumor was poorly differentiated focally.
- The tumor cells are typically immunoreactive for cytokeratins and occasionally for vimentin. Six of 11 tumors were immunoreactive for inhibin in one study.
- Distinction from the more common well-differentiated Sertoli–Leydig cell tumor (SLCT) is based on an absence of Leydig cells.

References

Ferry JA, Young RH, Engel G, Scully RE. Oxyphil Sertoli cell tumor of the ovary: a report of three cases, two in patients with the Peutz-Jeghers syndrome. Int J Gynecol Pathol 13:259–266, 1994.

Kommoss F, Oliva E, Bhan A, et al. Inhibin expression in ovarian neoplasms. Mod Pathol 11:656–664, 1998.

Tavassoli FA, Norris HJ. Sertoli tumors of the ovary: a clinicopathologic study of 28 cases with ultrastructural observations. Cancer 46:2281–2297, 1980.

Tracy SL, Askin FB, Reddick RL, et al. Progesterone secreting Sertoli cell tumor of the ovary. Gynecol Oncol 22:85–96, 1985.

Young RH, Scully RE. Ovarian Sertoli cell tumors: a report of ten cases. Int J Gynecol Pathol 2:349–363, 1984.

Sertoli–Leydig Cell Tumors

General Features

- SLCTs, which account for less than 0.5% of all ovarian tumors, typically occur in young women (75% of patients are younger than 30 years of age; mean age, 25 years) and only 10% occur in women older than 50 years of age. Well-differentiated SLCTs occur at a mean age of 35 years and retiform SLCTs at a mean age of 15 years.
- The patients present with abdominal swelling or pain and, in 50%, endocrine manifestations, usually virilization. There is a lower frequency of the latter feature with retiform tumors and those containing heterologous elements. Some patients have estrogenic manifestations.
- Elevated plasma levels of AFP have been found in some patients.
- Rare familial cases have been reported; some of these women have also had thyroid disease.
- The tumors are stage Ib in fewer than 2%, Ic in 12%, and II or III in 2% to 3%, with the remainder stage Ia.

Gross Features

- SLCTs have a mean maximal dimension of 13.5 cm, with typically solid, lobulated, and yellow sectioned surfaces.
- Tumors with heterologous or retiform components are often cystic, and rare tumors lacking these components are strikingly cystic. Tumors with a large heterologous mucinous component may grossly mimic a mucinous cystic tumor.
- The cysts in the retiform tumors may contain papillary or polypoid excrescences, potentially resembling a serous tumor or a hydatidiform mole.
- Poorly differentiated tumors, including those with mesenchymal heterologous elements, often are focally hemorrhagic and necrotic.

Microscopic Features of Well-Differentiated SLCTs

- Well-differentiated SLCTs are characterized by Sertoli cells arranged in a predominantly tubular pattern, with lobules composed of hollow or, less often, solid tubules and Leydig cells.
- The hollow tubules are typically round to oval and small, but they may be cystic or rarely have an endometrioid-like appearance. Luminal secretion is usually absent, but occasionally an eosinophilic, mucicarminophilic fluid is present. The solid tubules are typically elongated but may be round or oval.
- The Sertoli cells lining the hollow tubules are typically cuboidal or columnar, with usually moderate amounts of dense cytoplasm, but in some cases the cytoplasm is abundant, pale, and lipid rich.
- The Sertoli cell nuclei are round or oblong and without prominent nucleoli. Nuclear atypicality is usually absent or minimal, and mitotic figures are rare.
- The stroma consists of bands of mature fibrous tissue

with variable but usually conspicuous numbers of Leydig cells. The latter contain variable amounts of lipid and occasionally abundant lipochrome pigment and, in 20% of tumors, rare Reinke crystals.

Microscopic Features of Intermediate SLCTs

- The typical low-power appearance is that of lobulated cellular masses. The most obvious differentiation into Sertoli cell aggregates and Leydig cell clusters is often at the periphery of the lobules.
- The cellular masses are composed of immature, darkly staining Sertoli cells with small, round, oval, or angular nuclei admixed with Leydig cells. Nests, solid and hollow tubules, thin and usually short cords, or occasionally broad columns are also common.
- Small or large cysts are conspicuous in some tumors, sometimes containing eosinophilic secretion and creating a thyroid-like appearance.
- The stroma separating the Sertoli cell component ranges from fibromatous to densely cellular to edematous (often the latter) and typically contains Leydig cells. The stromal component may focally consist of immature, cellular mesenchymal tissue, resembling a nonspecific sarcoma.
- Other features of the Sertoli or Leydig cells include variable amounts of lipid and cells with bizarre nuclei in rare cases. Mitoses are typically present, particularly in the Sertoli cells.

Microscopic Features of Poorly Differentiated SLCTs

- Poorly differentiated SLCTs generally lack or exhibit only focally the lobulation or other evidence of an orderly arrangement of the Sertoli and stromal element seen in SLCTs of intermediate differentiation.
- The tumors are usually composed of solid sheets of poorly differentiated Sertoli cells, and may resemble a fibrosarcoma, an undifferentiated carcinoma, or even a primitive germ cell tumor. The mitotic rate is usually more than 10 MFs per 10 HPF.

Microscopic Features of Retiform SLCTS

- The patterns in retiform SLCTs, which resemble those of the rete testis, usually occur within otherwise typical intermediate and poorly differentiated SLCTs.
- Retiform SLCTs account for 15% of SLCTs. A retiform pattern predominates in 50% of them and is the exclusive or almost exlusive component in 15% of them.
- Low-power examination reveals irregularly branching, elongated, narrow, often slitlike tubules and cysts with intraluminal papillae or polypoid projections.
- The tubules and cysts are lined by epithelial cells with various degrees of stratification and nuclear atypicality. Columns or ribbons of immature Sertoli cells are common.
- The papillae and polyps are of three types: small and rounded or blunt and often hyalinized; large and bulbous, often with edematous cores; and delicate and branching and lined by stratified cells and cellular buds, simulating the papillae of a serous tumor.
- The stroma varies from hyalinized or edematous (most common) to moderately cellular or densely cellular and immature.

Microscopic Features of SLCTs With Heterologous Elements

- SLCTs with heterologous elements account for 20% of SLCTs, most of which are of intermediate differentiation, but occasionally they are poorly differentiated or retiform.
- In 80% of cases, the heterologous elements consist of mucinous epithelium, and in 25% of cases, there are stromal heterologous elements; 5% of cases have both types of heterologous tissue.
- The mucinous epithelium resembles gastric-type or intestinal-type mucinous epithelium with goblet cells, argentaffin cells, and rarely Paneth cells. The appearance of the epithelium may vary from benign to borderline to low-grade adenocarcinoma.
  - Insular or goblet cell carcinoids, usually of microscopic size, arise from the mucinous epithelium in more than 50% of the cases with argentaffin cells.
- Stromal heterologous elements consist of islands of cartilage arising on a sarcomatous background, areas of embryonal rhabdomyosarcoma, or both.
- Rare tumors have contained foci of neuroblastoma or AFP-immunoreactive hepatocytes. The presence of the latter accounts for at least some (or possibly all) of the SLCTs associated with elevated serum AFP levels.

Imunohistochemical Findings

- SLCTs, in contrast to most of the tumors in the differential diagnosis, are typically immunoreactive for inhibin.
- SLCTs typically lack immunoreactivity for EMA, in contrast to endometrioid carcinomas and some of the other epithelial tumors in the differential diagnosis.

Differential Diagnosis

- AGCT. SLCTs lack Call-Exner bodies and easily found nuclear grooves, have more primitive nuclei in their epithelial component, and have different patterns, although there is overlap. Their stroma tends to be less cellular.
- Endometrioid carcinomas with sex cord–like patterns (page 315).
- Tubular Krukenberg tumor. Features supportive or diagnostic of this diagnosis include bilaterality, marked atypicality of the cells forming tubules, and signet-ring cells filled with mucin.
- Trabecular carcinoid tumors (page 357).
- Struma ovarii with tubular patterns. Identification of more typical patterns of struma and immunohistochemical staining for thyroglobulin facilitate the differential diagnosis.

- Ovarian wolffian tumors. Wolffian tumors usually lack Leydig cells, are rarely associated with endocrine manifestations, and virtually always have other distinctive patterns in addition to tubular (page 393).
- Sarcomas or undifferentiated tumors. The diagnosis of poorly differentiated SLCT should be excluded by thorough sampling in an attempt to document more differentiated areas of SLCT, particularly in young women with androgenic manifestations.
- Teratomas (versus heterologous SLCTs). Gonadal teratomas lack Sertoli or Leydig cells and, in contrast to SLCTs, usually exhibit prominent ectodermal elements.
- Mucinous tumors (versus heterologous SLCTs with prominent mucinous epithelium). The distinction depends on thorough sampling to demonstrate the intermediate or, less often, poorly differentiated sertoliform elements in heterologous SLCTs.
- Serous tumors (versus retiform SLCTs) (page 300).
- Malignant mesodermal mixed tumor (versus SLCTs with sarcomatoid areas or with skeletal muscle or cartilage) (page 322).

Prognosis

- All well-differentiated tumors were benign in one large series, whereas 11% of SLCTs of intermediate differentiation, 59% of poorly differentiated SLCTs, and 19% of SLCTs with heterologous elements were malignant. Tumors in the last group were usually poorly differentiated and contained skeletal muscle, cartilage, or both.
- Retiform SLCTs are associated with a higher frequency of malignant behavior (25% of stage I tumors) compared with nonretiform SLCTs (10%).
- Tumor rupture is associated with a higher frequency of malignant behavior. Thirty percent of stage I tumors of intermediate differentiation with rupture were malignant, compared with 7% without rupture; the parallel figures for the poorly differentiated tumors were 86% and 45%.
- The rare SLCTs that are stage II or higher are almost always associated with a fatal outcome.
- SLCTs typically recur early, in contrast to granulosa cell tumors: 66% of clinically malignant tumors in one series recurred within 1 year, and only 6.6% recurred after 5 years.
- Recurrent tumor is usually confined to the pelvis and abdomen. The recurrent tumor often is less differentiated than the primary tumor and may resemble a soft tissue sarcoma.

References

Costa MJ, Ames PF, Walls J, Roth LM. Inhibin immunohistochemistry applied to ovarian neoplasms: a novel, effective, diagnostic tool. Hum Pathol 28:1247–1254, 1997.

Hammad A, Jasnosz KM, Olson PR. Expression of alpha-fetoprotein by ovarian Sertoli-Leydig cell tumors: case report and review of the literature. Arch Pathol Lab Med 119:1075–1079, 1995.

Mooney EE, Nogales FF, Tavassoli FA. Hepatocytic differentiation in retiform Sertoli-Leydig cell tumors: distinguishing a heterologous element from Leydig cells. Hum Pathol 30:611–617, 1999.

Prat J, Young RH, Scully RE. Ovarian Sertoli-Leydig cell tumors with heterologous elements. II. Cartilage and skeletal muscle: a clinicopathologic analysis of twelve cases. Cancer 50:2465–2475, 1982.

Riopel MA, Perlman EJ, Seidman JD, et al. Inhibin and epithelial membrane antigen immunohistochemistry assist in the diagosis of sex cord–stromal tumors and provide clues to the histogenesis of hypercalcemic small cell carcinomas. Int J Gynecol Pathol 17:46–53, 1998.

Young RH. Sertoli-Leydig cell tumors of the ovary: review with emphasis on historical aspects and unusual variants. Int J Gynecol Pathol 12:141–147, 1993.

Young RH, Prat J, Scully RE. Ovarian Sertoli-Leydig cell tumors with heterologous elements. I. Gastrointestinal epithelium and carcinoid: a clinicopathologic analysis of thirty-six cases. Cancer 50:2448–2456, 1982.

Young RH, Scully RE. Ovarian Sertoli-Leydig cell tumors with a retiform pattern: a problem in histopathologic diagnosis. A report of 25 cases. Am J Surg Pathol 77:755–771, 1983.

Young RH, Scully RE. Ovarian Sertoli-Leydig cell tumors: a clinicopathological analysis of 207 cases. Am J Surg Pathol 9:543–569, 1985.

Young RH, Scully RE. Ovarian sex cord stromal tumors with bizarre nuclei: a clinicopathological analysis of 17 cases. Int J Gynecol Pathol 1:325–335, 1983.

Young RH, Scully RE. Well-differentiated ovarian Sertoli-Leydig cell tumors: a clinicopathological analysis of 23 cases. Int J Gynecol Pathol 3:277–290, 1984.

Zaloudek C, Norris HJ. Sertoli-Leydig tumors of the ovary: A clinicopathologic study of 64 intermediate and poorly differentiated neoplasms. Am J Surg Pathol 8:405–418, 1984.

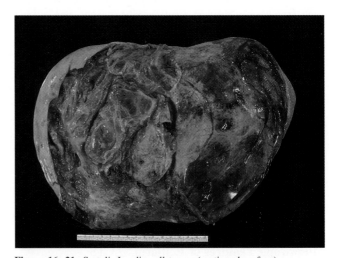

Figure 16–21. Sertoli–Leydig cell tumor (sectioned surface).

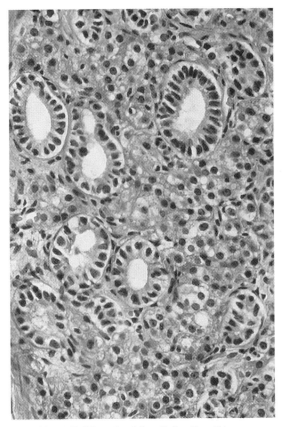

Figure 16–22. Well-differentiated Sertoli–Leydig cell tumor.

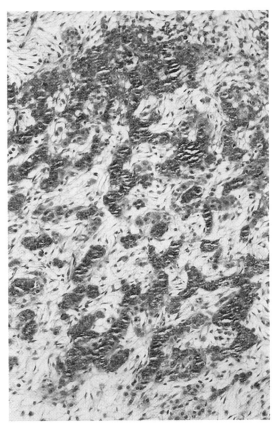

Figure 16–23. Sertoli–Leydig cell tumor of intermediate differentiation. Cords of Sertoli cells are admixed with small nests of Leydig-type cells. Notice the edematous stroma.

Figure 16–24. Poorly differentiated (sarcomatoid) Sertoli–Leydig cell tumor. Notice the microcystic change that is an occasional finding in these tumors and those of intermediate differentiation.

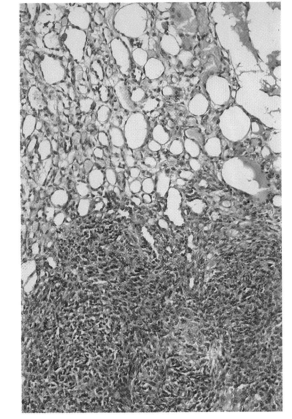

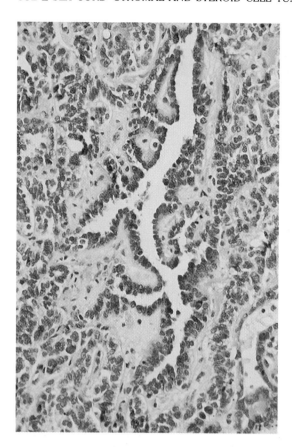

Figure 16–25. Retiform Sertoli–Leydig cell tumor. Papillae project into branching, slitlike spaces.

Figure 16–26. Sertoli–Leydig cell tumor with heterologous elements. Glands and cysts are lined by mucinous epithelium containing goblet cells. Cords of dark blue Sertoli cells are seen between them.

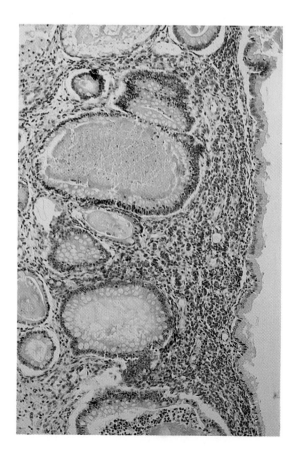

Gynandroblastoma

- Gynandroblastomas contain clearly recognizable, well-differentiated ovarian (granulosa-stromal) and testicular-type (Sertoli-stromal) cells, with the smaller component accounting for more than 10% of the tumor. Each component and its quantity should be specified in the pathology report.
- The tumors usually occur in young adults but may be encountered at any age. They may be associated with androgenic or estrogenic manifestations. They are almost always stage I and clinically benign.
- The differential diagnosis includes sex cord–stromal tumors that contain elements that are suggestive but not unequivocally diagnostic of ovarian or testicular differentiation and sex cord–stromal tumors that contain very minor foci (<10%) of another type.

References

Broshears JR, Roth LM. Gynandroblastoma with elements resembling juvenile granulosa cell tumor. Int J Gynecol Pathol 16:387–391, 1997.

Guo L, Liu T. Gynandroblastoma of the ovary: review of literature and report of a case. Int J Surg Pathol 3:137–140, 1995.

Neubecker RD, Breen JL. Gynandroblastoma: a report of five cases with a discussion of the histogenesis and classification of ovarian tumors. Am J Clin Pathol 38:60–69, 1962.

Sex Cord Tumor With Annular Tubules

General Features

- SCTATS have variable clinical manifestations depending on the presence (in one third of patients) or absence of the PJS. SCTATs are detected at an average age of 27 years in patients with PJS and at an average age of 34 years in those without PJS.
- SCTATs in women with the PJS are always incidental findings. Some tumors are associated with adenoma malignum of the cervix. In women without PJS, SCTATs usually present as palpable adnexal masses.
- Estrogenic manifestations occur in 40% of patients without PJS and in some patients with the syndrome. Progesterone secretion, which may result in decidual change of the endometrium, has been reported in a number of patients without PJS.
- Elevated serum levels of müllerian inhibiting substance, inhibin, or both have been found in some cases.

Pathologic Features

- SCTATs unassociated with PJS are almost always unilateral, typically moderately large, predominantly solid, and frequently yellow.
- In contrast, SCTATs associated with PJS are bilateral in at least two thirds of patients and are usually not recognized grossly; yellow nodules up to 3 cm in diameter have been observed in some cases.
- SCTATs are characterized microscopically by pure or predominant patterns of simple or complex annular tubules.
  - Ring-shaped simple tubules are composed of cells with nuclei oriented peripherally and around a central hyaline body containing basement membrane material. An intervening anuclear cytoplasmic zone forms the major component of the ring.
  - More numerous complex tubules forming rounded structures are composed of intercommunicating rings oriented around multiple hyaline bodies.
- PJS-associated SCTATs typically occur as tumorlets, varying from single tubules to clusters of tubules scattered within the ovarian stroma.
- Other findings in PJS-related tumors include islands of vacuolated lipid-rich sex cord cells, solid foci, and in more than 50% of cases, calcification, which is occasionally extensive.
- Findings in some SCTATs, usually unassociated with PJS, include extensive hyalinization of the tubules and stroma and foci of microfollicular granulosa cell tumor, well-differentiated Sertoli cell tumor, or both.
- The tumors are typically immunoreactive for inhibin.

Differential Diagnosis

- Gonadoblastoma. These tumors have similar patterns to those of SCTAT but also contain germ cells and almost always occur in patients with an underlying gonadal disorder and a Y chromosome.
- Other rare ovarian tumors occurring in PJS. These include the oxyphilic Sertoli cell tumor (page 378) and a distinctive sex cord–stromal tumor associated with sexual precocity that has a variable histologic appearance with solid, tubular, papillary, and cystic patterns and two predominant epithelial cell types.

Prognosis

- SCTATs unassociated with PJS are clinically malignant in at least 20% of cases, often spreading through lymphatics. Recurrences are often late, and multiple recurrences may occur over many years.
- PJS-associated SCTATs are clinically benign.

References

Hart WR, Kumar N, Crissman JD. Ovarian neoplasms resembling sex cord tumors with annular tubules. Cancer 45:2352–2363, 1980.

Kommoss F, Oliva E, Bhan A, et al. Inhibin expression in ovarian neoplasms. Mod Pathol 11:656–664, 1998.

Scully RE. Sex cord tumor with annular tubules: a distinctive ovarian tumor of the Peutz-Jeghers syndrome. Cancer 25:1107–1121, 1970.

Young RH, Dickersin GR, Scully RE. A distinctive ovarian sex cord–stromal tumor causing sexual precocity in the Peutz-Jeghers syndrome. Am J Surg Pathol 7:233–243, 1983.

Young RH, Welch WR, Dickersin GR, Scully RE. Ovarian sex cord tumor with annular tubules: review of 74 cases, including 27 with Peutz-Jeghers syndrome and 4 with adenoma malignum of the cervix. Cancer 50:1384–1402, 1982.

Unclassified Sex Cord–Stromal Tumors

- These tumors, which account for 10% of tumors in the sex cord–stromal category, have patterns and cell types intermediate between or common to granulosa–stromal cell tumors and Sertoli–stromal cell tumors.

- The tumors occur over a wide age range (means of 37 and 49 years in the two largest studies). Tumors in this category account for a disproportionate number of sex cord–stromal tumors removed during pregnancy.
- Rare tumors have been associated with hypertension secondary to renin or aldosterone production by the tumor.
- Many granulosa cell or Sertoli-stromal tumors removed during pregnancy have areas with an indifferent appearance, which can obscure the tumor architecture. These changes include prominent intercellular edema, increased luteinization in the granulosa cell tumors, and marked degrees of Leydig cell maturation in the Sertoli–stromal cell tumors.
- The tumors are typically immunoreactive for vimentin and sometimes for cytokeratin and inhibin.
- About 10% of cases have been associated with malignant behavior.

References

Kommoss F, Oliva E, Bhan A, et al. Inhibin expression in ovarian neoplasms. Mod Pathol 11:656–664, 1998.

Seidman JD. Unclassified ovarian gonadal stromal tumors: a clinicopathologic study of 32 cases. Am J Surg Pathol 20:699–706, 1996.

Simpson JL, Michael H, Roth LM. Unclassified sex cord–stromal tumors of the ovary: a report of eight cases. Arch Pathol Lab Med 122: 52–55, 1998.

Young RH, Dudley AG, Scully RE. Granulosa cell, Sertoli-Leydig cell and unclassified sex cord–stromal tumors associated with pregnancy: a clinicopathological analysis of thirty-six cases. Gynecol Oncol 18: 181–205, 1984.

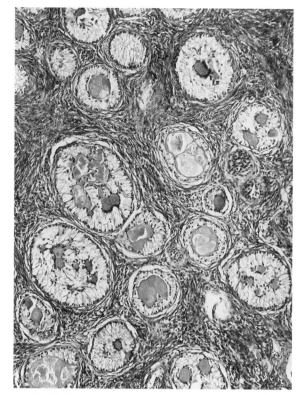

Figure 16–28. Sex cord tumor with annular tubules.

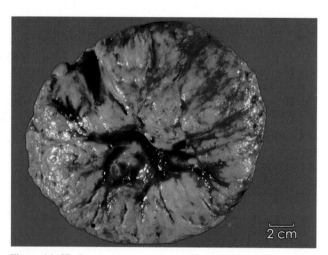

Figure 16–27. Sex cord tumor with annular tubules (sectioned surface). The tumor was not associated with the Peutz-Jeghers syndrome.

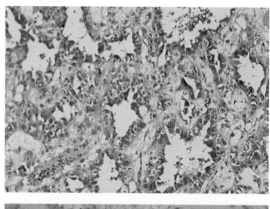

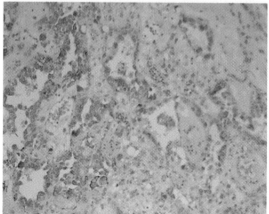

Figure 16–29. Unclassified sex cord tumor. The tumor cells are immunoreactive for inhibin.

STEROID CELL TUMORS

- Steroid cell tumors, formerly referred to as lipid or lipoid cell tumors, are composed entirely or almost entirely of cells resembling typical steroid hormone–secreting cells, i.e., lutein cells, Leydig cells, or adrenal cortical cells.
- These tumors, which account for only 0.1% of ovarian tumors, are subdivided into tumors of known origin, the stromal luteoma and the Leydig cell tumor, and tumors of uncertain lineage, steroid cell tumors not otherwise specified.

Stromal Luteoma

General Features

- These tumors, which account for 20% of steroid cell tumors, are typically small and occupy the ovarian stroma and are therefore assumed to arise from it.
- A stromal origin is also supported by the presence in 90% of cases of associated stromal hyperthecosis (SH) in the same or contralateral ovary. In some cases of SH, the nests of lutein cells form nodules (i.e., nodular SH) that, in contrast to stromal luteomas, are typically multiple and smaller than 0.5 cm in diameter.
- Eighty percent of the tumors are encountered in postmenopausal women. Abnormal vaginal bleeding, probably related to hyperestrinism, is the presenting feature in 60% of the cases. Androgenic manifestations are present in 12% of cases. Underlying SH may contribute to the clinical picture in some cases.
- All of the reported cases have been clinically benign.

Pathologic Features

- The tumors are, with rare exceptions, unilateral and are almost always less than 3 cm in diameter. The tumors have a well-circumscribed, solid sectioned surface that is usually gray-white or yellow, but one third of them have red or brown areas.
- Microscopic examination reveals a rounded nodule of cells of lutein type arranged diffusely or in small nests or cords. The nodule is completely or almost completely surrounded by ovarian stroma.
- The cells have lipid-poor cytoplasm, often with conspicuous intracytoplasmic lipochrome pigment and small round nuclei with single prominent nucleoli; mitotic figures are rare.

- A peculiar degenerative change occurs in 20% of cases characterized by irregular spaces that simulate glands or vessels. The spaces may contain lipid-laden cells and chronic inflammatory cells and may be separated by cells of those types as well as fibrotic tissue.
- The tumors are typically immunoreactive for inhibin.
- The differential is essentially the same as for steroid cell tumor not otherwise specified (page 387).

Reference

Hayes MC, Scully RE. Stromal luteoma of the ovary: a clinico-pathological analysis of 25 cases. Int J Gynecol Pathol 6:313–321, 1987.

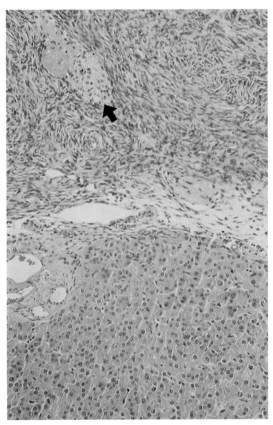

Figure 16–30. Stromal luteoma (*bottom*) abutting ovarian stroma (*top*) containing a nest of luteinized stromal cells (*arrow*) (i.e., stromal hyperthecosis).

Leydig Cell Tumor

General Features

- The diagnosis of these tumors, which account for 20% of steroid cell tumors, requires identification of Reinke crystals in the cytoplasm of the tumor cells.
- Most tumors are hilar (i.e., hilus cell tumor), but rare tumors arise in the ovarian stroma (i.e., Leydig cell tumor, nonhilar type).
- The tumors are detected at an average age of 58 years. Hirsutism or virilization, present in 75% of the cases and caused by testosterone production by the tumor, typically has a less abrupt onset and is milder than these symptoms associated with SLCTs. Estrogenic manifestations are present in rare cases.
- The tumors have been clinically benign in all well documented cases.

Pathologic Features

- The tumors are usually small (mean diameter, 2.4 cm), are red-brown to yellow but occasionally dark brown to black, and are typically centered in the hilus. Rare tumors are bilateral.
- Microscopic examination reveals a circumscribed mass composed of a predominantly solid proliferation of steroid cells in which the cell nuclei may cluster, separated by nucleus-free eosinophilic zones.
- The abundant cytoplasm varies from eosinophilic (most common) to spongy and lipid laden; sparse to abundant cytoplasmic lipochrome pigment is common. Reinke crystals are eosinophilic, rod-shaped inclusions of various lengths and often found only after prolonged search.
- The nuclei are typically round, are often hyperchromatic, and contain single small nucleoli. Slight to moderate nuclear pleomorphism, bizarre nuclei, and multinucleated cells are occasionally encountered; mitotic figures are rare.
- Other findings include a prominent fibrous stroma, imparting a nodular appearance; fibrinoid replacement of blood vessels in one third of tumors; and degenerative pseudovascular spaces (see Stromal Luteoma).
- The tumors are typically immunoreactive for inhibin.
- A diagnosis of "steroid cell tumor, probably Leydig cell tumor" is appropriate if a crystal-free steroid cell tumor is hilar, has a background of hilus cell hyperplasia, is associated with nonmedullated nerve fibers, has fibrinoid vascular change, or shows nuclear clustering.

References

Paraskevas M, Scully RE. Hilus cell tumor of the ovary: a clinico-pathological analysis of 12 Reinke crystal-positive and 9 crystal-negative cases. Int J Gynecol Pathol 8:299–310, 1989.

Roth LM, Sternberg WH. Ovarian stromal tumors containing Leydig cells. II. Pure Leydig cell tumor, non-hilar type. Cancer 32:952–960, 1973.

Sternberg WH, Roth LM. Ovarian stromal tumors containing Leydig cells. I. Stromal-Leydig cell tumors and non-neoplastic transformation of ovarian stroma to Leydig cells. Cancer 32:940–951, 1973.

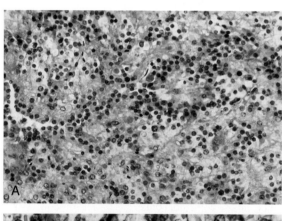
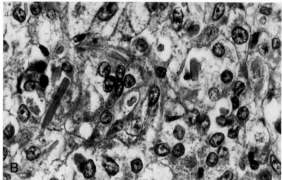

Figure 16–31. Leydig cell tumor. Notice the nuclear clustering (*A*) and Reinke crystals (*B*).

Steroid Cell Tumor, Not Otherwise Specified

General Features

- These tumors, which account for 60% of steroid cell tumors, occur at any age but typically at a younger age (mean, 43 years) than other types of steroid cell tumor. A few tumors occur before puberty.
- Fifty percent of the tumors are associated with androgenic changes, which may be of many years' duration. Estrogenic changes, including rare examples of isosexual pseudoprecocity, occur in 10% of the cases. Rarely, progestagenic changes have been documented.
- Rare tumors have been associated with Cushing's syndrome from cortisol production by the tumor, elevated cortisol levels in the absence of the syndrome, aldosterone secretion, hypercalcemia, erythrocytosis, or ascites.

Pathologic Features

- The tumors are typically grossly well circumscribed, with a mean diameter of 8.4 cm; 5% are bilateral. The sectioned surface is typically solid, yellow or orange (when lipid rich), red to brown (if lipid poor), or dark brown to black (if large quantities of intracytoplasmic lipochrome pigment are present). Necrosis, hemorrhage, and cystic degeneration can be seen.
- Microscopic examination reveals a predominantly solid growth pattern but occasionally shows large aggregates, small nests, irregular clusters, and thin cords or columns. Degenerative pseudovascular spaces (see Stromal Luteoma) may also be present.
- Polygonal to rounded tumor cells with distinct borders have moderate to abundant cytoplasm that varies from eosinophilic and granular (lipid free or lipid poor) to spongy (lipid rich). Cytoplasmic lipochrome pigment is present in about 50% of the cases.
- The nuclei are central and frequently contain prominent nucleoli. In one study, nuclear atypia was absent or slight in 60% of tumors and accompanied by a low mitotic rate (<2 MF per 10 HPF). Grade 1 to 3 nuclear atypia, usually associated with an increase in mitotic rate (up to 15 MF per 10 HPF), was present in the remaining cases.
- The stroma is usually inconspicuous but is prominent in 15% of cases and occasionally is focally fibromatous, edematous, myxoid, or calcified. Prominent necrosis and hemorrhage occur in some tumors, particularly in those with cytologic atypia.
- The tumors are typically immunoreactive for inhibin. One study revealed immunoreactivity for vimentin (75%), CAM 5.2 (46%) (globoid paranuclear staining), AE1/AE3/CK1 (37%), EMA (8%), S-100 protein (7%), and negative staining with carcinoembryonic antigen, chromogranin A, AFP, and HMB-45.

Differential Diagnosis

- Vascular tumors or adenocarcinoma (versus steroid cell tumors with degenerative spaces). Awareness of this degenerative change and its association with cellular debris, inflammatory cells, and fibrosis and the finding of typical areas elsewhere in the tumor facilitate the diagnosis.
- Other tumors containing oxyphilic cells (Appendix 4). These tumors, if well sampled, exhibit features that are absent in steroid cell tumors.
- Clear cell tumors (versus steroid cell tumors with lipid-rich cells). Steroid cell tumors lack the various patterns (other than diffuse) and mucin of primary clear cell carcinomas and the typical vascularity of metastatic renal cell carcinomas. Clear cell tumors also lack immunoreactivity for inhibin.

Prognosis

- Between 25% and 43% of the tumors are clinically malignant. These patients were, on average, 16 years older than those with probably benign tumors in one series. Most patients with Cushing's disease have had extensive intraabdominal spread of tumor at presentation.
- Features associated with malignant behavior include a size of 7 cm or greater (78% malignant); 2 MF or more per 10 HPF (92% malignant); necrosis (86% malignant); hemorrhage (77% malignant); and grade 2 or 3 nuclear atypia (64% malignant). Occasional tumors lacking these features, however, may be clinically malignant.

References

Hayes MC, Scully RE. Ovarian steroid cell tumor (not otherwise specified): a clinicopathological analysis of 63 cases. Am J Surg Pathol 11:835–845, 1987.

Kommoss F, Oliva E, Bhan A, et al. Inhibin expression in ovarian neoplasms. Mod Pathol 11:656–664, 1998.

Seidman JD, Abbondanzo SL, Bratthauer GL. Lipid cell (steroid cell) tumor of the ovary: immunophenotype with analysis of potential pitfall due to endogenous biotin-like activity. Int J Gynecol Pathol 14:331–338, 1995.

Young RH, Scully RE. Ovarian steroid cell tumors associated with Cushing's syndrome: a report of three cases. Int J Gynecol Pathol 6:40–48, 1987.

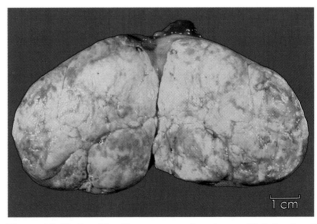

Figure 16–32. Steroid cell tumor, not otherwise specified (sectioned surface).

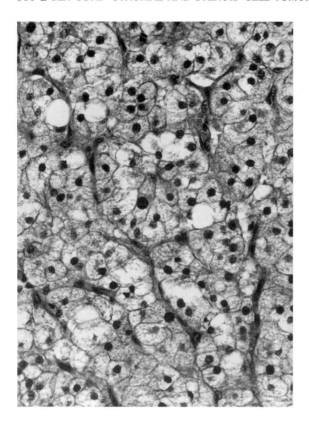

Figure 16–33. Steroid cell tumor, not otherwise specified. There is abundant, pale (lipid-rich) cytoplasm.

CHAPTER 17

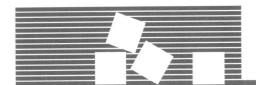

Miscellaneous Primary Tumors of the Ovary

MIXED GERM CELL–SEX CORD–STROMAL TUMORS

Gonadoblastoma

Clinical Features

- Gonadoblastomas are rare and occur almost exclusively in patients with an underlying gonadal disorder, accounting for two thirds of gonadal tumors in such individuals.
- The tumors typically occur in children or young adults, with about one third of the tumors detected before the age of 15 years. The clinical presentation depends on the presence of a mass, its occasional secretion of steroid hormones, the nature of the involved gonads, and the appearance of the secondary sex organs.
- A definite diagnosis of the gonadal abnormality may be impossible when one or both gonads are replaced by tumor. The sexual disorder, when identifiable, is almost always pure or mixed gonadal dysgenesis; a Y chromosome has been detected in more than 90% of cases.
- The patients are typically phenotypic females, who are usually virilized. A minority are phenotypic males with varying degrees of feminization.

Gross Features

- The tumors may be soft and fleshy, firm and cartilaginous, flecked with calcium, or totally calcified; they vary from brown to yellow to gray.
- Pure tumors are usually less than 8 cm in size, and 25% are microscopic; those with germinomatous overgrowth may be much larger.
- The contralateral gonad contains gonadoblastoma in about one third of cases; less often, it contains a malignant germ cell tumor, usually a germinoma, with no evidence of residual gonadoblastoma.
- The gonad in which the tumor develops is of unknown nature in 60%, an abdominal or inguinal testis in 20%, and a gonadal streak in 20% of the cases. Very rare tumors arise in an apparently normal ovary.

Microscopic Features

- Discrete cellular aggregates are composed of an intimate admixture of germ cells and smaller epithelial cells of sex cord type. The germ cells are similar to those of the dysgerminoma and usually exhibit mitotic activity.
- The smaller, round to oval epithelial cells have pale nuclei, are mitotically inactive, and resemble immature Sertoli or granulosa cells. They are immunoreactive for cytokeratin, vimentin, and, in some cases, inhibin.
- The sex cord–type cells surround round spaces filled with eosinophilic basement membrane material, line the periphery of nests that contain germ cells centrally, or surround individual germ cells.
- The epithelial nests are separated by a scanty to, less often, abundant fibrous stroma. Stromal Leydig cells or luteinized cells are present in two thirds of cases.
- The typical histologic appearance of gonadoblastomas can be altered or obliterated by:
  - Extensive deposition of hyalinized basement membrane material.
  - Calcification, present in more than 80% of tumors, typically as laminated plaques and mulberry-like masses.
  - Overgrowth by a malignant germ cell tumor in about 60% of cases, which in more than 80% of such cases is a germinoma that may vary from microscopic penetration into the stroma to massive replacement of the gonad. In the remaining cases, yolk sac tumor, embryonal carcinoma, choriocarcinoma, or immature teratoma overgrows the gonadoblastoma.
  - Overgrowth by a proliferation of the sex cord element; only one such case has been reported.
- Rare, otherwise typical gonadoblastomas exhibit focal histologic patterns of the types encountered within the unclassified mixed germ cell–sex cord–stromal tumors discussed in the next section.

Differential Diagnosis

- Dysgerminoma or seminoma. Either of these tumors in a patient with abnormal gonads should raise the suspicion of its origin in a gonadoblastoma; the only clue to the presence of the latter may be focal calcification or a rare nest of typical gonadoblastoma.
- Sex cord tumor with annular tubules. This tumor resembles the gonadoblastoma because of its similar growth pattern and the presence of basement membrane material and calcification, but it contains no germ cells.
- Unclassified germ cell–sex cord–stromal tumors (see next section).
- Microscopic gonadoblastoma-like foci occurring in 15% of normal fetuses and newborn infants.

Prognosis

- Pure gonadoblastomas are clinically benign, but because of the high frequency with which it gives rise to a malignant germ cell tumor, it should be regarded as an in situ malignant germ cell tumor.

References

Bhathena D, Haning RV Jr, Shapiro S. Coexistence of a gonadoblastoma and mixed germ cell–sex cord stroma tumor. Pathol Res Pract 180:203–206, 1985.

Hart WR, Burkons DM. Germ cell neoplasms arising in gonadoblastomas. Cancer 43:669–678, 1979.

Hussong J, Crussi FG, Chou PM. Gonadoblastoma: immunohistochemical localization of müllerian-inhibiting substance, inhibin, WT-1, and p53. Mod Pathol 10:1101–1105, 1997.

Nakashima K, Nagasaka T, Fukata S, et al. Ovarian gonadoblastoma with dysgerminoma in a woman with two normal children. Hum Pathol 20:814–816, 1989.

Nomura K, Matsui T, Aizawa S. Gonadoblastoma with proliferation resembling Sertoli cell tumor. Int J Gynecol Pathol 18:91–93, 1999.

Roth LM, Eglen DE. Gonadoblastoma: immunohistochemical and ultrastructural observations. Int J Gynecol Pathol 8:72–81, 1989.

Scully RE. Gonadoblastoma: a review of 74 cases. Cancer 25:1340–1356, 1970.

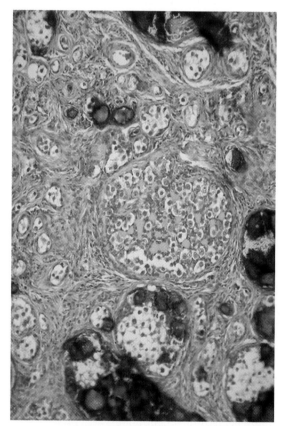

Figure 17–2. Gonadoblastoma. The nests of tumor are composed of large germ cells with clear cytoplasm and smaller sex cord–type cells that surround the germ cells and deposits of eosinophilic basement membrane material. Notice the calcification.

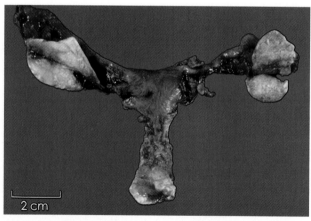

Figure 17–1. Bilateral gonadoblastoma. Each gonad has been bisected to reveal a small mass with white flecks that represent foci of calcification.

Unclassified Germ Cell–Sex Cord–Stromal Tumors

- This category includes all tumors that contain germ cells, sex cord elements, and occasionally, lutein or Leydig-type cells but that lack the distinctive patterns of the gonadoblastoma. These tumors are rare.
- The neoplasms usually occur in infants or girls younger than 10 years of age who have normal gonadal development and a normal karyotype. Occasional examples have caused isosexual precocity, and one bilateral tumor has been reported.
- The germ and sex cord cells may grow in diffuse masses, broad cords, or small solid tubules. Rarely, the sex cord cells grow in retiform patterns or in the form of annular tubules resembling those of the sex cord tumor with annular tubules.
- The sex cord cells may be less mature than in the gonadoblastoma. The germ cells usually have large round nuclei without prominent nucleoli in most cases, but occasionally they resemble closely the cells of a dysgerminoma.
- Two otherwise typical tumors in this category also contained a component that was interpreted as surface epithelial, although in one it was considered to be a retiform sex cord component by another observer. In the other case, glands and cysts were lined by mucinous epithelium of the intestinal type.
- Unlike gonadoblastomas, basement membrane material and calcified foci are scanty or absent.
- An associated dysgerminoma or, rarely, a more malignant germ cell tumor has been encountered in some cases.
- The tumors are usually clinically benign, but rare tumors have metastasized; one of the latter was fatal. The metastatic tumor has had a microscopic appearance similar to that of the primary tumor.

References

Arroyo JG, Harris W, Laden SA. Recurrent mixed germ cell–sex cord–stromal tumor of the ovary in an adult. Int J Gynecol Pathol 17:281–283, 1998.

Jacobsen GK, Braendstrup O, Talerman A. Bilateral mixed germ cell–sex cord–stromal tumour in a young adult woman: case report. APMIS Suppl 23:132–137, 1991.

Talerman A. A distinctive gonadal neoplasm related to gonadoblastoma. Cancer 30:1219–1224, 1972.

Tavassoli FA. A combined germ cell–gonadal stromal–epithelial tumor of the ovary. Am J Surg Pathol 7:73–84, 1983.

Zuntova A, Motlik K, Horejsi J, Eckschlager T. Mixed germ cell–sex cord–stromal tumor with heterologous structures. Int J Gynecol Pathol 11:227–233, 1992.

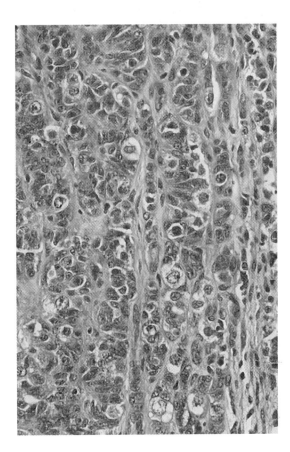

Figure 17–3. Mixed germ cell–sex cord–stromal tumor. Nests and trabeculae of tumor are composed of germ cells with large rounded nuclei (some with prominent nucleoli) that are admixed with oval to spindled sex cord–type cells.

HEPATOID CARCINOMA

■ Hepatoid carcinomas are rare tumors, and typically occur in postmenopausal women who present with nonspecific manifestations. Most of the tumors have spread beyond the ovary at the time of presentation.

■ The tumor has no distinctive gross features.

■ Microscopically, the tumor, at least focally, resembles hepatocellular carcinoma: sheets, trabeculae, and cords of cells have copious eosinophilic cytoplasm and round to oval, often pleomorphic, central nuclei. Mitotic figures and hyaline bodies may be numerous. Some tumor cells are alpha-fetoprotein (AFP) positive.

■ The additional finding of serous carcinoma (or less commonly, another surface epithelial tumor) supports a surface epithelial lineage.

Differential Diagnosis

■ Metastatic hepatocellular carcinoma. Features favoring or establishing this diagnosis include an age younger than 40 years, a liver mass compatible with a primary tumor, and the finding of bile in the tumor. An associated surface epithelial tumor strongly favors a primary tumor.

■ Other ovarian tumors with oxyphilic cells (Appendix 4), especially the hepatoid yolk sac tumor (YST). Features favoring or establishing a diagnosis of hepatoid YST include an age younger than 40 years, foci of more common patterns of YST, and absence of marked nuclear pleomorphism.

References

Ishikura H, Scully RE. Hepatoid carcinoma of the ovary: a report of five cases of a newly described tumor. Cancer 60:2775–2784, 1987.

Matsuta M, Ishikura H, Murakami K, et al. Hepatoid carcinoma of the ovary: a case report. Int J Gynecol Pathol 10:302–310, 1991.

Scurry JP, Brown RW, Jobling T. Combined ovarian serous papillary and hepatoid carcinoma. Gynecol Oncol 63:138–142, 1996.

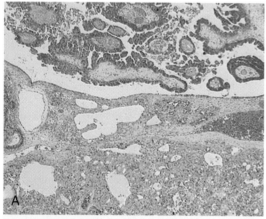

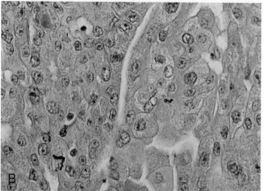

Figure 17–4. Hepatoid carcinoma. *A,* The hepatoid carcinoma abuts a papillary serous carcinoma. *B,* High-power view of the hepatoid carcinoma.

TUMOR OF PROBABLE WOLFFIAN ORIGIN

Clinical Features

- These tumors are thought to be of wolffian origin because they most commonly arise in the broad ligament, where wolffian remnants are present. The ovarian and broad ligament tumors have distinctive microscopic features that differ from tumors of surface epithelial origin.
- The ovarian tumors typically occur in adults and are associated with the usual symptoms of an ovarian tumor. In one case, adjacent stromal luteinization probably caused endometrial hyperplasia manifested clinically by irregular uterine bleeding.

Pathologic Findings

- The tumors are almost invariably unilateral, average 12 cm in diameter, and are solid or solid and cystic. The solid tissue is often lobulated, gray-white to tan or yellow, and rubbery to firm.
- The microscopic appearance is identical to that of the broad ligament tumors (page 261).
- Four of 10 tumors in one study were immunoreactive for inhibin.

Differential Diagnosis

- Sex cord tumors, particularly Sertoli cell tumors (page 378).
- Ovarian ependymomas. Differential features include perivascular pseudorosettes and immunoreactivity for glial fibrillary acidic protein.
- Endometrioid adenocarcinoma (page 317).

Prognosis

- A benign course is typical. One tumor with highly atypical microscopic features was clinically malignant.

References

Hughesdon PE. Ovarian tumours of wolffian or allied nature: their place in ovarian oncology. J Clin Pathol 35:526–535, 1982.

Kommoss F, Oliva E, Bhan A, et al. Inhibin expression in ovarian neoplasms. Mod Pathol 11:656–664, 1998.

Young RH, Scully RE. Ovarian tumors of probable wolffian origin: a report of 11 cases. Am J Surg Pathol 7:125–135, 1983.

RETE CYSTS AND TUMORS

Clinical Features

- Rete cysts and cystadenomas (cysts >1 cm in diameter) have occurred in women 23 to 80 years old (mean, 59 years). Patients with cystadenomas usually have a palpable mass on pelvic examination. Androgenic manifestations in several patients were caused by adjacent hilus hyperplasia and elevated testosterone levels.
- Because rete cystadenomas are often misdiagnosed as serous cystadenoma, their frequency is probably much higher than suggested by the small number of reported cases.
- Fewer than 10 rete adenomas, usually occurring in middle-aged or elderly patients, have been reported; most were incidental microscopic findings. The one well-documented rete adenocarcinoma occurred in a 52-year-old woman with ascites.

Pathologic Findings

- Rete cysts and rete cystadenomas are hilar, although the tumors may expand into the medulla. The cystadenomas, which may reach 24 cm in diameter (mean, 8.7 cm), are typically unilocular but may be multilocular and usually have thin walls and a smooth lining.
- The single patient with rete adenocarcinoma had nonspecific bilateral solid and cystic tumors.
- Rete cystadenomas have walls of fibrovascular tissue and smooth muscle and little or no stroma of ovarian type, and most of them have irregularly spaced, shallow crevices along their inner surfaces.
- Rete cysts and cystadenomas are typically lined by bland cells that are usually cuboidal but occasionally columnar or flattened; in rare cases, occasional ciliated cells have been observed. In about 50% of the cases, the cyst walls contain hilus cells that are typically hyperplastic.
- Rete adenomas are well-circumscribed, hilar proliferations of closely packed elongated small tubules; some tubules may be dilated and contain simple papillae. The tubules and papillae are lined by a single layer of cuboidal to columnar cells resembling that of the normal rete.
- The rete adenocarcinoma consisted of branching hollow or solid tubules and cysts containing papillae with fibrovascular or hyalinized cores. The tubules and papillae were lined by atypical cuboidal nonciliated cells and, focally, transitional-like cells; mitotic figures were numerous.

Differential Diagnosis

- Rete cysts and cystadenomas are distinguished from other benign ovarian and paraovarian cysts on the basis of their hilar location, mural smooth muscle or hilus cells, their characteristic crevices, and an absence or rarity of ciliated cells.
- Rete adenomas are similar to adnexal tumors of probable wolffian origin, but in contrast to the latter, the adenomas typically have a uniform tubular pattern without the sievelike and solid components of wolffian tumors.
- Rete adenocarcinomas are distinguished from retiform Sertoli-Leydig cell tumors by the presence of greater nuclear atypicality and an absence of other typical patterns of Sertoli-Leydig cell tumors. The retiform appearance of the tubules aids in the differential diagnosis with a transitional cell carcinoma.

References

Nogales FF, Carvia RE, Donné C, et al. Adenomas of the rete ovarii. Hum Pathol 26:1428–1433, 1997.

Rutgers JL, Scully RE. Cysts (cystadenomas) and tumors of the rete ovarii. Int J Gynecol Pathol 7:330–342, 1988.

ONCOCYTOMA

- An oncocytoma occurred in a 22-year-old woman and was composed of solid sheets of cells with oxyphilic cytoplasm. Numerous mitochondria were found by electron microscopy.
- Another tumor in a 39-year-old woman, interpreted as an oncocytic adenocarcinoma, was similar except for the additional presence of focal glandular and papillary differentiation.

- The differential diagnosis is with other ovarian tumors containing oxyphilic or oncocytic cells (Appendix 4). The "oncocytic adenocarcinoma" may be an oxyphilic (oncocytic) endometrioid adenocarcinoma (page 316). Before diagnosing ovarian oncocytoma, extensive sampling and immunohistochemical studies should be done to exclude a specific tumor type.

References

Takeda A, Matsuyama M, Sugimoto Y, et al. Oncocytic adenocarcinoma of the ovary. Virchows Arch 399:345–353, 1983.

Yoshida Y, Tenzaki T, Ishiguro T, et al. Oncocytoma of the ovary: light and electron microscopic study. Gynecol Oncol 18:109–114, 1984.

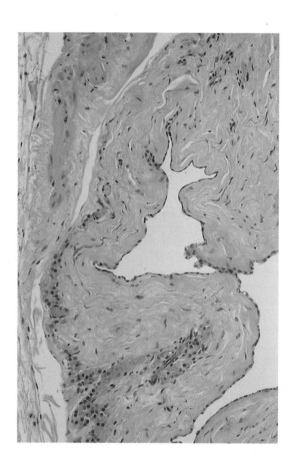

Figure 17–5. Rete cystadenoma. Notice the undulating contour of the cyst lining. The wall is composed of smooth muscle (*upper left*) with nests of Leydig-type cells (*lower left*).

PARAGANGLIOMA

- One paraganglioma, which occurred in a 15-year-old girl with hypertension, was large and unilateral and had the typical microscopic appearance of a pheochromocytoma. After removal of the tumor (which contained epinephrine and norepinephrine), the hypertension resolved.
- The tumor must be distinguished from other tumors containing oxyphil cells (Appendix 4). Immunohistochemical staining for chromogranin and the characteristic immunoreactivity for S-100 by sustentacular cells facilitate the diagnosis.

Reference

Fawcett FJ, Kimbell NKB. Phaeochromocytoma of the ovary. J Obstet Gynaecol Br Commonw 78:458–459, 1971.

WILMS' TUMOR

- One histologically typical Wilms' tumor, which was confined to the ovary, has been reported in a 56-year-old woman who was well 9 years later after postoperative adjuvant radiation therapy and chemotherapy.
- The differential diagnosis includes the retiform Sertoli-Leydig cell tumor, which is much more common than Wilms' tumor. It typically occurs in young females, is sometimes virilizing, usually contains more typical Sertoli-Leydig cell tumor, and lacks typical renal blastema.

Reference

Sahin A, Benda JA. Primary ovarian Wilms' tumor. Cancer 61:1460–1463, 1988.

GESTATIONAL TROPHOBLASTIC DISEASE

- Most reported cases of primary ovarian gestational trophoblastic disease (POGTD) have been choriocarcinomas, but some have been hydatidiform moles.
- Patients with choriocarcinoma typically have a symptomatic mass, which has sometimes ruptured with hemoperitoneum.
- Choriocarcinoma appears grossly as a solid hemorrhagic mass and the hydatidiform mole as a hemorrhagic mass containing vesicles.
- The microscopic findings are identical to their uterine counterparts (see Chapter 10).
- POGTD can be diagnosed only after excluding spread from an extraovarian lesion.
- Choriocarcinomas must be sectioned extensively to exclude a choriocarcinoma of germ cell origin (page 346) or of somatic cell origin (page 336). In a review of ovarian choriocarcinoma, 18 were gestational, 6 nongestational, and 11 of uncertain origin.
- Although the prognosis of the choriocarcinomas has been generally poor, 40% of patients with follow-up data in one review were free of disease 1 to 5.5 years postoperatively; a number of these patients were treated before the advent of modern chemotherapy.

References

Axe SR, Klein VR, Woodruff JD. Choriocarcinoma of the ovary. Obstet Gynecol 66:111–114, 1985.

D'Aguillo AF, Goldbert JI, Kamalamma M, et al. Primary ovarian hydatidiform mole. Hum Pathol 13:279–281, 1982.

Jacobs AJ, Newland JR, Green RK. Pure choriocarcinoma of the ovary. Obstet Gynecol Surv 37:603–609, 1982.

SOFT TISSUE–TYPE TUMORS

Leiomyoma

- Potential origins of these tumors include smooth muscle in the hilus, blood vessel walls, or smooth muscle metaplasia of the ovarian stroma. Ovarian leiomyomas are less common than paraovarian examples, and some tumors submitted as "ovarian" may on careful examination be shown not to originate in the ovary.
- About 50 cases have been reported, occurring in patients from the second to the eighth decades; about 80% of them are premenopausal women. The tumors are usually incidental findings, but larger ones may manifest as an adnexal mass.
- Rare associated findings have included Meigs' syndrome, adjacent hilus cell hyperplasia with elevated plasma testosterone and virilization, diffuse peritoneal leiomyomatosis, and intravenous leiomyomatosis in which the ovarian tumor was the probable source of the intravenous tumor.
- The tumors are usually smaller than 5 cm in diameter but are occasionally massive. They resemble their uterine counterparts grossly and microscopically, including many of the uterine leiomyoma variants, such as those with bizarre nuclei and epithelioid tumors (see Chapter 9).
- Mitotically active or unusually cellular tumors occur, but their rarity and lack of long-term follow-up preclude conclusions about their behavior. As with cellular fibromas (page 373), long-term follow-up to exclude late recurrence in cases of cellular leiomyoma is prudent.

Differential Diagnosis

- Fibroma. These tumors, which are much more common than leiomyomas, have (in contrast to the latter) fibroblastic cells, abundant intercellular collagen, and frequently, a storiform pattern.
- Neoplasms composed of oxyphilic (Appendix 4) or clear cells (Appendix 3) (versus epithelioid leiomyomas). Establishing the correct diagnosis may be difficult and require immunostaining for desmin and other markers.

References

Doss BJ, Wanek SM, Jacques SM, et al. Ovarian leiomyomas: clinicopathologic features in fifteen cases. Int J Gynecol Pathol 18:63–68, 1999.

Matamala MF, Nogales FF, Aneiros J, et al. Leiomyomas of the ovary. Int J Gynecol Pathol 7:190–196, 1988.

Prayson RA, Hart WR. Primary smooth-muscle tumors of the ovary: a clinicopathologic study of four leiomyomas and two mitotically active leiomyomas. Arch Pathol Lab Med 116:1068–1071, 1992.

Hemangioma

- Hemangiomas are uncommon tumors that may be associated with isolated hemangiomas elsewhere or with generalized hemangiomatosis. The tumors typically occur in the medulla and hilus and are usually of the cavernous type.
- Unusual associations have included thrombocytopenia (cured by removal of bilateral hemangiomas), a content of luteinized stromal cells with evidence of hormonal function, and contiguity with a mixed germ cell tumor in a patient with Turner's syndrome.
- The differential diagnosis includes the closely packed vessels in the ovarian medulla that are often a conspicuous normal finding in older women, as well as the pseudovascular spaces found in some steroid cell tumors (see Chapter 16).

References

Lawhead RA, Copeland LJ, Edwards CL. Bilateral ovarian hemangiomas associated with diffuse abdominopelvic hemangiomatosis. Obstet Gynecol 65:597–599, 1985.

Miyauchi J, Mukai M, Yamazaki K, et al. Bilateral ovarian hemangiomas associated with diffuse hemangioendotheliomatosis: a case report. Acta Pathol Jpn 37:1347–1355, 1987.

Savargaonkar PR, Wells S, Graham I, Buckley CH. Ovarian hemangiomas and stromal luteinization. Histopathology 25:185–188, 1994.

Tanaka Y, Sasaki Y, Tachibana K, et al. Gonadal mixed germ cell tumor combined with a large hemangiomatous lesion in a patient with Turner's syndrome and 45,X/46,X, +mar karyotype. Arch Pathol Lab Med 118:1135–1138, 1994.

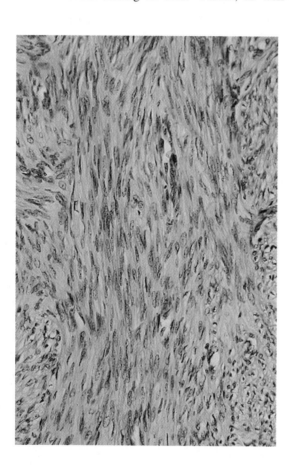

Figure 17–6. Cellular leiomyoma.

Other Benign Soft Tissue–Type Tumors

- Rare tumors, including benign neural tumors, lipomas, lymphangiomas, chondromas, osteomas, and ganglioneuromas, have resembled their extraovarian counterparts.
- Ovarian involvement by plexiform neurofibromatosis may be associated with synchronous involvement of other sites in the female genital tract.

References

Evans A, Lytwyn A, Urbach G, Chapman W. Bilateral lymphangiomas of the ovary: an immunohistochemical characterization and review of the literature. Int J Gynecol Pathol 18:87–90, 1999.

Gordon MD, Weilert M, Ireland K. Plexiform neurofibromatosis involving the uterine cervix, endometrium, myometrium, and ovary. Obstet Gynecol 88:699–701, 1996.

Hegg CA, Flint A. Neurofibroma of the ovary. Gynecol Oncol 37:437–438, 1990.

Nogales FF. Letter to the editor. Histopathology 6:376, 1982.

Prus D, Rosenberg AE, Blumenfeld A, et al. Infantile hemangioendothelioma of the ovary: a monodermal teratoma or a neoplasm of ovarian somatic cells? Am J Surg Pathol 21:1231–1235, 1997.

Sarcomas

- Rare pure sarcomas such as fibrosarcomas, leiomyosarcomas (including the myxoid variant), malignant schwannomas, lymphangiosarcomas, angiosarcomas, rhabdomyosarcomas, chondrosarcomas, and osteosarcomas may arise from the ovarian stroma or the nonspecific supporting tissue of the ovary.
- Some of these tumors may represent overgrowth of a component of a malignant mesodermal mixed tumor, mesodermal adenosarcoma, immature teratoma, dermoid cyst, or heterologous Sertoli-Leydig cell tumor. Thorough sampling in such cases is important.
- Rare sarcomas of various types have been associated with surface-epithelial stromal tumors, particularly serous, mucinous, and clear cell carcinomas, sometimes in the form of mural nodules.

Differential Diagnosis

- Cellular fibroma (versus fibrosarcoma) (page 373).
- Cellular leiomyoma (versus leiomyosarcoma). The differential criteria for these tumors in the ovary are not established because of their rarity. Most leiomyosarcomas, however, have obviously malignant microscopic features.
- YST with myxoid areas (versus myxoid leiomyosarcoma). The variety of patterns and primitive appearance of the YST and immunoreactivity for AFP should resolve this problem.
- Clear cell (Appendix 3) or oxyphilic tumors (Appendix 4) (versus epithelioid leiomyosarcoma).

References

Friedman HD, Mazur MT. Primary ovarian leiomyosarcoma: an immunohistochemical and ultrastructural study. Arch Pathol Lab Med 115:941–945, 1991.

Hines JF, Compton DM, Stacy CC, Potter ME. Pure primary osteosarcoma of the ovary presenting as an extensively calcified adnexal mass: a case report and review of the literature. Gynecol Oncol 39:259–263, 1990.

Kraemer BB, Silva EG, Sniege N. Fibrosarcoma of ovary: a new component in the nevoid basal-cell carcinoma syndrome. Am J Surg Pathol 8:231–236, 1984.

Nielsen GP, Oliva E, Young RH, et al. Primary ovarian rhabdomyosarcoma: a report of 13 cases. Int J Gynecol Pathol 17:113–119, 1998.

Nielsen GP, Young RH, Prat J, Scully RE. Primary angiosarcoma of ovary: a report of seven cases and a review of the literature. Int J Gynecol Pathol 16:378–382, 1997.

Nogales FF, Ayala A, Ruiz-Avila I, Sirvent JJ. Myxoid leiomyosarcoma of the ovary: analysis of three cases. Hum Pathol 22:1268–1273, 1991.

Nucci MR, Krausz T, Lifschitz-Mercer B, et al. Angiosarcoma of the ovary: clinicopathologic and immunohistochemical analysis of four cases with a broad morphological spectrum. Am J Surg Pathol 22:620–630, 1998.

Prat J, Scully RE. Cellular fibromas and fibrosarcomas of the ovary: a comparative clinicopathologic analysis of seventeen cases. Cancer 47:2663–2670, 1981.

Sahin A, Benda JA. An immunohistochemical study of primary ovarian sarcoma: an evaluation of nine tumors. Int J Gynecol Pathol 7:268–279, 1988.

Stone GC, Bell DA, Fuller A, et al. Malignant schwannoma of the ovary: report of a case. Cancer 58:1575–1582, 1986.

Talerman A, Auerbach WM, Van Meurs AJ. Primary chondrosarcoma of the ovary. Histopathology 5:319–324, 1981.

SMALL CELL CARCINOMAS AND NON–SMALL CELL–TYPE NEUROENDOCRINE CARCINOMAS

Hypercalcemic-Type Small Cell Carcinoma

Clinical Features

- Hypercalcemic-type small cell carcinoma has occurred in females 7 months to 46 years old (mean, 24 years). Rarely, it is familial, as exemplified by its occurrence in three sisters; the tumors in these women were all bilateral, in contrast to a 1% frequency of bilaterality in general.
- About 65% of the tumors are accompanied by paraendocrine hypercalcemia, accounting for one half of the ovarian tumors associated with the latter. Parathyroid-related polypeptide has been demonstrated immunohistochemically in some tumors.
- About 50% of the tumors have spread beyond the ovary at the time of laparotomy.

Pathologic Features

- Gross examination usually reveals a large, predominantly solid, cream-colored to gray mass resembling an ovarian lymphoma or dysgerminoma. Areas of necrosis, hemorrhage, and cystic degeneration are common; rare neoplasms are predominantly or entirely cystic.
- The most common microscopic pattern is a sheetlike arrangement of small, closely packed epithelial cells; small islands, cords, and trabeculae may also be seen. Follicle-like structures lined by tumor cells and usually containing eosinophilic fluid are present in 80% of cases.
- The tumors cells typically have scanty cytoplasm and small nuclei containing single small nucleoli; mitotic figures are common.

■ In about 50% of cases, a small or occasionally large proportion of the tumor cells have abundant eosinophilic cytoplasm, sometimes appearing globular (i.e., large cell variant). The large cells have larger, paler nuclei and more prominent nucleoli than the small cells.

■ Small foci of mucinous epithelium are present in about 10% of the tumors, ranging from glands or cysts lined by benign or atypical mucinous epithelium to signet-ring cells.

■ The tumor stroma is typically inconspicuous but is occasionally prominent and may be edematous, myxoid (particularly in areas with large cells), or hyalinized.

■ In most tumors, ultrastructural examination has shown an epithelial appearance of the tumor cells, usually with abundant, dilated rough endoplasmic reticulum. The large tumor cells may contain whorls of microfilaments; dense core granules are absent.

■ The cells are variably immunoreactive for vimentin, cytokeratin, and epithelial membrane antigen.

■ Flow cytometry on paraffin-embedded material has shown that the tumor cells are diploid.

Differential Diagnosis

■ Granulosa cell tumor of the adult (page 365) or juvenile type (page 368).

■ Other small cell carcinomas that may involve the ovary (Appendix 5). These include small cell carcinoma of the pulmonary type (page 400) and metastatic small cell carcinoma (page 419).

■ Malignant lymphomas. The presence of epithelial growth patterns, including follicle-like spaces, in the small cell carcinoma and the differing clinical, cytologic, immunohistochemical, and ultrastructural features of the two tumors enable their distinction.

■ Noncarcinomatous small cell malignant tumors that may involve the ovary (Appendix 5). These tumors are discussed under their respective headings. A variety of clinical and pathologic features facilitate the differential diagnosis.

Prognosis

■ The prognosis is poor: only one third of patients with stage Ia disease have disease-free follow-up periods of 1 to 13 years (mean, 5.7 years). Most patients with higher-stage tumors have died of disease, usually within 2 years, or had recurrent tumor at short postoperative intervals.

■ Rare patients with high-stage tumors who have received intensive chemotherapy, radiation therapy, or both were alive up to 6.5 years postoperatively.

■ Potentially favorable prognostic features in stage Ia cases include an age older than 30 years, a normal preoperative calcium level, a tumor size less than 10 cm, absence of large cells, an operation that included bilateral oophorectomy, and postoperative radiation therapy.

References

Aguirre P, Thor AD, Scully RE. Ovarian small cell carcinoma: histogenetic considerations based on immunohistochemical and other findings. Am J Clin Pathol 92:140–149, 1989.

Dickersin GR, Scully RE. An update on the electron microscopy of small cell carcinoma of the ovary with hypercalcemia. Ultrastruct Pathol 17:411–422, 1993.

Eichhorn JH, Bell DA, Young RH, et al. DNA content and proliferative activity in ovarian small cell carcinomas of the hypercalcemic type: implications for diagnosis, prognosis, and histogenesis. Am J Clin Pathol 98:579–586, 1992.

Matias-Guiu X, Prat J, Young RH, et al. Human parathyroid hormone-related protein in ovarian small cell carcinoma: an immunohistochemical study. Cancer 73:1878–1881, 1994.

McMahon JR, Hart WR. Ultrastructural analysis of small cell carcinomas of the ovary. Am J Clin Pathol 90:523–529, 1988.

Young RH, Oliva E, Scully RE. Small cell carcinoma of the ovary, hypercalcemic type: a clinicopathologic analysis of 150 cases. Am J Surg Pathol 18:1102–1116, 1994.

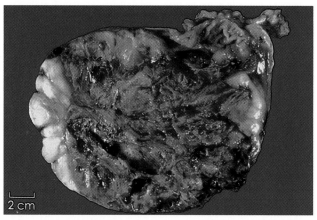

Figure 17–7. Hypercalcemic-type of small cell carcinoma (sectioned surface). Large areas of hemorrhage and necrosis are surrounded by a rim of solid, white, fleshy tumor.

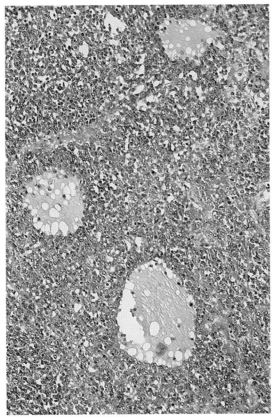

Figure 17–8. Hypercalcemic-type of small cell carcinoma. Sheets of tumor cells are interrupted by follicle-like spaces.

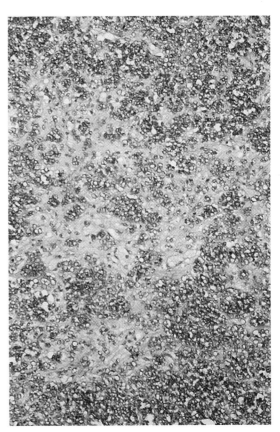

Figure 17–9. Hypercalcemic-type of small cell carcinoma. Small nests and individual tumor cells are separated by a hyalinized stroma.

Figure 17–10. Hypercalcemic-type of small cell carcinoma ("large cell variant"). The tumor cells have moderate amounts of eosinophilic cytoplasm. More typical small cell areas were present in other areas of the tumor.

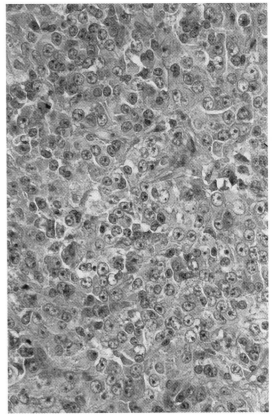

Pulmonary-Type Small Cell Carcinoma

Clinical Features

- The 11 reported tumors, which occurred in women 28 to 85 years old (mean, 59 years), were associated with a presentation similar to that of the usual ovarian cancer.
- At laparotomy almost one half of the tumors were bilateral and most had extraovarian spread.

Pathologic Features

- Most of the tumors are large (mean diameter, 13.5 cm) and solid; some have had a minor cystic component.
- Microscopically, sheets, closely packed islands, and trabeculae are composed of small to medium-sized, round to spindle-shaped cells with scanty cytoplasm, hyperchromatic nuclei with stippled chromatin and inconspicuous nucleoli.
- Most of the tumors are associated with a differentiated epithelial component, which has included endometrioid carcinoma, a focus of squamous differentiation, a cyst lined by atypical mucinous cells, and Brenner tumor.
- The tumors contain argyrophil granules in a minority of cases. Most are immunoreactive for keratin and neuron-specific enolase; less commonly, there is staining for epithelial membrane antigen, chromogranin, and Leu-7 but not for vimentin.
- Five of 8 tumors tested were aneuploid, and three were diploid.

Differential Diagnosis

- Small cell carcinomas of hypercalcemic type (page 397). The older age group and association with a surface epithelial tumor point to the correct diagnosis.
- Metastatic small cell carcinomas from the lung and rarely other sites (page 419). The distinction is facilitated by the usual association of the primary form with surface epithelial tumor and clinical identification of an extraovarian primary tumor.
- Other primary and metastatic ovarian tumors that are characterized by small cells with scanty cytoplasm (Appendix 5).

Prognosis

- Five of seven patients who had long term follow-up observation died of or with disease at 1 to 13 months (mean, 8 months); only one was alive after a long interval (7.5 years).

Reference

Eichhorn JH, Young RH, Scully RE. Primary ovarian small cell carcinoma of pulmonary type: a clinicopathologic, immunohistologic and flow cytometric analysis of 11 cases. Am J Surg Pathol 16:926–938, 1992.

Non−Small Cell Neuroendocrine−Type Undifferentiated Carcinoma

- Eight of these tumors, each of which was admixed with a surface epithelial tumor (seven mucinous, one endometrioid), have been reported in women 22 to 77 years of age. Six of the tumors were stage I, one, stage II and one, stage III. Most of them were unilateral.
- The neuroendocrine component is composed predominantly of sheets, closely packed islands, cords and trabeculae of epithelial cells with little stroma.
- Medium to large sized tumor cells contain scanty to moderate amounts of eosinophilic, sometimes granular, cytoplasm and large nuclei, which in some cases contain macronuclei.
- The cytoplasm of the neuroendocrine cells is argyrophilic and most of the cells are immunoreactive for chromogranin, neuron-specific enolase, and serotonin. Several tumors have contained neuropeptide hormones.
- The prognosis is poor.

Differential Diagosis

- Carcinoid tumors. These tumors have a more regular architecture and much less atypicality and less mitotic activity.
- Small cell carcinoma of the pulmonary type. This distinction is based on the differing sizes of the cells but does not appear to have prognostic significance.
- Metastatic non−small cell neuroendocrine carcinoma. The association with a surface epithelial tumor is a strong clue to the primary nature of the neoplasm in most cases, but in the absence of such a component, use of other criteria (page 405) to exclude a metastasis is necessary.

References

Eichhorn JH, Lawrence WD, Young RH, Scully RE. Ovarian neuroendocrine carcinomas of non−small cell type associated with surface epithelial adenocarcinomas: a study of five cases and review of the literature. Int J Gynecol Pathol 15:303–314, 1996.

Jones K, Diaz JA, Donner LR. Neuroendocrine carcinoma arising in an ovarian mucinous cystadenoma. Int J Gynecol Pathol 15:167–170, 1996.

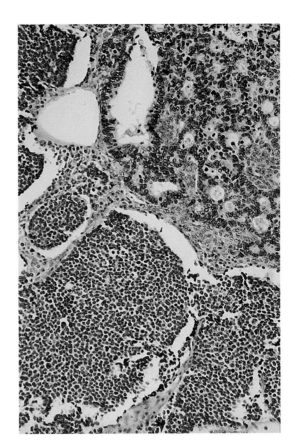

Figure 17–11. Pulmonary-type small cell carcinoma. The small cell carcinoma is admixed with an endometrioid carcinoma.

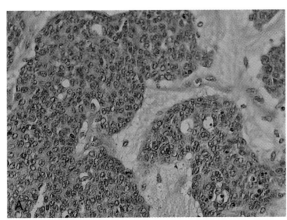

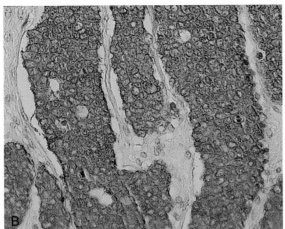

Figure 17–12. *A,* Non–small-cell, neuroendocrine-type, undifferentiated carcinoma. *B,* The tumor cells are immunoreactive for chromogranin.

ADENOID CYSTIC AND BASALOID CARCINOMAS

■ These rare tumors have an exclusive or conspicuous component resembling either adenoid cystic carcinoma (ACC) or basal cell carcinoma. These tumors are probably variants of surface epithelial carcinomas.

Adenoid Cystic Carcinoma

■ Six of the eight reported patients were in the seventh or eighth decades. Five had stage III disease.
■ Five of the tumors contained a component of surface epithelial neoplasia (serous, endometrioid, clear cell), which was usually carcinomatous but occasionally borderline.
■ "Adenoid cystic-like" is the appropriate term for most of these tumors because of the usual absence of myoepithelial cells (as shown by lack of immunoreactivity for S-100 and actin). At least one of the eight tumors, however, contained myoepithelial cells and was considered a true ACC.
■ All of the patients with high-stage tumors with follow-up were dead of disease or alive with disease at the time of reporting.

Basaloid Carcinomas

■ The six reported patients presented over a wide age range (19 to 65 years). Two had extraovarian spread at presentation.
■ In addition to the basaloid carcinoma, three tumors had an ameloblastoma-like pattern. Rarer findings have included foci of endometrioid carcinoma, squamous differentiation, or nonspecific glands.
■ The prognosis was excellent with relatively limited follow-up data (16 to 71 months).

References

Eichhorn JH, Scully RE. "Adenoid cystic" and basaloid carcinomas of the ovary: evidence for a surface epithelial lineage. A report of 12 cases. Mod Pathol 8:731–740, 1995.

Feczko JD, Jentz DL, Roth LM. Adenoid cystic ovarian carcinoma compared with other adenoid cystic carcinomas of the female genital tract. Mod Pathol 9:413–417, 1996.

Russell P, Wills EJ, Watson G, et al. Monomorphic (basal cell) salivary adenoma of ovary: report of a case. Ultrastruct Pathol 19:431–438, 1995.

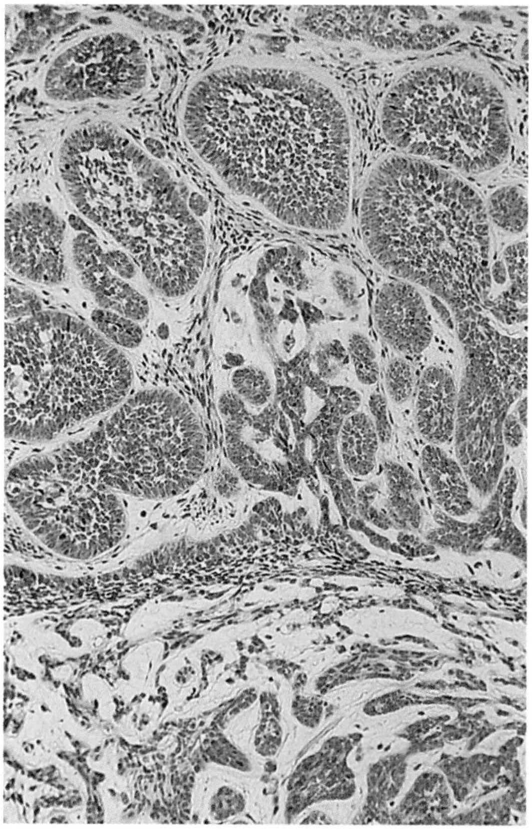

Figure 17–13. Basaloid carcinoma.

MESOTHELIAL TUMORS

Adenomatoid Tumor

- Only 10 well-documented examples of this benign tumor of mesothelial cell origin have been reported, all in adults; only two were symptomatic.
- Most of them were hilar and were less than 3 cm in diameter, but two were 6 and 8 cm. They were typically solid, but one was multicystic. The microscopic appearance is identical to that encountered in the uterus (page 229).

Differential Diagnosis

- Multilocular peritoneal inclusion cyst (page 450).
- Lymphangioma (page 229).

Reference

Young RH, Silva EG, Scully RE. Ovarian and juxtaovarian adenomatoid tumors: a report of six cases. Int J Gynecol Pathol 10:364–371, 1991.

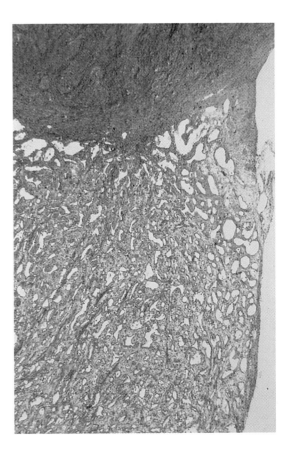

Figure 17–14. Adenomatoid tumor of the ovary. The tumor (*bottom*) abuts the ovarian stroma (*top*).

Malignant Mesothelioma

- Although secondary involvement of the ovary by well-differentiated papillary and malignant peritoneal mesothelioma is common (see Chapter 20), extensive ovarian involvement (with the clinical presentation that of an ovarian cancer) is rare. In 3 of 10 such cases, the tumor was confined to the ovary and interpreted as primary ovarian mesothelioma.

- When there is prominent ovarian involvement, the tumor may be misinterpreted as a type of primary ovarian tumor, usually serous carcinoma, the differential diagnosis of which is discussed on page 456.

References

Clement PB, Young RH, Scully RE. Malignant mesotheliomas presenting as ovarian masses: a report of nine cases, including two primary ovarian mesotheliomas. Am J Surg Pathol 20:1067–1080, 1996.

Goldblum J, Hart WR. Localized and diffuse mesotheliomas of the genital tract and peritoneum in women: a clinicopathological study of nineteen true mesothelial neoplasms, other than adenomatoid tumors, multicystic mesotheliomas and localized fibrous tumors. Am J Surg Pathol 19:1124–1137, 1995.

Stamatakos MD, Tavassoli FA. Mesotheliomas involving the ovary [Abstract]. Mod Pathol 11:115A, 1998.

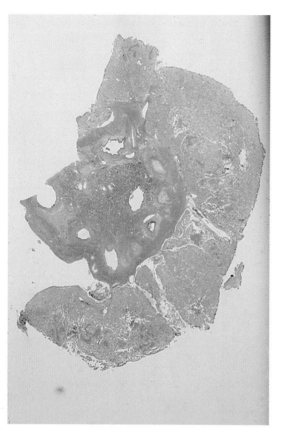

Figure 17–15. Diffuse malignant mesothelioma with prominent ovarian involvement. Tumor encases an otherwise normal ovary.

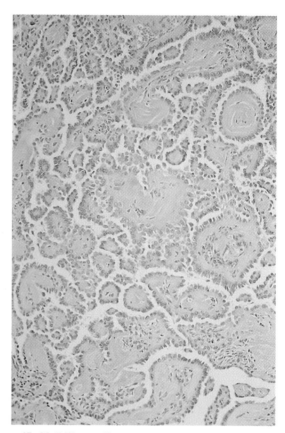

Figure 17–16. Diffuse malignant mesothelioma with prominent ovarian involvement. The tumor has a papillary pattern and cellular buds, an appearance potentially mimicking that of a serous borderline tumor.

CHAPTER 18

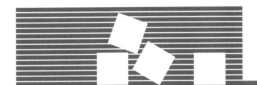

Secondary Tumors of the Ovary

GENERAL FEATURES

- Metastases to the ovary account for 6% to 7% of ovarian cancers found at laparotomy for a pelvic or abdominal mass.
- For the most common cancers that spread to the ovary (i.e., intestinal, gastric, and mammary), the average age of patients with ovarian involvement is significantly lower than that of those without ovarian spread, presumably because of the greater vascularity of the ovary of younger women.
- Tumors spread to the ovary by blood vessels, through lymphatics, transcoelomically, by direct extension (i.e., tumors of the tube and uterus, mesotheliomas, occasional colonic and appendiceal carcinomas), and through the tubal lumen (from genital tract carcinomas).
- Metastases are bilateral in about 70% of cases, and the possibility of metastasis increases with bilateral cancers. Almost 10% of the latter that manifest as adnexal masses are metastatic. Other gross findings that suggest metastasis, but are not diagnostic, are serosal deposits and multiple discrete nodules within the ovary.
- Some ovarian metastases are predominantly cystic, including cases in which the primary tumor is solid. These tumors may be grossly indistinguishable from a cystic surface epithelial tumor.
- Microscopic features that suggest metastases include surface implants (often with a desmoplastic stroma), growth as multiple nodules, lymphatic or blood vessel invasion, invasion of normal follicular structures, and variation in growth pattern from one nodule to another (e.g., benign-appearing glands and cysts in one nodule and small but irregular, infiltrating glands haphazardly arranged within a reactive stroma in an adjacent nodule).
- Well-formed tubules or follicle-like spaces are found in many types of metastatic tumor, simulating patterns of a variety of primary ovarian tumors, particularly those in the sex cord–stromal category.
- Recognition of an ovarian tumor as metastatic depends on an adequate clinical history, a thorough clinical and operative search by the gynecologist for an extraovarian primary, and a careful evaluation of the gross and microscopic features of the ovarian tumor. Special stains for mucins and immunostains help in some cases, and rarely, electron microscopy is a diagnostic aid.
- A primary extraovarian tumor may not be discovered until several years have elapsed since removal of the metastatic ovarian tumor. In one series of the latter, the primary tumors were not discovered until autopsy in almost 14% of cases.
- In rare cases, removal of a metastatic tumor in an ovary is associated with a prolonged survival, suggesting that isolated spread to an ovary occurs occasionally.

References

Demopoulos RI, Touger L, Dubin N. Secondary ovarian carcinoma: a clinical and pathological evaluation. Int J Gynecol Pathol 16:166–175, 1987.

Mazur MT, Hsueh S, Gersell DJ. Metastases to the female genital tract: analysis of 325 cases. Cancer 53:1978–1984, 1985.

Petru E, Pickel H, Heydarfadai M, et al. Nongenital cancers metastatic to the ovary. Gynecol Oncol 44:83–86, 1992.

Ulbright TM, Roth LM, Stehman FB. Secondary ovarian neoplasia: a clinicopathologic study of 35 cases. Cancer 53:1164–1174, 1984.

Yazigi R, Sandstad J. Ovarian involvement in extragenital cancer. Gynecol Oncol 34:84–87, 1989.

Young RH, Scully RE. Metastatic tumors in the ovary: a problem-oriented approach and review of the recent literature. Semin Diagn Pathol 8:250–276, 1991.

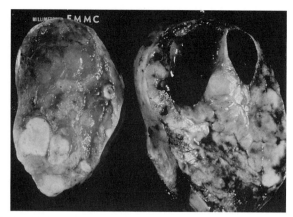

Figure 18–1. Sectioned surfaces of both ovaries showing bilateral involvement and multinodularity of metastatic tumor. The primary tumor was a goblet cell carcinoid of the appendix.

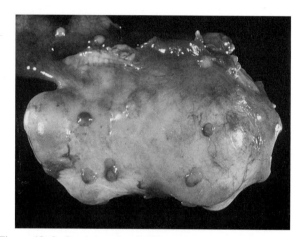

Figure 18–2. Ovarian surface implants of metastatic carcinoma. The primary tumor was carcinoma of the breast.

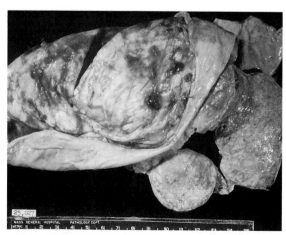

Figure 18–3. Metastatic tumor in an ovary that, unlike the primary colonic adenocarcinoma, was extensively cystic (one large locule has been opened) and necrotic.

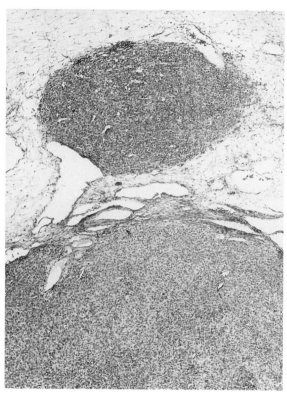

Figure 18–4. Multinodular growth pattern of metastatic tumor in the ovary. The primary tumor was malignant melanoma.

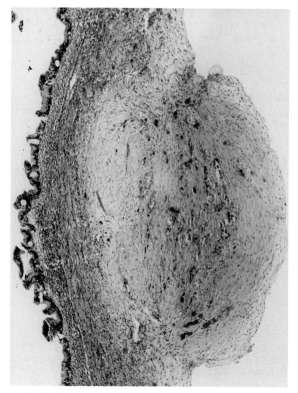

Figure 18–5. Tumor metastatic to the ovarian surface formed a discrete desmoplastic implant. The primary tumor was pancreatic adenocarcinoma. Notice the lining of a large cyst (*extreme left*) contrasting with the infiltrating small glands in the implant, findings reflecting the diversity of patterns that occurs in many metastatic tumors.

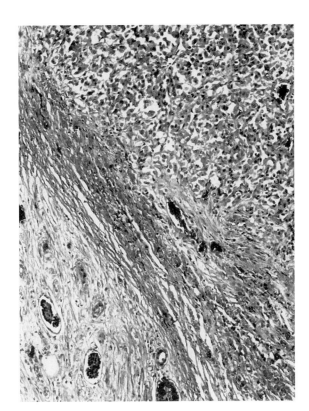

Figure 18–6. Carcinoma metastatic to the ovary exhibits prominent lymphatic invasion (*lower left*). The primary tumor was carcinoma of the breast.

GASTRIC CARCINOMA, INCLUDING KRUKENBERG TUMOR

General Features

- Most ovarian metastases of gastric origin are Krukenberg tumors: carcinomas with a prominent component of mucin-filled signet-ring cells typically but not invariably lying within a cellular stroma.
- About 70% of Krukenberg tumors arise in the stomach, usually in the pylorus. Other sources of Krukenberg tumors, in descending order of frequency, are carcinomas of the breast, colon, appendix, pancreas, gallbladder, biliary tract, urinary bladder, and cervix.
- Gastric signet-ring cell carcinomas metastasize to the ovary more than twice as often as gastric intestinal-type carcinomas, and signet-ring cell carcinomas of the breast and intestine more frequently spread to the ovaries than do carcinomas of these organs without signet-ring cells.
- The average age of patients with a Krukenberg tumor is about 45 years. It is the most common form of ovarian metastatic carcinoma in young women and is encountered often in the fourth decade and occasionally in the third decade or rarely even earlier.

- Almost 90% of patients with Krukenberg tumors have symptoms related to ovarian involvement (i.e., abdominal pain and swelling). Other symptoms in some cases include abnormal uterine bleeding, androgenic manifestations (particularly during pregnancy) as a result of stromal luteinization, and symptoms related to the primary tumor.
- The gastric carcinoma is usually diagnosed preoperatively, during the oophorectomy, or within a few months thereafter, but often a small primary tumor remains occult until 5 or more years after the oophorectomy. Very small gastric and breast primaries in women with Krukenberg tumors may require exhaustive sectioning to detect them, even at autopsy.
- Almost all the patients die within a year of the diagnosis of ovarian metastasis, but there have been rare long-term survivors with no clinical evidence of tumor after gastrectomy and bilateral oophorectomy.

Gross Features

- Gross examination reveals bilateral tumors in 80% of cases. They are usually rounded or reniform, white to pale yellow, solid, occasionally bosselated masses.
- The sectioned surfaces are white to pale yellow, often

with foci that are purple, red, or brown and with a firm, fleshy, gelatinous, or spongy cut surface. Occasionally, large, thin-walled cysts contain mucinous or watery fluid.

■ Metastatic gastric adenocarcinomas other than Krukenberg tumors may be predominantly solid or cystic.

Microscopic Features

■ Mucin-rich signet-ring cells occur singly, in clusters, or in large aggregates within an often cellular ovarian stroma that may have a storiform pattern.

■ The cytoplasm of the signet-ring cells may be granular and eosinophilic (rather than pale and vacuolated) or may contain a clear vacuole containing a central eosinophilic body. The mucin in the signet-ring cells is usually easily demonstrable by the periodic acid–Schiff (PAS) stain.

■ Other frequent findings include small glands, a prominent tubular architecture, mucin-poor tumor cells, cysts lined by minimally atypical mucinous epithelium, abundant collagen, marked stromal edema, pools of mucin, and blood vessel and lymphatic invasion. Luteinized stromal cells are often present, particularly in pregnant patients.

■ Metastatic gastric carcinomas of the non–signet-ring cell type are composed of glands and cysts of the intestinal type and sheets and irregular aggregates of poorly differentiated epithelial cells.

Differential Diagnosis

■ Fibroma. Careful search for typical signet-ring cells establishes the diagnosis.

■ Sertoli-Leydig cell tumor (SLCT) (versus tubular Krukenberg tumor, especially with luteinized stromal cells). Signet-ring cells, however, are not a feature of SLCTs (except heterologous tumors containing a goblet-cell carcinoid), and typical patterns of SLCT are also usually present.

■ Clear cell carcinomas with signet-ring cells. Other characteristic features of clear cell carcinoma are almost always present (page 326).

■ Mucinous carcinoid tumors with signet-ring cells. These tumors also contain a component of carcinoid tumor, the presence of which can be confirmed by argyrophil or chromogranin staining.

■ Sclerosing stromal tumor. Signet-ring cells in these tumors contain lipid not mucin.

■ Signet-ring stromal tumor. The vacuolated cells in this tumor are mucin negative.

■ Mucicarminophilic histiocytosis. The lesional cells are PAS negative.

■ Surface epithelial cystic or solid inclusions in the ovarian cortex with a vacuolar, presumably hydropic cytoplasmic change. The vacuolar material is mucin negative.

■ Other ovarian lesions containing signet-ring cells as listed in Appendix 14.

References

Bullon A, Arseneau J, Prat J, et al. Tubular Krukenberg tumor: a problem in histopathologic diagnosis. Am J Surg Pathol 5:225–232, 1981.

Holtz F, Hart WR. Krukenberg tumors of the ovary: a clinicopathologic analysis of 27 cases. Cancer 50:2438–2447, 1982.

Wong PC, Ferenczy A, Fan L-D, McCaughey WTE. Krukenberg tumors of the ovary: ultrastructural, histochemical, and immunohistochemical studies of 15 cases. Cancer 57:751–760, 1986.

Woodruff JD, Novak ER. The Krukenberg tumor: study of 48 cases from the Ovarian Tumor Registry. Obstet Gynecol 15:351–360, 1960.

Yakushiji M, Tazaki T, Nishimura H, Kato T. Krukenberg tumors of the ovary: a clinicopathologic analysis of 112 cases. Acta Obstet Gynaecol Jpn 39:479–485, 1987.

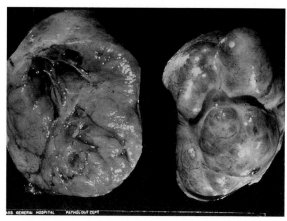

Figure 18–7. Krukenberg tumor: serosal (*right*) and sectioned surfaces (*left*).

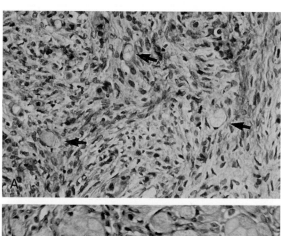

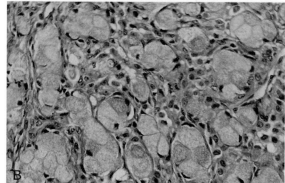

Figure 18–8. Krukenberg tumor. *A,* On low power, the appearance of the tumor simulates that of an ovarian fibroma, but rare, scattered signet-ring cells (*arrows*) are present. *B,* Numerous signet-ring cells from another case.

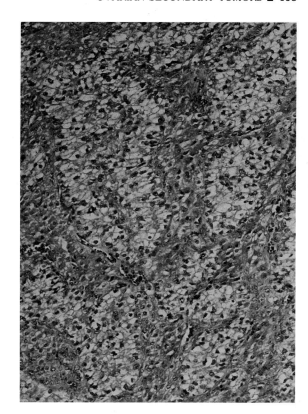

Figure 18–9. Tubular Krukenberg tumor has a prominent tubular pattern resembling that of lipid-rich Sertoli cell tumors.

INTESTINAL CARCINOMA

General Features

- About 4% of women with colonic cancer have ovarian metastases during the course of their disease; women about 40 years of age have them more frequently than older women.
- Almost one half of colorectal cancers metastatic to the ovary are misinterpreted clinically or microscopically as primary ovarian tumors, even when the existence of a colonic cancer is known.
- The site of the primary tumors in one study was 77% in the rectosigmoid, 5% descending colon, 9% ascending colon, and 9% cecum. Rare tumors occur in the transverse colon or the small intestine. Small primary tumors may account for large, bilateral ovarian tumors.
- The clinical picture may include:
  - Presentation with an intestinal carcinoma (50% to 75% of cases) that antedates the diagnosis of the ovarian tumor by up to 3 years in 90% of the cases
  - Unexpected ovarian involvement found during resection of a colonic carcinoma (15% to 20% of cases)
  - Presentation as an ovarian tumor (3% to 20% of the cases).
- Metastatic colonic carcinomas are among the most common ovarian tumors, excluding those in the sex cord–stromal category, that are associated with estrogenic or androgenic manifestations (a result of functioning stroma).
- Almost all patients with colonic carcinoma metastatic to the ovary die within 3 years of detection of ovarian involvement; the mean survival in one series was 16 months.

Gross Features

- The ovarian tumors, which are bilateral in about 60% of cases, may form solid masses but are more often predominantly cystic. They are frequently large (median largest dimension of 11 cm in one series) and commonly rupture preoperatively or during their removal.
- Sectioning typically reveals friable or mushy, yellow, red, or gray tissue and cysts with necrotic, mucinous, clear, or bloody contents. Multiple, thin-walled cysts

with mucinous contents may simulate a mucinous cystadenoma or cystadenocarcinoma.

Microscopic Features

- The characteristic low-power appearances include small or large glands often arranged in a cribriform pattern, extensive "dirty" necrosis (eosinophilic material with nuclear debris within cyst and gland lumens), a garland appearance (glands at the edge of the necrotic material), and focal segmental necrosis of the glandular epithelium.
- The glands are typically lined by stratified cells with moderate to severe cytologic atypia and frequent mitotic figures. Mucin-containing goblet cells may be scattered among mucin-free cells but are often absent. Cysts lined by well-differentiated, mucin-rich epithelium occur in up to 20% of the cases.
- Rarely, the appearance is that of a colloid carcinoma, or when the primary intestinal tumor is of the rare clear cell type, a clear cell carcinoma or endometrioid carcinoma of secretory type is simulated.
- Lymphovascular space invasion is common. The stroma may be desmoplastic, edematous, or mucoid but often simulates ovarian stroma, containing luteinized cells in about 30% of cases.
- The tumors, in contrast to primary surface epithelial tumors in the differential diagnosis, some of which may also exhibit dirty necrosis (DeConstanza et al), have a typical immunoprofile: cytokeratin (CK) 7 negative, CK 20 positive, and carcinoembryonic antigen (CEA) positive (CK 7−/CK 20+/CEA+).

Differential Diagnosis

- Primary endometrioid adenocarcinoma. Features favoring or establishing a diagnosis of metastatic colonic carcinoma include:
  - A known primary intestinal cancer, bilaterality, prominent dirty necrosis (particularly when extensive and associated with one or more of the other features listed here), segmental necrosis, and higher-grade nuclei and mitotic activity compared with endometrioid carcinomas with similar degrees of glandular differentiation
  - An absence of squamous metaplasia, adenofibromatous areas, and associated endometriosis
  - The immunoprofile of CK 7−/CK 20 + /CEA+
- Primary mucinous adenocarcinomas. These tumors have a much lower frequency of bilaterality, multinodularity, dirty necrosis, vascular space invasion, and surface involvement than metastatic intestinal cancer.
  - Small areas of carcinoma on the background of an extensive benign-appearing mucinous tumor strongly favor a primary carcinoma. However, metastatic intestinal carcinomas may focally have a deceptive appearance that may simulate a benign or borderline mucinous tumor.
- Clear cell adenocarcinoma and secretory endometrioid carcinoma (versus metastatic colonic carcinoma of the

clear cell type). Bilaterality, prominent dirty necrosis, and the immunoprofile of CK 7−/CK 20+/CEA+ all favor or establish a diagnosis of metastatic colonic clear cell carcinoma.

References

Daya D, Nazerali L, Frank GL. Metastatic ovarian carcinoma of large intestinal origin simulating primary ovarian carcinoma: a clinicopathologic study of 25 cases. Am J Clin Pathol 97:751–758, 1992.

DeConstanzo DC, Elias JM, Chumas JC. Necrosis in 84 ovarian carcinomas: a morphologic study of primary versus metastatic colonic carcinoma with a selective immunohistochemical analysis of cytokeratin subtypes and carcinoembryonic antigen. Int J Gynecol Pathol 16: 245–249, 1997.

Fowler LJ, Maygarden SJ, Novotny DB. Human alveolar macrophage-56 and carcinoembryonic antigen monoclonal antibodies in the differential diagnosis between primary ovarian and metastatic gastrointestinal carcinomas. Hum Pathol 25:666–670, 1994.

Lash RH, Hart WR. Intestinal adenocarcinomas metastatic to the ovaries: a clinicopathological evaluation of 22 cases. Am J Surg Pathol 11:114–121, 1987.

Loy TS, Calaluce RD, Keeney GL. Cytokeratin immunostaining in differentiating primary ovarian carcinoma from metastatic colonic adenocarcinoma. Mod Pathol 9:1040–1044, 1996.

Young RH, Hart WR. Metastatic intestinal carcinomas simulating primary ovarian clear cell carcinoma and secretory endometrioid carcinoma: a clinicopathologic and immunohistochemical study of five cases. Am J Surg Pathol 22:805–815, 1998.

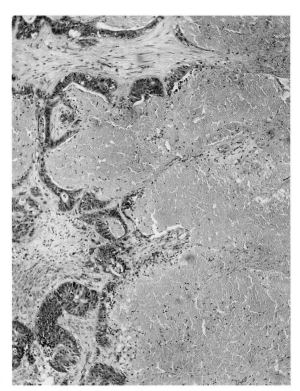

Figure 18–10. Colonic adenocarcinoma metastatic to the ovary. Notice the extensive, dirty luminal necrosis and focal necrosis of neoplastic epithelium lining the cysts.

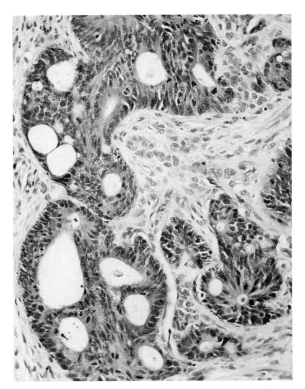

Figure 18–11. Typical high-power appearance of colonic adenocarcinoma metastatic to the ovary. Notice the cribriform pattern and moderate to high-grade nuclear features with numerous mitotic figures.

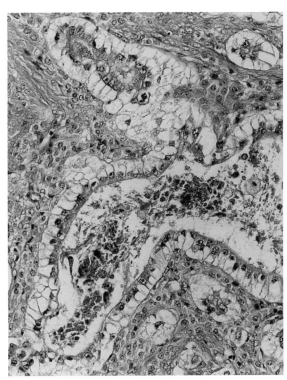

Figure 18–12. Colonic clear cell adenocarcinoma metastatic to the ovary mimicking the appearance of a primary ovarian endometrioid adenocarcinoma of the secretory type.

APPENDICEAL TUMORS

- Low-grade mucinous epithelial tumors are the most common appendiceal tumors that spread to the ovary, although some pathologists interpret the ovarian tumors in such cases as independent primaries.
  - The appendiceal tumors, which may be associated with a mucocele or no gross abnormality, are associated with similar tumors in one or both ovaries, accompanied by pseudomyxoma peritonei.
  - The ovarian tumors in such cases are often large, multicystic, and bilateral. This subject is discussed in Chapter 13.
- Appendiceal adenocarcinomas that metastasize to the ovaries include those of typical intestinal, colloid, and signet-ring cell types. About 40 such cases have been reported. In about one third of them, the ovarian involvement accounted for the presenting manifestations.
- Carcinoid tumors, which are almost always of the mucinous type (adenocarcinoids), also may spread to the ovaries (page 412), where they are more common than primary mucinous ovarian carcinoid tumors.

References

Merino MJ, Edmonds P, LiVolsi V. Appendiceal carcinoma metastatic to the ovaries and mimicking primary ovarian tumors. Int J Gynecol Pathol 4:110–120, 1985.

Prayson RA, Hart WR, Petras RE. Pseudomyxoma peritonei: a clinicopathologic study of 19 cases with emphasis on site of origin and nature of associated ovarian tumors. Am J Surg Pathol 18:591–603, 1994.

Ronnett BM, Kurman RJ, Shmookler BM, et al. The morphological spectrum of ovarian metastases of appendiceal adenocarcinomas: a clinicopathologic and immunohistochemical analysis of tumors often misinterpreted as primary ovarian tumors or metastatic tumors from other gastrointestinal sites. Am J Surg Pathol 21:1144–1155, 1997.

Seidman JD, Elsayed AM, Sobin LH, Tavassoli FA. Association of mucinous tumors of the ovary and appendix: a clinicopathologic study of 25 cases. Am J Surg Pathol 17:22–34, 1993.

Young RH, Gilks CB, Scully RE. Mucinous tumors of the appendix associated with mucinous tumors of the ovary and pseudomyxoma peritonei: a clinicopathological analysis of 22 cases supporting an origin in the appendix. Am J Surg Pathol 15:415–429, 1991.

CARCINOID TUMORS

General Features

- Carcinoid tumors metastatic to the ovary occur over a wide age range (21 to 82 years, with a median of 57 years in the largest series). Rare tumors are found at autopsy.

- Forty percent of women in whom metastases are found at operation have the carcinoid syndrome; some of them also have signs and symptoms referable to intestinal or ovarian involvement. Extraovarian metastases are found in at least 90% of cases.
- One third of patients die within 1 year, and 75% die within 5 years. As many as 25% of patients, however, may remain asymptomatic for years postoperatively, including relief of the carcinoid syndrome.
- Most of the primary tumors are found in the small intestine but rarely in the colon, stomach, pancreas, or bronchus.
- Appendiceal mucinous carcinoid tumors spread to the ovary in about one third of cases and in more than 50% of such cases the patient presents with an ovarian mass. Typical appendiceal carcinoids almost never spread to the ovary.

Gross Features

- The ovarian tumors, most of which are bilateral, are typically predominantly solid, with smooth or bosselated surfaces. Sectioning reveals single or confluent firm, white or yellow nodules.
- Scattered cysts in some tumors, typically filled with watery fluid, may create an appearance similar to that of a cystadenofibroma; rare tumors are predominantly cystic. Focal necrosis and hemorrhage may occur.

Microscopic Features

- Patterns similar to those in primary carcinoid tumors (see Chapter 15) are encountered, most commonly insular, but trabecular, mixed, and rarely, solid tubular patterns are also seen.
- Acini, typically small and round, are common and often contain a homogeneous eosinophilic secretion that may undergo calcification, which is sometimes psammomatous.
- Cysts and follicle-like spaces lined by tumor cells are sometimes seen. Occasionally, nests of tumor cells disintegrate, with the cells separating from one another.
- Carcinoids, with rare exceptions, are the only metastatic tumor that often elicits an extensive fibromatous stromal proliferation; occasionally, the stroma is extensively hyalinized.
- The cytologic features of the tumors are as seen elsewhere; in some tumors, the cells have abundant eosinophilic cytoplasm, resembling oxyphilic tumors of other types (Appendix 4).
- In metastatic mucinous carcinoids, nests and glands containing goblet cells and argentaffin or argyrophil cells are present. Foci of signet-ring cell carcinoma (simulating a Krukenberg tumor), cystic glands filled with mucin, or foci resembling colloid carcinoma also occur.

Differential Diagnosis of Usual Metastatic Carcinoid Tumors

- Primary ovarian carcinoid tumors. The differential diagnosis is discussed on page 356.
- Adult granulosa cell tumors; this differential is discussed in Chapter 16.
- Sertoli or Sertoli-Leydig cell tumors (SLCTs). The trabeculae of carcinoids are usually longer, thicker, and more orderly than the sex-cord–like structures of SLCTs. Rarely, however, carcinoid tumorlets may arise in a SLCT with mucinous heterologous elements. The finding of other distinctive patterns of SLCT, even if minor, facilitate the diagnosis.
- Epithelial tumors.
  - The epithelial nests of the Brenner tumor contain cells of urothelial type with oval, pale, grooved nuclei rather than the cells of carcinoid tumors with their characteristic round nuclei containing stippled chromatin.
  - Benign and borderline adenofibromas and endometrioid adenocarcinomas containing small acini are distinguished from carcinoids by their different patterns and cytologic features. Abortive or obvious squamous differentiation is common in endometrioid tumors but not a feature of carcinoids.
  - A metastatic breast carcinoma with a prominent insular pattern may simulate a carcinoid tumor.
- In difficult cases, more thorough sampling; histochemical staining for argentaffin and argyrophil granules; immunostaining for chromogranin, neuron-specific enolase, synaptophysin, peptide hormones, and serotonin; and ultrastructural search for dense core granules should be diagnostic. Surface epithelial tumors may contain neuroendocrine cells but not diffusely as in carcinoids.

Differential Diagnosis of Metastatic Mucinous Carcinoid Tumors

- Metastatic adenocarcinomas. This differential diagnosis requires recognizing the characteristic pattern of mucinous carcinoid and confirmation of a neuroendocrine cell population using immunostains.
- Primary mucinous carcinoid. These tumors are rarer than the metastatic form. The differential diagnosis depends on the distribution of tumor and the presence or absence of a dermoid or epidermoid cyst or mucinous cystic tumor, lesions that may be associated with primary mucinous carcinoids. Bilaterality and extraovarian spread strongly favor metastasis.

References

Chen KT. Appendiceal adenocarcinoid with metastasis. Gynecol Oncol 38:286–288, 1990.

Hirschfield LS, Kahn LB, Winkler B, et al. Adenocarcinoid of the appendix presenting as bilateral Krukenberg's tumor of the ovaries: immunohistochemical and ultrastructural studies and literature review. Arch Pathol Lab Med 109:930–933, 1985.

Robboy SJ, Scully RE, Norris HJ. Carcinoid metastatic to the ovary: a clinicopathologic analysis of 35 cases. Cancer 33:798–811, 1974.

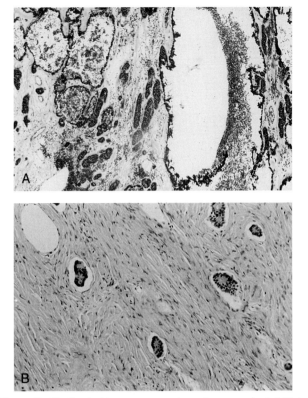

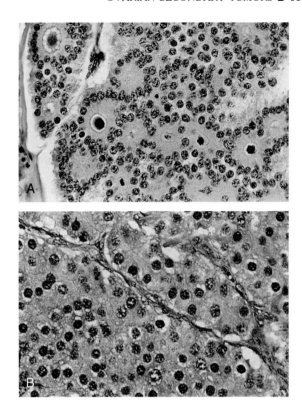

Figure 18–13. Carcinoid tumor metastatic to the ovary. *A,* A follicle-like pattern is seen. *B,* A prominent fibrotic stroma separates several acini.

Figure 18–14. Carcinoid tumor metastatic to the ovary. *A,* Cells forming acini (some with calcified luminal material) exhibit the typical nuclear features of carcinoid tumors. *B,* In a different metastatic carcinoid, the tumor cells contain abundant oxyphilic cytoplasm.

Figure 18–15. Goblet cell carcinoid metastatic to the ovary.

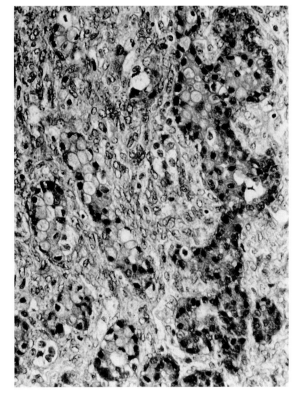

TUMORS OF THE PANCREAS, BILIARY TRACT, AND LIVER

■ Metastatic pancreatic adenocarcinoma, which accounts for up to 10% of ovarian metastases that manifest clinically as an ovarian tumor, are typically bilateral, large, cystic, and multiloculated, mimicking primary mucinous tumors of the ovary.

■ Microscopically, the tumors are variably differentiated, with cysts resembling those of mucinous cystadenomas, borderline tumors, and well-differentiated cystadenocarcinomas, as well as areas of infiltrating small glands and single cells, including signet-ring cells.

■ Clues to the metastatic nature of the tumor are similar to those used for recognizing metastatic carcinomas in general (see page 405), especially surface implantation. Pancreatic adenocarcinomas with a small acinar pattern spreading to the ovary may mimic a primary or metastatic carcinoid tumor but do not contain argyrophil cells.

■ The rare metastatic tumors from the gallbladder and bile ducts encountered intraoperatively are typically solid. Microscopically, the small irregular glands characteristic of the primary tumor may be seen or the appearance may simulate a primary endometrioid or mucinous carcinoma or even a cystadenofibroma. Rarely, the metastases take the form of a Krukenberg tumor.

■ The rare hepatocellular carcinoma involving the ovary is usually an incidental autopsy finding, but a few cases with clinical manifestations have been reported. Rare cholangiocarcinomas have metastasized to the ovaries as has a hepatoblastoma.

■ Metastatic hepatocellular carcinoma (HCC) must be distinguished from hepatoid yolk sac tumors (which usually have foci of typical yolk sac tumor), primary hepatoid carcinomas (which may have a component of serous carcinoma that excludes HCC), and hepatoid carcinomas metastatic from extraovarian sites. The finding of bile in the ovarian tumor favors the diagnosis of metastatic HCC.

References

Green LK, Silva EG. Hepatoblastoma in an adult with metastasis to the ovary. Am J Clin Pathol 92:110–115, 1989.

Young RH, Gersell DJ, Clement PB, Scully RE. Hepatocellular carcinoma metastatic to the ovary: a report of three cases discovered during life with discussion of the differential diagnosis of hepatoid tumors of the ovary. Hum Pathol 23:574–580, 1992.

Young RH, Hart WR. Metastases from carcinomas of the pancreas simulating primary mucinous tumors of the ovary: a report of seven cases. Am J Surg Pathol 13:748–756, 1989.

Young RH, Scully RE. Ovarian metastases from carcinoma of the gallbladder and extrahepatic bile ducts simulating primary tumors of the ovary: a report of six cases. Int J Gynecol Pathol 9:60–72, 1990.

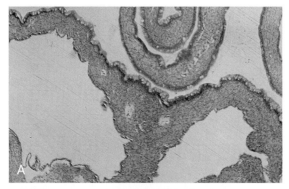
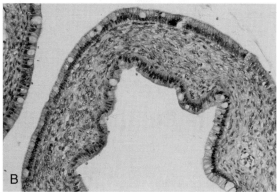

Figure 18–16. Pancreatic adenocarcinoma metastatic to ovary at low-(*A*) and high-power (*B*) magnifications. Cysts are lined by a single layer of bland, mucinous epithelium mimicking a primary mucinous cystadenoma of the ovary.

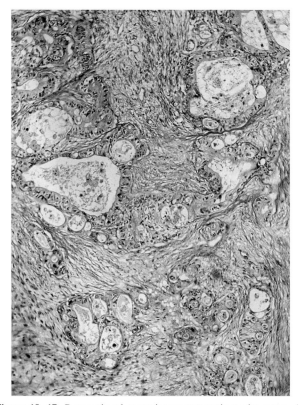

Figure 18–17. Pancreatic adenocarcinoma metastatic to the ovary. An obviously invasive mucinous adenocarcinoma is shown.

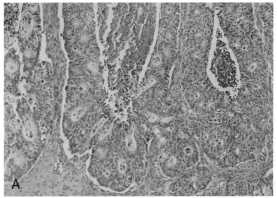

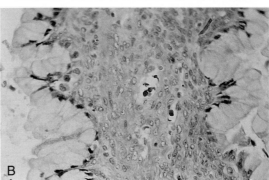

Figure 18–18. Gallbladder adenocarcinoma metastatic to the ovary. *A,* A poorly differentiated adenocarcinoma grows in a cribriform pattern with foci of dirty necrosis. *B,* In another case, glands are lined by benign-appearing to mildly atypical mucinous cells.

BREAST CARCINOMA

General Features

- The frequency with which ovarian metastases are found in women with breast cancer varies from 10% to 20% at autopsy to about 30% in therapeutic oophorectomy specimens.
- Signs or symptoms related to ovarian metastases in these patients are unusual, although breast cancer accounted for 17% of metastatic tumors that simulated a primary ovarian tumor in one series. Occasionally, the ovarian metastases are evident before the primary tumor is detected.
- Although ovarian metastases of breast cancer are usually accompanied by other intraabdominal metastases, involvement is limited to the ovary in about 15% of cases.
- Lobular carcinomas, including those of the signet-ring cell type, spread to the ovary more frequently than ductal carcinomas, but about 75% of ovarian metastases from breast cancer are of the ductal type because of the greater frequency of that subtype.

Pathologic Features

- The metastatic tumors, which are usually less than 5 cm in maximal dimension and bilateral in about two thirds of cases, have sectioned surfaces replaced by firm or gritty, white and discrete or confluent nodules. Cysts are prominent in about 20% of the cases, and rarely, the tumor is entirely cystic. Exceptionally, papillae are grossly visible.
- Metastatic ductal carcinoma appears as tubular glands, islands, and small clusters of cells. Other patterns include cribriform, solid, and papillary.
- Metastatic lobular carcinomas often grow in cords or may have an insular or solid pattern. Occasionally, the tumor cells of either type grow as single cells. Admixtures of patterns may be seen.
- Signet cells are usually inconspicuous unless the primary tumor contains them, but rarely, a metastatic breast cancer is a Krukenberg tumor.
- In premenopausal women, tumor often involves the theca interna of a graafian follicle or the granulosa or theca layer of a corpus luteum.
- The stroma of the tumor varies from sparse to abun-

dant; it is rarely luteinized. Lymphatic invasion in the ovary is seen in many cases.

Differential Diagnosis

- Surface epithelial adenocarcinomas (particularly endometrioid and undifferentiated carcinomas), carcinoid tumor, a metastatic desmoplastic small round cell tumor with divergent differentiation, and granulosa cell tumor.
- Awareness of a primary breast cancer is helpful in the differential diagnosis, but an ovarian tumor (Curtin et al) arising in a woman with breast cancer is more likely to be an independent primary surface epithelial tumor.
- Immunoreactivity for gross cystic disease fluid protein-15 (GCDFP-15) strongly favors a diagnosis of metastatic breast carcinoma and is present in about 50% of lobular carcinomas and in about 75% of ductal carcinomas. Surface epithelial tumors of the ovary are almost always GCDFP-15 negative.
- GCDFP-15 positivity and desmin negativity establishes the diagnosis of metastatic breast carcinoma over a desmoplastic small round cell tumor with divergent differentiation.
- Rarely, the diffuse patterns and occasional cordlike growth pattern of malignant lymphoma and leukemic infiltration of the ovary cause a problem in the differential diagnosis. Immunoreactivity for epithelial antigens and GCDFP-15 and negativity for lymphoid and myeloid markers are diagnostic.

References

Curtin JP, Barakat RR, Hoskins WJ. Ovarian disease in women with breast cancer. Obstet Gynecol 84:449–452, 1994.

Gagnon Y, Tetu B. Ovarian metastases of breast carcinoma: a clinicopathologic study of 59 cases. Cancer 64:892–898, 1989.

Harris M, Howell A, Chrissohou M, et al. A comparison of the metastatic pattern of infiltrating lobular carcinoma and infiltrating duct carcinoma of the breast. Br J Cancer 50:23–30, 1984.

Monteagudo C, Merino MJ, Laporte N, Neumann RD. Value of gross cystic disease fluid protein-15 in distinguishing metastatic breast carcinomas among poorly differentiated neoplasms involving the ovary. Hum Pathol 22:368–372, 1991.

Wick MR, Lillemoe TJ, Copland GT, et al. Gross cystic disease fluid protein-15 as a marker for breast cancer: immunohistochemical analysis of 690 human neoplasms and comparison with alpha-lactalbumin. Hum Pathol 20:281–287, 1989.

Young RH, Carey RW, Robboy SJ. Breast carcinoma masquerading as a primary ovarian neoplasm. Cancer 48:210–212, 1981.

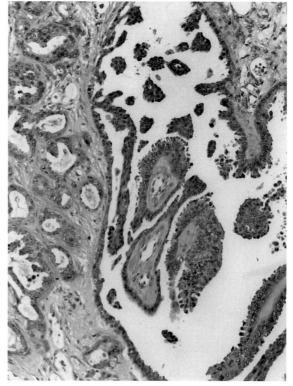

Figure 18–19. Breast carcinoma metastatic to the ovary. The appearance mimics that of a primary ovarian serous carcinoma.

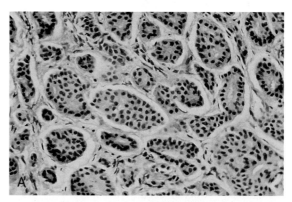

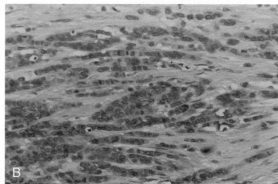

Figure 18–20. Breast carcinoma metastatic to the ovary. Ovarian metastases from a ductal carcinoma (*A*) and a lobular carcinoma (*B*) are shown. The appearance of the ductal carcinoma may be confused with a carcinoid tumor, whereas that of the lobular tumor brings to the differential diagnosis other tumors that may grow in the ovary as cords, such as malignant lymphoma (see Fig. 18–26*C*).

FEMALE GENITAL TRACT TUMORS

Endometrial Carcinoma

- Although endometrial endometrioid carcinomas have often involved the ovaries by the time of autopsy and ovarian metastases are occasionally found during life, endometrioid carcinomas involving the endometrium and ovary appear to be independently primary in most cases (see Tables 14–1 through 14–3).
- Involvement of both sites by serous carcinomas is less common, and involvement of both sites by other surface epithelial carcinomas is rare. In some such cases, fragments of tumor within the tubal lumen or ovarian surface involvement suggests spread of the tumor from one organ to another. Many of the criteria used for determining the site of origin of endometrioid carcinoma with combined organ involvement (see Tables 14–1 through 14–3) can be used for other types.
- Rarely, ovarian surface lesions secondary to an endometrial endometrioid adenocarcinoma with squamous differentiation take the form of deposits of keratin or ghosts of mature squamous cells associated with a foreign-body giant cell response (page 452).

Cervical Carcinoma

- Squamous cell carcinomas of the cervix have spread to the ovaries by the time of autopsy in approximately 3% of cases; the figure for adenocarcinomas is somewhat higher. Ovarian spread is rarely discovered during life, however, and most such cases are adenocarcinomas.
- When cervical and ovarian mucinous adenocarcinomas coexist, evaluating the different features of primary and metastatic ovarian tumors in general (page 405) is usually but not always helpful in determining whether the tumors are independent or the ovarian tumor is metastatic from the cervical tumor.
- When both sites are involved by squamous cell carcinoma, thorough sampling is crucial because many primary ovarian squamous cell carcinomas arise from a dermoid cyst or an endometriotic cyst. The possibility of metastasis from an occult carcinoma arising in the cervix or elsewhere should be investigated before a pure primary ovarian squamous cell carcinoma is diagnosed.
- In rare cases, an in situ or microinvasive cervical squamous cell carcinoma spreads upward to involve the endometrial and tubal mucosae and, exceptionally, the ovarian surface and the ovarian stroma.

Uterine Sarcomas and Choriocarcinoma

- Endometrial stromal sarcomas are the most common uterine sarcoma to metastasize to the ovary. The ovarian metastases sometimes are the initial manifestation of the uterine tumor, which are not discovered until months later. Uterine leiomyosarcomas may rarely spread to the ovaries.
- The differentiation of metastatic endometrial stromal sarcomas from primary endometrioid stromal sarcomas

and sex cord–stromal tumors of the ovary is discussed on page 324.

- Ovarian metastasis of uterine choriocarcinoma is rare and must be distinguished from a primary ovarian choriocarcinoma of gestational (page 395) or germ cell origin (page 346).

Fallopian Tube Tumors

- Tubal carcinomas may spread to the ovary directly or by surface implantation. The distinction between a tubal carcinoma with spread to the ovary and vice versa is sometimes difficult (page 251).

References

Eifel P, Hendrickson M, Ross J, et al. Simultaneous presentation of carcinoma involving the ovary and uterine corpus. Cancer 50:163–170, 1982.

Kaminski PF, Norris HJ. Coexistence of ovarian neoplasm and endocervical adenocarcinoma. Obstet Gynecol 64:553–556, 1984.

LiVolsi VA, Merino MJ, Schwartz PE. Coexistent endocervical adenocarcinoma and mucinous adenocarcinoma of ovary: a clinicopathological study of four cases. Int J Gynecol Pathol 1:391–402, 1983.

Pins MR, Young RH, Crum CP, et al. Cervical squamous cell carcinoma in situ with intraepithelial extension to the upper genital tract and invasion of tubes and ovaries: report of a case with human papillomavirus analysis. Int J Gynecol Pathol 16:272–278, 1997.

Ulbright TM, Roth LM. Metastatic and independent cancers of the endometrium and ovary: a clinicopathologic study of 34 cases. Hum Pathol 16:28–34, 1985.

Young RH, Gersell DJ, Roth LM, Scully RE. Ovarian metastases from cervical carcinomas other than pure adenocarcinomas: a report of 12 cases. Cancer 71:407–418, 1993.

Young RH, Scully RE. Mucinous tumors of the ovary associated with mucinous adenocarcinomas of the cervix: a clinicopathological analysis of 16 cases. Int J Gynecol Pathol 7:99–111, 1988.

Young RH, Scully RE. Sarcomas metastatic to the ovary: a report of 21 cases. Int J Gynecol Pathol 9:231–252, 1990.

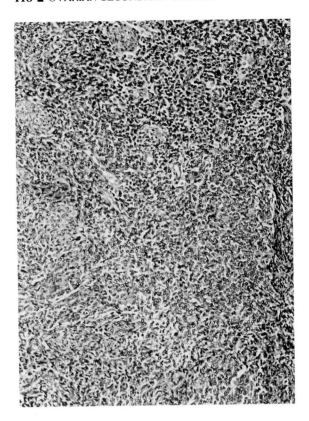

Figure 18–21. Endometrial stromal sarcoma metastatic to the ovary. The appearance mimics that of a primary ovarian sex cord–stromal tumor.

MISCELLANEOUS TUMORS

Renal and Urinary Tract Tumors

- Of the 10 reported cases of clinically detected ovarian metastases of renal cell carcinoma, the ovarian tumor was discovered first in six of them, leading to an initial misdiagnosis of primary ovarian clear cell carcinoma in three cases. The renal tumors were discovered at short intervals in these patients, except in one case in which the interval was 8 years.
- The ovarian metastases consisted of diffuse sheets or nests or tubules formed by clear cells; the tubules contained eosinophilic material or blood. A prominent sinusoidal vascular pattern was almost always present.
- Transitional cell carcinomas (TCCs) arising from the renal pelvis or urinary bladder can rarely spread to the ovaries. The metastases may be found synchronously with the urinary tract tumor, although in other women, not until several years later.
- Three signet-ring cell carcinomas of the bladder have been the source of Krukenberg tumors.

Differential Diagnosis

- Features favoring or establishing a diagnosis of primary ovarian clear cell carcinoma (versus metastatic renal cell carcinoma) include the presence of mixed patterns typical of ovarian clear cell carcinoma (i.e., tubulocystic, papillary, solid), stromal basement membrane deposition, hobnail cells, and intraluminal mucin; an absence of the typical sinusoidal vascular framework of renal cell carcinoma; and exclusion of a prior or concomitant renal cell carcinoma.
- The distinction between metastatic TCC of urothelial origin and a borderline or malignant Brenner tumor (BT) or a primary ovarian TCC can be difficult, or in the case of TCC, impossible.
  - Borderline and malignant BTs, however, contain foci of benign BT and frequently benign mucinous epithelium. Primary ovarian TCCs are often admixed with other epithelial carcinomas, usually serous.
  - The extent of the urinary tract TCC (if present) and the general features that favor an independent primary or metastatic nature of the ovarian tumor must also be considered (page 405).

References

Oliva E, Musulen E, Prat J, Young RH. Transitional cell carcinoma of the renal pelvis with symptomatic ovarian metastases. Int J Surg Pathol 2:231–236, 1995.

Young RH, Hart WR. Renal cell carcinoma metastatic to the ovary: a report of three cases emphasizing possible confusion with ovarian clear cell adenocarcinoma. Int J Gynecol Pathol 11:96–104, 1992.

Young RH, Scully RE. Urothelial and ovarian carcinomas of identical cell types: problems in interpretation: a report of three cases and review of the literature. Int J Gynecol Pathol 7:197–211, 1988.

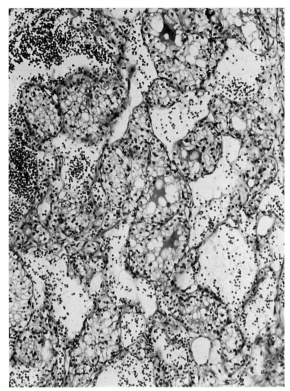

Figure 18–22. Renal clear cell adenocarcinoma metastatic to the ovary. Notice the diagnostically helpful sinusoidal vascular pattern.

Pulmonary and Mediastinal Tumors

- About 5% of women with lung cancer have ovarian metastases at autopsy. Much less commonly, ovarian metastasis precedes the clinical discovery of the pulmonary tumor or is found simultaneously. Small cell carcinoma accounts for most metastatic tumors from the lung, followed by adenocarcinoma and large cell carcinoma.
- When synchronous pulmonary and ovarian neoplasms are present, determining which tumor is primary can be difficult.
  - When the histologic features are typical of a lung carcinoma, a pulmonary origin is probable.
  - Primary ovarian small cell carcinomas of the pulmonary type are usually unassociated with pulmonary involvement and contain an associated component of surface epithelial tumor.
- Three patients with mediastinal small cell carcinomas (apparently of thymic origin) had ovarian metastases at presentation. Rare thymomas and neuroblastomas of the posterior mediastinum have metastasized to the ovary.

References

Eichhorn JH, Young RH, Scully RE. Non-pulmonary small cell carcinomas of extragenital origin metastatic to the ovary: a report of seven cases. Cancer 71:177–186, 1993.

Eichhorn JH, Young RH, Scully RE. Primary ovarian small cell carcinoma of pulmonary type: a clinicopathologic, immunohistologic, and flow cytometric analysis of 11 cases. Am J Surg Pathol 16:926–938, 1992.

Yoshida A, Shigematsu T, Mori H, et al. Non-invasive thymoma with wide spread blood-borne metastasis. Virchows Arch (Pathol Anat) 390:121–126, 1981.

Young RH, Kozakewich HPW, Scully RE. Metastatic ovarian tumors in children: a report of 14 cases and review of the literature. Int J Gynecol Pathol 12:8–19, 1993.

Young RH, Scully RE. Ovarian metastases from cancer of the lung: problems in interpretation—a report of seven cases. Gynecol Oncol 21:337–350, 1985.

Malignant Melanoma

- Patients with malignant melanoma have ovarian metastases at autopsy in about 20% of cases, but ovarian involvement detected clinically is rare. Although most such patients have a known primary tumor with extraovarian metastases, isolated ovarian spread may occur, often with a negative or remote history of a primary melanoma.

■ The ovarian metastases, which are bilateral in about 50% of the cases, have no specific gross features other than occasional pigmentation.

■ Typically, there is solid growth of large cells with abundant eosinophilic cytoplasm, although rarely there is a predominant or even exclusive population of small cells with scanty cytoplasm. Other patterns include discrete aggregates with a nevoid appearance and, in about 40% of cases, follicle-like spaces.

■ The variably pleomorphic nuclei usually contain prominent nucleoli. Spindle cells may be seen but are generally inconspicuous. Cytoplasmic intranuclear pseudoinclusions are present in 25% of the tumors. Melanin pigment is inconspicious or absent in about 50% of the cases.

Differential Diagnosis

■ Primary malignant melanoma. These tumors usually arise in the wall of a dermoid cyst; other teratomatous elements, such as struma, may be present. A diagnostic feature is the presence of junctional activity beneath the squamous lining of the cyst.

  • In cases of apparently pure ovarian melanoma without junctional activity, a meticulous search for an occult primary tumor should be conducted, although a regressed primary cutaneous melanoma may be the source of the ovarian tumor in some such cases.

  • Bilaterality, multinodular growth, or both strongly suggest metastasis even in the absence of a known primary tumor.

■ Undifferentiated or poorly differentiated carcinoma (such as TCC) of the ovary. Careful search for pigment and immunostains are indicated in tumors in which the histologic pattern is consistent with carcinoma or melanoma.

■ Juvenile granulosa cell tumor. This differential diagnosis is discussed on page 368.

■ Lipid-poor steroid cell tumor or pregnancy luteoma (when the cells have abundant cytoplasm and the melanin pigment is mistaken for lipochrome pigment). Bilaterality and multinodularity strongly favor melanoma over steroid cell tumor, although both these features can occur in pregnancy luteomas. Immunoreactivity for inhibin and negative staining for S-100 and HMB-45 facilitate the diagnosis.

References

Fitzgibbons PL, Martin SE, Simmons TJ. Malignant melanoma metastatic to the ovary. Am J Surg Pathol 11:959–964, 1987.
Young RH, Scully RE. Malignant melanoma metastatic to the ovary: a clinicopathologic analysis of 20 cases. Am J Surg Pathol 15:849–860, 1991.

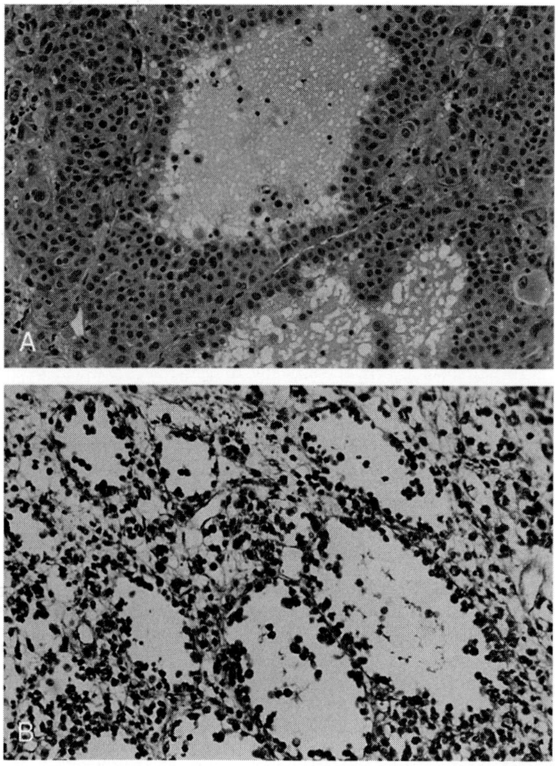

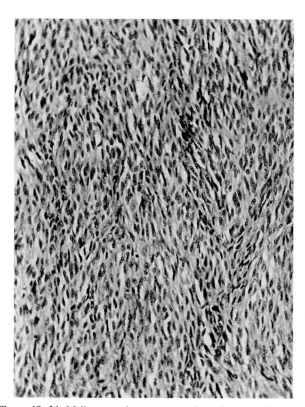

Figure 18–23. Malignant melanoma metastatic to the ovary with follicular patterns. *A,* The tumor cells have moderate amounts of cytoplasm that was eosinophilic, an appearance that may simulate a juvenile granulosa cell tumor. *B,* The tumor cells have scanty cytoplasm, which resulted in an initial misdiagnosis of small cell carcinoma of the hypercalcemic type.

Figure 18–24. Malignant melanoma metastatic to the ovary. Neoplastic spindle cells have only mildly atypical nuclear features, an appearance simulating that of a primary ovarian stromal tumor or low-grade sarcoma.

Neuroblastoma

■ Between 25% and 50% of females with adrenal neuroblastoma have ovarian involvement at autopsy, but clinically significant ovarian metastases are comparatively uncommon, and those responsible for the presenting clinical manifestations of the neuroblastoma are rare.

■ Bilaterality, absence of an association with a teratoma, and the presence of a known extraovarian primary tumor help establish the metastatic nature of the tumor.

■ A fibrillary background and the presence of Wright pseudorosettes facilitate the distinction of neuroblastoma from other small cell tumors (Appendix 5). Immunohistochemical staining and electron microscopic examination may be helpful in difficult cases.

Reference

Young RH, Kozakewich HPW, Scully RE. Metastatic ovarian tumors in children: a report of 14 cases and review of the literature. Int J Gynecol Pathol 12:8–19, 1993.

Rhabdomyosarcoma

■ Of the approximately 10 reported cases of rhabdomyosarcomas metastatic to the ovary, more than one half were of the alveolar type. The metastases have been only rarely symptomatic. Rarely, the clinical picture simulates that of acute leukemia.

■ Rhabdomyosarcoma metastatic to the ovary must be distinguished from the primary form. Features indicating metastatic rhabdomyosarcoma to the ovary include a known extraovarian primary, bilaterality, and multinodularity.

■ The differential diagnosis also includes other malignant primary and metastatic small cell tumors of the ovary, most of which occur in young patients (Appendix 5).

References

Nunez C, Abboud SL, Lemon NC, Kemp JA. Ovarian rhabdomyosarcoma presenting as leukemia. Cancer 52:297–300, 1983.

Young RH, Scully RE. Alveolar rhabdomyosarcoma metastatic to the ovary: a report of two cases and discussion of the differential diagnosis of small cell malignant tumors of the ovary. Cancer 64:899–904, 1989.

Other Sarcomas

■ Sarcomas that have rarely metastasized to the ovary include hemangiosarcomas (some primary in the breast), Ewing's sarcoma, leiomyosarcomas (most from the gastrointestinal tract), fibrosarcoma, osteosarcoma, chondrosarcoma, and chordoma.

■ Although the tumors in this group do not usually cause diagnostic difficulty, the clinical findings and immunoprofile of the tumors may be helpful in the differential diagnosis.

References

Sedgely MG, Östör AG, Fortune DW. Angiosarcoma of breast metastatic to the ovary and placenta. Aust N Z J Obstet Gynaecol 25:299–302, 1985.

Young RH, Scully RE. Sarcomas metastatic to the ovary: a report of 21 cases. Int J Gynecol Pathol 9:231–252, 1990.

Zukerberg LR, Young RH. Chordoma metastatic to the ovary: report of a case. Arch Pathol Lab Med 114:208–210, 1990.

Miscellaneous Carcinomas

■ Isolated examples of head and neck carcinomas, including rare thyroid carcinomas, metastatic to the ovary have been documented. Two cases of cutaneous Merkel cell tumor of the groin have metastasized to the ovary.

■ In some cases, the interval between removal of the primary and discovery of the ovarian tumors has been as long as 10 years (an adenoid cystic carcinoma of the submandibular gland) or 12 years (a thyroid carcinoma).

References

Eichhorn JH, Young RH, Scully RE. Non-pulmonary small cell carcinomas of extragenital origin metastatic to the ovary. Cancer 71:177–186, 1993.

Longacre TA, O'Hanlan K, Hendrickson MR. Adenoid cystic carcinoma of the submandibular gland with symptomatic ovarian metastases. Int J Gynecol Pathol 15:349–355, 1996.

Young RH, Jackson A, Wells M. Ovarian metastasis from thyroid carcinoma twelve years after partial thyroidectomy mimicking struma ovarii: report of case. Int J Gynecol Pathol 13:181–185, 1994.

Peritoneal Tumors

■ Secondary ovarian involvement by low-grade papillary mesotheliomas and diffuse malignant mesothelioma (DMM) is common (see Chapter 17).

  • The tumor is usually confined to the surface of the ovary, but parenchymal invasion may be prominent in some DMMs.

  • In most cases, the distribution of the tumor and its characteristic appearance facilitate the diagnosis.

  • The distinction of DMM from serous carcinoma is discussed on page 456.

■ The intraabdominal desmoplastic small round cell tumor with divergent differentiation may be associated with ovarian involvement at presentation, potentially mimicking a primary ovarian tumor.

  • The associated extensive extraovarian tumor at the time of presentation, the typical young age of the patient, and the characteristic histologic and immunohistochemical findings facilitate the diagnosis from other small cell malignant tumors that involve the ovary (Appendix 5).

References

Clement PB, Young RH, Scully RE. Malignant mesotheliomas presenting as ovarian masses: a report of nine cases, including two primary ovarian mesotheliomas. Am J Surg Pathol 20:1067–1080, 1996.

Goldblum J, Hart WR. Localized and diffuse mesotheliomas of the genital tract and peritoneum in women: a clinicopathologic study of nineteen true mesothelial neoplasms, other than adenomatoid tumors, multicystic mesotheliomas, and localized fibrous tumors. Am J Surg Pathol 19:1124–1137, 1995.

Stamatakos MD, Tavassoli FA. Mesotheliomas involving the ovary [Abstract]. Mod Pathol 11:115A, 1998.

Young RH, Eichhorn JH, Dickersin GR, Scully RE. Ovarian involvement by the intra-abdominal desmoplastic small round cell tumor with divergent differentiation: a report of three cases. Hum Pathol 23: 454–464, 1991.

HEMATOPOIETIC TUMORS

Malignant Lymphoma

General Features

- Although up to 25% of women with lymphoma have ovarian involvement at autopsy, lymphoma rarely presents clinically as an ovarian mass, and in most such cases, there is more extensive intraabdominal or generalized lymphoma. The long-term survival of a patient with ovarian lymphoma after oophorectomy indicates that rarely such tumors are primary in the ovary.
- An exception to the foregoing is ovarian involvement in countries where Burkitt's lymphoma is endemic, where it accounts for about 50% of the cases of malignant ovarian tumors in childhood. In these cases, ovarian enlargement is second only to jaw involvement as the presenting manifestation of the disease.
- Lymphomatous ovarian involvement may occur at any age, but the peak age is in the fourth and fifth decades. The most common presenting manifestations are similar to those of most ovarian masses; some patients have generalized symptoms or abnormal vaginal bleeding.
- At laparotomy the ovarian involvement is bilateral in about 50% of the cases and is confined to the ovaries in 10% to 20% of the cases. Extraovarian disease most often involves the pelvic or paraaortic lymph nodes or both and occasionally involves the peritoneum, the fallopian tubes, the uterus, and miscellaneous other sites. Ascites is common.

Gross Features

- Ovarian lymphomas, which have a mean diameter of 10 to 15 cm, typically have an intact external surface, which may be smooth or nodular, and a soft, fleshy to firm or rubbery consistency.
- The sectioned surfaces are usually white, tan, or gray-pink, with occasional foci of cystic degeneration, hemorrhage, or necrosis.

Microscopic Features

- The appearance is similar to that in extraovarian sites, except for a tendency for the tumor cells to form islands, cords, trabeculae, and follicle-like spaces and to be separated by sclerotic fibrous tissue. The tumor may surround follicles and their derivatives or obliterate all the underlying tissue.
- The most common subtypes presenting with ovarian involvement are diffuse large cell type (usually immunoblastic), small noncleaved cell type (Burkitt or non-Burkitt), and follicular lymphomas (small cleaved, mixed small cleaved and large cell, and large cell types). Involvement by Hodgkin's disease is unusual, even at autopsy. Almost all ovarian lymphomas are of B-cell type.

- In patients in the first two decades, the small noncleaved cell type is the most common. In contrast to adults in whom lymphomas of many types (follicular and diffuse) are encountered, younger patients almost always have aggressive diffuse lymphomas.

Differential Diagnosis

- Dysgerminoma (page 339), undifferentiated carcinomas (page 336), small cell carcinoma of hypercalcemic type (page 398), metastatic breast carcinomas (page 416), and granulocytic sarcoma (page 422). Other tumors in the differential diagnosis are listed in Appendix 5.

Prognosis

- Malignant lymphoma presenting with ovarian involvement is associated with a poor prognosis. Fewer than 10% of patients in one series and fewer than 25% in another series who were treated by oophorectomy, irradiation, or both survived more than 5 years. The survival rate in a more recent series was 47%.
- Features associated with a good prognosis have included unilateral involvement, focal ovarian involvement, FIGO stage Ia, and a follicular pattern. Features associated with a poor prognosis have included a rapid onset of symptoms related to a mass, the presence of systemic symptoms, bilaterality, and an advanced stage.

Leukemia

- Leukemic involvement of the ovaries at autopsy in one large study was present in 11% of cases of acute myelogenous leukemia (AML), with corresponding figures of 9% for chronic myelogenous leukemia, 21% for acute lymphoblastic leukemia, and 22% for chronic lymphocytic leukemia.
- Patients with AML only rarely present with an ovarian tumor, with or without hematologic evidence of leukemia. Most of the reported patients, some of whom were infants or children, were dead or alive with disease after chemotherapy. The ovary also can be a clinically apparent but usually not isolated site of relapse after chemotherapy for AML.
- The ovarian tumors in AML can be unilateral or bilateral, with a mean diameter of 12 to 14 cm, and are typically solid, soft, and white, yellow, or red-brown, but cystic degeneration, hemorrhage, or necrosis may be seen. Only a minority of tumors have been green (i.e., chloroma).
- The microscopic patterns are similar to those of malignant lymphoma, which is the most important tumor in the differential diagnosis. Differential features include the following:
  - The cells of granulocytic sarcoma usually have more finely dispersed nuclear chromatin and more abundant cytoplasm, which may be deeply eosinophilic.
  - The identification of eosinophilic myelocytes, staining for chloroacetate esterase, or immunohistochemical staining for lysozyme confirms the diagnosis.

■ We are unaware of documented cases of acute lymphoblastic or chronic lymphocytic leukemia presenting as an ovarian mass, but about 10 cases of acute lymphoblastic leukemia that relapsed in the ovaries (and in other sites) during bone marrow remission have been reported.

Plasmacytoma

■ Five females, 12 to 63 years of age, have had unilateral ovarian plasmacytomas, which ranged up to 24 cm in diameter and were white, pale yellow, or gray. Overt multiple myeloma developed in one woman 2 years after the oophorectomy.

References

Barcos M, Lane W, Gomez GA, et al. An autopsy study of 1206 acute and chronic leukemias (1958–1982). Cancer 60:827–837, 1987.

Ferry JA, Young RH. Malignant lymphoma of the genitourinary tract. Curr Diagn Pathol 4:145–169, 1997.

Fox H, Langley FA, Govan ADT, et al. Malignant lymphoma presenting as an ovarian tumour: a clinicopathological analysis of 34 cases. Br J Obstet Gynaecol 95:386–390, 1988.

Halpin TF. Gynecologic implications of Burkitt's tumor: review. Obstet Gynecol Surv 30:351–358, 1975.

Linden MD, Tubbs RR, Fishleder AJ, Hart WR. Immunotypic and genotypic characterization of non-Hodgkin's lymphoma of the ovary. Am J Clin Pathol 89:156–162, 1988.

Monterroso V, Jaffe ES, Merino MJ, Medeiros LJ. Malignant lymphomas involving the ovary: a clinicopathologic analysis of 39 cases. Am J Surg Pathol 17:154–170, 1993.

Oliva E, Ferry JA, Young RH, et al. Granulocytic sarcoma of the female genital tract: a clinicopathologic study of 11 cases. Am J Surg Pathol 21:1156–1165, 1997.

Osborne BM, Robboy SJ. Lymphomas or leukemia presenting as ovarian tumors: an analysis of 42 cases. Cancer 52:1933–1943, 1983.

Paladugu RR, Bearman RM, Rappaport H. Malignant lymphoma with primary manifestation in the gonad: a clinicopathologic study of 38 patients. Cancer 45:561–571, 1980.

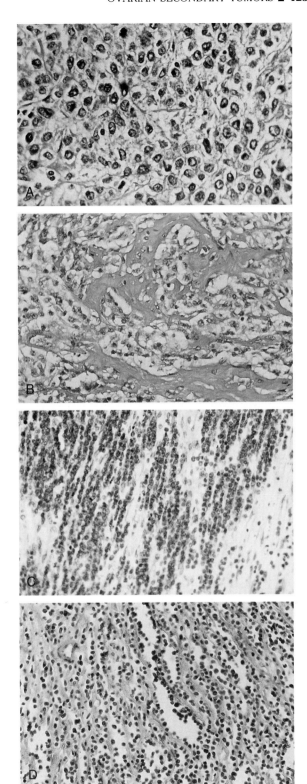

Figure 18–26. Malignant lymphoma involving the ovary. Sheets (*A*), nests separated by a hyalinized stroma (*B*), cords (*C*), and irregular, focally slitlike spaces (*D*) are illustrated.

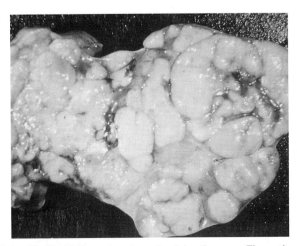

Figure 18–25. Malignant lymphoma involving the ovary. The sectioned surface of the tumor consists of numerous, well-circumscribed, white, fleshy nodules. This gross appearance in a young woman suggests a dysgerminoma.

CHAPTER 19

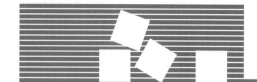

Pathology of Endometriosis and Lesions of the Secondary Müllerian System

GENERAL FEATURES

- The lesions considered in this chapter are characterized by müllerian differentiation on microscopic examination and reflect the metaplastic potential of the pelvic and lower abdominal mesothelium and the subjacent mesenchyme of females (i.e., secondary müllerian system).
- The müllerian potential of these tissues is consistent with their close embryonic relation to the müllerian ducts that arise by invagination of the coelomic epithelium. Displacement of coelomic epithelium and subcoelomic mesenchyme during embryonic development may account for the presence of identical lesions within pelvic and abdominal lymph nodes.
- Other histogenetic mechanisms may also exist for some of these lesions, such as spread of cells (e.g., implantation, lymphatic or hematogenous embolization) from the uterus (e.g., endometriosis, "benign metastasizing leiomyoma"), or fallopian tubes (e.g., endosalpingiosis).

References

Clement PB. Diseases of the peritoneum. In Kurman RJ (ed): Blaustein's Pathology of the Female Genital Tract, 4th ed. New York: Springer-Verlag, 1994:647–703.
Lauchlan SC. The secondary müllerian system. Obstet Gynecol Surv 27: 133–146, 1972.

ENDOMETRIOSIS

Clinical Features

- Endometriosis, defined as the presence of endometrial tissue outside the endometrium and myometrium, occurs in as many as 10% to 15% of women of reproductive age.
- More than 80% of affected patients are in the reproductive age group, approximately 10% of patients are adolescents, and fewer than 5% of cases are in postmenopausal women.

- The typical symptoms are dysmenorrhea; lower abdominal, pelvic, and back pain; dyspareunia; irregular bleeding; and infertility. Involvement of less common sites may be associated with localized clinical manifestations, which are occasionally catamenial.
- Pelvic examination may reveal tender nodules in the cul-de-sac and uterosacral ligments; tender, semifixed, cystic ovaries; a fixed, retroverted uterus; and sometimes, a tender and indurated rectovaginal septum.
- Serum CA-125 levels may be elevated and correlate with the severity and the clinical course of the disease.
- Rare complications include ascites (sometimes accompanied by a right pleural effusion), infection of an endometriotic cyst, hemoperitoneum, and rupture of an ovarian endometriotic cyst, which may result in an acute abdomen.

Sites

COMMON	LESS COMMON	RARE
Ovaries	Large bowel, small	Lungs, pleura
Uterosacral,	bowel, appendix	Soft tissues,
round, and	Mucosa of cervix,[a]	breast
broad	vagina, and	Bone
ligaments	fallopian tubes[b]	Upper abdominal
Rectovaginal	Skin (scars,	peritoneum
septum	umbilicus, vulva,	Stomach,
Cul-de-sac	perineum,	pancreas, liver
Peritoneum of	inguinal region)	Kidney, urethra,
uterus, tubes,	Ureter, bladder	prostate,
rectosigmoid,	Omentum, pelvic	paratesticular
ureter, and	lymph nodes	Sciatic nerve,
bladder	Inguinal region	subarachnoid
		space, brain

[a] Discussed in Chapter 4.
[b] Discussed in Chapter 11.

424

Gross Findings

- Endometriotic foci may appear as punctate, red, blue, brown or white spots, patches, or nodules with a slightly raised or puckered surface; the lesions are frequently associated with dense fibrous adhesions.
- Endometriotic cysts (i.e., endometriomas), which most commonly involve the ovaries, usually have fibrotic walls, a smooth or shaggy, brown to yellow lining, and semifluid or inspissated, chocolate-colored cyst contents. Mural nodules or intraluminal polypoid projections should be sampled histologically to exclude a neoplasm originating in the cyst.
- Intestinal endometriosis typically forms a solid, tumor-like mural mass that may impinge on the lumen or cause kinking of the involved segment.
- Rarely, pelvic peritoneal or mucosal endometriosis (e.g., bowel, bladder) may form multiple, polypoid masses of soft, gray tissue that may simulate a neoplasm (i.e., polypoid endometriosis).

Typical Microscopic Findings

- Endometrial epithelium and stroma are usually present, the appearance of which may reflect, albeit imperfectly, that of the eutopic endometrium, or they may have a relatively inactive appearance.
- The stromal component is usually obvious and resembles typical endometrial stroma, including a network of arterioles. In other cases, the endometriotic stromal cells are sparse and confined to thin periglandular rims; some glands may lack an investment of endometriotic stroma. The stromal cells are sometimes more spindled and fibroblastic in appearance than typical endometrial stromal cells.
- The lining of an endometriotic cyst may be attenuated, with a single layer of cuboidal epithelial cells that appear endometrioid or nonspecific. In the latter situation, a diagnosis of unequivocal endometriosis may be possible only if a rim of subjacent endometrial stroma persists.
- Hemorrhage within endometriosis is common and may by itself provide a clue to the diagnosis of endometriosis. The hemorrhage often elicits an infiltrate of histiocytes (i.e., pseudoxanthoma cells) that typically contain lipid and two types of brown granular pigment, ceroid (i.e., lipofuscin and hemofuscin) and hemosiderin.
- The cyst lining may be totally replaced by granulation tissue, fibrous tissue, and pseudoxanthoma cells, an appearance that strongly suggests endometriosis, although a similar appearance rarely may be seen with other lesions.
- Occasionally, the epithelial cells lining the cyst may contain abundant eosinophilic cytoplasm and large atypical nuclei.
  - This change may be reactive in some cases, but in other cases, it merges with neoplasms arising within the cyst, suggesting it may be a premalignant change in at least some cases.
  - Seidman studied 20 women with this change and no

adjacent neoplasm: no endometriosis-associated tumor developed during a mean follow-up of 8.9 years.
- Progestational changes (during pregnancy or progestin therapy) include:
  - A decidual reaction, sometimes with cytoplasmic vacuoles in the decidual cells or a stromal myxoid change, potentially mimicking a signet-ring adenocarcinoma (the vacuoles, however, contain acid rather than neutral mucin, and the cells are cytokeratin negative)
  - Atrophy of the endometriotic glands or, occasionally, an Arias-Stella reaction
- Inactive or atrophic changes in endometriosis are usual after menopause and are seen in premenopausal patients treated with oral contraceptives or danazol.
- Endometriosis involving smooth muscle (e.g., uterine ligaments, walls of hollow viscera) is typically associated with a proliferation of the smooth muscle that may be striking, creating an appearance similar to that of adenomyosis.

Unusual Microscopic Findings

- Hyperplastic changes (similar to those occurring in the endometrium) occur in endometriotic glands, sometimes related to an endogenous or exogenous estrogenic stimulus or resulting from tamoxifen therapy. These hyperplastic changes in endometriosis may precede or coexist with an adenocarcinoma (usually endometrioid or clear cell carcinoma) in the same area.
- Necrotic pseudoxanthomatous nodules, probably representing "burned-out" endometriotic foci, have a central necrotic zone surrounded by pseudoxanthoma cells, often in a palisaded arrangement, hyalinized fibrous tissue, or both; typical endometriotic glands and stroma are usually absent or sparse.
- Stromal endometriosis refers to rare endometriotic lesions with an absence or rarity of glands (the same term was used in the older literature to refer to low-grade endometrial stromal sarcoma).
  - The finding is most common in the ovarian stroma and the superficial stroma of the uterine cervix (see page 72), where it is usually an incidental microscopic finding unassociated with pelvic endometriosis.
  - In occasional examples of peritoneal endometriosis, rounded aggregates of endometrial stromal cells, which we refer to as micronodular stromal endometriosis, are present. In some cases, this finding may represent the only evidence of underlying endometriosis, particularly in a scanty biopsy specimen.
- Metaplastic changes in endometriotic glands include tubal (ciliated), hobnail, and rarely, squamous and mucinous metaplasia. Metaplasias are more common in cases of ovarian endometriosis associated with an ovarian epithelial tumor than in cases without an ovarian tumor. Mucinous metaplasia may abut an endocervical-type borderline mucinous tumor.
- Smooth muscle metaplasia of the endometriotic stroma (usually within the walls of endometriotic cysts) can, if extensive, form uterus-like masses (i.e., endomyome-

triosis). Some uterus-like masses in the region of the ovary (see Chapter 12), however, may represent a congenital malformation.

■ Myxoid change in the endometriotic stroma, which may be more common during pregnancy, rarely mimics metastatic mucinous or colloid adenocarcinoma or pseudomyxoma peritonei.

■ A striking stromal elastotic response is a not uncommon finding in our experience and occasionally can focally obliterate the typical endometriotic stroma.

■ Other rare findings include numerous neutrophils within an endometriotic cyst, usually reflecting a bacterial infection; endometrial polyp-like structures associated with tamoxifen therapy; associated foci of peritoneal leiomyomatosis, glial implants of ovarian teratomas, or nodules of splenosis; perineural and vascular invasion; and Liesegang rings.

Differential Diagnosis

■ Endosalpingiosis (see page 431). The absence of a stromal component and the usual absence of a stromal response facilitate the diagnosis.

■ Necrotic pseudoxanthomatous nodules (NPNs) should be distinguished from other ovarian and peritoneal necrotic nodules, such as infectious granulomas, isolated palisading granulomas of the ovary, and granulomas related to diathermy. These granulomas have characteristic features and lack the numerous pseudoxanthoma cells of NPNs.

■ Rare, low-grade endometrial stromal sarcomas (ESSs) with benign-appearing or atypical endometrial glands may be confused with endometriosis. These tumors, however, contain foci of more typical ESS devoid of glands and, in some cases, prominent mitotic activity of the stromal cells, sex-cord–like elements, and prominent vascular invasion.

Neoplasms Arising From Endometriosis

■ Malignant tumors have arisen in up to 0.8% of cases of ovarian endometriosis, but the exact frequency of cancer originating in pelvic endometriosis is unknown, because the frequency of endometriosis in the general population is unknown and because some cancers that arise in endometriosis may overgrow and obliterate the endometriosis from which the tumor arose.

■ Other studies have found evidence of associated endometriosis (sometimes with hyperplastic changes) in up to 30% of stage I epithelial ovarian cancers (typically endometrioid, clear cell, or a mixture of the two types).

■ Approximately 75% of tumors complicating endometriosis arise within the ovary. The most common extraovarian site is the rectovaginal septum; less frequent sites include the vagina, colon, rectum, urinary bladder, and other sites in the pelvis and abdomen.

■ Endometrioid carcinomas account for approximately 75% of carcinomas arising within endometriosis and clear cell carcinoma for approximately 15% of such cases.

■ Rare tumors arising in endometriosis include adenomyomas; ovarian serous cystadenomas of low malignant potential; benign, borderline, and malignant mucinous tumors; squamous cell carcinomas; endometrioid stromal sarcomas; malignant mesodermal mixed tumors; and adenosarcomas.

References

Bergqvist A, Ljungberg O, Myhre E. Human endometrium and endometriotic tissue obtained simultaneously: a comparative histological study. Int J Gynecol Pathol 3:135–145, 1984

Clement PB. Pathology of endometriosis. Pathol Annu 25(1):245–295, 1990.

Clement PB, Young RH, Scully RE. Necrotic pseudoxanthomatous nodules of the ovary and peritoneum in endometriosis. Am J Surg Pathol 12:390–397, 1988.

Clement PB, Young RH, Scully RE. Stromal endometriosis of the uterine cervix: a variant of endometriosis that may simulate a sarcoma. Am J Surg Pathol 14:449–455, 1990.

Clement PB, Granai CO, Young RH, Scully RE. Endometriosis with myxoid change: a case simulating pseudomyxoma peritonei. Am J Surg Pathol 18:849–853, 1994.

Dadmanesh F, Young RH, Clement PB. Polypoid endometriosis: a clinicopathologic analysis of 15 cases [Abstract]. Mod Pathol 12:115A, 1999.

Fukunaga M, Nomura K, Ishikawa E, Ushigome S. Ovarian atypical endometriosis: its close association with malignant epithelial tumors. Histopathology 30:249–255, 1997.

Fukunaga M, Ushigome S. Epithelial metaplastic changes in ovarian endometriosis. Mod Pathol 11:784–788, 1998.

Hitti IF, Glasberg SS, Lubicz S. Clear cell carcinoma arising in extravarian endometriosis: report of three cases and review of the literature. Gynecol Oncol 39:314–320, 1990.

LaGrenade A, Silverberg SG. Ovarian tumors associated with atypical endometriosis. Hum Pathol 19:1080–1084, 1988.

Mostoufizadeh M, Scully RE. Malignant tumors arising in endometriosis. Clin Obstet Gynecol 23:951–963, 1980.

Perrotta PL, Ginsburg FW, Siderides CI, Parkash V. Liesegang rings and endometriosis. Int J Gynecol Pathol 17:358–362, 1998.

Sainz de la Cuesta R, Eichhorn JH, Rice LW, et al. Histologic transformation of benign endometriosis to early epithelial ovarian cancer. Gynecol Oncol 60:238–244, 1996.

Schlesinger C, Silverberg SG. Tamoxifen-associated polyps (basalomas) arising in multiple endometriotic foci: a case report and review of the literature. Gynecol Oncol 73:305–311, 1999.

Schmidt CL, Demopoulos RI, Weiss G. Infected endometriotic cysts: clinical characterization and pathogenesis. Fertil Steril 36:27–30, 1981.

Seidman JD. Prognostic importance of hyperplasia and atypia in endometriosis. Int J Gynecol Pathol 15:1–9, 1996.

Shiraki M, Otis CN, Powell JL. Endometrial stromal sarcoma arising from ovarian and extraovarian endometriosis—report of two cases and review of the literature. Surg Pathol 4:333–343, 1991.

Toki T, Fujii S, Silverberg SG. A clinicopathologic study of the association of endometriosis and carcinoma of the ovary using a scoring system. Int J Gynecol Cancer 6:68–75, 1996.

Yantiss RK, Clement PB, Young RH. Neoplastic and pre-neoplastic changes in gastrointestinal endometriosis: a study of 17 cases. Am J Surg Pathol (in press).

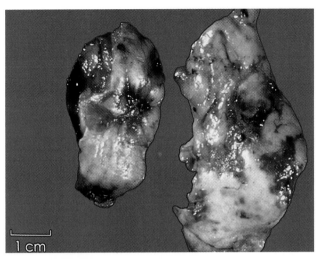

Figure 19–1. Ovarian endometriosis. The serosal surfaces of both ovaries are involved by multiple hemorrhagic and pigmented lesions, some of which are retracted.

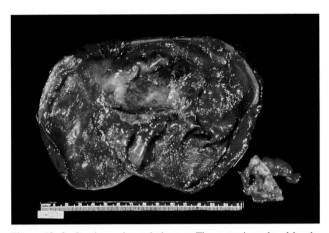

Figure 19–2. Ovarian endometriotic cyst. The ovary is replaced by the cyst, which has been opened to reveal its contents of old blood.

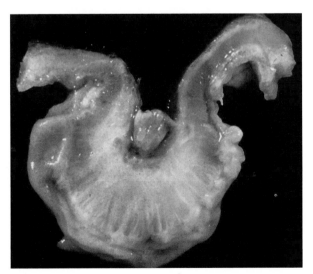

Figure 19–3. Colonic endometriosis. The bowel wall is markedly thickened, with kinking of the lumen. Most of the thickening results from endometriosis-induced hyperplasia of smooth muscle of the muscularis.

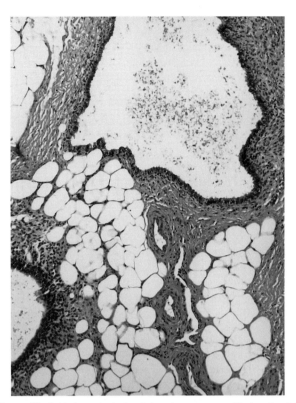

Figure 19–4. Endometriosis involving the omentum. Notice the thin cuffs of endometriotic stroma around cystic endometrial glands.

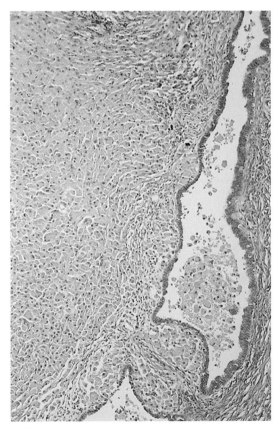

Figure 19–5. Endometriosis with a prominent infiltrate of pseudoxanthoma cells and occasional pigmented histiocytes.

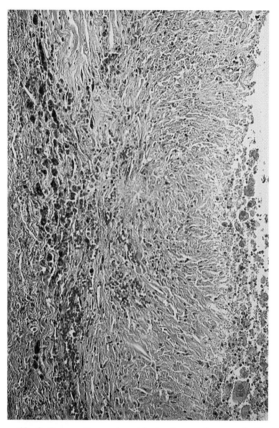

Figure 19–6. Presumptive endometriosis. An ovarian cyst is lined by fibrous tissue infiltrated by pigmented histiocytes. No diagnostic endometriotic epithelium or stroma is present. The cyst lumen is present on the extreme right.

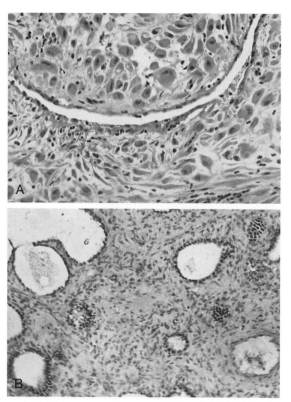

Figure 19–8. Hormonal changes in endometriosis. *A,* Pregnancy-related changes. Decidualized endometriotic stroma surrounds an atrophic gland with a slitlike lumen and flattened lining cells. *B,* Atrophic endometriosis in a postmenopausal woman. Fibrotic stroma surrounds atrophic cystic glands.

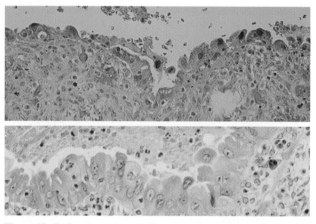

Figure 19–7. Ovarian endometriotic cysts with reactive atypia of lining epithelial cells. Two different cases are shown. In both cysts, the cells have eosinophilic cytoplasm and atypical nuclei. In the upper panel, the nuclei are hyperchromatic and have a smudged appearance.

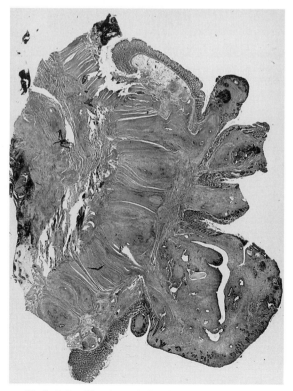

Figure 19–9. Polypoid endometriosis of the colon. The endometriosis forms mucosal polyps and has resulted in marked thickening of the muscularis.

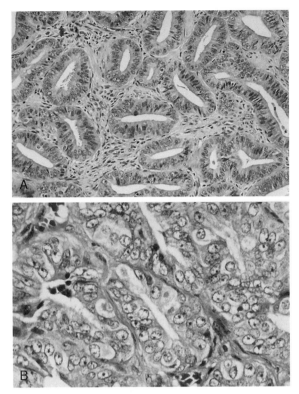

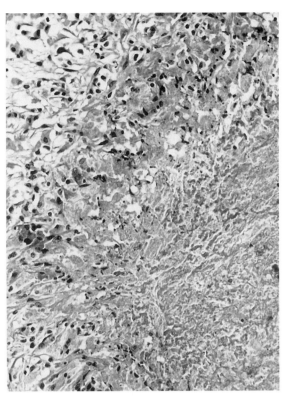

Figure 19–10. Atypical hyperplasia (*A*) and grade 1 endometrioid adenocarcinoma (*B*) arising in pelvic endometriosis. The patient had been on unopposed estrogen therapy for 10 years.

Figure 19–11. Necrotic pseudoxanthomatous nodule of endometriosis. A necrotic center is lined by pseudoxanthoma cells.

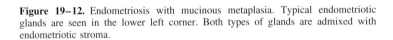

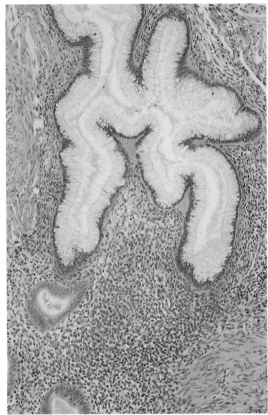

Figure 19–12. Endometriosis with mucinous metaplasia. Typical endometriotic glands are seen in the lower left corner. Both types of glands are admixed with endometriotic stroma.

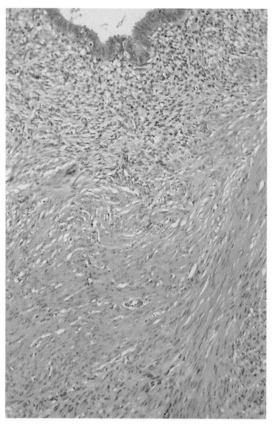

Figure 19–13. Endometriosis with prominent smooth muscle metaplasia (i.e., endomyometriosis).

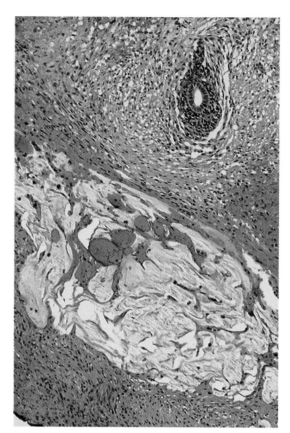

Figure 19–14. Endometriosis with prominent myxoid stroma. A typical endometriotic gland with surrounding endometriotic stroma is present in the upper right. This lesion was misdiagnosed as pseudomyxoma peritonei on frozen section examination.

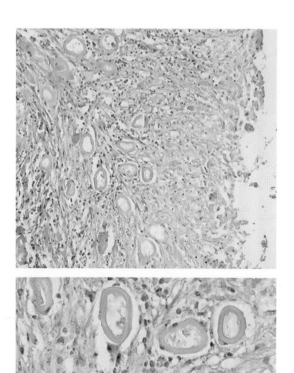

Figure 19–15. Endometriotic cyst with numerous Liesegang rings within its lining (low- and high-power magnifications).

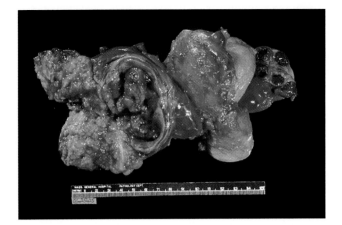

Figure 19–16. Endometrioid carcinoma arising in an endometriotic cyst.

PERITONEAL ENDOMETRIOID LESIONS OTHER THAN ENDOMETRIOSIS

- Benign endometrioid glands (lacking associated endometrial stroma) that rarely involve the peritoneum may represent foci of endometriosis in which the stromal component has atrophied. Similar glands have been associated with a borderline ovarian endometrioid tumor.
- A variety of peritoneal endometrioid neoplasms occur in the absence of demonstrable endometriosis and probably arise from the mesothelium or submesothelial stroma. These have included endometrioid cystadenofibromas and cystadenocarcinomas, endometrioid stromal sarcomas, malignant mesodermal mixed tumors, and adenosarcomas.

References

Chang KL, Crabtree GS, Lim-Tan SK, et al. Primary extrauterine endometrial stromal neoplasms: a clinicopathological study of 20 cases and a review of the literature. Int J Gynecol Pathol 12:282–286, 1993.

Chen KTK. Malignant mixed müllerian tumor of the peritoneum. Int J Surg Pathol 3:155–162, 1996.

Clement PB, Scully RE. Extrauterine mesodermal (müllerian) adenosarcoma: a clinicopathologic analysis of five cases. Am J Clin Pathol 69:276–283, 1978.

Hafiz MA, Toker C. Multicentric ovarian and extraovarian cystadenofibroma. Obstet Gynecol 68:94S–98S, 1986.

PERITONEAL SEROUS LESIONS

- Peritoneal lesions of serous type include endosalpingiosis (a nonneoplastic lesion) and the full spectrum of serous neoplasms seen in the ovary.

Endosalpingiosis

Clinical Features

- Endosalpingiosis refers to the presence of benign glands lined by tubal-type epithelium involving the peritoneum and subperitoneal tissues and retroperitoneal lymph nodes.
- This lesion occurs typically during the reproductive era (mean age of 29.7 years in one study), although occasional cases occur in postmenopausal women.
- Endosalpingiosis is almost always an incidental finding on microscopic examination. It was found in 12.5% of surgically removed omenta in a retrospective study, but this figure doubled when omenta were more thoroughly examined prospectively (Zinsser and Wheeler).
- Unusual presentations include a mass when the glands are cystic, fine pelvic calcifications on x-ray examination, or psammoma bodies within cul-de-sac fluid, peritoneal washings, the lumen of the fallopian tube, or cervical smears.

Pathologic Findings

- The most common sites are the serosa of the uterus, fallopian tubes, cul-de-sac, and omentum. An identical finding, common in the ovary, is by convention referred to as surface epithelial inclusion glands. Less frequent sites include the pelvic parietal peritoneum and serosa of the urinary bladder and bowel.
- Although usually microscopic, multiple, usually less than 5 mm in diameter, opaque or translucent, fluid-filled cysts may be seen. Rare cases may form cystic masses involving the peritoneum or the wall of the uterus, potentially mimicking a neoplasm on gross examination.

- On microscopic examination, glands of variable size and shape, sometimes cystic, are lined by a single layer of benign-appearing, mitotically inactive, tubal-type epithelium, which may include ciliated cells, nonciliated secretory cells, and "peg" cells. Periglandular stroma consists of scanty loose or dense fibrous tissue, occasionally with a sparse mononuclear inflammatory infiltrate.
- Psammoma bodies are common within the lumens or the stroma, and in some cases, numerous psammoma bodies within subserosal fibrous tissue in the absence of epithelium may indicate atrophic endosalpingiosis.
- Periodic acid–Schiff–positive, diastase-resistant material is often present at the luminal tips of the cells and within the glandular lumens. Estrogen and progesterone receptors have been identified immunohistochemically within the cells.
- "Atypical endosalpingiosis" refers to endosalpingiosis with cellular stratification and cellular atypia (see below).

Differential Diagnosis

- Atypical endosalpingiosis merges microscopically with peritoneal serous tumors of borderline malignancy. Bell and Scully use the latter term if the "lesions composed of tubal-type epithelium exhibit papillarity, tufting, or detachment of cell clusters . . . even when they arise on a background of endosalpingiosis."
- Mesonephric remnants, which are common incidental microscopic findings in the region of the fallopian tube, may be confused with endosalpingosis. Mesonephric tubules are typically located more deeply than endosalpingiosis and typically have a collar of smooth muscle and an epithelial lining that consists of a single layer of nonciliated, low columnar to cuboidal cells.

References

Clement PB, Young RH. Tumor-like manifestations of florid cystic endosalpingiosis: a report of four cases including the first reported cases of mural endosalpingiosis of the uterus. Am J Surg Pathol 23:166–175, 1999.

Copeland LJ, Silva EG, Gershenson DM, et al. The significance of müllerian inclusions found at second-look laparotomy in patients with epithelial ovarian neoplasms. Obstet Gynecol 71:763–770, 1988.

Sidaway MK, Silverberg SG. Endosalpingiosis in female peritoneal washings: a diagnostic pitfall. Int J Gynecol Pathol 6:340–346, 1987.

Sneige M, Fernandez T, Copeland LJ, et al. Müllerian inclusions in peritoneal washings. Acta Cytol 30:271–276, 1986.

Zinsser KR, Wheeler JE. Endosalpingiosis in the omentum: a study of autopsy and surgical material. Am J Surg Pathol 6:109–117, 1982.

Peritoneal Serous Borderline Tumors

- Peritoneal serous borderline tumors (PSBLTs) are characterized by usually widespread extraovarian peritoneal involvement and normal-sized ovaries that are free of disease or that have serosal involvement similar to that involving the extraovarian peritoneum.

Clinical Features

- The patients are typically in the reproductive age group (range, 16 to 67 years) and present with infertility and chronic pelvic or abdominal pain; less commonly, the presentation is related to an adnexal mass or small bowel obstruction. Many cases, however, are discovered incidentally at laparotomy for other conditions.
- At operation, focal or diffuse miliary granules, fibrous adhesions, or both involve the pelvic peritoneum and omentum and, less commonly, the abdominal peritoneum.

Pathologic Features

- The peritoneal lesions are superficial and resemble non-invasive epithelial or desmoplastic implants of ovarian serous borderline tumors (SBLTs); the diagnosis of PSBLT is appropriate only when the ovaries are uninvolved or only minimally involved by similar tumor or harbor a benign serous tumor.
- Coexistent endosalpingiosis is present in more than 80% of cases.

Behavior

- Eighty-five percent of the patients have had no clinical evidence of persistent or progressive disease on follow-up, and most of the rest are well after resection of recurrent tumor. In rare cases, the tumors transform to an invasive, low-grade peritoneal serous carcinoma.
- These data indicate that patients with PSBLTs have a good prognosis, similar to that of patients with ovarian serous borderline tumors with noninvasive implants, even when the patients are treated conservatively in order to preserve fertility.

References

Bell DA, Scully RE. Serous borderline tumors of the peritoneum. Am J Surg Pathol 14:230–239, 1990.

Biscotti CV, Hart WR. Peritoneal serous micropapillomatosis of low malignant potential (serous borderline tumors of the peritoneum): a clinicopathologic study of 17 cases. Am J Surg Pathol 16:467–475, 1992.

Weir M, Bell DA, Young RH. Grade 1 peritoneal serous carcinomas: a report of 14 cases and comparison with 7 peritoneal serous psammocarcinomas and 19 peritoneal serous borderline tumors. Am J Surg Pathol 22:849–862, 1998.

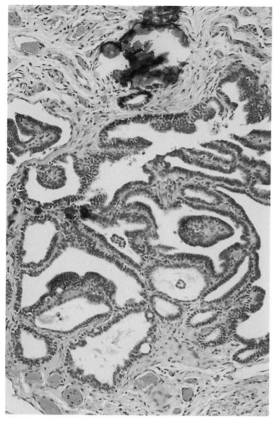

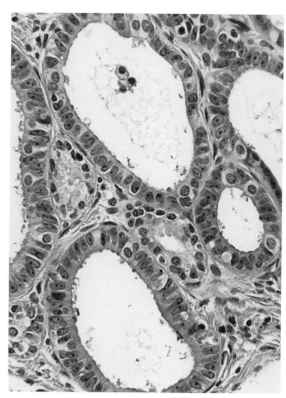

Figure 19–18. Endosalpingiosis. Notice the admixture of cell types, including ciliated cells.

Figure 19–17. Endosalpingiosis. Notice the psammomatous calcification (*top*).

Figure 19–19. Atypical endosalpingiosis. The epithelial cells are focally stratified and have mildly atypical nuclei.

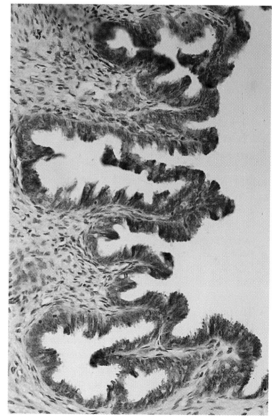

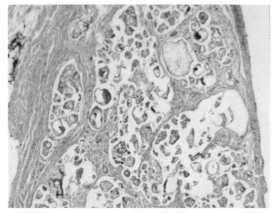

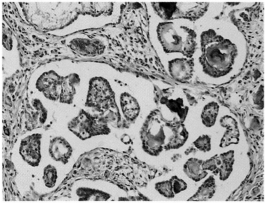

Figure 19–20. Peritoneal serous borderline tumor (low- and high-power magnifications).

Low-Grade Peritoneal Serous Carcinomas, Including Psammocarcinomas

■ Low-grade peritoneal serous carcinomas (LGPSCs) resemble invasive implants of serous borderline tumors. They lack high-grade nuclear atypia, show tissue or lymphovascular space invasion or both, and have appreciable solid epithelial proliferation.

■ Peritoneal psammocarcinomas are a subtype of LGPSCs with a predominance of psammoma bodies and absent or rare solid epithelial proliferation (see Chapter 13 for definition).

■ The average age of patients in one study was 57 years (LGPSC of usual type) and 40 years (peritoneal psammocarcinomas). Presenting features in both tumors are usually abdominal pain, a mass, or both, but about 40% are incidental findings. Operative and gross findings vary from nodules to adhesions to a dominant mass.

■ Short-term outcomes for patients with LGPSCs and peritoneal psammocarcinomas are favorable, but follow-up is too limited in the reported cases to determine long-term outcomes.

■ These tumors should be distinguished from PSLBTs, which are similar except for an absence of invasion. Adequate sampling is necessary to identify invasion, with highest yields of invasive foci in the omentum.

References

Gilks CB, Bell DA, Scully RE. Serous psammocarcinoma of the ovary and peritoneum. Int J Gynecol Pathol 9:110–121, 1990.

Weir M, Bell DA, Young RH. Grade 1 peritoneal serous carcinomas: a report of 14 cases and comparison with 7 peritoneal serous psammocarcinomas and 19 peritoneal serous borderline tumors. Am J Surg Pathol 22:849–862, 1998.

High-Grade Peritoneal Serous Carcinomas

■ These tumors, which resemble high-grade ovarian serous carcinomas and exhibit invasion, are much more common than low-grade peritoneal serous carcinomas.

- In some cases, the ovaries are involved with exclusively surface involvement or by small parenchymal nodules (<5 mm in maximal size), but the ovaries retain their normal size and shape (i.e., normal-sized ovary cancer syndrome).
- The typical intraoperative appearance, with widespread, often bulky peritoneal tumor and ovaries of normal size may mimic that of a diffuse malignant mesothelioma or peritoneal carcinomatosis with an unknown primary.
- Some tumors have occurred in women who have had bilateral oophorectomy performed as prophylactic treatment for familial ovarian cancer.
- The prognosis is similar to that for high-stage serous ovarian carcinomas in most series.

Differential Diagnosis

- Primary ovarian serous surface carcinoma (POSSC). Criteria for primary peritoneal serous carcinoma (PPSC) (versus POSSC) proposed by the Gynecologic Oncology Group (GOG) are as follows:
  - Both ovaries are normal in size or enlarged by a benign process. In the judgment of the surgeon and the pathologist, the bulk of the tumor is in the peritoneum, and the extent of tumor involvement at one or more extraovarian sites is greater than on the surface of either ovary.
  - Microscopic examination of the ovaries reveals no tumor; tumor confined to the surface epithelium with no evidence of cortical invasion; tumor involving the ovarian surface and the underlying cortical stroma but less than 5 × 5 mm; and tumor less than 5 × 5 mm within the ovarian substance, with or without surface involvement.
  - The histologic and cytologic characteristics of the tumor are predominantly serous and similar or identical to those of ovarian serous papillary adenocarcinomas of any grade.
  - Cases in which an oophorectomy had been performed before the diagnosis of the peritoneal tumor should have one of the following: a pathology report to document the absence of carcinoma in the specimen, with review of all the slides of the ovarian specimen if the oophorectomy had been performed within 5 years of the diagnosis of the peritoneal serous carcinoma; or if the oophorectomy had been performed more than 5 years before the diagnosis of PPSC, the pathology report of the specimen is required, and an attempt to review the slides should be made.
- Diffuse malignant mesotheliomas (see Chapter 20).

References

Ben-Baruch G, Sivan E, Moran O, et al. Primary peritoneal serous papillary carcinoma: a study of 25 cases and comparison with stage III–IV ovarian papillary serous carcinoma. Gynecol Oncol 60:393–396, 1996.

Bloss JD, Liao S, Buller RE, et al. Extraovarian peritoneal serous papillary carcinoma: a case-control retrospective comparison to papillary adenocarcinoma of the ovary. Gynecol Oncol 50:347–351, 1993.

Fromm G, Gershenson DM, Silva EG. Papillary serous carcinoma of the peritoneum. Obstet Gynecol 75:89–95, 1990.

Killackey MA, Davis AR. Papillary serous carcinoma of the peritoneal surface: matched-case comparison with papillary serous ovarian carcinoma. Gynecol Oncol 51:171–174, 1993.

Mills SE, Andersen WA, Fechner RE, Austin MB. Serous surface papillary carcinoma: a clinicopathologic study of 10 cases and comparison with stage III–IV ovarian serous carcinoma. Am J Surg Pathol 12:827–834, 1988.

Mulhollan TJ, Silva EG, Tornos C, et al. Ovarian involvement by serous surface papillary carcinoma. Int J Gynecol Pathol 13:120–126, 1994.

Piver MS, Jishi MF, Tsukada Y, Nava G. Primary peritoneal carcinoma after prophylactic oophorectomy in women with a family history of ovarian cancer: a report of the Gilda Radner Familial Ovarian Cancer Registry. Cancer 71:2751–2755, 1993.

Truong LD, Maccato ML, Awalt H, et al. Serous surface carcinoma of the peritoneum: a clinicopathologic study of 22 cases. Hum Pathol 21:99–110, 1990.

Wick MR, Mills SE, Dehner LP, et al. Serous papillary carcinomas arising from the peritoneum and ovaries: a clinicopathologic and immunohistochemical comparison. Int J Gynecol Pathol 8:179–188, 1989.

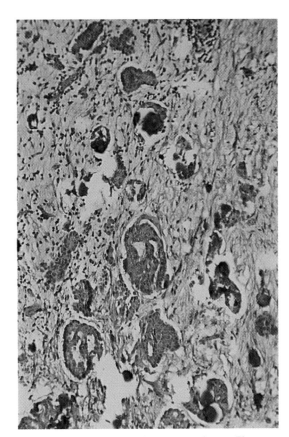

Figure 19–21. Peritoneal low-grade serous carcinoma. The tumor was invasive. Although psammoma bodies are conspicuous, there are many large groups of epithelial cells that lack psammoma bodies, an appearance that excludes psammocarcinoma (compare with Fig. 19–22).

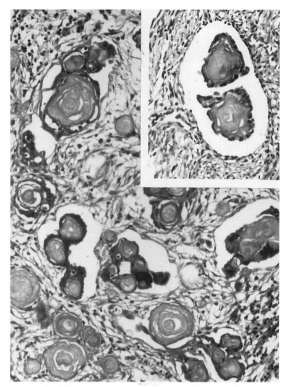

Figure 19–22. Peritoneal low-grade serous carcinoma of the psammo-carcinoma type. Notice the paucity of epithelial cells (compare with Fig. 19–20). *Inset,* The tumor was invasive and extensively involved myometrial lymphatics.

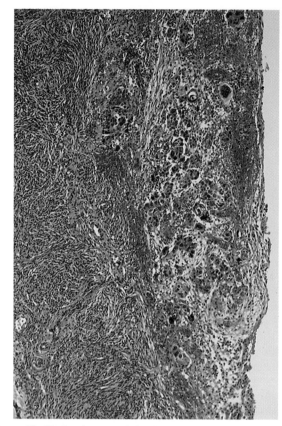

Figure 19–24. Ovarian serosal involvement by high-grade peritoneal serous carcinoma.

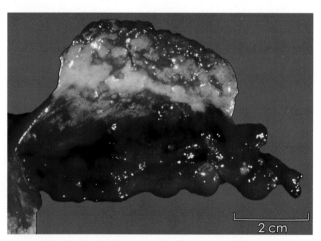

Figure 19–23. Ovarian serosal involvement by high-grade peritoneal serous carcinoma. The ovary is of normal size and shape and is involved by only small surface nodules of tumor. The pelvic and abdominal peritoneum was extensively involved by bulky tumor deposits.

PERITONEAL MUCINOUS LESIONS

Endocervicosis

- Endocervicosis refers to benign glands of endocervical type involving the peritoneum, a finding that is much less common than endometriosis or endosalpingiosis.
- Involved sites have included the uterine serosa, the cul-de-sac, and the urinary bladder. In the latter site, the lesions form tumor-like masses in the posterior wall or posterior dome in women of reproductive age.
- On microscopic examination of the vesical lesions, the benign endocervical-type glands extensively involve the muscularis propria and occasionally involve the mucosa. Rare tubal-type or endometrioid glands (sometimes with associated endometriotic stroma) may also be present.
- In several cases, the infiltrative gland pattern, mild epithelial atypia, and a reactive periglandular stroma, alone or in combination, resulted in an initial misdiagnosis of well-differentiated mucinous adenocarcinoma.

- The differential diagnosis includes otherwise similar bladder lesions characterized by an admixture of müllerian glandular epithelia (e.g., tubal, endocervical, endometrioid, with tubal glands usually predominating) and designated "müllerianosis."

References

Clement PB, Young RH. Endocervicosis of the urinary bladder: a report of six cases of a benign müllerian lesion that may mimic adenocarcinoma. Am J Surg Pathol 16:533–542, 1992.

Nazeer T, Ro JY, Tornos C, et al. Endocervical type glands in urinary bladder: a clinicopathologic study of six cases. Hum Pathol 27: 816–820, 1996.

Ruffolo R, Suster S. Diffuse histiocytic proliferation mimicking mesothelial hyperplasia in endocervicosis of the female pelvic peritoneum. Int J Surg Pathol 1:101–106, 1993.

Young RH, Clement PB. Müllerianosis of the urinary bladder. Mod Pathol 9:731–737, 1996.

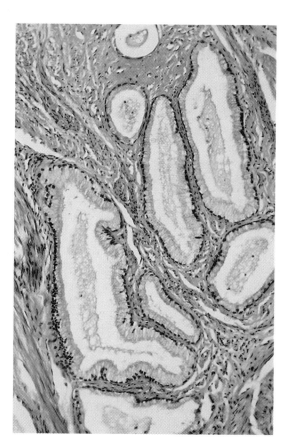

Figure 19–25. Endocervicosis of the urinary bladder.

Extraovarian Mucinous Tumors of Ovarian Type

■ Ovarian-type extraovarian mucinous tumors usually form large cystic masses in the retroperitoneum; a single inguinal case has been described.

■ Cystadenomas, borderline tumors, and cystadenocarcinomas have been described; some contain ovarian-type stroma and even luteinized stromal cells in their walls.

■ Some of these tumors may originate within a supernumerary ovary, but the great rarity of the latter, the absence of follicles or their derivatives within the ovarian-like stroma, and the rare occurrence of similar tumors in males strongly support a peritoneal origin.

References

de Peralta MN, Delahoussaye PM, Tornos CS, Silva EG. Benign retroperitoneal cysts of müllerian type: a clinicopathologic study of three cases and review of the literature. Int J Gynecol Pathol 13:273–278, 1994.

Lee I, Ching K, Pang M, Ho T. Two cases of primary retroperitoneal mucinous cystadenocarcinoma. Gynecol Oncol 63:145–150, 1996.

Pearl ML, Valea F, Chumas J, Chalas E. Primary retroperitoneal mucinous cystadenocarcinoma of low malignant potential: a case report and literature review. Gynecol Oncol 61:150–152, 1996.

PERITONEAL TRANSITIONAL, SQUAMOUS, AND CLEAR CELL LESIONS

■ Nests of transitional (urothelial) epithelium (Walthard nests) commonly involve the serosa of the fallopian tubes, mesosalpinx, and mesovarium in women of all ages.

• Cystification of the nests often results in grossly visible cysts. On microscopic examination, the cysts usually contain a distinctive flocculent eosinophilic material. The transitional nature of the compressed cells lining the cysts may not be apparent.

■ Squamous metaplasia of the peritoneum has been described but is rare compared with transitional cell metaplasia.

■ Two clear cell carcinomas of apparent peritoneal origin have been described. One was a mass within the sigmoid mesocolon, and the other diffusely involved the peritoneum. No endometriosis was identified in either case.

References

Bransilver BR, Ferenczy A, Richart RM. Brenner tumors and Walthard cell nests. Arch Pathol Lab Med 98:76–86, 1974.

Evans H, Yates WA, Palmer WE, et al. Clear cell carcinoma of the sigmoid mesocolon: a tumor of the secondary müllerian system. Am J Obstet Gynecol 162:161–163, 1990.

Hampton HL, Huffman HT, Meeks GR. Extraovarian Brenner tumor. Obstet Gynecol 79:844–846, 1992.

Lee KR, Verma U, Belinson J. Primary clear cell carcinoma of the peritoneum. Gynecol Oncol 41:259–262, 1991.

Roth LM. The Brenner tumor and the Walthard cell nest: an electron microscopic study. Lab Invest 31:15–23, 1974.

Schatz JE, Colgan TJ. Squamous metaplasia of the peritoneum. Arch Pathol Lab Med 115:397–398, 1991.

Teoh TB. The structure and development of Walthard nests. J Pathol 66:433–439, 1953.

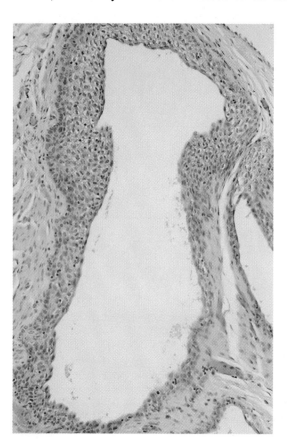

Figure 19–26. Cystic Walthard nests.

SUBPERITONEAL MESENCHYMAL LESIONS

Peritoneal Decidual Reaction

Clinical and Operative Findings

- Frequent sites of involvement include the submesothelial stroma of the fallopian tubes, uterus and uterine ligaments, appendix and omentum, and within pelvic adhesions.
- The ectopic decidua is typically an incidental microscopic finding but may be visible at cesarean section or postpartum tubal ligation as gray-white peritoneal nodules or plaques that may mimic a malignant tumor. Intraperitoneal (occasionally fatal) hemorrhage during the third trimester, labor, or the puerperium is a rare complication.

Microscopic Findings

- Submesothelial decidual cells are disposed individually or arranged in nodules or plaques. The decidual foci are typically vascular and contain a sprinkling of lymphocytes.
- Smooth muscle cells, probably derived from submesothelial myofibroblasts, may be admixed.
- Unusual findings that may raise the possibility of a tumor include hemorrhagic necrosis, myxoid stroma, signet-ring–like decidual cells, and nuclear pleomorphism and hyperchromasia.
- In contrast to adenocarcinomas, the vacuoles in the decidual cells contain acid, rather than neutral, mucin, and the cytoplasm is cytokeratin negative.
- The finding must be distinguished from deciduoid malignant mesotheliomas (page 456).

References

Buttner A, Bassler R, Theele C. Pregnancy-associated ectopic decidua (deciduosis) of the greater omentum: an analysis of 60 biopsies with cases of fibrosing deciduosis and leiomyomatosis peritonealis disseminata. Pathol Res Pract 189:352–359, 1993.

Nascimento AG, Keeney GL, Fletcher CDM. Deciduoid peritoneal mesothelioma: an unusual phenotype affecting young females. Am J Surg Pathol 18:439–445, 1994.

Sabatelle R, Winger E. Postpartum intraabdominal hemorrhage caused by ectopic deciduosis. Obstet Gynecol 41:873–875, 1973.

Zaytsev P, Taxy JB. Pregnancy-associated ectopic decidua. Am J Surg Pathol 11:526–530, 1987.

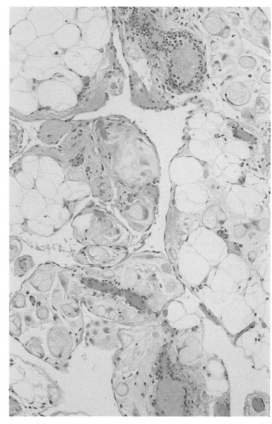

Figure 19–27. Ectopic decidua involving the omentum removed at cesarean section. Most of the decidual cells contain mucin-filled cytoplasmic vacuoles and eccentric nuclei, the appearance potentially mimicking metastatic signet-ring cell adenocarcinoma.

Diffuse Peritoneal Leiomyomatosis

Clinical Findings

- Patients with diffuse peritoneal leiomyomatosis (DPL) are usually of reproductive age but occasionally have been postmenopausal. Approximately 70% of the patients are pregnant or puerperal or use oral contraceptives.
- DPL is often an incidental finding during cesarean section or postpartum tubal ligation, but patients occasionally present with palpable pelvic nodules or symptoms caused by uterine leiomyomas.
- Several to innumerable, firm nodules, most of which are usually smaller than 0.5 cm, are scattered over the pelvic peritoneum and omentum, potentially mimicking metastatic tumor. Rarely, synchronous nodules have been found in pelvic lymph nodes and, in one case, the lungs (see Benign Metastasizing Leiomyoma, page 190).

Pathologic Features

- The nodules resemble typical or cellular leiomyomas, usually with no significant nuclear pleomorphism or mitotic activity, but as many as 3 mitotic figures per 10 high-power-fields have been recorded. In a unique case, epithelioid smooth muscle cells in a pseudoglandular pattern were found in a recurrence.
- Decidual cells and cells transitional in form between muscle and decidual cells may be found in the nodules in pregnant patients.
- Endometriosis or endosalpingiosis has been in continuity with the nodules in 10% of cases.

Behavior

- Although usually self-limiting despite incomplete excision, DPL has occasionally recurred; the recurrence has sometimes been synchronous with a subsequent pregnancy.
- Occasional cases of persistent DPL have been successfully treated with gonadotropin-releasing hormone agonists.
- Five cases of leiomyosarcomatous transformation of DPL have been reported. In each case, rapidly growing intraabdominal tumor (and metastatic tumor in one) with the histologic appearance of leiomyosarcoma appeared within a year of a diagnosis of typical DPL. Four of the women died of disease within 2 years of their initial presentations.

Histogenesis

- DPL appears to arise from metaplastic transformation of submesothelial mesenchymal cells into smooth muscle cells.
- The association with pregnancy or exogenous hormones, the reduction in size of the lesions after pregnancy or surgical castration, the usual presence of progesterone receptors within the lesional cells, and the production in guinea pigs of similar lesions by the administration of estrogen or estrogen and progesterone suggest a hormonal cause in at least some cases.

References

Abulafia O, Angel C, Sherer DM, et al. Computed tomography of leiomyomatosis peritonealis disseminata with malignant transformation. Am J Obstet Gynecol 169:52–54, 1995.

Akkersdijk GJM, Flu PK, Giard RWM, et al. Malignant leiomyomatosis peritonealis disseminata. Am J Obstet Gynecol 163:591–593, 1990.

Butnor KJ, Burchette JL, Robboy SJ. Progesterone receptor activity in leiomyomatosis peritonealis disseminata. Int J Gynecol Pathol 18: 259–264, 1999.

Buttner A, Bassler R, Theele C. Pregnancy-associated ectopic decidua (deciduosis) of the greater omentum: an analysis of 60 biopsies with cases of fibrosing deciduosis and leiomyomatosis peritonealis disseminata. Pathol Res Pract 189:352–359, 1993.

Clavero PA, Nogales FF, Ruiz-Avila I, et al. Regression of peritoneal leiomyomatosis after treatment with gonadotropin releasing hormone analogue. Int J Gynecol Cancer 2:52–54, 1992.

Hales HA, Peterson CM, Jones KP, Quinn JD. Leiomyomatosis peritonealis disseminata treated with a gonadotropin-releasing hormone agonist. Am J Obstet Gynecol 167:515–516, 1992.

Ma KF, Chow LTC. Sex cord–like pattern leiomyomatosis peritonealis disseminata: a hitherto undescribed feature. Histopathology 21:389–391, 1992.

Raspagliesi F, Quattrone P, Grosso G, et al. Malignant degeneration in leiomyomatosis peritonealis disseminata. Gynecol Oncol 61:272–274, 1996.

Tavassoli FA, Norris HJ. Peritoneal leiomyomatosis (leiomyomatosis peritonealis disseminata): a clinicopathologic study of 20 cases with ultrastructural observations. Int J Gynecol Pathol 1:59–74, 1982.

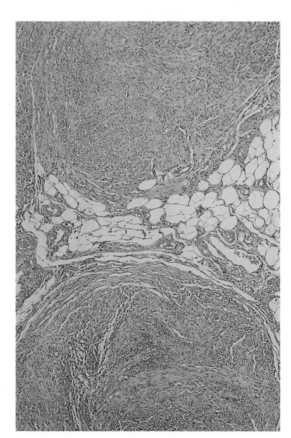

Figure 19–29. Peritoneal leiomyomatosis involving the omentum. Two nodules are seen.

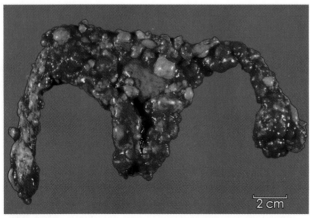

Figure 19–28. Peritoneal leiomyomatosis involving the omentum.

RETROPERITONEAL LYMPH NODE LESIONS

Benign Glands of Müllerian Type

Clinical Features

- Almost all of the patients with benign, müllerian-type glands have been adults, although rare examples have been reported in children.
- The glands are usually found within pelvic and para-aortic lymph nodes and rarely in inguinal and femoral lymph nodes.
- The frequency of the finding (from 2% to 41% of patients undergoing lymphadenectomy) depends on the number of lymph nodes removed and the extent of the histologic sampling.
- Although typically without clinical or intraoperative manifestations, rare cases have been associated with a false-positive lymphangiogram, ureteral obstruction from lymph node enlargement, or visible enlargement at the time of operation.
- Associated findings have included peritoneal endosalpingiosis, salpingitis isthmica nodosa, and acute and chronic salpingitis. Other patients have had coexistent ovarian serous tumors, which have been benign, borderline, or carcinomas.

Pathologic Findings

- The glands are grossly apparent in only rare cases, recognizable as cysts several millimeters in diameter.
- The usual location is the periphery of the node, most commonly within its capsule or between the lymphoid follicles in the superficial cortex. In florid cases, a diffuse distribution throughout the lymph node has been described.
- The glands are almost always of endosalpingiotic type (page 431), often with intraglandular or periglandular psammoma bodies. The glands may be surrounded by a thin rim of fibrous tissue, or they may abut directly on lymphoid cells.
- In some cases, atypical endosalpingiotic glands merge

with intranodal SBLT, suggesting that the SBLT has originated within the lymph node (see Chapter 13). In other cases, benign glands are present in a node that also contains SBLT metastatic from the ovary.
- Rarely, the intranodal glands have been endometrioid, mucinous (endocervical or of goblet-cell type), or are partly replaced by metaplastic squamous epithelium.

Differential Diagnosis

- Intranodal endometriosis is distinguished by the presence of periglandular endometriotic stroma; rarely, endometriosis and endosalpingiotic glands are present in the same lymph node.
- The distinction from metastatic adenocarcinoma is usually not difficult, because the latter usually exhibits malignant nuclear features and at least focal involvement of subcapsular sinuses.
- Similarly, metastatic SBLT, in contrast to primary intranodal SBLT, usually focally involves the subcapsular sinuses and lacks obvious merging with intranodal endosalpingiotic glands.

References

Bell DA, Scully RE. Clinicopathological features of lymph node involvement with ovarian serous borderline tumors [Abstract]. Mod Pathol 5:61A, 1992.

Ehrmann RL, Federschneider JM, Knapp RC. Distinguishing lymph node metastases from benign glandular inclusions in low-grade ovarian carcinoma. Am J Obstet Gynecol 136:737–746, 1980.

Horn L-C, Bilek K. Frequency and histogenesis of pelvic retroperitoneal lymph node inclusions of the female genital tract: an immunohistochemical study of 34 cases. Pathol Res Pract 191:991–996, 1995.

Karp LA, Czernobilsky B. Glandular inclusions in pelvic and abdominal para-aortic lymph nodes. Am J Clin Pathol 52:212–218, 1969.

Kheir SM, Mann WJ, Wilkerson JA. Glandular inclusions in lymph nodes: the problem of extensive involvement and relationship to salpingitis. Am J Surg Pathol 5:353–359, 1981.

Mills SE. Decidua and squamous metaplasia in abdominopelvic lymph nodes. Int J Gynecol Pathol 2:209–215, 1983.

Prade M, Spatz A, Bentley R, et al. Borderline and malignant serous tumor arising in pelvic lymph nodes: evidence of origin in benign glandular inclusions. Int J Gynecol Pathol 14:87–91, 1995.

Yoonessi M, Satchindanand SK, Ortinez CG, et al. Benign glandular elements and decidual reaction in retroperitoneal lymph nodes. J Surg Oncol 19:81–86, 1982.

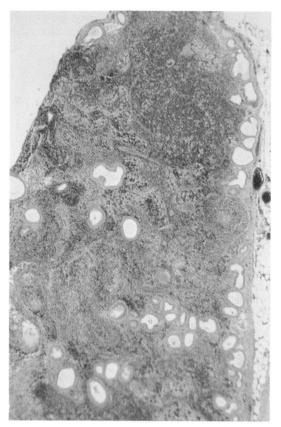

Figure 19–30. Extensive nodal involvement by benign müllerian (endosalpingiotic) glands.

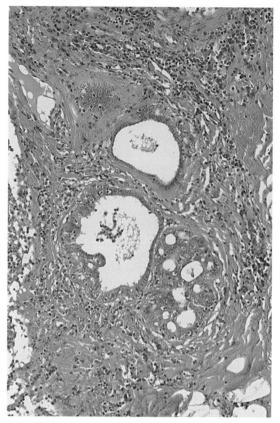

Figure 19–31. Benign endosalpingiotic glands within the capsule of a pelvic lymph node. A cribriform pattern is present in one of the glands (i.e., atypical endosalpingiosis).

Intranodal Decidua

- Ectopic decidua is a rare, incidental microscopic finding in paraaortic and pelvic lymph nodes in pregnancy. Rarely, the decidual tissue is grossly visible as tiny, gray, subcapsular nodules.
- An associated peritoneal decidual reaction also may be present.
- The decidual nests typically occupy the subcapsular sinus and superficial cortex and, less commonly, the central part of the lymph node.
- The decidual cells usually appear benign but occasionally have atypical, hyperchromatic nuclei, potentially mimicking metastatic squamous cell carcinoma. The absence of mitotic activity, keratinization, and negativity for cytokeratin facilitate this differential diagnosis. Metastatic squamous cell carcinoma, however, has rarely coexisted with decidual cells in the same node.

References

Ashraf M, Boyd CB, Beresford WA. Ectopic decidual reaction in paraaortic and pelvic lymph nodes in the presence of cervical squamous cell carcinoma during pregnancy. J Surg Oncol 26:6–8, 1984.

Burnett RA, Millan D. Decidual change in pelvic lymph nodes: a source of possible diagnostic error. Histopathology 10:1089–1092, 1986.

Cobb CJ. Ectopic decidua and metastatic squamous carcinoma: presentation in a single pelvic lymph node. J Surg Oncol 38:126–129, 1988.

Covell LM, Disciullo AJ, Knapp RC. Decidual change in pelvic lymph nodes in the presence of cervical squamous cell carcinoma during pregnancy. Am J Obstet Gynecol 127:674–676, 1977.

Mills SE. Decidua and squamous metaplasia in abdominopelvic lymph nodes. Int J Gynecol Pathol 2:209–215, 1983.

Yoonessi M, Satchindanand SK, Ortinez CG, et al. Benign glandular elements and decidual reaction in retroperitoneal lymph nodes. J Surg Oncol 19:81–86, 1982.

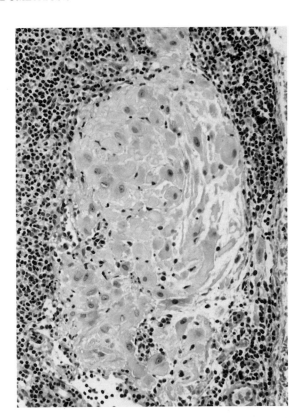

Figure 19–32. Ectopic decidua within a pelvic lymph node.

Leiomyomatosis

■ Rarely, nodules of benign-appearing smooth muscle have been found within pelvic or paraaortic lymph nodes. In pregnant patients, the process may merge with intranodal decidua.

■ The affected women usually also have typical uterine leiomyomas or, rarely, disseminated peritoneal leiomyomatosis (page 439) or pulmonary nodules of similar smooth muscle (page 190).

■ The possible histogenesis of the lesion includes an origin from entrapped subcoelomic mesenchyme, myofibroblastic organization of intranodal decidua, and lymphatic spread from uterine leiomyomas.

■ The differential diagnosis includes nodal involvement by lymphangioleiomyomatosis. In cases of the latter, however, the appearance is typically that of a lymphangiomyoma, and there is usually tuberous sclerosis and associated pulmonary involvement.

References

Abell MR, Littler ER. Benign metastasizing uterine leiomyoma: multiple lymph nodal metastases. Cancer 36:2206–2213, 1975.

Horie A, Ishii N, Matsumoto M, et. al. Leiomyomatosis in the pelvic lymph node and peritoneum. Acta Pathol Jpn 34:813–819, 1984.

Hsu YK, Rosenshein NB, Parmley TH, et al. Leiomyomatosis in pelvic lymph nodes. Obstet Gynecol 57:91S–93S, 1981.

Mazzoleni G, Salerno A, Santini D, et al. Leiomyomatosis in pelvic lymph nodes. Histopathology 21:588–589, 1992.

CHAPTER 20

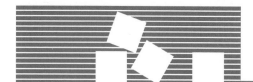

Tumor-like Lesions and Tumors of the Peritoneum, Excluding Secondary Müllerian Lesions

TUMOR-LIKE LESIONS (Table 20–1)

Inflammatory Lesions

Granulomatous Peritonitis

- A variety of infectious and noninfectious agents can cause granulomatous peritonitis. The peritoneum may be studded with nodules, which can mimic disseminated tumor at operation or on gross examination. The diagnosis rests on the microscopic and, in some cases, microbiologic identification of the causative agent.
- Infectious causes include tuberculosis and, rarely, fungal infections (i.e., histoplasmosis, coccidioidomycosis, cryptococcosis) and parasitic infestations (i.e., schistosomiasis, oxyuriasis, echinococcosis, ascariasis, strongyloidiasis).
- Noninfectious causes in women include sebaceous material and keratin from ruptured dermoid cysts; spillage of amniotic fluid at cesarean section, with its content of vernix caseosa (keratin, squames, sebum, lanugo hair) and meconium (bile, pancreatic, intestinal secretions); and keratin derived from uterine and ovarian adenoacanthomas (page 452). Rare cases of meconium peritonitis are associated with disseminated intravascular spread of the meconium.
- Other noninfectious causes include foreign material such as starch granules from surgical gloves, douche fluid, and lubricants, talc (from surgical gloves, in drug abusers), cellulose and cotton fibers from surgical pads and drapes, microcrystalline collagen hemostat (Avitene), oily materials (e.g., hysterosalpingographic contrast medium, mineral oil, paraffin), escaped bowel contents, or bile.
- Granulomatous peritonitis can result from Crohn's disease, sarcoidosis, silicosis, and Whipple's disease. Necrotizing peritoneal granulomas may occur after diathermy ablation of endometriosis.

Nongranulomatous Histiocytic Lesions

- Aggregates of nonpigmented histiocytes as a nonspecific inflammatory response may be visible as small nodules at operation and have been initially misinterpreted microscopically as metastatic granulosa cell tumor. In one case, a diffuse histiocytic proliferation of the pelvic peritoneum was associated with endocervicosis.
- Ceroid-rich histiocytes, a response to endometriosis or a peritoneal decidual reaction, can involve the peritoneum, usually representing a microscopic finding.
- Peritoneal melanosis (i.e., melanin-laden histiocytes) is a rare complication of ovarian dermoid cysts; some had ruptured preoperatively.
  - Tan to black peritoneal staining or pigmented tumor-like nodules involving the pelvic peritoneum and omentum may mimic metastatic tumor at laparotomy. Locules within the dermoid cysts also had pigmentation of their contents and lining.
  - The lesions are distinguished from malignant melanoma by the presence of melanin within bland histiocytes rather than in atypical melanocytes, a differential facilitated by immunohistochemical staining.
- Mucicarminophilic histiocytosis is characterized by histiocytes that contain polyvinylpyrrolidone (PVP), a substance that has been used as a blood substitute.
  - The histiocytes are found within and outside the female genital tract, including pelvic lymph nodes and the omentum.
  - The vacuolated basophilic to lavender cytoplasm and an eccentric nucleus may suggest the diagnosis of signet-ring cell adenocarcinoma. The histiocytes are mucicarminophilic, but in contrast to neoplastic signet-ring cells, are periodic acid–Schiff (PAS) negative.
- A peritoneal reaction similar to mucicarminophilic his-

Table 20–1
TUMOR-LIKE REACTIVE LESIONS OF THE PERITONEUM

Granulomatous Lesions

    Vernix caseosa and meconium peritonitis
    Granulomatous peritonitis secondary to foreign material, including keratin
    Necrotic pseudoxanthomatous nodules
    Postcautery granulomas

Nongranulomatous Histiocytic Lesions

    Ceroid-rich histiocytic infiltrates
    Peritoneal melanosis
    Mucicarminophilic histiocytosis
    Other histiocytic infiltrates

Fibrosing Lesions

    Sclerosing peritonitis
    Peritoneal fibrous nodules

Mesothelial Lesions

    Mesothelial hyperplasia
    Peritoneal inclusion cysts

tiocytosis has been described in response to oxidized regenerated cellulose, a topical hemostatic agent. The histiocytes have abundant, granular, basophilic, and mucinocarminophilic cytoplasm.

- The histiocytes in all of the lesions should be distinguished from mesothelial cells, a distinction that can be aided by the different immunoreactivities of the cell types.

Peritoneal Fibrosis

- Reactive peritoneal fibrosis, fibrous adhesions, or both are common sequelae of prior peritoneal inflammation and a surgical procedure.
- Localized hyaline plaques are a common incidental finding on the splenic capsule, and fibrous thickening of the peritoneum has been described as a histologic finding in patients with hepatic cirrhosis and ascites.
- Sclerosing peritonitis, which is a reactive proliferation of the submesothelial mesenchymal cells to a variety of stimuli, often encases the small bowel (i.e., abdominal cocoon), causing bowel obstruction. Some cases are idiopathic, whereas others result from practolol therapy, chronic ambulatory peritoneal dialysis, the use of a peritoneovenous shunt, bacterial or mycobacterial infection, sarcoidosis, the carcinoid syndrome, familial Mediterranean fever, foreign materials, lupus erythematosus, and rare luteinized thecomas.
- Rarely, reactive fibrous proliferations of the peritoneum can form tumor-like nodules, in contrast to the more widespread peritoneal thickening of sclerosing peritonitis.
- Reactive peritoneal fibrosis may be difficult to distinguish from a desmoplastic mesothelioma, particularly in a small biopsy specimen. Features favoring or indicating the latter diagnosis include nuclear atypia, necrosis, organized patterns of collagen deposition (i.e., fascicular, storiform), frankly sarcomatoid areas, and infiltration of adjacent tissues.

References

Clarke TJ, Simpson RHW. Necrotizing granulomas of peritoneum following diathermy ablation of endometriosis. Histopathology 16:400–402, 1990.

Clement PB. Reactive tumor-like lesions of the peritoneum [Editorial]. Am J Clin Pathol 103:673–676, 1995.

Clement PB, Young RH, Hanna W, Scully RE. Sclerosing peritonitis associated with luteinized thecomas of the ovary: a clinicopathological analysis of six cases. Am J Surg Pathol 18:1–13, 1994.

George E, Leyser S, Zimmer HL, et al. Vernix caseosa peritonitis: an infrequent complication of cesarean section with distinctive histopathologic features. Am J Clin Pathol 103:681–684, 1995.

Kershisnik MM, Ro JY, Cannon GH, et al. Histiocytic reaction in pelvic peritoneum associated wtih oxidized regenerated cellulose. Am J Clin Pathol 103:27–31, 1994.

Kolker SE, Ferrell LD, Bollen AW, Ursell PC. Disseminated intravascular meconium in a newborn with meconium peritonitis. Hum Pathol 30:592–594, 1999.

Kuo T, Hsueh S. Mucicarminophilic histiocytosis: a polyvinylpyrrolidone (PVP) storage disease simulating signet-ring cell carcinoma. Am J Surg Pathol 8:419–428, 1984.

Mangano WE, Cagle PT, Churg A, et al. The diagnosis of desmoplastic malignant mesothelioma and its distinction from fibrous pleurisy: a histologic and immunohistochemical analysis of 31 cases including p53 immunostaining. Am J Clin Pathol 110:191–199, 1998.

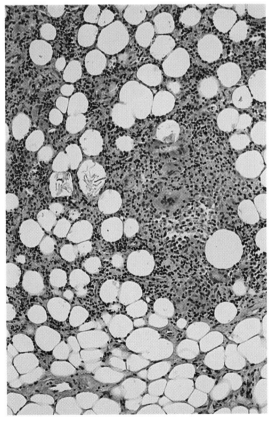

Figure 20–1. Vernix caseosa peritonitis. Granulomatous inflammation and flakes of keratin are seen in the center of the field.

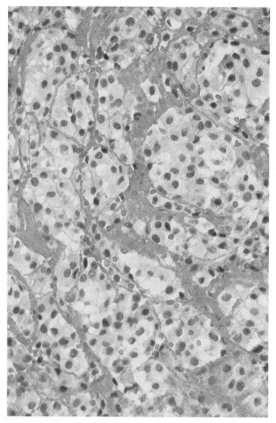

Figure 20–2. Peritoneal histiocytic nodule. The cells were immunoreactive for KP-1.

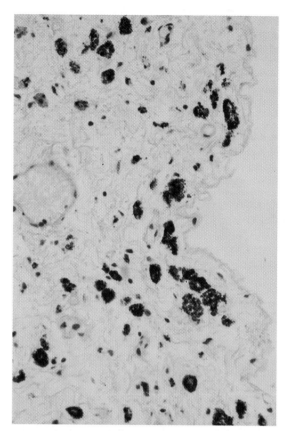

Figure 20–3. Peritoneal melanosis.

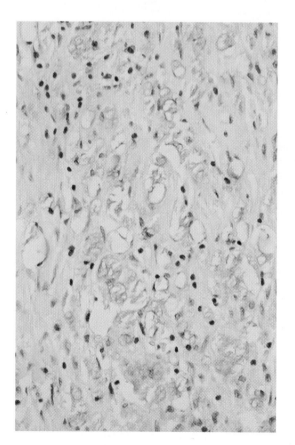

Figure 20–4. Mucicarminophilic histiocytosis (mucicarmine stain). Some of the cells resemble signet-ring cells.

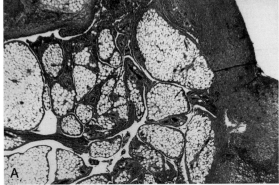

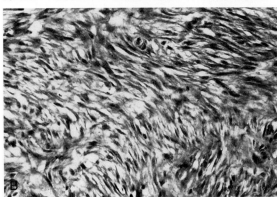

Figure 20–5. *A,* Sclerosing peritonitis involving the omentum in a woman with a luteinized thecoma of the ovary. *B,* On high-power examination, the proliferation consists of spindle cells of fibroblastic or myofibroblastic type.

Mesothelial Lesions

Mesothelial Hyperplasia

■ Mesothelial hyperplasia is a common response to chronic effusions, inflammation (e.g., pelvic inflammatory disease), endometriosis, and ovarian tumors (see Table 20–1). Mesothelial hyperplasia confined to a hernia sac may reflect trauma or incarceration.

■ Solitary or multiple, small nodules may be visible at operation, but more commonly the process is an incidental microscopic finding.

■ Florid examples may form solid, trabecular, tubular, papillary, or tubulopapillary patterns that may superficially extend into the underlying tissues. The cells may be focally disposed in linear, sometimes parallel arrangement with fibrin or reactive fibrous tissue. The same finding within the walls of ovarian tumors, endometriotic cysts, and peritoneal inclusion cysts (i.e., mural mesothelial proliferation) can sometimes be mistaken for invasive tumor.

■ The mesothelial cells may contain cytoplasmic vacuoles that stain for acid mucin (predominantly hyaluronic acid) and may exhibit mild to moderate nuclear pleomorphism, multinucleation, and occasional mitotic fig-

ures. Uncommon findings include psammoma bodies and eosinophilic strap-shaped cells resembling rhabdomyoblasts.

■ Mesothelial cells in abdominal lymph nodes may be misinterpreted as metastatic tumor, especially in women with a known primary pelvic cancer. There may be comcomitant mesothelial hyperplasia of the pelvic and abdominal peritoneum. The appearance of the cells on routine stains suggests the correct diagnosis and can be confirmed by histochemical and immunohistochemical staining.

Differential Diagnosis

■ Diffuse malignant mesothelioma (DMM). Features that favor or indicate DMM include grossly visible nodules, deep infiltration, necrosis, large "empty" cytoplasmic vacuoles, marked nuclear atypia, atypical mitotic figures, and strong membranous immunoreactivity for epithelial membrane antigen (EMA). Some of these features, such as marked nuclear atypia, may be absent or present only focally within a DMM.

■ Borderline serous tumors (BSTs) of primary peritoneal or ovarian origin. Grossly visible ovarian or peritoneal tumor, columnar cells with or without cilia, neutral mucin, numerous psammoma bodies, and immunohistochemical markers for epithelial differentiation (page 456) all favor a BST.

References

Clement PB, Young RH. Florid mesothelial hyperplasia associated with ovarian tumors: a possible source of error in tumor diagnosis and staging. Int J Gynecol Pathol 12:51–58, 1993.

Clement PB, Young RH, Oliva E, et al. Hyperplastic mesothelial cells within abdominal lymph nodes: a mimic of metastatic ovarian carcinoma and serous borderline tumor—a report of two cases associated with ovarian neoplasms. Mod Pathol 9:879–886, 1996.

Daya D, McCaughey WTE. Pathology of the peritoneum: a review of selected topics. Semin Diagn Pathol 8:277–289, 1991.

Henderson DW, Shilkin KB, Whitaker D. Reactive mesothelial hyperplasia vs mesothelioma, including mesothelioma in situ. Am J Clin Pathol 110:397–404, 1998.

Kerner H, Gaton E, Czernobilsky B. Unusual ovarian, tubal and pelvic mesothelial inclusions in patients with endometriosis. Histopathology 5:277–282, 1981.

McCaughey WTE, Al-Jabi M. Differentiation of serosal hyperplasia and neoplasia in biopsies. Pathol Annu 21(1):271–292, 1986.

Rosai J, Dehner LP. Nodular mesothelial hyperplasia in hernia sacs: a benign reactive condition stimulating a neoplastic process. Cancer 35:165–175, 1975.

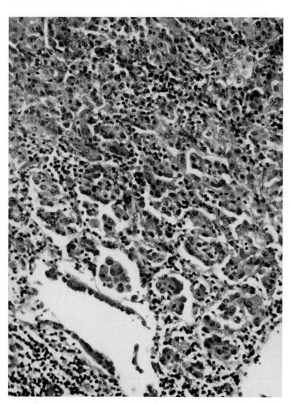

Figure 20–6. Papillary mesothelial hyperplasia. Notice the admixed chronic inflammatory cells.

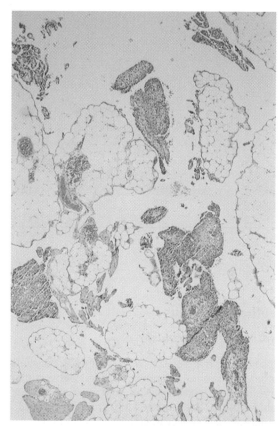

Figure 20–7. Nodular mesothelial hyperplasia involving the omentum.

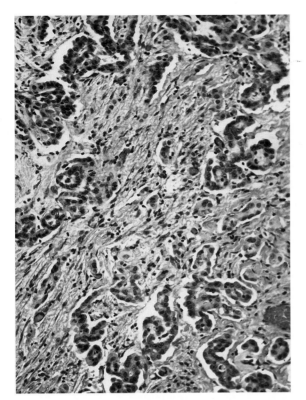

Figure 20–8. Mesothelial hyperplasia within the wall of a borderline ovarian tumor. The nests of mesothelial cells are surrounded by spaces due to retraction artifact. The process was initially misdiagnosed as invasive carcinoma with stromal and lymphatic invasion.

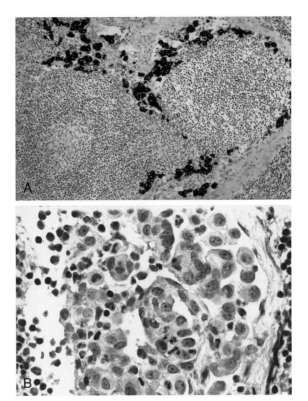

Figure 20–9. Hyperplastic mesothelial cells within a pelvic lymph node. *A,* A cytokeratin stain reveals darkly staining mesothelial cells in a sinusoidal pattern. *B,* Hyperplastic mesothelial cells occupy a sinusoid (hematoxylin and eosin stain).

Peritoneal Inclusion Cysts

- Peritoneal inclusion cysts (PICs) typically occur in women of reproductive age; rarely, the lesions occur in males and in the pleural cavity.

Unilocular Peritoneal Inclusion Cysts

- Unilocular PICs are usually an incidental intraoperative finding. Single or multiple, small, thin-walled, translucent, unilocular cysts are attached or free floating.
- The cysts have a smooth lining, yellow and watery to gelatinous contents, and a lining composed of a single layer of flattened, benign mesothelial cells.
- Most unilocular PICs are probably reactive, whereas some of those in the mesocolon, mesentery of the small intestine, retroperitoneum, and splenic capsule may be developmental.

Multilocular Peritoneal Inclusion Cysts

- Multilocular PICs (MPICs) are also referred to as benign cystic mesotheliomas, inflammatory cysts of the peritoneum, and postoperative peritoneal cysts.
- MPICs, which may reach 20 cm in maximal dimension, are usually associated with clinical manifestations, most commonly lower abdominal pain, a palpable mass, or both.
- MPICs are usually adherent to pelvic organs and may simulate a cystic ovarian tumor on clinical examination, at laparotomy, or even on pathologic examination; the upper abdominal cavity, the retroperitoneum, or hernia sacs may also be involved.
- Unlike unilocular PICs, the septa and walls of MPICs may contain considerable amounts of fibrous tissue. Their contents may resemble those of the unilocular cysts or be serosanguineous or bloody.
- MPICs are typically lined by a single layer of flat to

cuboidal, occasionally hobnail-shaped mesothelial cells with nuclear features that vary from bland to mildly atypical.

■ Unusual findings include squamous metaplasia, intracystic papillae, cribriform patterns, and mural proliferations of typical or atypical mesothelial cells arranged singly, as glandlike structures or nests, or in patterns resembling those in adenomatoid tumors. Occasional vacuolated mesothelial cells in the stroma may simulate signet-ring cells.

■ The septa typically consist of fibrovascular connective tissue but occasionally contain a marked acute and chronic inflammatory cell infiltrate, abundant fibrin, granulation tissue, and evidence of recent and remote hemorrhage.

■ History of a prior abdominal operation, pelvic inflammatory disease, or endometriosis can be found in as many as 84% of patients, suggesting a role for inflammation in the pathogenesis of the cysts.

■ In cases that we consider MPICs, follow-up has not disclosed malignant behavior. In as many as one half of the cases, however, the MPICs have recurred months to many years postoperatively. At least some of these "recurrences" are probably the result of newly formed postoperative adhesions.

■ Differential diagnosis:
  • "True" cystic mesotheliomas (page 455).
  • Multilocular cystic lymphangiomas. In contrast to MPICs, these lesions typically occur in children (especially boys), are usually extrapelvic (i.e., mesentery of the small intestine, omentum, mesocolon, or retroperitoneum), contain chylous fluid, have mural lymphoid aggregates and smooth muscle, and lining cells that are immunoreactive for endothelial markers.
  • Multicystic adenomatoid tumor. In contrast to MPICs, these tumors typically involve the myometrium, contain foci of typical adenomatoid tumor, and lack prominent numbers of inflammatory cells.

References

Carpenter HA, Lancaster JR, Lee RA. Multilocular cysts of the peritoneum. Mayo Clin Proc 57:634–638, 1982.

McFadden DE, Clement PB. Peritoneal inclusion cysts with mural mesothelial proliferation: a clinicopathological analysis of six cases. Am J Surg Pathol 10:844–854, 1986.

Ross MJ, Welch WR, Scully RE. Multilocular peritoneal inclusion cysts (so-called cystic mesotheliomas). Cancer 64:1336–1346, 1989.

Weiss SW, Tavassoli FA. Multicystic mesothelioma: an analysis of pathologic findings and biologic behavior in 37 cases. Am J Surg Pathol 12:737–746, 1988.

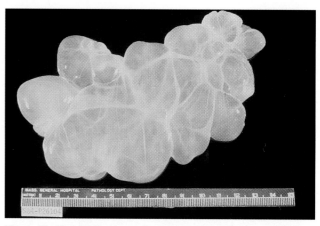

Figure 20–10. Multilocular peritoneal inclusion cyst.

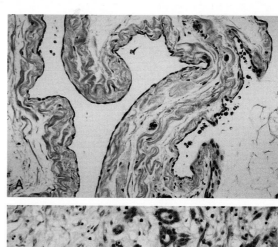

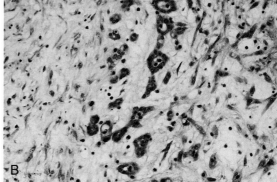

Figure 20–11. Multilocular peritoneal inclusion cyst. *A,* Spaces are lined by flattened mesothelial cells. *B,* In a different case, the walls and septa of the cysts are formed by reactive fibrous tissue containing focal nests and glandlike arrangements of hyperplastic mesothelial cells.

Splenosis

- Splenosis, which results from implantation of splenic tissue, is typically an incidental finding at laparotomy or autopsy months to years after splenectomy for traumatic splenic rupture.
- A few to innumerable, red-blue, peritoneal nodules, ranging up to 7 cm in diameter, are scattered widely thoughout the abdominal and, less commonly, the pelvic cavity.
- The intraoperative appearance may mimic endometriosis, benign or malignant vascular tumors, or metastatic cancer.

References

Carr NJ, Turk EP. The histological features of splenosis. Histopathology 21:549–553, 1992.

Fleming CR, Dickson ER, Harrison EG Jr. Splenosis: autotransplantation of splenic tissue. Am J Med 61:414–419, 1976.

Trophoblastic Implants

- Implants of trophoblast on the pelvic or omental peritoneum are a complication of the operative treatment of tubal pregnancy.
- The implants are more likely to occur in cases managed by laparoscopy than those managed by laparotomy and are more likely to occur after salpingotomy than salpingectomy.
- There is an initial postoperative decline in the serum chorionic gonadotropin level, followed by a rising level, abdominal pain, and in some cases, intraabdominal hemorrhage.
- Microscopic examination of the implants reveals viable trophoblastic tissue that may include chorionic villi. We have also seen a peritoneal trophoblastic implant that resembled a placental site nodule.

References

Cartwright PS. Peritoneal trophoblastic implants after surgical management of tubal pregnancy. J Reprod Med 36:523–524, 1991.

Reich H, De Caprio J, McGlynn F, et al. Peritoneal trophoblastic tissue implants after laparoscopic treatment of tubal ectopic pregnancy. Fertil Steril 52:337, 1989.

Thatcher SS, Grainger DA, True LD, DeCherney AH. Pelvic trophoblastic implants after laparoscopic removal of a tubal pregnancy. Obstet Gynecol 74:514–515, 1989.

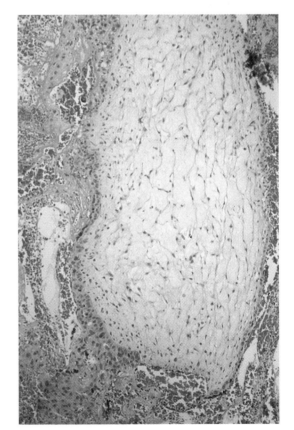

Figure 20–12. Trophoblastic peritoneal implant after treatment of a tubal pregnancy. The implant, which consists of a chorionic villus, was found near the spleen.

Peritoneal Keratin Granulomas

- Peritoneal granulomas may form in response to implants of keratin usually derived from endometrioid carcinomas with squamous differentiation of the endometrium or ovary or, less commonly, squamous cell carcinomas of the cervix or atypical polypoid adenomyomas of the uterus.
- Laminated deposits of keratin, sometimes with ghost squamous cells, are surrounded by foreign-body giant cells and fibrous tissue.
- Follow-up data suggest that the granulomas have no prognostic significance, although they should be thoroughly sampled by the gynecologist and carefully examined microscopically to exclude viable tumor.
- The differential diagnosis includes peritoneal granulomas in reponse to keratin derived from other sources, as discussed earlier.

Reference

Kim K, Scully RE. Peritoneal keratin granulomas with carcinomas of endometrium and ovary and atypical polypoid adenomyoma of endometrium. Am J Surg Pathol 14:925–932, 1990.

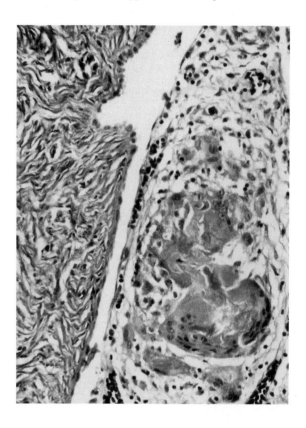

Figure 20–13. Peritoneal keratin granuloma on the serosal surface of the ovary. The ovary was removed at the time of a hysterectomy performed for an endometrial endometrioid adenocarcinoma with squamous differentiation.

Infarcted Appendix Epiploica

- Torsion, infarction, and subsequent calcification of an appendix epiploica can result in a hard, tumor-like mass attached or loose in the peritoneal cavity.
- In the late stages, layers of hyalinized connective tissue surround a central necrotic and calcified zone in which infarcted adipose tissue is usually recognizable.

References

Elliott GB, Freigang B. Aseptic necrosis, calcification and separation of appendices epiploicae. Ann Surg 155:501–505, 1962.
Vuong PN, Guyot H, Moulin G, et al. Pseudotumoral organization of a twisted epiploic fringe or "hard-boiled egg" in the peritoneal cavity. Arch Pathol Lab Med 114:531–533, 1990.

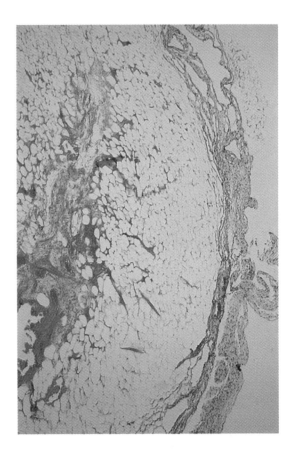

Figure 20–14. Infarcted appendix epiploica.

MESOTHELIAL NEOPLASMS

Solitary Fibrous Tumor

- Localized fibrous tumors of the peritoneum of the type that involve the pleura are rare. Although once referred to as fibrous mesotheliomas, they are now designated solitary fibrous tumors and are thought to originate from submesothelial fibroblasts.
- The clinical and pathologic features are similar to those of their pleural counterparts, including immunoreactivity for CD34 and lack of immunoreactivity for cytokeratin, an immunoprofile that is useful in distinguishing these tumors from desmoplastic mesotheliomas.
- One malignant peritoneal solitary fibrous tumor has been reported.

References

Flint A, Weiss SW. CD-34 and keratin expression distinguishes solitary fibrous tumor (fibrous mesothelioma) of pleura from desmoplastic mesothelioma. Hum Pathol 26:428–431, 1995.

Fukunaga M, Naganuma H, Ushigome S, et al. Malignant solitary fibrous tumour of the peritoneum. Histopathology 28:463–466, 1996.

Young RH, Clement PB, McCaughey WTE. Solitary fibrous tumors ("fibrous mesotheliomas") of the peritoneum: a report of three cases. Arch Pathol Lab Med 114:493–495, 1990.

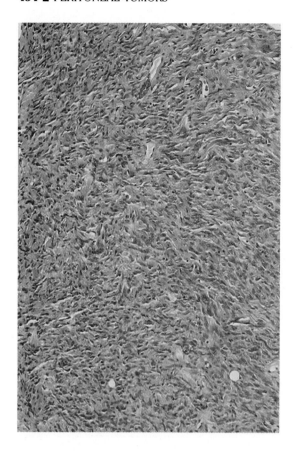

Figure 20–15. Solitary fibrous tumor of the peritoneum.

Adenomatoid Tumor

- Adenomatoid tumor is benign and of mesothelial origin, although it rarely arises from extragenital peritoneum, such as the omentum or mesentery. It is much more commonly encountered within the fallopian tube and myometrium and, in the male, the epididymis.
- Its pathologic features are discussed in Chapter 10.

Well-Differentiated Papillary Mesothelioma

- Well-differentiated papillary mesotheliomas (WDPMs) of the peritoneum are uncommon tumors, 80% of which have occurred in females, who are usually of reproductive age but some of whom are postmenopausal.
- WDPMs are usually an incidental finding at laparotomy, but rare tumors have been associated with abdominal pain or ascites. Occasional patients, including two sisters, have had possible asbestos exposure.

- WDPMs are solitary or, more often, multiple, and are typically grey to white, firm, papillary or nodular lesions less than 2 cm in the maximal dimension. The omental and pelvic peritoneum is typically involved or, rarely, the gastric, intestinal, or mesenteric peritoneum.
- Fibrous papillae are lined by a single layer of flattened to cuboidal mesothelial cells with occasional basal vacuoles. The nuclear features are benign, and mitotic figures are rare or absent.
- Uncommon patterns include tubulopapillary, adenomatoid-like areas, branching cords, and solid sheets. The stroma may be extensively fibrotic. Multinucleated stromal giant cells and psammoma bodies are encountered in some cases.
- Follow-up studies indicate that solitary WDPMs are clinically benign; occasional tumors, however, have persisted for decades.
- When multiple tumors are present, they should each be removed for microscopic examination, because lesions with the appearance of a WDPM may be associated with other lesions that have the appearance of a diffuse

malignant mesothelioma and progressive disease on fol-low-up.

References

Daya D, McCaughey WTE. Well-differentiated papillary mesothelioma of the peritoneum: a clinicopathologic study of 22 cases. Cancer 65: 292–296, 1990.

Goldblum J, Hart WR. Localized and diffuse mesotheliomas of the genital tract and peritoneum in women: a clinicopathological study of nineteen true mesothelial neoplasms, other than adenomatoid tumors, multicystic mesotheliomas and localized fibrous tumors. Am J Surg Pathol 19:1124–1137, 1995.

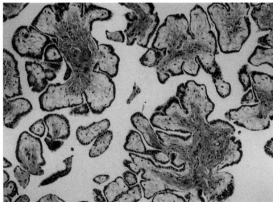

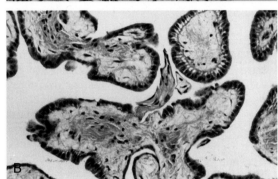

Figure 20–16. Well-differentiated papillary mesothelioma at low (*A*) and higher (*B*) magnifications.

Low-Grade Cystic Mesothelioma

- Although most multilocular cystic mesothelial lesions are MPICs by our criteria, rare multicystic mesotheliomas do occur.
- In contrast to MPICs, the cysts in multicystic mesotheliomas are lined, at least focally, by markedly atypical mesothelial cells, and the tumors may contain areas of conventional malignant mesothelioma on histologic examination.

Reference

DeStephano DB, Wesley JR, Heidelberger KP, et al. Primitive cystic hepatic neoplasm of infancy with mesothelial differentiation: report of a case. Pediatr Pathol 4:291–302, 1985.

Diffuse Malignant Mesothelioma

Clinical Features

- DMMs of the peritoneal cavity (PDMMs) account for only 10% to 20% of all mesotheliomas. PDMMs in women are much less common than extraovarian papillary serous carcinomas (see Chapter 19).
- About two thirds of patients with PDMM are male who are usually middle-aged or elderly. PDMMs occasionally occur in young adults and children.
- The presenting manifestations are usually nonspecific, including abdominal discomfort and distention, digestive disturbances, and weight loss. Ascites occurs in most cases, and cytologic examination of the ascitic fluid may be diagnostic.

■ Occasionally, the tumor may be localized to a hernia or hydrocele sac; present as a retroperitoneal, umbilical, intestinal, or pelvic tumor; or occur as cervical or inguinal lymphadenopathy. Rarely, there is prominent ovarian involvement, with the intraoperative appearance mimicking that of a primary ovarian tumor (see Chapter 17).

■ More than 80% of the patients in one series had a history of asbestos exposure, but most of these patients were identified because of an occupational exposure to asbestos. In contrast, two series of PDMMs in women found no association with a history of asbestos exposure. Asbestos fibers, however, have been identified with special techniques in some of these women.

■ Aside from asbestos, irradiation, chronic inflammation, organic chemicals, and nonasbestos mineral fibers may be etiologic agents.

■ Most males with PDMMs in the literature survived less than 2 years after diagnosis, although there are occasional long-term survivors. Preliminary findings in a study of women with PDMMs (Turnnir and coworkers) suggest that a greater proportion of them have a longer survival than men with PDMMs.

Pathologic Findings

■ The visceral and parietal peritoneum is usually diffusely thickened by nodules and plaques. The viscera are often encased by tumor, but visceral invasion and lymphatic and hematogenous spread are less common than in carcinomas with comparable degrees of peritoneal involvement. Some tumors incite a striking desmoplastic reaction. Rare PDMMs form localized solitary masses.

■ Most PDMMs are of the epithelial type, with tumor cells arranged in tubulopapillary and solid patterns; areas of necrosis may be present. There is usually evidence of invasion of subperitoneal tissues, such as the omentum. Intraabdominal lymph nodes may be involved.

■ The tumor cells usually retain some resemblance to mesothelial cells, with a cuboidal shape and eosinophilic cytoplasm. Usually, there are mild to moderate degrees of nuclear atypicality and variably prominent nucleoli. Mitotic figures are usually present but not numerous.

■ Rare tumors with an exclusively solid pattern of polygonal cells, abundant eosinophilic cytoplasm, and prominent nucleoli (i.e., deciduoid DMMs) have all occurred in adolescent or young adult women.

■ Biphasic and sarcomatoid PDMMs occur but are less common than their pleural counterparts.

■ Some PDMMs contain a prominent inflammatory infiltrate that may include a dense lymphocytic infiltrate with lymphoid follicles or granulomas or large numbers of foamy lipid-rich histiocytes.

■ The histochemical and immunohistochemical features are indicated in the differential diagnosis section.

Differential Diagnosis

■ Atypical mesothelial hyperplasia (page 447).
■ Adenocarcinoma with diffuse peritoneal involvement, including metastatic adenocarcinomas and adenocarcinomas of primary peritoneal origin (see Chapter 19).

• Features favoring a diagnosis of DMM include a prominent tubulopapillary pattern, polygonal cells with moderate amounts of eosinophilic cytoplasm, only mild to moderate nuclear atypia, a paucity of mitotic figures, and the presence of acid mucin (alcianophilic material) rather than neutral (PAS-positive) mucin.

• DMMs usually lack immunoreactivity for a variety of epithelial antigens, including carcinoembryonic antigen, B72.3, Leu-M1 (CD15), MOC-31, CA19-9, S-100 protein, Ber-EP4, and placental alkaline phosphatase. Of these, B72.3, Leu-M1 (CD15), MOC-31, and CA19-9 are the most useful in the differential diagnosis with primary peritoneal serous carcinoma, which are usually positive for these markers.

• Antigens that are usually present in epithelial DMMs but not primary peritoneal serous carcinomas include cytokeratin 5/6, thrombomodulin, calretinin, and Wilms' tumor gene product.

• No single immunohistochemical stain is diagnostic in the separation of PDMM from adenocarcinoma, and the results of a panel of antibodies should be interpreted in conjunction with the hematoxylin and eosin stain and mucin stain results.

■ Ectopic decidua (versus deciduoid PDMM). The prominent nucleoli, often brisk mitotic activity, and immunoreactivity of the tumor cells for cytokeratin exclude an ectopic decidual reaction.

■ Malignant vascular tumors of the peritoneum.

• Lin and colleagues reported peritoneal epithelioid hemangioendotheliomas or epithelioid angiosarcomas that mimicked DMM. Features that suggested the diagnosis of DMM in some cases included epithelioid cells in a tubulopapillary pattern and the presence of reactive or neoplastic spindle cells, resulting in a focal biphasic pattern.

• Various degrees of vascular differentiation and immunoreactivity of the neoplastic cells for endothelial antigens (and negative or weak cytokeratin staining) excluded the diagnosis of DMM.

■ Reactive fibrosis (versus desmoplastic DMM) (page 445).

References

Attanoos R, Gibbs AR. Pathology of malignant mesothelioma. Histopathology 30:403–418, 1997.

Bollinger DJ, Wick MR, Dehner LP, et al. Peritoneal malignant mesothelioma versus serous papillary adenocarcinoma: a histochemical and immunohistochemical comparison. Am J Surg Pathol 13:659–670, 1989.

Brainard JA, Goldblum JR. An immunohistocemical analysis of the Wilms' tumor as a discriminator of peritoneal mesothelioma from primary peritoneal serous adenocarcinoma in women [Abstract]. Mod Pathol 11:101A, 1998.

Clement PB, Young RH, Scully RE. Malignant mesotheliomas presenting as ovarian masses. Am J Surg Pathol 20:1067–1080, 1996.

Daya D, McCaughey WTE. Pathology of the peritoneum: a review of selected topics. Semin Diagn Pathol 8:277–289, 1991.

Goldblum J, Hart WR. Localized and diffuse mesotheliomas of the genital tract and peritoneum in women: a clinicopathological study of nineteen true mesothelial neoplasms, other than adenomatoid tumors, multicystic mesotheliomas and localized fibrous tumors. Am J Surg Pathol 19:1124–1137, 1995.

Kannerstein M, Churg J. Peritoneal mesothelioma. Hum Pathol 8:83–94, 1977.

Kannerstein M, Churg J, McCaughey WTE, Hill DP. Papillary tumors of the peritoneum in women: mesothelioma or papillary carcinoma. Am J Obstet Gynecol 127:306–314, 1977.

Khoury N, Raju U, Crissman JD, et al. A comparative immunohistochemical study of peritoneal and ovarian serous tumors, and mesotheliomas. Hum Pathol 21:811–819, 1990.

Lin BT-Y, Colby T, Gown AM, et al. Malignant vascular tumors of the serous membranes mimicking mesothelioma: a report of 14 cases. Am J Surg Pathol 20:1431–1439, 1996.

McCaughey WTE, Colby TV, Battifora H, et al. Diagnosis of diffuse malignant mesothelioma: experience of a US/Canadian mesothelioma panel. Mod Pathol 4:342–353, 1991.

Nascimento AG, Keeney GL, Fletcher CDM. Deciduoid peritoneal mesothelioma: an unusual phenotype affecting young females. Am J Surg Pathol 18:439–445, 1994.

Ordonez NG. Role of immunohistochemistry in distinguishing epithelial peritoneal mesotheliomas from peritoneal and ovarian serous carcinomas. Am J Surg Pathol 22:1203–1214, 1998.

Sheibani K, Esteban JM, Bailey A, et al. Immunopathologic and molecular studies as an aid to the diagnosis of malignant mesothelioma. Hum Pathol 23:107–116, 1992.

Sussman J, Rosai J. Lymph node metastasis as the initial manifestation of malignant mesothelioma: report of six cases. Am J Surg Pathol 14:818–828, 1990.

Turrnir R, Young RH, Churg A, et al. Peritoneal mesotheliomas in women—a clinicopathologic analysis of 36 cases [Abstract]. Mod Pathol 12:126A, 1999.

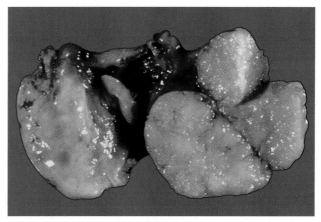

Figure 20–18. Localized malignant mesothelioma. The tumor forms a paraovarian mass.

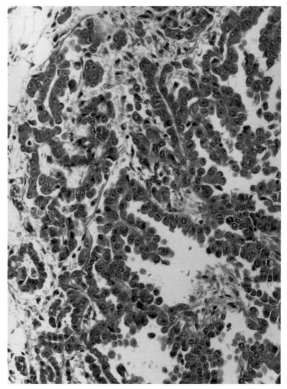

Figure 20–19. Malignant mesothelioma with a tubulopapillary pattern.

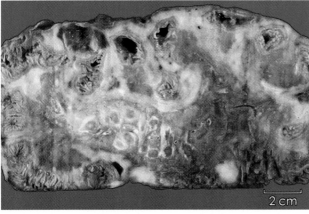

Figure 20–17. Desmoplastic malignant mesothelioma. (Courtesy of J. Prat, MD, Barcelona, Spain).

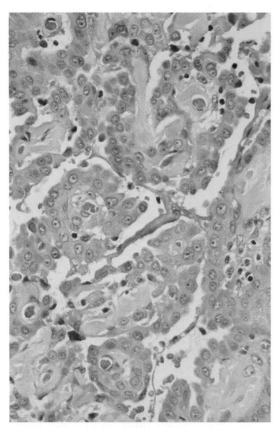

Figure 20–20. Malignant mesothelioma. The cells have conspicuous eosinophilic cytoplasm and malignant nuclear features. Some of the papillae have hyalinized cores.

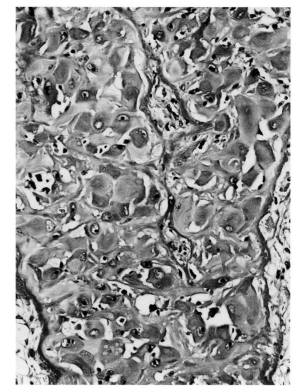

Figure 20–21. Malignant mesothelioma of the "deciduoid" type.

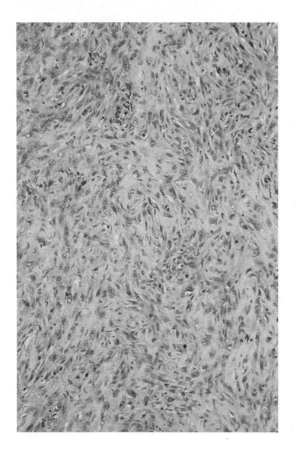

Figure 20–22. Sarcomatoid component of a biphasic malignant mesothelioma.

MISCELLANEOUS PRIMARY TUMORS

Intraabdominal Desmoplastic Small Round Cell Tumor

Clinical Features

- Desmoplastic small round cell tumors (DSRCTs) are of uncertain histogenesis, but they may prove to be a primitive tumor of mesothelial origin (i.e., mesothelioblastoma). Although most are intraabdominal, similar tumors have also been described in the pleura and rarely at a distance from a mesothelium-lined surface (e.g., parotid gland, tentorium).
- DSRCTs have a strong male predilection (male to female ratio 4:1) and are most common in adolescents and young adults (range, 5 to 76 years), who usually have abdominal distention, pain, and a palpable abdominal, pelvic, or scrotal mass, sometimes in association with ascites. Some patients have had an elevated serum level of CA-125 or neuron-specific enolase.
- DSRCTs exhibit a reciprocal translocation [t(11;22)(p13;q12)], resulting in fusion of the *EWS1* gene on chromosome 22 and the Wilms' tumor suppressor gene (*WT1*) on chromosome 11, which appears to be unique for this tumor. This fusion results in the expression of the EWS/WT1 chimeric transcript detectable by reverse transcriptase polymerase chain reaction.
- The *EWS/ERG* fusion gene characteristic of Ewing's sarcoma and peripheral neuroectodermal tumors has been found in rare DSRCTs, suggesting some overlap between the two groups of tumors.
- Laparotomy typically discloses variably sized but usually large, intraabdominal masses associated with smaller peritoneal "implants" of similar appearance. The tumor is sometimes confined to the pelvis, and prominent involvement of the tunica vaginalis or the ovaries may mimic a primary testicular or ovarian tumor. The retroperitoneum is involved in some cases. One tumor appeared to originate within the liver.
- After initial treatment (i.e., debulking and postoperative chemotherapy, irradiation, or both), there may be an initial response, but more than 90% of patients die of tumor progression. The bulk of the tumor tends to remain within the peritoneal cavity, although extraabdominal metastases occur in some patients.

Pathologic Features

- On gross examination, the tumors, which may reach 40 cm in maximal dimension, have smooth or bosselated outer surfaces and firm to hard, gray-white, focally myxoid and necrotic sectioned surfaces. Direct invasion of intraabdominal or pelvic viscera may occur.
- Microscopic examination reveals sharply circumscribed aggregates of small epithelioid cells delimited by a cellular desmoplastic stroma. The aggregates vary from tiny clusters (or even single cells) to rounded or irregularly shaped islands.
- Other common features include rounded, rosette-like or glandlike spaces; peripheral palisading of basaloid cells in some of the nests; and central necrosis with or without calcification.
- The tumor cells are typically uniform with scanty cytoplasm and indistinct cell borders, although tumor cells with eosinophilic cytoplasmic "inclusions" and an eccentric nucleus, resulting in a rhabdoid appearance, are common.
- Small to medium-sized, round, oval, or spindle-shaped hyperchromatic nuclei have clumped chromatin and nucleoli that are usually inapparent. Mitotic figures and single necrotic cells are numerous.
- Architectural features seen in a minority of cases, which can occasionally predominate and lead to diagnostic problems, include tubules, glands (sometimes with luminal mucin), cysts, papillae, anastomosing trabeculae, cords of cells mimicking lobular breast carcinoma, adenoid cystic-like foci, and only a sparse desmoplastic stroma.
- Cytologic features identified in a minority of cases, which can occasionally predominate, include spindle cells, cells with abundant eosinophilic or clear cytoplasm, signet-ring–like cells, and cells with marked nuclear pleomorphism.
- Invasion of vascular spaces, especially lymphatics, is a common feature. Lymph nodes are occasionally involved by tumor.

Immunohistochemical and Ultrastructural Features

- The usual immunoreactivity for epithelial (low-molecular-weight cytokeratins, EMA), neural/neuroendocrine (NSE, CD57/Leu-7), and muscle (desmin) markers, as well as vimentin, suggests divergent differentiation. Desmin and vimentin immunoreactivity is typically paranuclear and globular and is particularly intense in the rhabdoid cells.
- Immunoreactivity for other antigens has occurred in a variable proportion of cases, including Wilms' tumor protein (WT1), Leu-M1 (CD15), S-100, B72.3, CA-125, MIC2 protein, actin (muscle-specific and smooth muscle actin), desmoplakin, CD99, MOC-31, NB84, Ber-EP4, chromogranin, and synaptophysin, although not HBA 71 (i.e., Ewing's sarcoma peripheral neuroectodermal tumor antigen). The stroma is typically immunoreactive for vimentin and muscle-specific actin.
- Ultrastructural variability suggests a range of differentiation. Cell junctions have varied from scant and primitive to more prominent ones, including intermediate, desmosomal, and tight types. Paranuclear intermediate cytoplasmic filaments and basal lamina surrounding the nests of tumor have been prominent features in most of the cases.

Differential Diagnosis

- The typical age of the patient, the absence of an extraperitoneal primary tumor, the distribution of the tumor, and its typical microscopic features and immunoprofile facilitate the distinction from other malignant small cell tumors (Appendix 5) in most cases. Identification of the unique reciprocal translocation is diagnostic in problem cases.

References

Gerald W, Ladanyi M, de Alava E, et al. Clinical, pathological and molecular spectrum of desmoplastic small round cell tumor based on a review of 100 cases [Abstract]. Mod Pathol 10:10A, 1997.

Gerald WL, Miller HK, Battifora H, et al. Intra-abdominal desmoplastic small round cell tumor. Am J Surg Pathol 15:499–513, 1991.

Ordi J, de Alava E, Torne A, et al. Intraabdominal desmoplastic small round cell tumor with EWS/ERG fusion transcript. Am J Surg Pathol 2:1026–1032, 1998.

Ordonez NG. Desmoplastic small round cell tumor. I. A histopathologic study of 39 cases with emphasis on unusual histologic patterns. Am J Surg Pathol 22:1303–1313, 1998.

Ordonez NG. Desmoplastic small round cell tumor. II. An ultrastructural and immunohistochemical study with emphasis on new histochemlcal markers. Am J Surg Pathol 22:1314–1327, 1998.

Wolf AN, Ladanyi M, Paull G, et al. The expanding clinical spectrum of desmoplastic small round-cell tumor: a report of two cases with molecular confirmation. Hum Pathol 30:430–435, 1999.

Young RH, Eichhorn JH, Dickersin GR, Scully RE. Ovarian involvement by the intra-abdominal desmoplastic small round cell tumor with divergent differentiation: a report of three cases. Hum Pathol 23:454–464, 1991.

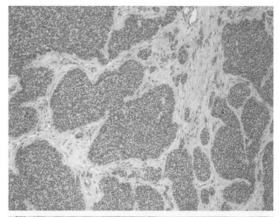
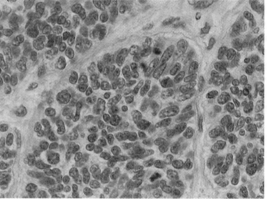

Figure 20–24. Typical appearance of an intraabdominal desmoplastic small round cell tumor at low and high magnifications.

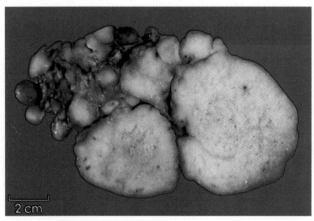

Figure 20–23. Peritoneal intraabdominal desmoplastic small round cell tumor (sectioned surface). Two predominant masses have multiple smaller satellite nodules.

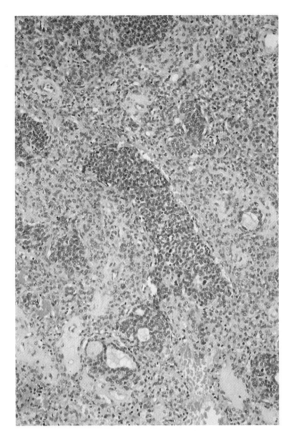

Figure 20–25. Atypical appearance of an intraabdominal desmoplastic small round cell tumor. Some of the tumor cells have moderate amounts of eosinophilic cytoplasm, resulting in a biphasic pattern. Notice the occasional glandlike spaces with luminal secretions.

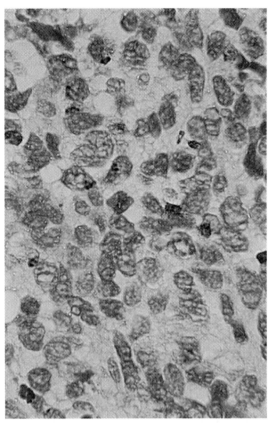

Figure 20–26. Intraabdominal desmoplastic small round cell tumor (desmin stain). Notice the paranuclear globular pattern of staining.

Inflammatory Myofibroblastic Tumor

- Tumors variously referred to as inflammatory pseudotumor, plasma cell granuloma, or inflammatory myofibroblastic tumor may involve the abdomen.
- The lesions usually occur in patients younger than 20 years of age who present with a mass, fever, growth failure or weight loss, hypochromic anemia, thrombocytosis, and polyclonal hypergammaglobulinemia. Laparotomy typically reveals a solid mesenteric mass.

- Microscopic examination reveals myofibroblastic spindle cells, mature plasma cells, and small lymphocytes.
- All of the patients have had an uneventful postoperative course with disappearance of the clinical manifestations.

Reference

Day DL, Sane S, Dehner LP. Inflammatory pseudotumor of the mesentery and small intestine. Pediatr Radiol 16:210–215, 1986.

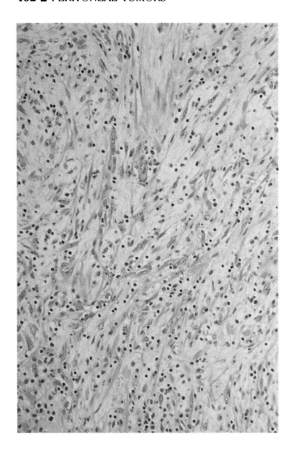

Figure 20–27. Peritoneal inflammatory myofibroblastic tumor (inflammatory pseudotumor).

Omental-Mesenteric Myxoid Hamartoma

■ The designation of omental-mesenteric myxoid hamartoma was applied by Gonzalez-Crussi and colleagues to a lesion in infants characterized by multiple omental and mesenteric nodules composed of plump mesenchymal cells in a myxoid, vascularized stroma.

■ The initial pathologic diagnosis was usually that of some type of sarcoma, but the follow-up was uneventful. The lesions may be hamartomatous.

Reference

Gonzalez-Crussi F, deMello DE, Sotelo-Avila C. Omental-mesenteric myxoid hamartomas. Am J Surg Pathol 7:567–578, 1983.

METASTATIC TUMORS

■ Peritoneal involvement by metastatic tumor usually reflects spread from a primary tumor arising within the abdomen or pelvis, most commonly the ovary. Peritoneal serous tumors in which the ovaries are normal or only minimally involved may arise directly from the peritoneum (see Chapter 19) or are metastatic from a serous papillary carcinoma of the endometrium or fallopian tube.

■ Other tumors particularly associated with peritoneal spread include carcinomas of the breast and gastrointestinal tract, especially the colon and stomach, and the pancreas.

• These tumors may have a prominent or exclusive component of signet-ring adenocarcinoma. The signet-ring tumor cells may be widely scattered in a fibrous stroma and have deceptively bland nuclear features. Such tumors can be misdiagnosed as a benign process, particularly at the time of frozen section.

• Peritoneal involvement by low-grade mucinous tumors (i.e., pseudomyxoma peritonei) is discussed with ovarian mucinous tumors in Chapter 13. Pseudomyxoma peritonei in males is a result of peritoneal spread from a low-grade mucinous carcinoma, usually of appendiceal origin. In such cases, the presenting manifestation may be involvement of a hernia sac.

References

Abu-Rustum NR, Aghajanian CA, Venkatraman ES, et al. Metastatic breast carcinoma to the abdomen and pelvis. Gynecol Oncol 66:41–44, 1997.

Merino MJ, Livolsi VA. Signet ring carcinoma of the female breast: a clinicopathologic analysis of 24 cases. Cancer 48:1830–1837, 1981.

Young RH, Rosenberg AE, Clement PB. Mucin deposits presenting within inguinal hernia sacs: a presenting finding of low grade mucinous cystic tumors of the appendix—a report of two cases and review of the literature. Mod Pathol 10:1228–1232, 1997.

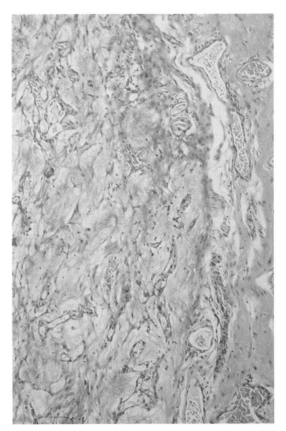

Figure 20–29. Pseudomyxoma peritonei presenting in an inguinal hernia sac in a man. This finding prompted an appendectomy that disclosed a low-grade malignant mucinous cystic tumor of the appendix. Similar findings have been described in women.

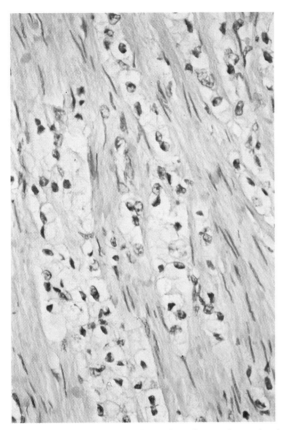

Figure 20–28. Metastatic gastric signet-ring adenocarcinoma involving the peritoneum.

APPENDIX 1

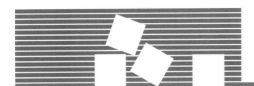

Ovarian Tumors With Mucinous Epithelium

Primary Tumors

Mucinous cystic tumors of intestinal and endocervical-like type

Surface epithelial tumors of mixed cell type with a minor mucinous component

Mucinous carcinoid

Teratomas

Sertoli-Leydig cell tumor with heterologous elements

Small cell carcinomas of the hypercalcemic type

Brenner tumors

Other

Metastatic Tumors

Mucinous carcinoma arising elsewhere in female genital tract, especially the cervix

Mucinous carcinomas from the colon, appendix, small bowel, stomach, pancreas, biliary tract, urinary bladder, and urachus

Low-grade mucinous tumors from the appendix

Mucinous carcinoid

Other

APPENDIX 2

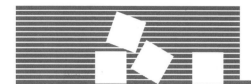

Ovarian Tumors That May Have an Endometrioid-like Glandular Pattern

Primary Tumors

Endometrioid carcinoma
Mucin-poor mucinous adenocarcinoma
Endometrioid-like yolk sac tumor
Sertoli-Leydig cell tumor
Tumors of probable wolffian origin
Ependymoma
Other

Metastatic Tumors

Endometrioid carcinoma arising elsewhere in female genital tract
Intestinal adenocarcinoma of typical and clear cell type
Other gastrointestinal, pancreatic, and biliary adenocarcinomas
Mucin-poor mucinous adenocarcinomas from other sites
Breast carcinoma
Other

APPENDIX 3

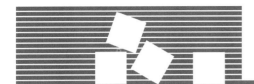

Ovarian Tumors and Tumor-like Lesions That May Be Composed of Clear Cells

Primary Tumors

Clear cell carcinoma
Endometrioid carcinoma
Brenner tumor
Dysgerminoma
Yolk sac tumor
Struma ovarii
Malignant melanoma
Sertoli cell tumor (particularly those in the not otherwise specified category)
Steroid cell tumors
Epithelioid smooth muscle tumors
Other

Metastatic Tumors

Clear cell carcinoma arising elsewhere in the female genital tract
Renal cell carcinoma
Clear cell intestinal carcinoma
Malignant melanoma
Other

Tumor-like Lesions

Arias-Stella reaction
Epithelial inclusion glands and cysts with hydropic change

APPENDIX 4

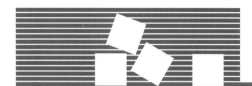

Oxyphilic Tumors and Tumor-like Lesions of the Ovary

Primary Carcinomas

Clear cell
Endometrioid
Hepatoid
Anaplastic carcinoma
   In mucinous cystic tumor
   In squamous cell carcinoma
Small cell carcinoma, large cell variant

Germ Cell Tumors (pure or associated with dermoid cyst)

Struma ovarii
Pituitary-type tumor in dermoid cyst
Malignant melanoma
Apocrine carcinoma in dermoid cyst
Squamous cell carcinoma
Hepatoid yolk sac tumor

Sex Cord–Stromal Tumors

Luteinized granulosa cell tumors, adult and juvenile
Luteinized thecoma
Oxyphilic Sertoli cell tumor

Steroid Cell Tumors

Paraganglioma

Mesenchymal Tumors

Epithelioid smooth muscle tumors
Other

Secondary Tumors

Malignant melanoma
Hepatocellular carcinoma
Breast adenocarcinoma
Large cell carcinoma of lung
Carcinoid tumor
Malignant mesothelioma

Tumor-like Lesions

Pregnancy luteoma
Nodular hyperthecosis
Hilus cell hyperplasia
Malacoplakia
Mesothelial hyperplasia

APPENDIX 5

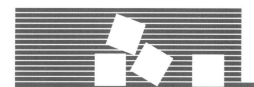

Tumors That Occur in the Ovary as Small Round Cell Tumors

Primary Tumors

Small cell carcinoma, hypercalcemic type
Small cell carcinoma, pulmonary type
Undifferentiated carcinoma, not otherwise specified
Adult granulosa cell tumor
Sertoli-Leydig cell tumor of intermediate and poor differentiation
Endometrioid stromal sarcoma
Malignant melanoma
Primitive neuroectodermal tumors
Embryonal and alveolar rhabdomyosarcoma
Other

Metastatic Tumors

Lymphoma and leukemia
Small cell carcinomas, pulmonary type, from diverse sites
Endometrial stromal sarcoma
Merkel cell tumor
Malignant melanoma
Desmoplastic small round cell tumor with divergent differentiation
Alveolar and embryonal rhabdomyosarcoma
Ewing's sarcoma
Neuroblastoma
Other

APPENDIX 6

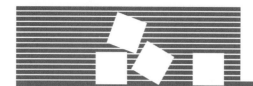

Ovarian Tumors That May Have an Insular Pattern

Primary Tumors

Granulosa cell tumors
Endometrioid carcinomas
Carcinoid tumors
Brenner tumors and transitional cell carcinomas
Squamous carcinoma
Undifferentiated carcinoma
Malignant melanoma
Other

Metastatic Tumors

Carcinoid tumors
Breast adenocarcinoma
Pancreatic "microadenocarcinoma," neuroendocrine neo-
  plasms, and acinar cell carcinomas
Small cell carcinomas from lung, cervix, and other sites
Malignant melanoma
Other

APPENDIX 7

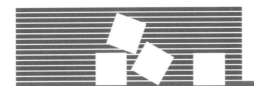

Ovarian Tumors That May Have a Tubular or Pseudotubular Pattern

Primary Tumors

Endometrioid adenocarcinoma
Sertoli and Sertoli-Leydig cell tumors
Sex cord tumor with annular tubules
Granulosa cell tumor (rare foci)
Sex cord tumor, unclassified
Carcinoid tumor
Struma ovarii
Tumor of probable wolffian origin
Other

Metastatic Tumors

Krukenberg tumor
Carcinoid tumor
Breast adenocarcinoma
Endometrioid adenocarcinoma
Other

APPENDIX 8

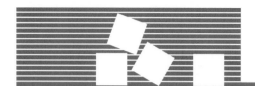

Ovarian Tumors That May Have Cords and Columns

Primary Tumors

Endometrioid adenocarcinoma
Endometrioid stromal sarcoma
Brenner tumor
Granulosa cell tumor
Sertoli-Leydig cell tumors
Dysgerminoma
Trabecular carcinoid
Strumal carcinoid
Other

Metastatic Tumors

Metastatic carcinoid
Metastatic lobular carcinoma of breast
Lymphoma and leukemia
Other

APPENDIX 9

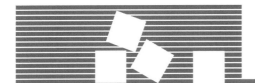

Ovarian Tumors With Small Acini

Primary Tumors

Endometrioid carcinoma
Brenner tumor
Sertoli-Leydig cell tumor
Carcinoid tumor
Struma ovarii
Other

Metastatic Tumors

Carcinoid tumor
Breast adenocarcinoma
Gastric adenocarcinoma
Other

APPENDIX 10

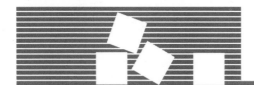

Ovarian Tumors That May Have Follicles or Follicle-like Spaces

Primary Tumors

Granulosa cell tumors
Sertoli-Leydig cell tumor
Small cell carcinoma of hypercalcemic type
Carcinoid tumors
Struma ovarii
Pituitary adenoma arising in a dermoid cyst
Malignant melanoma
Other

Metastatic Tumors

Carcinoid tumors
Malignant melanoma
Small cell carcinomas from diverse sites
Intraabdominal desmoplastic small round cell tumor
Malignant lymphoma
Alveolar rhabdomyosarcoma
Other

Tumor-like Lesions

Pregnancy luteoma

APPENDIX 11

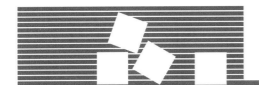

Ovarian Lesions Containing Spaces With Colloid or Colloid-like Material (Struma-like)

Primary Tumors

Struma ovarii
Endometrioid carcinoma
Mucinous carcinoma
Clear cell carcinoma
Sertoli-Leydig cell tumor
Juvenile granulosa cell tumor
Yolk sac tumor
Pituitary adenoma arising in a dermoid cyst
Small cell carcinoma of the hypercalcemic type
Ovarian tumor of probable wolffian origin
Other

Metastatic Tumors

Renal cell carcinoma
Intestinal clear cell adenocarcinoma
Other

Tumor-like Lesions

Pregnancy luteoma

APPENDIX 12

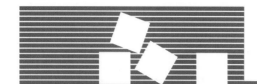

Ovarian Tumors That May Have a Focal Fibromatous or Thecomatous Appearance Other Than Fibroma and Thecoma

Primary Tumor

Surface epithelial adenofibromas with a predominant
   fibromatous component
Brenner tumor
Endometrioid stromal sarcoma
Mesodermal adenosarcoma
Carcinoid tumor
Granulosa cell tumor
Sex cord tumor, unclassified
Fibrosarcoma
Stromal tumor with minor sex cord elements
Sclerosing stromal tumor
Other

Metastatic Tumors

Endometrial stromal sarcoma
Krukenberg tumor
Carcinoid tumor
Other

APPENDIX 13

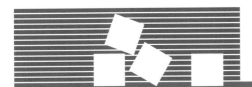

Ovarian Sarcomatoid Tumors*

Primary Tumors

Endometrioid carcinoma with spindle cells
Sarcomatoid Sertoli–Leydig cell tumor
Sarcomatoid adult granulosa cell tumor
Spindle cell squamous carcinoma
Malignant melanoma
Other

Metastatic Tumors

Malignant melanoma
Intraabdominal desmoplastic small round cell tumor with
    spindle cells
Spindle cell carcinomas from diverse sites
Other

---

*Malignant mesodermal mixed tumors are excluded.

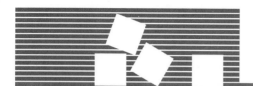

APPENDIX 14

Ovarian Lesions Containing Signet-Ring Cells

Tumors

Metastatic signet-ring cell carcinoma (Krukenberg tumor)
Clear cell carcinoma
Mucinous carcinoma
Mucinous carcinoid
    Primary, pure or associated with epidermoid cyst, mucinous tumor, teratoma, or Sertoli–Leydig cell tumor
    Metastatic
Sclerosing stromal tumor
Signet-ring stromal tumor
Adenomatoid tumor
Malignant mesothelioma
Signet-ring cell melanoma
Signet-ring cell lymphoma
Epithelioid leiomyoma
Other

Tumor-like Lesions

Mucicarminophilic histiocytosis
Surface epithelial glands and cysts with hydropic change
Eutopic and ectopic decidua
Normal endocervical glandular cells
Microglandular hyperplasia

APPENDIX 15

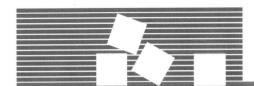

Ovarian Tumors That May Mimic a Mixed Epithelial-Stromal Tumor*

Primary Tumors

Endometrioid carcinoma with a prominent spindle cell epithelial component

Other surface epithelial tumors (e.g., squamous carcinoma, undifferentiated carcinoma) with a spindle cell epithelial component (i.e., sarcomatoid carcinoma)

Endometrioid stromal sarcoma with epithelial-like elements

Endometrioid-like yolk sac tumors with cellular stroma

Carcinoid tumor with prominent fibrous stroma

Malignant melanoma with spindle cells

Other

Metastatic Tumors

Krukenberg tumor

Other adenocarcinomas with a prominent fibrous stroma

Carcinoid tumor

Endometrioid stromal sarcoma with epithelial-like elements

Malignant melanoma with spindle cells

Malignant mesothelioma with spindle cells

Other

---

*For most of these tumors, the differential diagnosis is with a malignant mesodermal mixed tumor.

APPENDIX 16

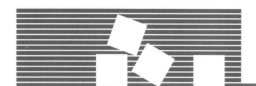

Ovarian Tumors With Functioning Stroma

The term *tumor with functioning stroma* was coined by Robert E. Scully and first used in the literature in 1957.[1] In the 1958 publication by Scully and Morris, *Endocrine Pathology of the Ovary*,[2] the phenomenon received detailed coverage. The process may be associated with metastatic[3] or primary tumors of the ovary. Elevated levels of chorionic gonadotropin explain this phenomenon for tumors in pregnant patients and some of those with germ cell tumors.[4] The luteinized stromal cells in these cases usually have, at the routine light microscopic level, features of steroid hormone–secreting cells with appreciable eosinophilic or pale, lipid-rich cytoplasm. Occasionally, cells without these features, the so-called enzymatically active stromal cells,[5] are responsible for steroid hormone secretion. Although the luteinized stromal cells or, rarely, the Leydig cells in these cases usually are dispersed within the neoplasm, they occasionally have a distinct peripheral disposition.[6] Most tumors responsible for that phenomenon have been monodermal teratomas, usually of large size. Nonneoplastic lesions that cause the phenomenon have been rete cysts. Approximately one third of virilizing ovarian tumors with functioning stroma have been from pregnant patients. Most tumors in pregnant and nonpregnant patients with virilization have been Krukenberg tumors, with lesser numbers of mucinous cystic tumors and rare examples of tumors of other types. Estrogenic manifestations in cases in this overall category are usually seen in postmenopausal patients.[7]

References

1. Scully RE, Morris JM. Functioning ovarian tumors. In Meigs J, Sturgis SH (eds): Progress in Gynecology, III. New York: Grune & Stratton, 1957:31–33.
2. Morris JM, Scully RE. Endocrine pathology of the ovary. St. Louis: CV Mosby, 1958.
3. Scully RE, Richardson GS. Luteinization of the stroma of metastatic cancer involving the ovary and its endocrine significance. Cancer 14:827–840, 1961.
4. Herrington JB, Scully RE. Endocrine aspects of germ cell tumors. In Damjanov I, Knowles B (eds): The Human Teratomas. Totowa, NJ: Humana Press, 1983:215–229.
5. Scully RE, Cohen RB. Oxidative-enzyme activity in normal and pathological human ovaries. Obstet Gynecol 24:667–681, 1964.
6. Rutgers JL, Scully RE. Ovarian tumors with peripheral steroid cell proliferation: a report of 24 cases. Int J Gynecol Pathol 5:319–337, 1986.
7. Scully RE. Functioning ovarian tumors with functioning stroma. In Fox H (ed): Haines and Taylor Obstetrical and Gynecological Pathology, 4th ed. Edinburgh: Churchill Livingstone, 1995.

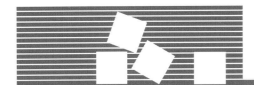

APPENDIX 17

Nontrophoblastic Pregnancy-Associated Findings

Diverse Sites

Fibroepithelial polyps of the lower genital tract
Microglandular hyperplasia
   Of endocervical glands
   Within vaginal adenosis
Arias-Stella reaction and clear cell change
   Within eutopic endometrium
   Within adenomyosis
   Within fallopian tube mucosa
   Within endocervical glands
   Within endometriosis
Optically clear nuclei
   Within eutopic endometrium
   Within endometriosis
Eutopic and ectopic decidua
Pregnancy-related changes in leiomyomas

Site Specific

Ovary
   Pregnancy luteoma
   Hyperreactio luteinalis
   Large solitary luteinized follicle cyst
   Granulosa cell proliferations
   Hilus cell hyperplasia
   Pregnancy-related changes in sex cord–stromal tumors
   Ovarian tumors with functioning stroma (see Appendix 16)
Metaplastic papillary "tumor" of the fallopian tube
Peritoneum
   Peritoneal leiomyomatosis
   Maternal vernix caseosa peritonitis

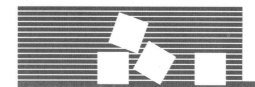

Clinical Syndromes Reported in Association With Tumors of the Female Genital Tract

TUMORS ASSOCIATED WITH UNUSUAL ENDOCRINE AND PARAENDOCRINE SYNDROMES

Tumors Associated With Ectopic Chorionic Gonadotropin Production

Germ cell tumors containing syncytiotrophoblastic cells
Ovarian and uterine adenocarcinomas with trophoblastic differentiation

Tumors Associated With Thyroid Hyperfunction

Ovarian tumors
    Struma ovarii
    Strumal carcinoid
Gestational trophoblastic disease

Tumors Associated With the Carcinoid Syndrome

Ovarian tumors
    Insular carcinoid tumor
    Strumal carcinoid tumor
    Metastatic carcinoid tumor
Extraovarian tumors
    Small cell carcinoma of the uterine cervix

Ovarian Tumors Associated With the Zollinger-Ellison Syndrome

Ovarian mucinous tumors (benign, borderline, and malignant)

Tumors Associated With Hypercalcemia

Ovarian tumors (in descending order of frequency)
    Small cell carcinoma
    Clear cell carcinoma
    Serous carcinoma
    Squamous cell carcinoma arising in a dermoid cyst
    Dysgerminoma
    Mucinous carcinoma
    Other epithelial and undifferentiated carcinomas
    Steroid cell tumor
Extraovarian tumors
    Squamous cell carcinomas of the vulva, cervix, and vagina
    Endometrial adenosquamous, clear cell, and serous carcinomas
    Others (e.g., uterine leiomyosarcoma, endometrial stromal sarcoma, malignant juxtaovarian tumor of wolffian origin)

Tumors Associated With Cushing's Syndrome

Ovarian tumors
    Steroid cell tumor
    Malignant Sertoli cell tumor
    Endometrioid carcinoma, poorly differentiated adenocarcinoma
    Trabecular carcinoid, "atypical carcinoid"
    Dermoid cyst with pituitary tissue
Other tumors
    Small cell carcinoma of the cervix

Tumors Associated With Hypoglycemia

Ovarian tumors
  Serous cystadenocarcinoma
  Dysgerminoma
  Carcinoid tumor
  Fibroma
  Malignant schwannoma
Extraovarian tumors
  Small cell carcinoma of the cervix
  Uterine leiomyomas

Tumors Associated With Renin and Aldosterone Production

Ovarian tumors
  Sex cord–stromal tumors
  Steroid cell tumors
  Others (e.g., leiomyosarcoma, mucinous adenocarcinoma)
Nonovarian tumors
  Adenocarcinoma of the fallopian tube
  Uterine leiomyosarcoma

Ovarian Tumors Associated With Hyperprolactinemia

Squamous cell carcinoma of the cervix
Dermoid cyst with pituitary tissue
Gonadoblastoma

Tumors Associated With Antidiuretic Hormone Secretion

Small cell carcinoma of the cervix
Ovarian epithelial carcinomas

Ovarian Carcinoid Tumors Associated With Constipation

Paraovarian Nodular Hyperplasia of Steroid-Type Cells Associated With Nelson's Syndrome

Virilizing Placental Site Trophoblastic Tumor

TUMORS ASSOCIATED WITH PARANEOPLASTIC SYNDROMES

Tumors Associated With Subacute Cerebellar Degeneration

Serous and other ovarian carcinomas
Carcinomas of endometrium, fallopian tube, and pelvic peritoneum

Tumors Associated With Retinal Degeneration

Undifferentiated small cell carcinomas of the endometrium and cervix
Malignant müllerian mixed tumor of uterus

Tumors Associated With Connective Tissue Disorders

Dermatomyositis-polymyositis
  Epithelial carcinomas of ovary (usually serous)
  Carcinomas of endometrium, cervix, and vagina
  Other
Polyarthritis and palmar fasciitis
  Ovarian epithelial carcinomas (endometrioid, serous, undifferentiated)
  Other
Hypertrophic pulmonary osteoarthropathy
  Ovarian epithelial carcinomas
Rheumatoid-like arthritis
  Carcinomas of ovary and cervix
Scleroderma
  Carcinomas of ovary, endometrium, cervix, vulva
Shoulder-hand syndrome
  Tubo-ovarian carcinoma
Systemic lupus erythematosus
  Carcinoma of the cervix
Digital gangrene
  Carcinomas of ovary, endometrium, cervix
Raynaud's phenomenon
  Ovarian epithelial carcinomas

Tumors Associated With Hematologic Disorders

Autoimmune hemolytic anemia
  Dermoid cysts
  Other
Disseminated intravascular coagulation (including nonbacterial thrombotic endocarditis, microangiopathic hemolytic anemia; migratory thombophlebitis [Trousseau's syndrome])
  Ovarian epithelial carcinomas
  Other
Erythrocytosis
  Uterine leiomyoma
  Other
Reactive thrombocytosis
  Ovarian and cervical carcinomas
  Other
Nonthrombocytopenic purpura
  Mucinous cystadenoma
Granulocytosis
  Clear cell carcinoma
Thrombocytopenia
  Serous carcinoma
  Other
Pancytopenia
  Granulosa cell tumor

Tumors Associated With Cutaneous Disorders*

Acanthosis nigricans
    Polycystic ovary disease (PCOD) stromal hyperthecosis, HAIR-AN syndrome (i.e., hyperandrogenemia, insulin resistance, and acanthosis nigricans)
    Ovarian epithelial carcinomas
    Other
Torre-Muir (Muir-Torre) syndrome
    Endometrial and ovarian adenocarcinoma
    Other
Sweet's syndrome
    Clear cell carcinoma of ovary
Erythema nodosum
    Carcinoma of cervix
Cutaneous melanosis
    Strumal carcinoid tumor

Tumors Associated With the Nephrotic Syndrome

Serous carcinoma of the ovary
Placental site trophoblastic tumor

HERITABLE AND OTHER CONGENITAL SYNDROMES

Familial Ovarian Cancer

Breast and ovarian cancer syndrome
Site-specific ovarian cancer
Lynch syndrome II (i.e., hereditary nonpolyposis colorectal cancer and other cancers [endometrial, stomach, pancreas]

Peutz-Jeghers Syndrome

Ovarian tumors
    Sex cord tumor with annular tubules
    Rare distinctive ovarian sex cord–stromal tumor
    Lipid-rich variant of Sertoli cell tumor
    Mucinous cystic tumors (benign, borderline, or malignant)
Nonovarian tumors
    Adenoma malignum (minimal deviation adenocarcinoma) of the uterine cervix

---

*Excluding cutaneous manifestations of the Peutz-Jeghers and the nevoid basal cell carcinoma syndromes (see Heritable and Other Congenital Syndromes)
From Clement PB, Young RH, Scully RE. Clinical syndromes associated with tumors of the female genital tract. Semin Diagn Pathol 8:204–233, 1991.

Nevoid Basal Cell Carcinoma Syndrome (Basal Cell Nevus Syndrome, Gorlin's Syndrome)

Ovarian fibroma
Ovarian fibrosarcoma
Sclerosing stromal tumor

Ollier's Disease and Maffucci's Syndrome

Juvenile granulosa cell tumor
Ovarian fibroma and fibrosarcoma

Other Abnormalities Associated With Juvenile Granulosa Cell Tumors

Goldenhar's syndrome
Potter's syndrome
Leprechaunism
Bone tumors and soft tissue tumors

Thyroid Abnormalities and Ovarian Tumors

Sertoli–Leydig cell tumor
Steroid cell tumor (associated with multiple endocrine adenomatosis, including thyroid and parathyroid adenomas)

Leiomyomatosis

Uterine leiomyomas associated with leiomyomatosis of the skin
Gastroesophageal leiomyomatosis (with or without tracheobronchial leiomyomatosis) associated with leiomyomatosis of the uterus, vulva, or both; Alport's syndrome is also present in most cases

Tuberous Sclerosis

Uterine and ovarian lymphangioleiomyomatosis
Uterine angiomyoma
Ovarian angiomyolipoma

Ataxia-Telangiectasia

Ovarian tumors
    Dysgerminoma
    Yolk sac tumor
    Gonadoblastoma
Uterine smooth muscle tumors

Von Hippel-Lindau Disease

Papillary cystadenoma of the broad ligament of wolffian duct origin

Carney's Complex

Uterine myxomas

Hereditary Hemorrhagic Telangiectasia and Klippel-Trenaunay-Weber Syndrome

Uterine hemangiomas

Cowden's Disease

Cancers of the endometrium, cervix, or ovary

OTHER SYNDROMES

Meigs' Syndrome

Fibroma or "predominantly fibrous tumor" of the ovary (including thecoma, granulosa cell tumor, and Brenner tumor)

Other benign pelvic tumors or tumor-like lesions

Sclerosing Peritonitis

Luteinized ovarian thecomas
Ovarian fibromatosis, massive ovarian edema

Tumors Associated With Hyperamylasemia

Ovarian epithelial tumors (serous or endometrioid)

Uveal Melanocytic Lesions

Ovarian carcinomas

Melkersson-Rosenthal Syndrome

Granulomatous vulvitis
Vulvar squamous cell carcinoma

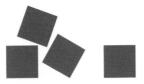

INDEX

Note: Page numbers in *italics* refer to illustrations; page numbers followed by t refer to tables.